Gastrointestinal Cancer

Hoon Jai Chun • Seun Ja Park
Yun Jeong Lim • Si Young Song

Gastrointestinal Cancer

A Comprehensive Guide to Diagnosis and Management

Springer

Hoon Jai Chun
Department of Internal Medicine
Korea University Anam Hospital
Seoul, Korea (Republic of)

Seun Ja Park
Department of Internal Medicine
Kosin University Gospel Hospital
Busan, Korea (Republic of)

Yun Jeong Lim
Department of Internal Medicine
Dongguk University Ilsan Hospital
Goyang, Kyonggi-do, Korea (Republic of)

Si Young Song
Department of Internal Medicine
Yonsei University Severance Hospital
Seoul, Korea (Republic of)

ISBN 978-981-99-0814-1 ISBN 978-981-99-0815-8 (eBook)
https://doi.org/10.1007/978-981-99-0815-8

This Springer imprint is published by the registered company Springer Nature Singapore Pte Ltd.
The registered company address is: 152 Beach Road, #21-01/04 Gateway East, Singapore 189721, Singapore

Contents

Part II Gastroesophageal Junction and Esophageal Cancer

Part V Colorectal Cancer

Part XII Special Clinical Considerations for Gastrointestinal Cancer

Part I

Gastric Cancer

Epidemiology, Risk Factors, and Clinical Manifestations

Key Points

- Gastric cancer has a high incidence and cancer-related mortality.
- Various factors are involved in the development of gastric cancer. Of these, *Helicobacter pylori* infection is the most important cause of gastric cancer.
- There are no specific symptoms or signs in early gastric cancer.
- Nevertheless, regular endoscopic screening has decreased the morbidity and mortality of gastric cancer in high-prevalent countries such as Korea and Japan.

Introduction

Gastric cancer is one of the cancers with the highest incidence rates and cancer-related mortality. Although the incidence and mortality of gastric cancer have been gradually declining in recent decades, the most recent epidemiological study reports that gastric cancer is the fifth most common cancer, accounting for 5.6% of all cancers worldwide, while gastric cancer-related mortality is the fourth most common, accounting for 7.7% of all cancer-related mortality [1].

Epidemiology

About 95% of gastric cancers consist of adenocarcinoma [2]. Therefore, gastric cancer is mainly described as gastric adenocarcinoma. The epidemiology of gastric cancer shows significant variability across populations due to its tumor properties.

Geographic and Population-Based Differences

Gastric cancer is most common in East Asia, Eastern Europe, and South America, and relatively rare in Western Europe, North America, and Africa (Fig. 1a) [3]. The incidence of gastric cancer is higher in developing countries. Furthermore, the incidence rate is approximately twice as high in men than in women. It is also higher in older adults and very low in individuals under the age of 40 [4, 5].

Histological Differences

Gastric cancer is traditionally classified as intestinal, diffuse, and mixed type according to the Lauren classification [6]. The intestinal type of gastric cancer is more common in high-risk areas, males, and older adults. The diffuse type is more

Yun Jeong Lim is the lead author of this chapter.

In this chapter, worldwide epidemiology and risk factors for gastric cancer are summarized. Although early gastric cancer has no specific symptoms or signs, the clinical features of advanced gastric cancer should be noted.

H. J. Chun et al., *Gastrointestinal Cancer*, https://doi.org/10.1007/978-981-99-0815-8_1

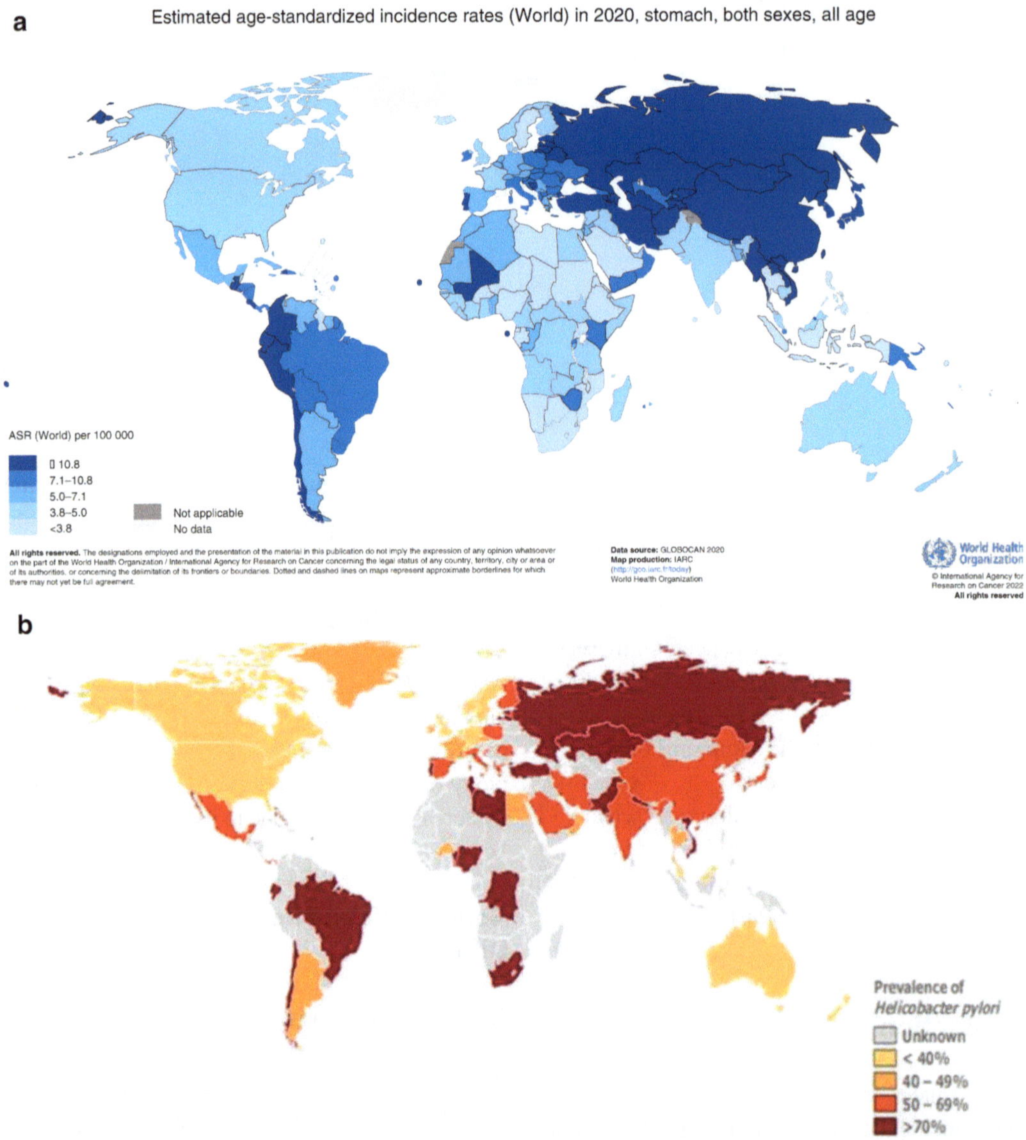

Fig. 1 Relationship between the incidence of gastric cancer. (**a**) and the prevalence of *Helicobacter pylori* infection (**b**). Regions with a high prevalence of *Helicobacter pylori* (darker red) tend to a high incidence of gastric cancer (*darker blue*). Adapted from (**a**) https://gco.iarc.fr/today and (**b**) https://people.ucalgary.ca/~ggkaplan/HP2016.html

common at younger ages and has a poor prognosis. In recent years, the intestinal type of gastric cancer has been on the decline.

Anatomical Differences

The incidence of gastric cancer also differs depending on the anatomy. Distal or noncardiac gastric cancer occurs in high-risk areas and is thought to be associated with *Helicobacter pylori* (*H. pylori*) infection and gastric atrophy. Proximal or cardiac gastric cancer is common in Western countries and has been reported to be related to gastroesophageal reflux or genetic factors [7]. Contrary to noncardiac gastric cancer, the incidence of cardiac gastric cancer has increased in the Western world.

Risk Factors

There are various factors that influence the development of gastric cancer and can be broadly divided into environmental factors and genetic factors. In the Correa cascade, a representative model of gastric cancer, various factors affect the development of gastric cancer [8]. The risk factors for gastric cancer are summarized (Table 1) and the main risk factors are described below [9, 10].

H. Pylori Infection

H. pylori infection is the strongest risk factor for gastric cancer and was announced as a Group 1 carcinogen by the International Agency on Research on Cancer in 1994 [11]. Chronic *H. pylori* infection is known to increase the incidence of gastric cancer and is associated with chronic atrophic gastritis, intestinal metaplasia, and dysplasia [12]. *H. pylori* infection has been particularly associated with the development of noncardiac gastric cancer. In areas where *H. pylori* infection is common, the incidence of gastric cancer tends to be proportional (Fig. 1b) [13]. Treatment of *H. pylori* is believed to reduce the risk of gastric cancer by about 40% [14]. Although *H. pylori* treatment and prevention of gastric cancer have not yet been fully established, a recent global consensus recommends *H. pylori* treatment for the prevention of gastric cancer in populations with high-risk areas [15].

It is estimated that about 50% of the world's population will have *H. pylori* infection [16]. However, only a small fraction of *H. pylori*-infected individuals progress to gastric cancer [17]. Therefore, among *H. pylori* strains, strains with specific virulence factors are considered to be associated with the occurrence of gastric cancer. To date, CagA (cytotoxin-associated gene A) and VacA (vacuolating cytotoxin A) are well-known main virulence factors [18].

The incidence of metachronous gastric cancer was lower in patients with early gastric cancer, who received *H. pylori* treatment. But in some patients, the risk of gastric cancer is not reduced even after the eradication of *H. pylori* [19]. In addition, *H. pylori*-negative gastric cancer, which is more commonly presented as an undifferentiated type, is known to occur in less than 5% cases of gastric cancer [20]. Therefore, although *H. pylori* infection plays a critical role in the development of gastric cancer, the relationship with other cofactors should also be carefully considered.

Table 1 Established and potential risk factors for gastric cancer

Environmental factors
Helicobacter pylori (*H. pylori*) infection
Epstein-Barr virus (EBV) infection
Smoking
Alcohol
Obesity
Salted/pickled food
Radiation exposure
Occupational exposures (metal, mining, rubber)
Low consumption of fruits and vegetables
Genetic factors
Familial or inherited factors
• Hereditary diffuse gastric cancer
• Hereditary cancer syndromes
Molecular factors
• *P53* mutation (chromosomal instability)
• *HER2* overexpression
• *PD-L1/2* overexpression
• *MLH1* hypermethylation (microsatellite instability)
• *PIK3CA* mutations (EBV infection)
• *CDH1* somatic mutations (diffuse histology)

Dietary or Social Factors

There have also been reports of an association of high nitrates in dried, smoked, and salted foods with gastric carcinogenesis. The hypothesis is that nitrites are converted into carcinogenic N-nitroso compounds by intragastric bacteria. The decrease in the incidence of gastric cancer has also been suggested to be related to the storage of fresh food. Smoking, heavy alcohol use, and obesity have also been reported to be associated with gastric carcinogenesis [21, 22]. Low consumption of fruits and vegetables is associated with the occurrence of gastric cancer [23].

Epstein–Barr Virus Infection

In addition to *H. pylori* infection, Epstein Barr virus (EBV) infection is also believed to be associated with the development of gastric cancer. Various mediators of EBV virus infection can act to induce aberrant DNA methylation [24].

Genetic and Molecular Factors

About 10% of gastric cancers are believed to have a familial predisposition. In particular, diffuse-type gastric cancers or early-onset gastric cancer are considered to occur due to genetic factors. Among them, less than 5% of cases with an inherited predisposition are known and most are inherited as autosomal dominant patterns. The representative types are as follows [25]:

1. Hereditary diffuse gastric cancer (HDGC): HDGC is an inherited form of diffuse-type gastric cancer with a poor prognosis. It is known to be associated with a mutation of the cadherin-1 (*CDH1*) gene related to the cell adhesion protein E-cadherin.
2. Familial intestinal gastric cancer (FIGC).
3. Gastric adenocarcinoma and proximal polyposis of the stomach (GAPPS).
4. Other hereditary polyposis syndromes: Lynch syndrome, familial adenomatous polyposis, Li–Fraumeni syndrome, Peutz–Jeghers syndrome, and MYH-associated polyposis also affect the development of gastric cancer.

Recently, several molecular factors related to the development of gastric cancer have been identified [10]. *P53*, a renowned tumor suppressor gene, presents mutations that are particularly well observed in gastric cancer with virulent *H. pylori* infection. In addition to microsatellite instability, PIK3CA mutations in EBV infection and CDH1 mutations are known to play an important role in gastric carcinogenesis.

Clinical Manifestations

Symptoms

Early gastric cancer is often detected during routine screening in an asymptomatic state. Patients with advanced gastric cancer can express nonspecific symptoms such as dyspepsia, nausea, anorexia, and abdominal pain. In addition, it is sometimes diagnosed in a late or incurable stage, accompanied with refractory vomiting, gastrointestinal bleeding, cachexia, weight loss, and ascites [26].

Physical Examination

There are no typical signs in patients with early gastric cancer. Most physical signs appear in later stages [27]. A palpable abdominal mass may appear due to regional growth, and biliary obstruction due to extension of the surrounding organs or jaundice may be observed due to hepatic metastasis. Characteristic signs of lymph node or peritoneal metastasis may appear.

- Virchow's node (left supraclavicular nodes).
- Sister Mary Joseph's nodule (nodule in the periumbilical area).
- Blumer's shelf (tumor on the cul-de-sac).
- Krukenberg's tumor (enlarged ovary).
- Malignant ascites (peritoneal carcinomatosis).

Rarely, paraneoplastic syndromes such as microangiopathic hemolytic anemia, the Leser–Trélat sign, acanthosis nigricans, and Trousseau's syndrome may also occur [28].

Conclusion

Although the incidence and cancer-related mortality of gastric cancer are declining worldwide, gastric cancer remains one of the most burdensome cancers. In addition, gastric cancer is still one of the most common cancers in East Asia.

Gastric cancer is developed by a combination of environmental and genetic factors. Among the various risk factors, *H. pylori* infection is the most important. Chronic *H. pylori* infection is related to noncardiac and intestinal type gastric cancer.

Since gastric cancer has no specific symptoms or signs, routine endoscopic screening and aggressive treatment to eradicate *H. pylori* infection may be necessary for the prevention of gastric cancer in high-risk areas.

References

1. Sung H, Ferlay J, Siegel RL, Laversanne M, Soerjomataram I, Jemal A, et al. Global cancer statistics 2020: GLOBOCAN estimates of incidence and mortality worldwide for 36 cancers in 185 countries. CA Cancer J Clin. 2021;71:209–49.
2. Dicken BJ, Bigam DL, Cass C, Mackey JR, Joy AA, Hamilton SM. Gastric adenocarcinoma: review and considerations for future directions. Ann Surg. 2005;241:27–39.
3. Ajani JA, Lee J, Sano T, Janjigian YY, Fan D, Song S. Gastric adenocarcinoma. Nat Rev Dis Primers. 2017;3:17036.
4. Fuchs CS, Mayer RJ. Gastric carcinoma. N Engl J Med. 1995;333:32–41.
5. Collaborators GBDSC. The global, regional, and national burden of stomach cancer in 195 countries, 1990-2017: a systematic analysis for the global burden of disease study 2017. Lancet Gastroenterol Hepatol. 2020;5:42–54.
6. Lauren P. The two histological Main types of gastric carcinoma: diffuse and so-called intestinal-type carcinoma. An attempt at a Histo-clinical classification. Acta Pathol Microbiol Scand. 1965;64:31–49.
7. Smyth EC, Nilsson M, Grabsch HI, van Grieken NC, Lordick F. Gastric cancer. Lancet. 2020;396:635–48.
8. Correa P, Piazuelo MB. The gastric precancerous cascade. J Dig Dis. 2012;13:2–9.
9. Sekiguchi M, Oda I, Matsuda T, Saito Y. Epidemiological trends and future perspectives of gastric cancer in eastern Asia. Digestion. 2021;7:1.
10. Cancer Genome Atlas Research N. Comprehensive molecular characterization of gastric adenocarcinoma. Nature. 2014;513:202–9.
11. Schistosomes, liver flukes and Helicobacter pylori. IARC Working Group on the Evaluation of Carcinogenic Risks to Humans. Lyon, 7–14 June 1994. IARC Monogr Eval Carcinog Risks Hum. 1994;61:1–241.
12. Uemura N, Okamoto S, Yamamoto S, Matsumura N, Yamaguchi S, Yamakido M, et al. Helicobacter pylori infection and the development of gastric cancer. N Engl J Med. 2001;345:784–9.
13. de Martel C, Ferlay J, Franceschi S, Vignat J, Bray F, Forman D, et al. Global burden of cancers attributable to infections in 2008: a review and synthetic analysis. Lancet Oncol. 2012;13:607–15.
14. Lee YC, Chiang TH, Chou CK, Tu YK, Liao WC, Wu MS, et al. Association between helicobacter pylori eradication and gastric cancer incidence: a systematic review and meta-analysis. Gastroenterology. 2016;150:1113–24.
15. Liou JM, Malfertheiner P, Lee YC, Sheu BS, Sugano K, Cheng HC, et al. Screening and eradication of helicobacter pylori for gastric cancer prevention: the Taipei global consensus. Gut. 2020;69:2093–112.
16. Hooi JKY, Lai WY, Ng WK, Suen MMY, Underwood FE, Tanyingoh D, et al. Global prevalence of helicobacter pylori infection: systematic review and meta-analysis. Gastroenterology. 2017;153:420–9.
17. Peek RM Jr, Blaser MJ. Helicobacter pylori and gastrointestinal tract adenocarcinomas. Nat Rev Cancer. 2002;2:28–37.
18. Graham DY. Helicobacter pylori update: gastric cancer, reliable therapy, and possible benefits. Gastroenterology. 2015;148:719–31.
19. Choi IJ, Kook MC, Kim YI, Cho SJ, Lee JY, Kim CG, et al. Helicobacter pylori therapy for the prevention of metachronous gastric cancer. N Engl J Med. 2018;378:1085–95.
20. Yamamoto Y, Fujisaki J, Omae M, Hirasawa T, Igarashi M. Helicobacter pylori-negative gastric cancer: characteristics and endoscopic findings. Dig Endosc. 2015;27:551–61.
21. Machlowska J, Baj J, Sitarz M, Maciejewski R, Sitarz R. Gastric cancer: epidemiology, risk factors, classification, genomic characteristics and treatment strategies. Int J Mol Sci. 2020;21:4012.
22. Sung H, Siegel RL, Torre LA, Pearson-Stuttard J, Islami F, Fedewa SA, et al. Global patterns in excess body weight and the associated cancer burden. CA Cancer J Clin. 2019;69:88–112.
23. Tsugane S, Sasazuki S. Diet and the risk of gastric cancer: review of epidemiological evidence. Gastric Cancer. 2007;10:75–83.
24. Yau TO, Tang CM, Yu J. Epigenetic dysregulation in Epstein-Barr virus-associated gastric carcinoma: disease and treatments. World J Gastroenterol. 2014;20:6448–56.

25. Smyth EC, Verheij M, Allum W, Cunningham D, Cervantes A, Arnold D, et al. Gastric cancer: ESMO clinical practice guidelines for diagnosis, treatment and follow-up. Ann Oncol. 2016;27:38–49.
26. Wanebo HJ, Kennedy BJ, Chmiel J, Steele G Jr, Winchester D, Osteen R. Cancer of the stomach. A patient care study by the American College of Surgeons. Ann Surg. 1993;218:583–92.
27. Jemal A, Siegel R, Ward E, Murray T, Xu J, Thun MJ. Cancer statistics, 2007. CA Cancer J Clin. 2007;57:43–66.
28. Feldman M, Friedman LS, Brandt LJ. Sleisenger and Fordtran's gastrointestinal and liver disease : pathophysiology, diagnosis, management. 11th ed. Philadelphia, PA: Saunders/Elsevier; 2021. p. 834.

Screening of Gastric Cancer

Key Points

- Gastric cancer screening in the general population is controversial even in areas with a high prevalence of gastric cancer.
- The two main methods used for screening gastric cancer are upper endoscopy and upper gastrointestinal imaging series.
- Endoscopic screening might reduce the gastric cancer mortality rate, but radiographic screening has no impact on the gastric cancer mortality rate.
- Further large, randomized trials are needed to demonstrate lower gastric cancer mortality in screened populations.

Introduction

Gastric cancer is the fifth most common cancer in the world, with over 1,000,000 new cases in 2018. It is the third leading cause of cancer death worldwide, with an estimated 783,000 deaths in 2018 alone [1]. The incidence of gastric cancer is decreasing around the world, but the incidence and mortality of gastric cancer are still high in East Asia. Early detection is crucial for reducing the mortality rate of gastric cancer, and screening tests are required for the general population. Population-based screening for gastric cancer has been performed in countries such as Japan, Korea, Chile, and Venezuela, where the incidence of gastric cancer is high [2–4]. Some observational studies have shown that screening tests increase the detection of gastric cancer in the early stages and lower gastric cancer mortality in areas with a high incidence of gastric cancer [2, 5–12]. However, there have been no randomized controlled studies showing that the mortality rate of gastric cancer has decreased in screened populations. The detection of gastric cancer in asymptomatic people is controversial even in areas with a high prevalence of gastric cancer [13]. This chapter will focus on the types of screening tests for gastric cancer and will discuss the advantages and risks of each method (Table 1).

Table 1 Screening modalities for gastric cancer

Tests	Characteristics
Upper gastrointestinal imaging series	Less invasive, less sensitive, high false negative rate
Upper endoscopy	More invasive, more sensitive, high false positive rate, higher cost
Other tests	Further studies are needed
Serum pepsinogen	Low sensitivity, low specificity
Serum trefoil factor 3	Low sensitivity, low specificity
MicroRNAs[a]	Experimental
Multianalyte blood tests[b]	Experimental

[a] miRNA-421, miRNA 18a, and miR-106a
[b] Combinations of tumor-specific circulating proteins and mutations in cell-free DNA in the blood

Moo In Park is the lead author of this chapter.

H. J. Chun et al., *Gastrointestinal Cancer*, https://doi.org/10.1007/978-981-99-0815-8_2

Screening Tests for Gastric Cancer

There are two main screening tests for gastric cancer, upper gastrointestinal endoscopy, and upper gastrointestinal imaging series. In Japan, gastric cancer screening has been performed in the general population using an upper gastrointestinal imaging series as a national screening program since 1983, and has contributed to a reduction in gastric cancer mortality to some extent [14]. In Korea, gastric cancer screening has been performed by upper gastrointestinal endoscopy and upper gastrointestinal imaging series since 2000 [15].

Upper Gastrointestinal Imaging Series

The upper gastrointestinal imaging series can identify malignant gastric ulcers, infiltrating lesions, and in some cases, early gastric cancers. Although upper gastrointestinal imaging series can identify early gastric cancer, the sensitivity of a barium study may be as low as 14% [16].

Upper Gastrointestinal Endoscopy

Upper gastrointestinal endoscopy allows direct observation of the gastric mucosa and allows to obtain a tissue biopsy and the diagnosis of gastric cancer as well as atrophic gastritis, intestinal metaplasia, and gastric dysplasia, which are precursor lesions of gastric cancer. Upper gastrointestinal endoscopy is more invasive than other diagnostic modalities, but it is more sensitive for the diagnosis of gastric cancer.

Other Tests

Various modalities, including serum pepsinogen [17], serum trefoil factor [3, 18], microRNAs [19], and combinations of tumor-specific circulating proteins and mutations in cell-free DNA [20] in the blood have been proposed to detect gastric cancer or precursor lesions of gastric cancer. More studies are needed to introduce these modalities for the detection of gastric cancer.

Benefits and Harms of Gastric Cancer Screening

Endoscopic and radiological methods have been used as screening tests for gastric cancer in Japan and Korea, and only observational studies have been conducted for evaluating the performance and effectiveness of these two methods. Evidence on the benefits and harms of endoscopic and radiological methods has been obtained from cohort and case-control studies mainly conducted in Japan and Korea.

Effectiveness

Although some studies have shown that radiological screening reduces the mortality rate from gastric cancer by 40% [21–23], careful attention is required in the interpretation of their findings. A nested case-control study using data from the Korean National Cancer Screening Program for gastric cancer since 2002 included a total of 16,584,283 Korean men and women, aged 40 years and older, comprising the cancer-free cohort [24]. The overall rate of gastric cancer mortality decreased to 21% and endoscopic screening reduced the gastric cancer mortality rate by 47%, but radiographic screening did not reduce the gastric cancer mortality rate in this study.

A meta-analysis of observational studies, including six cohort studies and four nested case-control studies comprising 342,013 individuals, all from Asia, suggested that gastric cancer mortality could be reduced by 40% after endoscopic screening [25]. There was no association between endoscopic screening and the incidence of gastric cancer. However, due to the different biases, including lead time bias, length bias, and selection bias of observational studies, considerable caution is needed when interpreting the results.

Endoscopic screening for gastric cancer may be cost-effective for high-risk subgroups, but not low-risk populations [26, 27]. A one-time upper endoscopy at age 50 in the general US population for upper gastrointestinal cancers was not shown to be cost-effective [28]. Instead, a one-time upper endoscopy at age 50 for gastric cancer with ongoing surveillance of gastric intestinal metaplasia was shown to be cost-effective for Asian Americans aged 50 years or older in the US [29].

Test Performance

Although there are no studies comparing radiographic and endoscopic screening for gastric cancer directly, several studies have suggested that upper endoscopy is slightly more sensitive than an upper gastrointestinal imaging series [2–4, 30, 31]. A population-based study in Korea showed that the sensitivity rates for upper endoscopy versus upper gastrointestinal imaging series in detecting gastric cancer were 69 and 37 percent, respectively. Both diagnostic tests had a specificity of 96% [32].

Harms of Gastric Cancer Screening

The main harmful effects of radiographic and endoscopic screenings are complications, false positive cases, and overdiagnosis [30]. The complications of gastric cancer screening are radiation exposure from upper gastrointestinal imaging series and infection from upper endoscopy. Endoscopic screening can cause serious harms such as infection and overdiagnosis.

Strategies for the Detection of Gastric Cancer

Gastric cancer screening in the general population is controversial, and recommendations vary depending on the incidence of gastric cancer. Population-based screening for gastric cancer has been performed in some countries with a high incidence of gastric cancer, such as Japan, Korea, Venezuela, and Chile. In Japan, upper gastrointestinal imaging series every 3 years or upper endoscopy every 2–3 years is recommended for individuals aged 50 years and older [33]. In Korea, upper endoscopy or upper gastrointestinal imaging series are recommended every 2 years for people aged 40–75 years [34].

Conclusion

Gastric cancer is one of the most common cancers in the world. The incidence of gastric cancer is decreasing around the world, but the incidence and mortality of gastric cancer are still high in East Asia. Early detection is essential to reduce the mortality rate of gastric cancer, so screening tests are required for the general population. The two main methods of gastric cancer screening are upper endoscopy and upper gastrointestinal imaging series. Endoscopic screening might reduce the gastric cancer mortality rate, but radiographic screening does not reduce the gastric cancer mortality rate. Furthermore, endoscopic screening might not reduce the incidence of gastric cancer. Further large, randomized trials are needed to verify lower gastric cancer mortality in screened populations.

References

1. Bray F, Ferlay J, Soerjomataram I, Siegel RL, Torre LA, Jemal A. Global cancer statistics 2018: GLOBOCAN estimates of incidence and mortality worldwide for 36 cancers in 185 countries. CA Cancer J Clin. 2018;68(6):394–424.
2. Mizoue T, Yoshimura T, Tokui N, Hoshiyama Y, Yatsuya H, Sakata K, et al. Prospective study of screening for stomach cancer in Japan. Int J Cancer. 2003;106(1):103–7.
3. Llorens P. Gastric cancer mass survey in Chile. Semin Surg Oncol. 1991;7(6):339–43.
4. Pisani P, Oliver WE, Parkin DM, Alvarez N, Vivas J. Case-control study of gastric cancer screening in Venezuela. Br J Cancer. 1994;69(6):1102–5.
5. Murakami R, Tsukuma H, Ubukata T, Fujimoto I, Kawashima T, Yamazaki H, et al. Estimation of validity of mass screening program for gastric cancer in Osaka. Japan Cancer. 1990;65(1):1255–60.
6. Hisamichi S, Sugawara N, Fukao A. Effectiveness of gastric mass screening in Japan. Cancer Detect Prev. 1988;11(3–6):323–9.

7. Fukao A, Tsubono Y, Tsuji I, HIsamichi S, Sugahara N, Takano A, et al. The evaluation of screening for gastric cancer in Miyagi prefecture, Japan: a population-based case-control study. Int J Cancer. 1995;60(1):45–8.
8. Oshima A, Hirata N, Ubukata T, Umeda K, Fujimoto I. Evaluation of a mass screening program for stomach cancer with a case-control study design. Int J Cancer. 1986;38(6):829–33.
9. Tsuji I, Fukao A, Sugawara N, Shoji T, Kuwajima I, Hisamichi S, et al. Cost-effectiveness analysis of screening for gastric cancer in Japan. Tohoku J Exp Med. 1991;164(4):279–84.
10. Kunisaki C, Ishino J, Nakajima S, Motohashi H, Akiyama H, Nomura M, et al. Outcomes of mass screening for gastric carcinoma. Ann Surg Oncol. 2006;13(2):221–8.
11. Inaba S, Hirayama H, Nagata C, Kurisu Y, Takatsuka N, Kawakami N, et al. Evaluation of a screening program on reduction of gastric cancer mortality in Japan: preliminary results from a cohort study. Prev Med. 1999;29(2):102–6.
12. Choi KS, Jun JK, Suh M, Park B, Noh DK, Song SH, et al. Effect of endoscopy screening on stage at gastric cancer diagnosis: results of the National Cancer Screening Programme in Korea. Br J Cancer. 2015;112(3):608–12.
13. Leung WK, Wu MS, Kakugawa Y, Kim JJ, Yeoh K, Goh KL, et al. Screening for gastric cancer in Asia: current evidence and practice. Lancet Oncol. 2008;9(3):279–87.
14. Oshima A. A critical review of cancer screening programs in Japan. Int J Technol Assess Health Care. 1994;10(3):346–58.
15. Kim Y, Jun JK, Choi KS, Lee HY, Park EC. Overview of the national cancer screening programme and the cancer screening status in Korea. Asian Pac J Cancer Prev. 2011;12(3):725–30.
16. Longo WE, Zucker KA, Zdon MJ, Modlin IM. Detection of early gastric cancer in an aggressive endoscopy unit. Am Surg. 1989;55(2):100–4.
17. Miki K. Gastric cancer screening using the serum pepsinogen test method. Gastric Cancer. 2006;9(4):245–53.
18. Aikou S, Ohmoto Y, Gunji T, Matsuhashi N, Ohtsu H, Miura H, et al. Tests for serum levels of trefoil factor family proteins can improve gastric cancer screening. Gastroenterology. 2011;141(3):837–45.
19. Liu HN, Wu H, Tseng YJ, Chen YJ, Zhang DY, Zhu L, et al. Serum microRNA signatures and metabolomics have high diagnostic value in gastric cancer. BMC Cancer. 2018;18(1):415–33.
20. Cohen JD, Li L, Wang Y, Thoburn C, Afsari B, Danilova L, et al. Detection and localization of surgically resectable cancers with a multi-analyte blood test. Science. 2018;359(6378):926–30.
21. Lee KJ, Inoue M, Otani T, Iwasaki M, Sasazuki S, Tsugane S, et al. Gastric cancer screening and subsequent risk of gastric cancer: a large-scale population-based cohort study, with a 13-year follow-up in Japan. Int J Cancer. 2006;118(9):2315–21.
22. Miyamoto A, Kuriyama S, Nishino Y, Tsubono Y, Nakaya N, Ohmori K, et al. Lower risk of death from gastric cancer among participants of gastric cancer screening in Japan: a population-based cohort study. Prev Med. 2007;44(1):12–9.
23. Rosero-Bixby L, Sierra R. X-ray screening seems to reduce gastric cancer mortality by half in a community-controlled trial in Costa Rica. Br J Cancer. 2007;97(7):837–43.
24. Jun JK, Choi KS, Lee HY, Suh M, Park B, Song SH, et al. Effectiveness of the Korean national cancer screening program in reducing gastric cancer mortality. Gastroenterology. 2017;152(6):1319–28.
25. Zhang X, Li M, Chen S, Hu J, Guo Q, Liu R, et al. Endoscopic screening in Asian countries is associated with reduced gastric cancer mortality: A meta-analysis and systematic review. Gastroenterology. 2018;155(2):347–54.
26. Dan YY, So JB, Yeoh KG. Endoscopic screening for gastric cancer. Clin Gastroenterol Hepatol. 2006;4(6):709–16.
27. Yeh JM, Hur C, Ward Z, Schrag D, Goldie SJ. Gastric adenocarcinoma screening and prevention in the era of new biomarker and endoscopic technologies: a cost-effectiveness analysis. Gut. 2016;65(4):563–74.
28. Gupta N, Bansal A, Wani SB, Gaddam S, Rastogi A, Sharma P. Endoscopy for upper GI cancer screening in the general population: a cost-utility analysis. Gastrointest Endosc. 2011;74(3):610–24.
29. Shah SC, Canakis A, Peek RM Jr, Saumoy M. Endoscopy for gastric cancer screening is cost effective for Asian Americans in the United States. Clin Gastroenterol Hepatol. 2020;18(13):3026–39.
30. Hamashima C, Shibuya D, Yamazaki H, Inoue K, Fukao A, Saito H, et al. The Japanese guidelines for gastric cancer screening. Jpn J Clin Oncol. 2008;38(4):259–67.
31. Hamashima C, Saito H, Nakayama T, Nakayama T, Sobue T. The standardized development method of the Japanese guidelines for cancer screening. Jpn J Clin Oncol. 2008;38(4):288–95.
32. Choi KS, Jun JK, Park EC, Park S, Jung KW, Han MA, et al. Performance of different gastric cancer screening methods in Korea: a population-based study. PLoS One. 2012;7(11):e50041–14.
33. Hamashima C. Update version of the Japanese guidelines for gastric cancer screening. Jpn J Clin Oncol. 2018;48(7):673–83.
34. Park HA, Nam SY, Lee SK, Kim SG, Shim KN, Park SM, et al. The Korean guideline for gastric cancer screening. J Korean Med Assoc. 2015;58(5):373–84.

Pathologic and Molecular Characteristics

Key Points

- The main histological subtypes of gastric adenocarcinoma are tubular, papillary, poorly cohesive, mucinous, and mixed adenocarcinoma.
- Immunohistochemistry (mismatch repair proteins, E-cadherin, and p53) plus in situ hybridization for small EBV-encoded RNA could possibly classify molecular subtypes of gastric adenocarcinoma in the routine pathologic laboratory.
- The HER2 test is important in patients with advanced and/or metastatic HER2-positive gastric adenocarcinoma and it is assessed primarily by immunohistochemistry.

Introduction

Gastric cancer develops from the lining of the stomach. In particular, gastric adenocarcinoma is a malignant epithelial tumor of the gastric mucosa. The intratumoral and intertumoral heterogeneity of gastric cancer are a challenge to overcome to better understand its underlying pathophysiology.

Histopathology

The overwhelming majority (about 95%) of malignant stomach tumors are adenocarcinoma that form glandular structures. Although various classifications for gastric adenocarcinoma have been proposed, the Lauren, Japanese Gastric Cancer Association (JGCA), and World Health Organization (WHO) classification system are used the most [1, 2]. The Lauren classification divides gastric adenocarcinoma into intestinal and diffuse subtypes [2]. The intestinal subtype is characterized by well-formed glands lined with cuboidal to columnar epithelial cells. In contrast, the diffuse subtype is composed of individual or poorly formed nests of tumor cells that grow in an infiltrative form. However, some cases show features of both intestinal and diffuse subtypes: these are classified as mixed subtypes. Five main histological subtypes of gastric adenocarcinoma are noted in the WHO schemes: tubular, papillary, poorly cohesive (including signet-ring cell and other subtypes), mucinous, and mixed adenocarcinoma. The intestinal subtype of the Lauren classification is similar to papillary adenocarcinoma and well/moderately differentiated tubular adenocarcinoma of the WHO scheme. Conversely, the diffuse subtype is similar to poorly cohesive carcinoma (signet-ring cell phenotype and other cell phenotypes). The morphological classification of differentiation, which is based on the architecture of gland or tubule for-

An Na Seo is the lead author of this chapter.

H. J. Chun et al., *Gastrointestinal Cancer*, https://doi.org/10.1007/978-981-99-0815-8_3

mation, is only applicable to tubular and papillary adenocarcinoma subtypes, but not to other gastric adenocarcinoma subtypes.

Tubular adenocarcinoma: This subtype is the most common histological subtype of gastric adenocarcinoma and consists of large and small glandular structures of simple or complex nature. Individual tumor cells can be cuboidal, columnar, or flattened by prominent intraluminal mucin or cell debris. Tumors with solid growth structures with an indistinguishable tubular shape are considered to be of this subtype. Poorly differentiated tubular adenocarcinoma is similar to por1 in the JGCA classification.

Papillary adenocarcinoma: This subtype is a relatively rare subtype characterized by an exophytic growth pattern of tumor cells in elongated finger-like processes supported by fibrovascular connective tissue cores (Fig. 1). As the tumor progresses gradually, it may exhibit the form of tubulopapillary adenocarcinoma, in which papillary adenocarcinoma and tubular adenocarcinoma are mixed.

Poorly cohesive carcinoma (PCC), including signet-ring cell carcinoma and other subtypes: This subtype has been reported to be relatively common in Asian patients. It is characterized by a diffuse distribution of tumor cells that are isolated or arranged in small aggregates without well-formed glands. PCCs can be either of the signet-ring cell type or the non-signet-ring cell type (PCC-NOS). The signet-ring cell type shows large amounts of cytoplasmic mucin with crescent-shaped peripherally displaced nuclei (Fig. 2a). This signet-ring cell type can rarely form a lace-like glandular or delicate microtrabecular structures. Non-signet-ring cell type (PCC-NOS) may resemble histiocytes, lymphocytes, or plasma cells (Fig. 2b). PCC can be accompanied by a desmoplastic reaction of the stroma. PCC appears to be resistant to chemotherapy [3]. The signet-ring cell type and PCC-NOS are classified as signet-ring cell carcinoma and as Por2 (non-solid type) in JGCA classification, respectively [1]. Some researchers have suggested that tumors with more than 90% signet-ring cell morphology should be recognized as signet-ring cell carcinoma [4].

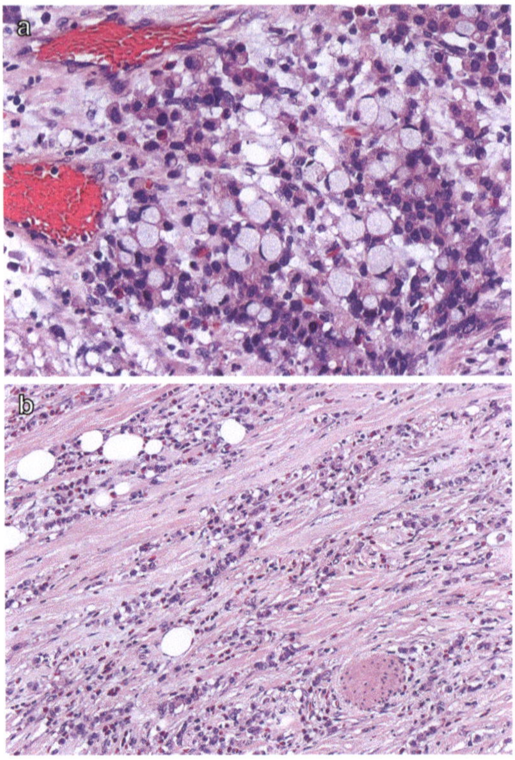

Fig. 2 Poorly cohesive carcinoma (PCC). (**a**) The nucleus of tumor cells is displaced to one side because of abundant mucin in the cytoplasm (signet ring cell type) (40× objective). (**b**) Tumor cells are scattered and infiltrated and resemble plasma cells and/or lymphocytes (non-signet ring cell type, PCC, NOS) (20× objective)

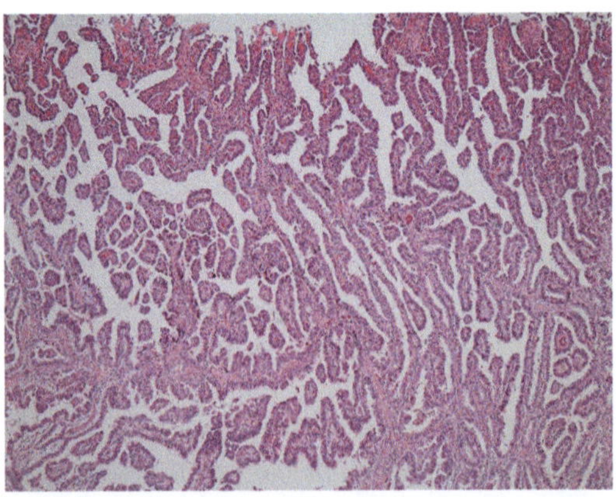

Fig. 1 Papillary adenocarcinoma. Gastric cancer showing elongated finger-like processes with fibrovascular cores (4× objective)

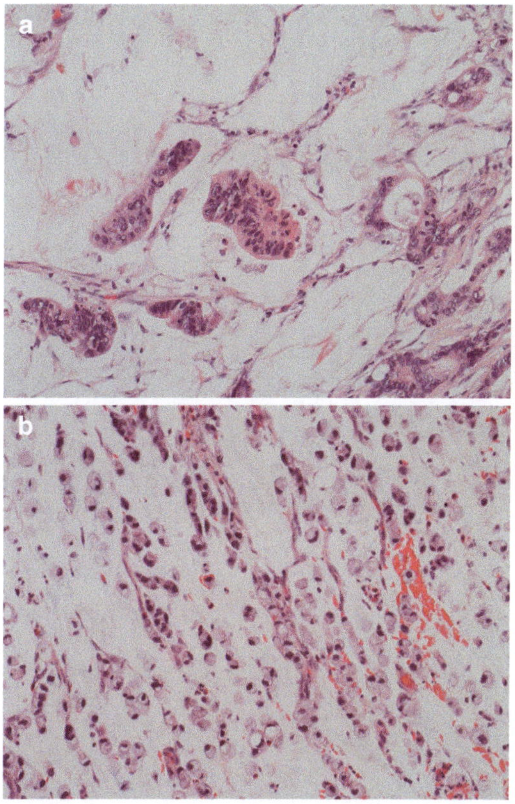

Fig. 3 Mucinous adenocarcinoma. (**a**) Malignant glands and tubules lined by columnar epithelium floating in extracellular mucin pool; (**b**) Scattered floating signet-ring cells in an extracellular mucin pool (20× objective)

Mucinous adenocarcinoma: This subtype accounts for ~2.6–8.1% of gastric cancers and is characterized by malignant tumor cells with more than 50% of the tumor volume showing extracellular mucin pools [5, 6]. These tumor cells can be composed of two main growth patterns: (1) glands and tubules lined by columnar epithelium floating in background mucin (Fig. 3a); (2) nest or single tumor cells (signet-ring cell features) floating in background mucin (Fig. 3b).

Mixed adenocarcinoma: This subtype is characterized by showing two or more distinct histological components: glandular (tubular/papillary) and PCC (Fig. 4).

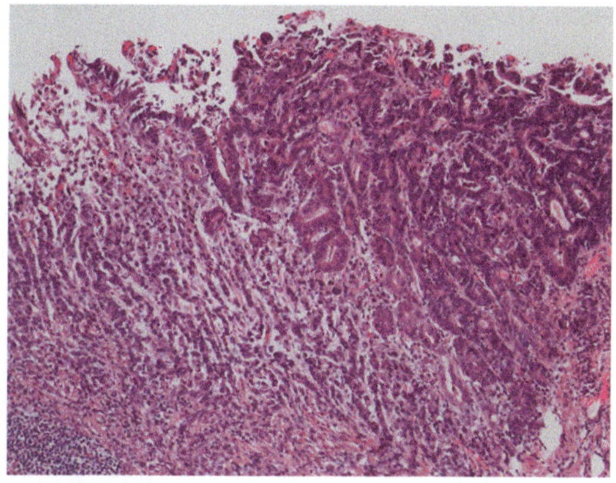

Fig. 4 Mixed carcinoma. This image shows a mixed tubular adenocarcinoma (right) and poorly cohesive carcinoma (left) (10× objective)

Unusual Histologic Variants

Gastric carcinoma with lymphoid stroma: This subtype has been referred to as lymphoepithelioma-like carcinoma and medullary carcinoma. This tumor accounts for 1–7% of gastric cancers and is characterized by irregular sheets, poorly defined tubules, lace-like pattern, and prominent lymphocytic infiltration (Fig. 5). It is strongly associated with Epstein-Barr virus (EBV) infection, which is identified in ~22.5–100% of this subtype. This subtype can also show gastric cancers with mismatch repair deficiency, although EBV and microsatellite instability (MSI) are mutually exclusive in gastric cancer (Fig. 6) [7, 8].

Hepatoid adenocarcinoma: This subtype is predominantly composed of large polygonal eosinophilic hepatocyte-like tumor cells. Immunohistochemistry for AFP can be identified in hepatoid differentiation.

Micropapillary adenocarcinoma: This subtype is an aggressive variant of gastric cancer, characterized by small clusters of tumor cells with inside-out growth patterns in clear lacunar spaces, simulating lymphatic or vascular channels (Fig. 7) [9].

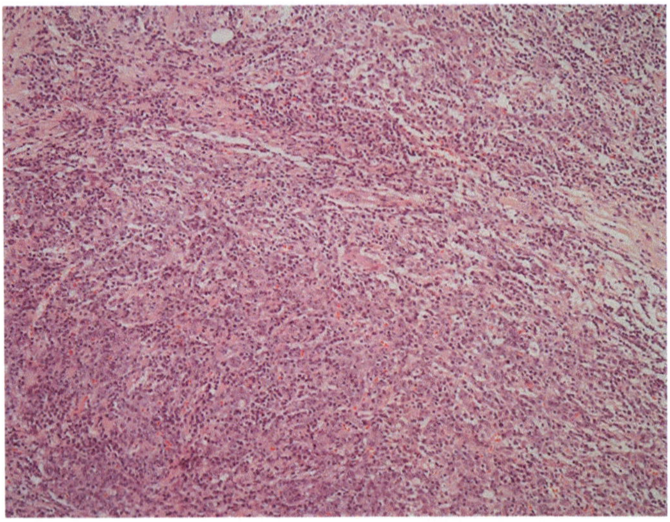

Fig. 5 Gastric carcinoma with lymphoid stroma. This example displays lace-like pattern of tumor cells and prominent lymphocytic infiltration (10× objective)

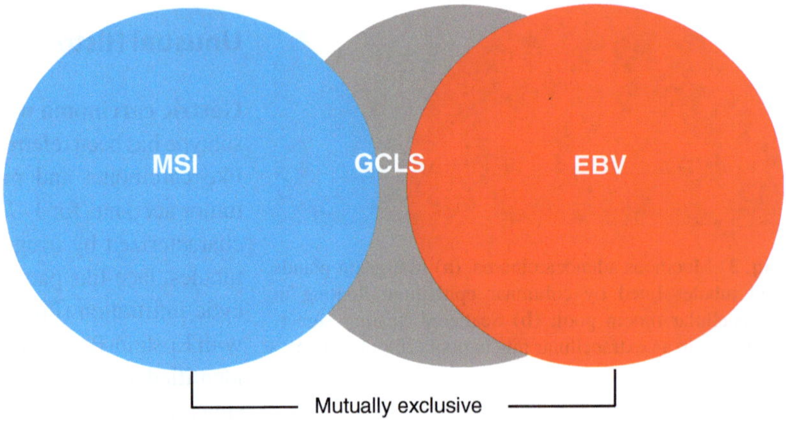

Fig. 6 Venn Diagram of gastric carcinoma with lymphoid stroma (GCLS). GCLS is an unusual variant enriched for mutually exclusive Epstein-Barr virus (EBV) positivity and mismatch repair (MMR) deficiency

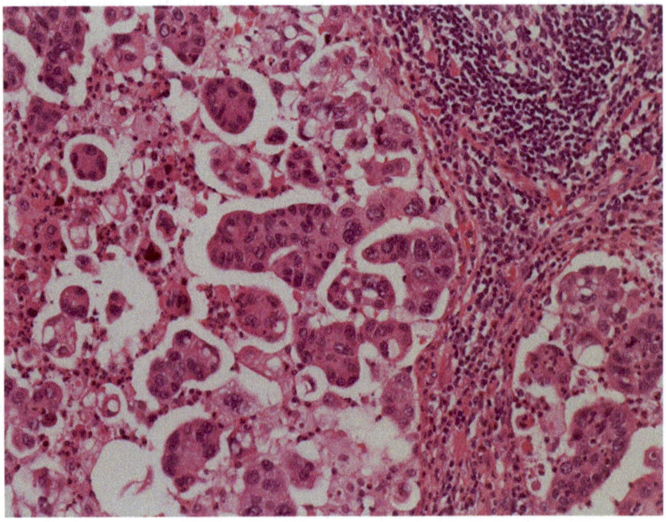

Fig. 7 Micropapillary adenocarcinoma. The tumor cluster was characterized by small tufts without fibrovascular core (20× objective)

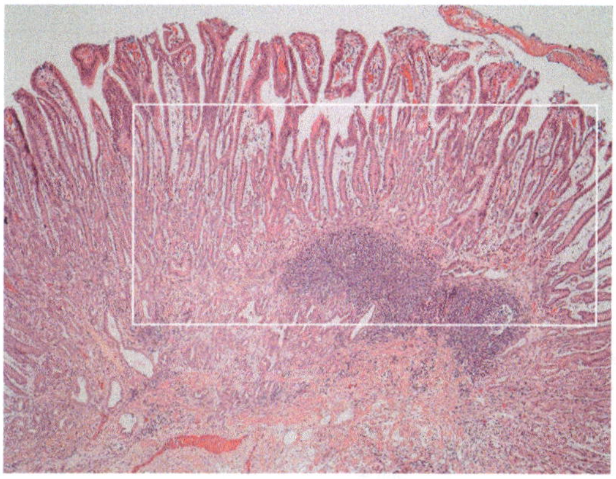

Fig. 8 Gastric adenocarcinoma of fundic-gland type. Tumor cells composed of irregular anastomosing cords and glands that are similar to the fundic glands with invasion into the submucosal layer (white rectangle) (4× objective)

Gastric adenocarcinoma of fundic-gland type: This subtype is a new rare variant of gastric cancer, and it has been added to the 5th Edition of the WHO classification [10] and accounts for 1% of patients with early gastric cancer who underwent esophagogastroduodenoscopy [11]. This tumor differentiates toward the fundic gland and commonly involves dominant cell-predominant differentiation (~99% of reported cases) with low-grade cytology [10]. Submucosal invasion is reported in approximately 60% of this subtype [12]. Due to the lack of awareness of this subtype, a correct diagnosis can be difficult to achieve (Fig. 8).

Molecular Classification of Gastric Cancer

The molecular genetic classification of gastric cancer may help define future personalized therapy plans by providing opportunities for patient stratification and the development of new biomarkers for clinical trials. Recently, advancements in genomic technology have allowed gastric cancer to be studied at a high-resolution molecular level [13]. Such molecular profiles have facilitated an improved understanding of driver alterations involved in gastric carcinogenesis and the identification of candidate driver alterations in gastric cancer [13]. Using high-throughput analysis, such as chromosomal alterations, gene mutations, epigenetic derangements, and transcriptional changes, several groups have proposed a genetic and epigenetic molecular classification of gastric cancer [14–18]. There are three well-known representative molecular genetic classifications as follows: 'Singapore-Duke' study, The Cancer Genome Atlas (TCGA) Research Network, and the Asian Cancer Research Group (ACRG) (Fig. 9) [14–16].

In 2013, the Singapore-Duke study classified gastric cancers into three subtypes according to particular biological properties and responses to chemotherapy and the targeted agents: proliferative, metabolic, and mesenchymal type.

In 2014, TCGA proposed a classification categorizing gastric cancer into four molecular subtypes. Epstein-Barr virus (EBV)-positive, microsatellite-unstable, genomically stable (GS), and chromosomal instability (CIN) gastric cancers [15]. Although this taxonomy did not confirm the association with the clinical outcome of the patient, it associates distinct clinical characteristics for each molecular subtype. CIN gastric cancers have been reported to achieve the greatest benefit from adjuvant chemotherapy among the four subtypes, whereas GS gastric cancers show the least benefit from adjuvant chemotherapy [19].

In 2015, ACRG proposed a molecular classification of gastric cancer into four different subtypes: microsatellite-unstable, microsatellite-stable (MSS) with epithelial–mesenchymal transition (EMT) gene signature; MSS; and *TP53*-active; and MSS and *TP53*-inactive gastric cancers. The ACRG classification shows a correlation with appropriate clinico-pathological findings and can predict clinical outcome by stratifying differences in survival rates according to molecular subtypes [16]. Microsatellite-unstable gastric cancers had the best overall survival rate among the four subtypes of ACRG classification [16]. Unfortunately, there was no agreement between the classified category pre-

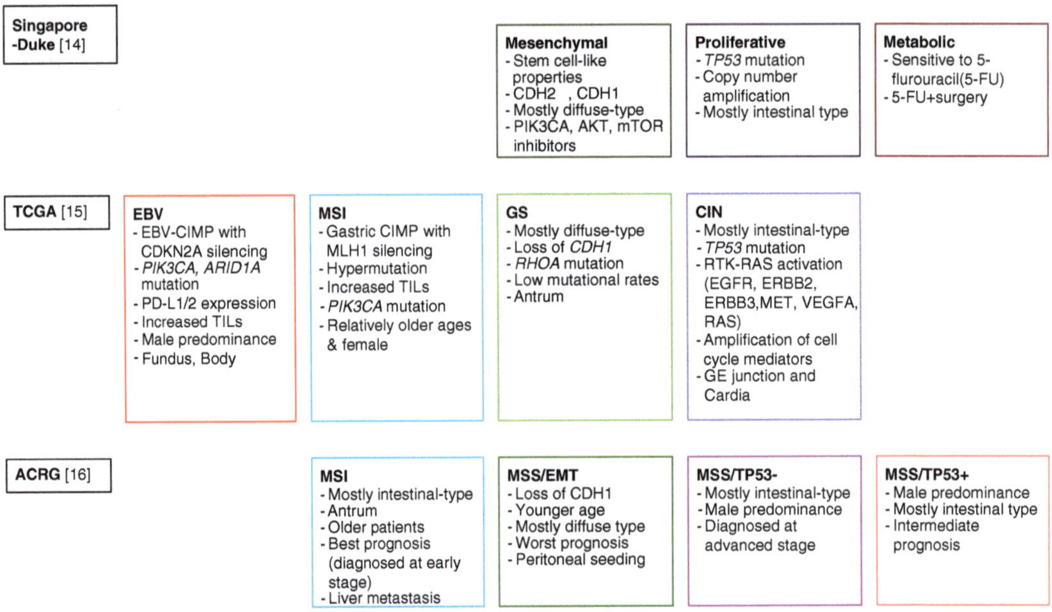

Fig. 9 Summary of famous molecular classification of gastric cancer

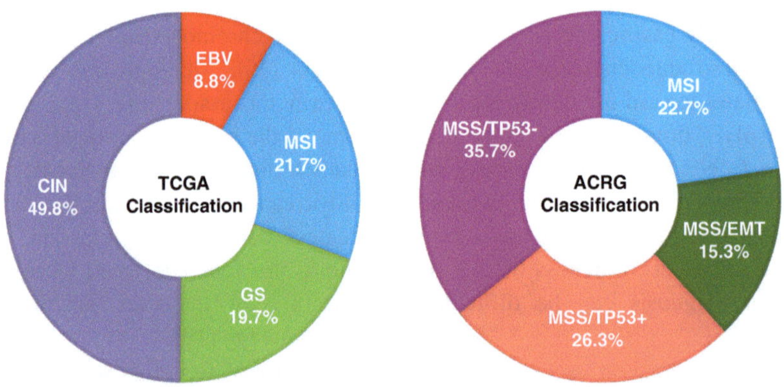

Fig. 10 Comparison between The Cancer Genome Atlas (TCGA) Research Network, and the Asian Cancer Research Group (ACRG) classification. Among subtypes of the TCGA and ACRG classifications, only microsatellite-instability (MSI) subtypes are common EBV (Epstein-Barr virus); GS (genomically stable); CIN (chromosomal instability); MSS (microsatellite-stable); EMT (epithelial–mesenchymal transition)

sented by the two datasets, TCGA and ACRG, except for subtype of MSI gastric cancer (Fig. 10).

In routine pathologic practice, it is possible to identify a protein and mRNA expression-based classification for the five subgroups of gastric cancer using immunohistochemistry for the expression of mismatch repair (MMR) proteins (MLH1, etc.), E-cadherin, and p53 combined with in situ hybridization for EBV-encoded small RNA (EBER) (five subtypes: EBV-positive, microsatellite-instability, aberrant E-cadherin, aberrant p53 expression, and normal p53 expression subtypes) [18, 20].

ERBB2 (Human Epidermal Growth Factor Receptor 2 [HER2])

Based on the randomized controlled Trastuzumab for Gastric Cancer (ToGA) study [21], anti-ERBB2 therapy (especially, trastuzumab) was approved for the treatment of unresectable locally advanced, metastatic, or recurrent HER2-positive gastric cancer [7]. Overall, 7–15% of gastric cancers have been reported to be HER2-positive, which is more closely related to the upper third location of the stomach and the intestinal type of Lauren classification. Furthermore, 24–38% of gastro-esophageal junction (GEJ) adenocarcinoma have been shown to be HER2-positive [22]. In routine practice, the HER2 test is performed according to the published guideline and is assessed primarily by immunohistochemistry (IHC) [7, 22–25].

In endoscopy biopsy specimens, at least four to six biopsy tissue fragments containing cancer cells are recommended for the proper HER2 IHC test [7, 23]. Surgical specimens from patients that were initially HER2-negative in biopsy specimens should be re-assessed to increase the chances of finding HER2-positive patients [26]. This is due to intratumoral heterogeneity of HER2, which has been reported in up to 30% of gastric cancers [27, 28]. If the HER2 immunohistochemistry results are equivocal (IHC 2+), ERBB2 in situ hybridization of ERBB2 (ISH) using fluorescence or silver is recommended [7, 22]. Dual-color ISH is recommended for HER2 amplification analysis, and at least 20 evaluable and non-overlapping cells should be initially counted [7]. If the HER2: chromosome enumeration probe 17 (CEP17) ratio is ≥2.0, it is defined as 'ISH positive' [7, 22].

Epstein-Barr Virus

Although laboratory detection of EBV has been performed by several published methods [29], the presence or absence of EBV is observed by EBER ISH, which are amplified EBER transcripts, and is regarded as the gold standard for identifying and localizing latent EBV in tissue samples [7, 30]. Interpretation of EBER ISH is made by microscopic examination, and only nuclear EBER-positivity (black or dark blue signals) in tumor cells is defined as EBV-positive (Fig. 11) [7].

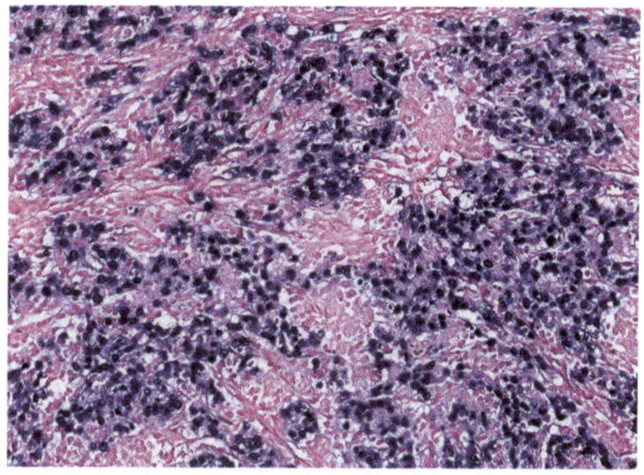

Fig. 11 Epstein–Barr virus (EBV)-encoded RNA in situ hybridization (ISH) in EBV-associated gastric cancer (EBVaGC). Black/dark blue signals are localized in the nuclei of infected tumor cells (20× objective)

Cancer Immunotherapy

Tumor mutation load, also known as tumor mutation burden, the density of intratumoral CD8-positive cytotoxic T cell infiltration (TIL), and PD-L1 expression have been suggested as predictors of response to immune checkpoint blockade therapy [31, 32]. Elevated expression of PD-L1 is associated with high TIL densities, MMR deficiency, and EBV positivity [15, 33]. Therefore, patients with EBV-positive and microsatellite-unstable gastric cancers, which are mutually exclusive, could benefit from immunotherapy targeting the PD1/PD-L1 axis [34].

Conclusion

Although molecular and genetic analysis is ongoing in gastric cancer, the interpretation of histopathologic features is still important. Because histopathologic features are well-known, a correlation with the molecular genetic characteristics is expected in the future.

References

1. Japanese Gastric Cancer A. Japanese gastric cancer treatment guidelines 2018 (5th edition). Gastric Cancer 2021;24:1–21.

2. Lauren P. The two histological main types of gastric carcinoma: diffuse and so-called intestinal-type carcinoma. An attempt at a histo-clinical classification. Acta Pathol Microbiol Scand. 1965;64:31–49.
3. Voron T, Messager M, Duhamel A, Lefevre J, Mabrut JY, Goere D, et al. Is signet-ring cell carcinoma a specific entity among gastric cancers? Gastric Cancer. 2016;19:1027–40.
4. Mariette C, Carneiro F, Grabsch HI, van der Post RS, Allum W, de Manzoni G. Consensus on the pathological definition and classification of poorly cohesive gastric carcinoma. Gastric Cancer. 2019;22:1–9.
5. Kunisaki C, Akiyama H, Nomura M, Matsuda G, Otsuka Y, Ono HA, et al. Clinicopathologic characteristics and surgical outcomes of mucinous gastric carcinoma. Ann Surg Oncol. 2006;13:836–42.
6. Hyung WJ, Noh SH, Shin DW, Yoo CH, Kim CB, Min JS, et al. Clinicopathologic characteristics of mucinous gastric adenocarcinoma. Yonsei Med J. 1999;40:99–106.
7. Lee HS, Kim WH, Kwak Y, Koh J, Bae JM, Kim K-M, et al. Molecular testing for gastrointestinal Cancer. J Pathol Transl Med. 2017;51:103–21.
8. Hissong E, Ramrattan G, Zhang P, Zhou XK, Young G, Klimstra DS, et al. Gastric carcinomas with lymphoid stroma: an evaluation of the histopathologic and molecular features. Am J Surg Pathol. 2018;42:453–62.
9. Eom DW, Kang GH, Han SH, Cheon GJ, Han KH, Oh HS, et al. Gastric micropapillary carcinoma: a distinct subtype with a significantly worse prognosis in TNM stages I and II. Am J Surg Pathol. 2011;35:84–91.
10. Li C, Wu X, Yang S, Yang X, Yao J, Zheng H. Gastric adenocarcinoma of the fundic gland type: clinicopathological features of eight patients treated with endoscopic submucosal dissection. Diagn Pathol. 2020;15:131.
11. Ueyama H, Matsumoto K, Nagahara A, Hayashi T, Yao T, Watanabe S. Gastric adenocarcinoma of the fundic gland type (chief cell predominant type). Endoscopy. 2014;46:153–7.
12. Benedict MA, Lauwers GY, Jain D. Gastric adenocarcinoma of the fundic gland type: update and literature review. Am J Clin Pathol. 2018;149:461–73.
13. Chia NY, Tan P. Molecular classification of gastric cancer. Ann Oncol. 2016;27:763–9.
14. Lei Z, Tan IB, Das K, Deng N, Zouridis H, Pattison S, et al. Identification of molecular subtypes of gastric cancer with different responses to PI3-kinase inhibitors and 5-fluorouracil. Gastroenterology. 2013;145:554–65.
15. Network CGAR. Comprehensive molecular characterization of gastric adenocarcinoma. Nature. 2014;513:202–9.
16. Cristescu R, Lee J, Nebozhyn M, Kim KM, Ting JC, Wong SS, et al. Molecular analysis of gastric cancer identifies subtypes associated with distinct clinical outcomes. Nat Med. 2015;21:449–56.
17. Oh SC, Sohn BH, Cheong JH, Kim SB, Lee JE, Park KC, et al. Clinical and genomic landscape of gastric cancer with a mesenchymal phenotype. Nat Commun. 2018;9:1777.
18. Setia N, Agoston AT, Han HS, Mullen JT, Duda DG, Clark JW, et al. A protein and mRNA expression-based classification of gastric cancer. Mod Pathol. 2016;29:772–84.
19. Sohn BH, Hwang JE, Jang HJ, Lee HS, Oh SC, Shim JJ, et al. Clinical significance of four molecular subtypes of gastric cancer identified by the cancer genome atlas project. Clin Cancer Res. 2017;23:4441–9.
20. Ahn S, Lee SJ, Kim Y, Kim A, Shin N, Choi KU, et al. High-throughput protein and mRNA expression-based classification of gastric cancers can identify clinically distinct subtypes, concordant with recent molecular classifications. Am J Surg Pathol. 2017;41:106–15.
21. Bang YJ, Van Cutsem E, Feyereislova A, Chung HC, Shen L, Sawaki A, et al. Trastuzumab in combination with chemotherapy versus chemotherapy alone for treatment of HER2-positive advanced gastric or gastro-oesophageal junction cancer (ToGA): a phase 3, open-label, randomised controlled trial. Lancet. 2010;376:687–97.
22. Bartley AN, Washington MK, Colasacco C, Ventura CB, Ismaila N, Benson AB 3rd, et al. HER2 Testing and Clinical Decision Making in Gastroesophageal Adenocarcinoma: Guideline From the College of American Pathologists, American Society for Clinical Pathology, and the American Society of Clinical Oncology. J Clin Oncol. 2017;35:446–64.
23. Hofmann M, Stoss O, Shi D, Büttner R, van de Vijver M, Kim W, et al. Assessment of a HER2 scoring system for gastric cancer: results from a validation study. Histopathology. 2008;52:797–805.
24. Kim KM, Bilous M, Chu KM, Kim BS, Kim WH, Park YS, et al. Human epidermal growth factor receptor 2 testing in gastric cancer: recommendations of an Asia-Pacific task force. Asia Pac J Clin Oncol. 2014;10:297–307.
25. Rüschoff J, Hanna W, Bilous M, Hofmann M, Osamura RY, Penault-Llorca F, et al. HER2 testing in gastric cancer: a practical approach. Mod Pathol. 2012;25:637–50.
26. Park SR, Park YS, Ryu MH, Ryoo BY, Woo CG, Jung HY, et al. Extra-gain of HER2-positive cases through HER2 reassessment in primary and metastatic sites in advanced gastric cancer with initially HER2-negative primary tumours: results of GASTric cancer HER2 reassessment study 1 (GASTHER1). Eur J Cancer. 2016;53:42–50.
27. Kaito A, Kuwata T, Tokunaga M, Shitara K, Sato R, Akimoto T, et al. HER2 heterogeneity is a poor prognosticator for HER2-positive gastric cancer. World J Clin Cases. 2019;7:1964–77.
28. Haffner I, Schierle K, Raimúndez E, Geier B, Maier D, Hasenauer J, et al. HER2 expression, test deviations, and their impact on survival in metastatic gastric Cancer: results from the prospective multicenter VARIANZ study. J Clin Oncol. 2021;39:1468–78.
29. Gulley ML. Molecular diagnosis of Epstein-Barr virus-related diseases. J Mol Diagn. 2001;3:1–10.

30. Ambinder RF, Mann RB. Epstein-Barr-encoded RNA in situ hybridization: diagnostic applications. Hum Pathol. 1994;25:602–5.
31. Topalian SL, Taube JM, Anders RA, Pardoll DM. Mechanism-driven biomarkers to guide immune checkpoint blockade in cancer therapy. Nat Rev Cancer. 2016;16:275–87.
32. Kwak Y, Seo AN, Lee HE, Lee HS. Tumor immune response and immunotherapy in gastric cancer. J Pathol Transl Med. 2020;54:20–33.
33. Kawazoe A, Kuwata T, Kuboki Y, Shitara K, Nagatsuma AK, Aizawa M, et al. Clinicopathological features of programmed death ligand 1 expression with tumor-infiltrating lymphocyte, mismatch repair, and Epstein-Barr virus status in a large cohort of gastric cancer patients. Gastric Cancer. 2017;20:407–15.
34. Kim ST, Cristescu R, Bass AJ, Kim KM, Odegaard JI, Kim K, et al. Comprehensive molecular characterization of clinical responses to PD-1 inhibition in metastatic gastric cancer. Nat Med. 2018;24:1449–58.

Diagnosis, Staging, and Prognosis

Key Points

- Gastric cancer is diagnosed by endoscopic examination, during which the tumor localization within the stomach and its macroscopic type are determined, and biopsies are obtained for confirmation of histological diagnosis.
- All patients with gastric cancer should be staged to determine the direction of treatment approach (curative or palliative) and evaluate the survival and prognosis.
- EUS is considered a diagnostic device for the locoregional staging of gastric cancer.
- The eighth AJCC cancer staging manual includes the clinical stage, pathologic stage, and post-neoadjuvant stage, and provides better critical guidance to clinicians in making informed decisions throughout the treatment course.

Introduction

Gastric cancer is the third leading cause of cancer mortality after lung and colorectal cancer and the fifth in incidence. Once gastric cancer is histologically diagnosed, the next important step is staging, which can determine the direction of the treatment approach (curative or palliative). In addition, survival and prognosis vary significantly depending on the stage of the disease at the time of diagnosis. Since the eighth Edition of the American Joint Committee on Cancer (AJCC) Cancer Staging manual including the clinical stage and post-neoadjuvant stage has been released, clinicians have received improved guidance on treatment-decision making and prognostic information throughout the treatment course. Here, we will review the diagnosis, staging, and prognosis prediction in patients with gastric cancer.

Diagnosis

Gastric cancer is diagnosed by endoscopic examination, during which tumor location within the stomach and its macroscopic type are determined and biopsies are obtained for histological confirmation. Diagnosis should be made from endoscopic or surgical biopsy and reviewed by an experienced pathologist. There are several classification systems in gastric cancer, including the Lauren classification, the Nakamura classification, and the World Health Organization (WHO) classification. The Lauren classification of gastric cancer was established in 1965 [1] and is still widely used. The Laruren classification distinguishes two histological subtypes of gastric can-

Seon-Young Park is the lead author of this chapter.

H. J. Chun et al., *Gastrointestinal Cancer*, https://doi.org/10.1007/978-981-99-0815-8_4

Table 1 Histological classification of gastric cancer

Lauren (1965)	Nakamura (1968)	JGCA (2017)	WHO (2018)
Intestinal	Differentiated	Papillary Tubular1, well-differentiated Tubular2, moderately-differentiated	Papillary Tubular, well-differentiated Tubular, moderately-differentiated
Intermediate	Undifferentiated	Poorly 1 (solid type): Por 1	Tubular, poorly-differentiated (solid)
Diffuse	Undifferentiated	Signet-ring cell carcinoma (SRC): Sig Poorly 2 (non-solid type): por2	Poorly cohesive, SRC type poorly cohesive, NOS
Intestinal/diffuse/indeterminate	Differentiated/undifferentiated	Mucinous	Mucinous
Mixed		Description according to the proportion (e.g. por2 > sig > tub2)	Mixed
Not defined	Not defined	**Specific type**: Adenosquamous carcinoma Squamous cell carcinoma Undifferentiated carcinoma Carcinoma with lymphoid stroma Hepatoid adenocarcinoma Adenocarcinoma with enteroblastic differentiation Adenocarcinoma of fundic gland type	**Histological variants**: Adenosquamous carcinoma Squamous cell carcinoma Undifferentiated carcinoma Carcinoma with lymphoid stroma Hepatoid carcinoma Adenocarcinoma with enteroblastic differentiation Adenocarcinoma of fundic gland type Micropapillary adenocarcinoma

JGCA Japanese gastric cancer association, *WHO* World health organisation

cer, intestinal and diffuse, and an indeterminate type was included to characterize infrequent histology. Signet-ring cell carcinoma is assigned to the diffuse subtype. The WHO classification is considered the most detailed classification. It also describes other types of gastric tumors with decreased incidence [2]. In this classification, gastric adenocarcinoma is divided into subtypes (tubular, parietal cell, papillary, micropapillary, mucoepidermoid, mucinous, poorly cohesive, signet-ring cell, medullary adenocarcinoma with lymphoid stroma, hepatoid, and Paneth cell type. Tubular adenocarcinoma is classified into three subcategories: well-differentiated adenocarcinoma, moderately-differentiated adenocarcinoma, and poorly differentiated adenocarcinoma. The Nakamura classification includes two major categories: differentiated and undifferentiated type. The former includes well-differentiated, moderately differentiated, and papillary adenocarcinoma. The latter undifferentiated type is considered to have a higher probability of lymph node metastasis than the differentiated type. Table 1 summarizes the histological classifications of gastric cancer.

Staging

All patients should be staged according to the latest edition of the Union for International Cancer Control (UICC) and the AJCC and staging should be reviewed by an experienced multidisciplinary tumor board before determining a treatment pathway [3]. Clinical staging includes computed tomography (CT) findings of the abdomen and chest, which provides information on the presence of metastasis in the liver, lung, or peritoneum and helps clinicians to determine clinical staging and whether the treatment approach will be curative or palliative. For patients who require curative resection, the physician must consider whether endoscopic resection or surgical resection would be more appropriate. As endoscopic resection can be considered as a definite treatment for most early gastric cancers without risk factors for lymph node metastasis, an important risk factor for lymph node metastasis is the presence of lymphovascular invasion, which can be identified in the pathological finding after endoscopic resection. Other risk factors include submucosal invasion (T1b), poor differentiation, ulceration, and large tumor size [4]. Among these risk factors, endoscopic ultrasound could be helpful in identifying the depth of the tumor. Endoscopic ultrasonography (EUS) is considered a diagnostic instrument for the locoregional staging of gastric cancer. Recent meta-analysis showed that EUS discriminated between T1a (mucosal) and T1b (submucosal) cancer with sensitivity of 0.87 (95% CI 0.81–0.92) and specificity of 0.75 (95% CI 0.62–0.84), suggesting lower diagnostic accuracy [5]. However, EUS could be helpful in identifying superficial lesions that do not penetrate further than the submucosa (T1) or muscularis propria (T2) from advanced cancers (T3-T4). Furthermore, EUS is able to discriminate between T1 and T2 cancers with a sensitivity and specificity of 0.85 (95% CI 0.75–0.91) for T1 and 0.90 (0.85–0.93) for T2 [5]. Positron emission tomography CT may be helpful in detecting CT-occult metastasis and preoperative lymph node staging, but is less sensitive in mucinous or diffuse cancers [6, 7]. Peritoneal relapse is common in patients with resected gastric cancer, especially in patients with diffuse-type cancers. Exploratory laparoscopy to detect peritoneal metastasis is recommended for patients with gastric cancer at stage 1B or greater, for whom surgical resection is planned [8].

Prognosis

Prognosis and survival vary significantly depending on the stage of the disease at the time of diagnosis. Early-stage gastric adenocarcinoma has a 5-year survival rate of >90%, while regional gastric adenocarcinoma has a 5-year survival rate of 29%, and metastatic adenocarcinoma 4% [9]. Staging is performed according to the AJCC TNM [tumor (T), node (N), and metastasis (M)] classification, eighth Edition (Tables 2 and 3)

Table 2 American Joint Committee on Cancer (AJCC) TNM staging classification of carcinoma of the stomach (8th ed. 2017) [10]

TNM stages	
Primary tumor (T)	
TX	Primary tumor cannot be assessed
T0	No evidence of primary tumor
Tis	Carcinoma in situ (intraepithelial tumor without invasion of the lamina propria)
T1	Tumor invades lamina propria, muscularis mucosa or submucosa
T1a	Tumor invades lamina propria or muscularis mucosa
T1b	Tumor invades submucosa
T2	Tumor invades muscularis propria[a]
T3	Tumor penetrates subserosa connective tissue without invasion of visceral peritoneum or adjacent structures[b,c]
T4	Tumor invades serosa (visceral peritoneum) or adjacent structures[b,c]
T4a	Tumor invades serosa
T4b	Tumor invades adjacent structures
Regional LN (N)	
N0	No nodal metastasis
N1	Metastasis in 1–2 regional lymph nodes
N2	Metastasis in 3–6 regional lymph nodes
N3	Metastasis in 7 or more regional lymph nodes
N3a	Metastasis in 7 to 15 regional lymph nodes
N3b	Metastasis in 16 or more regional lymph nodes
Distant metastasis (M)	
M0	No distant metastasis
M1	Distant metastasis

[a]A tumor may penetrate the muscularis propria with extension into the gastrocolic or gastrohepatic ligaments, or into the greater or lesser omentum, without perforation of the visceral peritoneum covering these structures. In this case, the tumor is classified as T3. If there is perforation of the visceral peritoneum covering the gastric ligaments or the omentum, the tumor should be classified as T4

[b]The adjacent structures of the stomach include the spleen, transverse colon, liver, diaphragm, pancreas, abdominal wall, adrenal gland, kidney, small intestine, and retroperitoneum

[c]Intramural extension to the duodenum or esophagus is not considered invasion of an adjacent structure, but is classified using the depth of the greatest invasion in any of these sites

Table 3 AJCC prognostic stage groups [10]

Stage grouping	
0	Tis N0 M0
IA	T1, N0, M0
IB	T1, N1, M0; T2, N0, M0
IIA	T3, N0, M0; T2, N1, M0; T1, N2, M0
IIB	T4a, N0, M0; T3, N1, M0; T2, N2, M0; T1, N3, M0
IIIA	T4a, N2, M0; T4b, N0, M0; T3, N1–2, M0; T2, N3a, M0
IIIB	T4b, N1–2, M0; T3, N3a, M0; T1–2, N3b, M0
IIIC	T4b, N3a-b, M0; T3-4a, N3b, M0
IV	Any T; any N; M1

[10]. This is the internationally accepted standard for cancer staging and influences the prognosis and treatment decisions. The AJCC cancer staging manual includes clinical staging, pathologic staging, and post-neoadjuvant staging, and provides better critical guidance to clinicians in making informed decisions throughout the treatment course. Until the seventh Edition, the staging system for gastric cancer had been based on pathological findings from resected specimens, which was an unmet need in staging patients under different situations. The prognostic information from the eighth Edition AJCC classification is based on datasets from the National Cancer Database (NCDB) in the United States (patients treated surgically and non-surgically) and the Shizuoka Cancer Center dataset in Japan (patients treated surgically) [10]. In the NCDB cohort, the 5-year survival rates for pathological Stage IA and IIA are 94% and 88%, respectively. However, for clinical stage I, that was 56%. Likewise, the 5 - year survival for pathologic stage IIb was 98%, whereas for clinical stage IIb, that was 33%. In the Shizuoka Cancer Center dataset cohort in Japan, 5-year survival rates for clinical stage IA, IB, IIA, and IIb were 94%, 84.7%, 71.7%, and 56.1%, respectively [11]. There are potential reasons for these survival disparities, including selection bias and differences in the population of patients (US vs. Japanese patient). However, the survival curves were clearly separated in two cohorts. The prognostic values of these two cohorts have been externally validated in a cohort of 4374 surgically- treated patients in Japan [9].

Conclusions

Gastric cancer is diagnosed by endoscopic examination, during which tumor location within the stomach and its macroscopic type are determined and biopsies are taken for histological confirmation. All patients with gastric cancer should be adequately staged to determine the direction of the treatment approach and to evaluate survival and prognosis. Since the proposed eighth AJCC Cancer Staging manual includes prognostic information for patients before treatment and for patients who have undergone surgery following neoadjuvant therapy, it provides improved guidance to clinicians for making informed decisions throughout the treatment course.

References

1. Lauren P. The two histological main types of gastric carcinoma: diffuse and so-called intestinal-type carcinoma. An attempt at a histo-clinical classification. Acta Pathol Microbiol Scand. 1965;64:31–49.
2. Smyth EC, Verheij M, Allum W, Cunningham D, Cervantes A, Arnold D. Gastric cancer: ESMO Clinical Practice Guidelines for diagnosis, treatment and follow-up. Ann Oncol. 2016;27:v38–49.
3. Amin MB, Greene FL, Edge SB, Compton CC, Gershenwald JE, Brookland RK, et al. The Eighth Edition AJCC Cancer Staging Manual: Continuing to build a bridge from a population-based to a more "personalized" approach to cancer staging. CA Cancer J Clin. 2017;67:93–9.
4. Hatta W, Gotoda T, Koike T, Masamune A. History and future perspectives in Japanese guidelines for endoscopic resection of early gastric cancer. Dig Endosc. 2020;32:180–90.
5. Mocellin S, Pasquali S. Diagnostic accuracy of endoscopic ultrasonography (EUS) for the preoperative locoregional staging of primary gastric cancer. Cochrane Database Syst Rev. 2015;2015:Cd009944.
6. Smyth E, Schöder H, Strong VE, Capanu M, Kelsen DP, Coit DG, et al. A prospective evaluation of the utility of 2-deoxy-2-[(18) F]fluoro-D-glucose positron emission tomography and computed tomography in staging locally advanced gastric cancer. Cancer. 2012;118:5481–8.
7. Lehmann K, Eshmuminov D, Bauerfeind P, Gubler C, Veit-Haibach P, Weber A, et al. (18)FDG-PET-CT improves specificity of preoperative lymph-node staging in patients with intestinal but not diffuse-type esophagogastric adenocarcinoma. Eur J Surg Oncol. 2017;43:196–202.

8. Jamel S, Markar SR, Malietzis G, Acharya A, Athanasiou T, Hanna GB. Prognostic significance of peritoneal lavage cytology in staging gastric cancer: systematic review and meta-analysis. Gastric Cancer. 2018;21:10–8.
9. In H, Ravetch E, Langdon-Embry M, Palis B, Ajani JA, Hofstetter WL, et al. The newly proposed clinical and post-neoadjuvant treatment staging classifications for gastric adenocarcinoma for the American Joint Committee on Cancer (AJCC) staging. Gastric Cancer. 2018;21:1–9.
10. Anonymous. American Joint Committee on Cancer. AJCC cancer staging manual. New York, NY: Springer International Publishing; 2017.
11. Bando E, Makuuchi R, Tokunaga M, Tanizawa Y, Kawamura T, Terashima M. Impact of clinical tumor-node-metastasis staging on survival in gastric carcinoma patients receiving surgery. Gastric Cancer. 2017;20:448–56.

Overview of Treatment

Key Points

- Endoscopic submucosal dissection (ESD) is recommended for stage 1A (cT1aN0M0) gastric cancer confined to the mucosa.
- After endoscopic resection, radical surgery is recommended in case of lymphatic vessel or vertical marginal invasion.
- Gastrectomy is recommended for cT1a, which is not included in the indication for ESD and ≥ cT1b or cN+ and M0 gastric cancers.
- Laparoscopic gastrectomy is recommended for early gastric cancer and can be adopted in locally advanced gastric cancer.
- Adjuvant chemotherapy (S-1 or capecitabine + oxaliplatin) is recommended for patients with pathological stage II or III gastric cancer after radical surgery including D2 lymph node dissection.

Introduction

In the treatment of gastric cancer, standard surgery forms the basis of treatment. Endoscopic resection can be performed for early gastric cancer and chemotherapy and supportive care can be used for stage IV patients with distant metastases, as recommended by the Korean [1] and Japanese [2] guidelines established in 2018. Table 1 shows the stages, and Table 2 summarizes the treatment plans according to the clinical and pathological stages. Figures 1 and 2 illustrate the treatment algorithm.

Endoscopic Resection

Endoscopic submucosal dissection (ESD) is recommended for stage 1 gastric cancer of T1a, N0, and M0 (cT1aM0) confined to the mucosa. Early gastric cancer with a tumor size of 2 cm or less, no ulcers, well or moderately differentiated or papillary adenocarcinoma with a limited depth of invasion to the mucosal layer has a very low risk of lymph node metastasis. After endoscopic resection, radical surgery is recommended if the pathological result is beyond the criteria for radical endoscopic resection or if there is invasion of the lymphatic vessel or vertical margin. In a meta-analysis study comparing ESD and surgery, there were no differences in overall survival (OS) and disease-specific survival between the two groups. Although ESD had a shorter hospital stay and fewer complications, it had a lower rate of en bloc resection, histologically complete resection, curative resection, and a higher rate of local recurrence, metachronous cancer, and synchronous cancer [3].

Jung-Hwan Oh is the lead author of this chapter.

H. J. Chun et al., *Gastrointestinal Cancer*, https://doi.org/10.1007/978-981-99-0815-8_5

Table 1 Stage grouping based on clinical and pathological stages[a]

	M0					M1
	N0		N(+)			Any N
Clinical stages						
T1/T2	I		IIA			IVB
T3/T4a	IIIB		III			
T4b	IVA					
	M0					M1
	N0	N1	N2	N3a	N3b	Any N
Pathologic stages						
T1a/T1b	IA	IB	IIA	IIB	IIIB	IV
T2	IB	IIA	IIB	IIIA	IIIB	
T3	IIA	IIB	IIIA	IIIB	IIIC	
T4a	IIB	IIIA	IIIA	IIIB	IIIC	
T4b	IIIA	IIIB	IIIB	IIIC	IIIC	

cStage, decided based on preoperative imaging, staging laparoscopy findings, and intraoperative findings
pStage, decided based on pathologic findings of resected specimen
N: the number of metastatic lymph nodes among the regional lymph nodes (No. 1–12. 14v), N1: 1–2, N2: 3–6, N3a: 7–15, N3b: ≥16
[a]Adapted from the Japanese Gastric Cancer Treatment Guidelines 2018 (5th Edition) [2]

Table 2 Treatment according to stage

	M0		M1
Clinical stages (cTNM, cStage)	N0	N(+)	Any N
T1a (mucosa)	ESD	Gastrectomy D2[a]	Palliative systemic therapypalliative radiotherapypalliative gastrectomy
T1b (submucosa)	ESD or gastrectomy D1+	Gastrectomy D2[a]	
T2	Gastrectomy D2	Gastrectomy D2[a]	
T3	Gastrectomy D2[a]	Gastrectomy D2[a]	
T4	Gastrectomy D2[a]	Gastrectomy D2[a]	

ESD endoscopic submucosal dissection
[a]Adjuvant chemotherapy or adjuvant chemo radiotherapy should be considered

Surgery

Standard surgery is defined as gastrectomy of more than two-thirds of the whole stomach with D2 lymph node dissection. Surgical treatment is recommended for cT1a, which are not eligible for ESD, ≥cT1b or cN+, and M0 gastric cancers. According to the location of the tumor and clinical stage, the extent of resection is determined as distal gastrectomy, proximal gastrectomy, or total gastrectomy. Regarding lymph node dissection, limited lymph node dissection such as D1 or D1+ lymph node dissection can be applied in clinically early gastric cancer in patients with cN0. For clinically advanced gastric cancer, standard gastrectomy is mandatory.

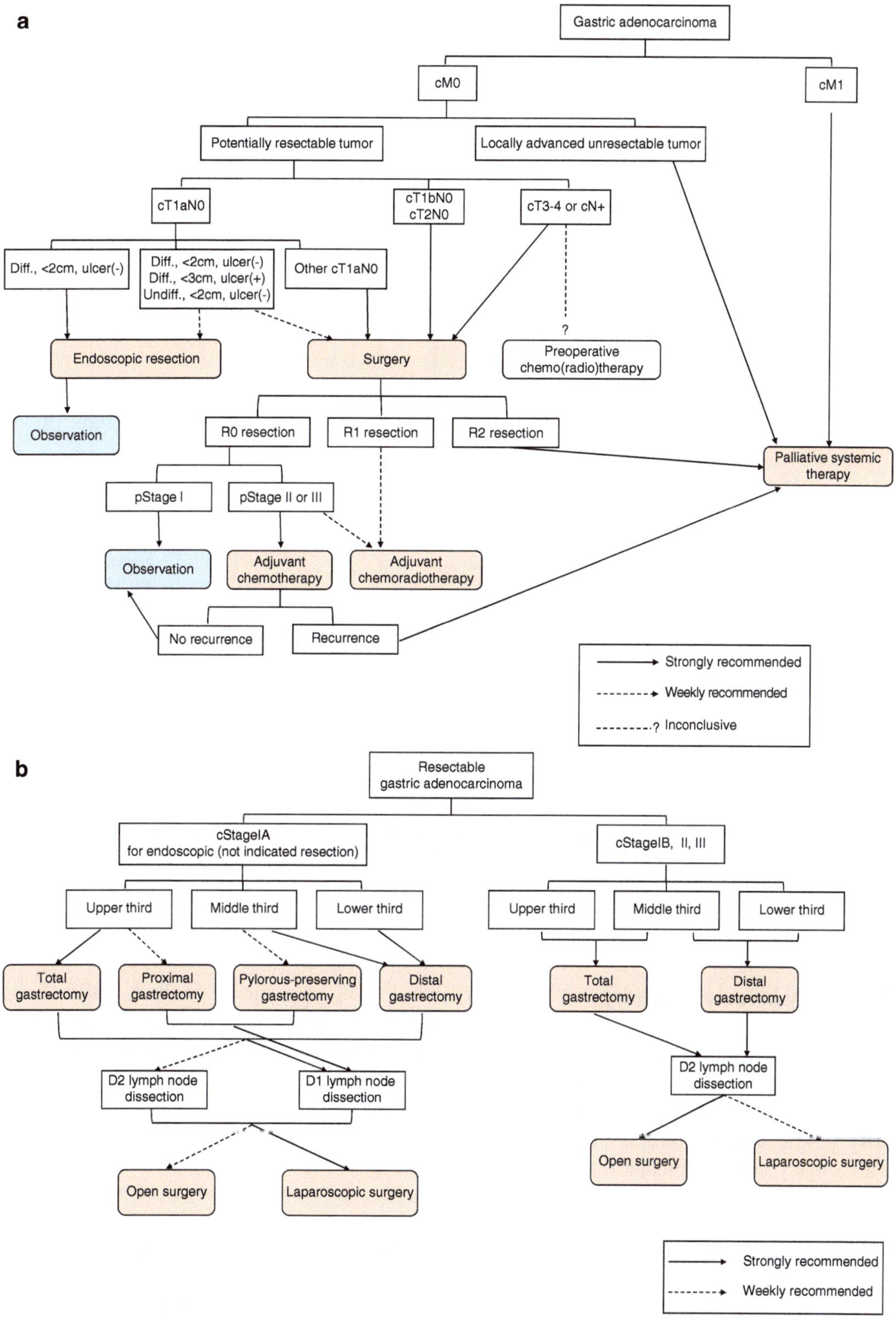

Fig. 1 (**a**) Overall treatment algorithm for gastric adenocarcinoma. (**b**) Treatment algorithm for resectable gastric adenocarcinoma. (Adapted from Korean Practice Guideline for Gastric Cancer 2018 [1])

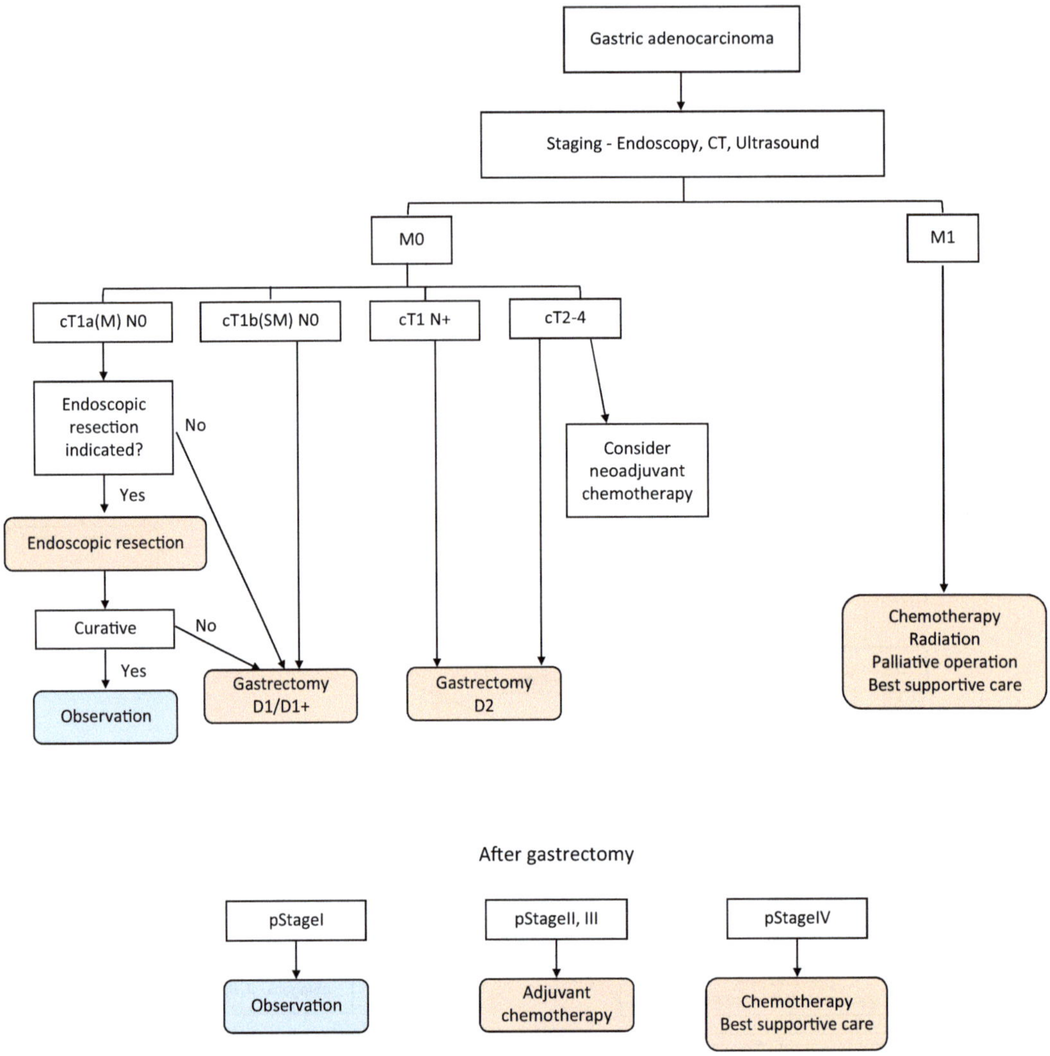

Fig. 2 Algorithm of standard treatments. (Adapted from Japanese gastric cancer treatment guidelines 2018 [2])

Minimally Invasive Surgery

In the past, open surgery was performed mainly for gastric cancer, but nowadays laparoscopic gastrectomy is being performed for the treatment of early gastric cancer. Clinical trials comparing open surgery and laparoscopic surgery for early gastric cancer were conducted in the early 2000s. Recently, in the KLASS-01 study conducted in Korea, the OS rates of the laparoscopic and laparotomy groups were compared in patients in clinical stage I gastric cancer. The 5-year OS rate was 94.2% in the laparoscopic group and 93.3% in the open surgery group. OS and cancer-specific survival rates were similar between patients who underwent open and laparoscopic distal gastrectomy. Therefore, laparoscopic distal gastrectomy is recommended for the treatment of clinical stage I gastric cancer [4]. The clinical studies KLASS-02 and CLASS-01 compared the 3-year relapse-free survival rate between laparoscopic and open gastrectomy for locally advanced gastric cancer. Since laparoscopic distal gastrectomy was comparable to open surgery in terms of relapse-free survival in patients with locally advanced gastric cancer, laparoscopic distal gastrectomy may be accepted as a standard treatment option for locally advanced gastric cancer [5, 6].

Systemic Therapy

Chemotherapy

- Currently used anticancer drugs include: capecitabine, carboplatin, cisplatin, docetaxel, fluorouracil, irinotecan, oxaliplatin, and paclitaxel.
- After gastrectomy: adjuvant chemotherapy (S-1 or capecitabine + oxaliplatin) is recommended for patients with pathological stage II or III gastric cancer after radical surgery, including D2 lymph node dissection.
- Neoadjuvant: when D2 lymph node dissection is being considered or the evidence of efficacy for prior chemotherapy for potentially resectable gastric cancer is inconclusive.
- Unresectable stage IV: systemic chemotherapy is the first-line treatment to consider for patients with locally advanced unresectable (irresectable T4b or extensive regional lymph node metastases), metastatic disease, or non-radical resection. Such palliative systemic chemotherapy should be decided based on the patient's systemic performance status, medical comorbidities, and organ function. Palliative first-line platinum+fluoropyrimidine combination therapy is recommended for patients with locally advanced unresectable or metastatic gastric cancer if the patient's systemic performance and major organ functions are preserved. Palliative first-line trastuzumab + capecitabine or fluorouracil + cisplatin is recommended for patients with locally advanced unresectable or metastatic gastric cancer.

Target Therapy

- Trastuzumab is a humanized monoclonal antibody targeting HER2, which is known as first-line therapy for patients with advanced gastric cancer. It would be an eligible option if the immunohistochemical intensity score of HER2 is 2+ or 3+ in fluorescence in situ hybridization.
- Ramucirumab, an antibody against vascular endothelial growth factor (VEGF), blocks VEGFR-2 to reduce tumor angiogenesis in advanced gastric cancer.
- Entrectinib and larotrectinib target the TRK protein. Some patients with stomach cancer harbor a mutation in one of the NTRK genes, which produces an abnormal TRK protein.

Immunotherapy

- Pembrolizumab and nivolumab are PD-1 inhibitors. PD-1 is a protein present on the surface of T cells. By binding to PD-1, these agents prevent the cancer cell from interacting with the PD-L1 protein, allowing T cells to attack the cancer cells.

Radiation Therapy

- Radiation therapy can be used to reduce the size of a tumor before surgery (neoadjuvant) or to destroy the remaining cancer cells after surgery.
- Neoadjuvant: When D2 lymph node dissection is considered, the evidence for the efficacy of prior chemoradiation for locally advanced gastric cancer is inconclusive.
- Unresectable stage IV: Palliative radiotherapy can be effective in alleviating symptoms caused by localized primary and metastatic lesions.
- Side effects include fatigue, mild skin reactions, nausea, vomiting, epigastric discomfort, and loose bowel movements.

Supportive Care

- In metastatic gastric cancer, gastrectomy can only be performed for the relief of emergency symptoms such as bleeding, perforation, and obstruction.
- Tumor bleeding can be controlled by hemostatic powder spray by endoscopy, embolization angiography, and radiotherapy.
- An endoscopic stent can be helpful when a patient cannot eat due to obstruction caused by a mass at the gastroesophageal junction or gastric pylorus.

Conclusion

Stomach cancer can be treated with endoscopic therapy, surgery, radiation therapy, chemotherapy, targeted therapy, or immunotherapy. It is important to detect and treat it as early as possible. Treatment options and recommendations should be determined according to the stage of cancer. ESD and minimally invasive surgery should be performed at the appropriate stage. Several treatments can be used together to treat stomach cancer.

References

1. Anonymous. Korean Practice Guideline for Gastric Cancer 2018: An evidence-based, multi-disciplinary approac. JGastric Cancer. 2019;19:1–48.
2. Japanese Gastric Cancer A. Japanese gastric cancer treatment guidelines 2018 (5th edition). Gastric Cancer. 2021(24):1–21.
3. Liu Q, Ding L, Qiu X, Meng F. Updated evaluation of endoscopic submucosal dissection versus surgery for early gastric cancer: a systematic review and meta-analysis. Int J Surg. 2020;73:28–41.
4. Kim HH, Han SU, Kim MC, Kim W, Lee HJ, Ryu SW, et al. Effect of laparoscopic distal gastrectomy vs open distal gastrectomy on long-term survival among patients with stage I gastric cancer: the KLASS-01 randomized clinical trial. JAMA Oncol. 2019;5:506–13.
5. Hyung WJ, Yang HK, Park YK, Lee HJ, An JY, Kim W, et al. Long-term outcomes of laparoscopic distal gastrectomy for locally advanced gastric Cancer: the KLASS-02-RCT randomized clinical trial. J Clin Oncol. 2020;38:3304–13.
6. Yu J, Huang C, Sun Y, Su X, Cao H, Hu J, et al. Effect of laparoscopic vs open distal gastrectomy on 3-year disease-free survival in patients with locally advanced gastric Cancer: the CLASS-01 randomized clinical trial. JAMA. 2019;321:1983–92.

Endoscopic Treatment

Key Points

- Endoscopic resection (ER) is a minimally invasive curative treatment for early gastric cancer (EGC) with negligible lymph node metastasis (LNM).
- Endoscopic submucosal dissection is the preferred technique, given the risk of incomplete resection with endoscopic mucosal resection.
- An appropriate selection of lesions, based on an accurate prediction of tumor margins and invasion depth, is crucial for successful outcomes.
- In cases of non-curative resection, stratified management can be applied depending on the risk of LNM.
- The long-term outcomes of ER for EGC, including overall survival and disease-specific survival, are comparable to those of gastrectomy with lymphadenectomy.
- After ER, careful endoscopic surveillance is necessary due to a high incidence rate of metachronous cancer in the remnant stomach.

Introduction

Endoscopic resection (ER) is an established curative treatment for early gastric cancer (EGC) with a negligible risk of lymph node metastasis (LNM). The widespread use of screening endoscopy has facilitated the early diagnosis of gastric cancer and subsequently increased the number of ERs for EGCs. ER is a minimally invasive procedure that preserves the entire stomach, improves the quality of life, requires a shorter hospital stay, and is more cost-effective than surgical resection. Endoscopic mucosal resection (EMR) was first reported in 1984 and has been used as an effective treatment for EGC [1]. Since EMR is not suitable for en bloc resection of lesions larger than 20 mm or non-lifting lesions. The endoscopic submucosal dissection (ESD) technique was established as a derivative of EMR in 1999 [2]. Although ESD requires a longer procedure time and endoscopic skill and expertise, it enables complete resection for large lesions with or without fibrosis, resulting in more precise histological evaluation and a lower likelihood of local recurrence. With the development of high-frequency electric generators and dedicated electrocautery knives, ESD is now recommended as the preferred method for endoscopic treatment of EGC [3–5].

Indications for Endoscopic Treatment

The indications for ER were established using a combination of the risk factors for LNM from a retrospective analysis of surgically resected samples and are classified as absolute and expanded

Bong Eun Lee is the lead author of this chapter.

H. J. Chun et al., *Gastrointestinal Cancer*, https://doi.org/10.1007/978-981-99-0815-8_6

Fig. 1 Indications of endoscopic treatment [5]

Histology	Depth					
	M cancer				SM cancer	
	Ulcer (-)		Ulcer (+)		SM1	SM2
	≤ 20 mm	> 20 mm	≤ 30 mm	> 30 mm	≤ 30 mm	Any size
Differentiated	A	B	B	C	B	C
Undifferentiated	B	C	C	C	C	C

A : Absolute indication, B : Expanded indication, C : Out of indication

indications [6] (Fig. 1). Absolute indications, initially accepted as a standard for EMR, include differentiated T1a cancers without ulcerative findings ≤20 mm. Afterward, the ESD technique allowed us to resect a wider range of EGCs termed 'expanded indications'. Expanded indications include: (1) differentiated T1a cancers without ulcerative findings, regardless of tumor size; (2) differentiated T1a cancers with ulcerative findings ≤30 mm; (3) differentiated minute T1b cancers (submucosal invasion depth ≤500 μm from the muscularis mucosa) ≤30 mm; and (4) undifferentiated T1a cancers without ulcerative findings ≤20 mm.

Preprocedural Considerations for Successful Outcomes

Accurate prediction of the tumor, especially for tumor margins and depth of invasion, is critical to determine whether the lesion is eligible for ER. Delineation of tumor margins can be assessed with conventional white light endoscopy (WLE), chromoendoscopy (CE), or magnifying endoscopy (ME) with narrow-band imaging (NBI) [7–9]. To predict the depth of invasion, endoscopic ultrasound (EUS) can be performed, although it has limited accuracy in EGC. To reduce the overestimation of tumor depth, some studies have suggested that EUS could be considered for lesions with suspicion of submucosal invasion in WLE [10, 11].

Techniques of Endoscopic Treatment

Commonly used EMR techniques can be classified as injection-, cap-, and ligation-assisted EMR (Fig. 2) [12]. However, these EMR techniques are not feasible for EGCs larger than 1.5–2.0 cm, resulting in incomplete resection and possibly an increased risk of local recurrence [13].

ESD consists of five cardinal steps: marking, injection, incision, dissection, and en bloc retrieval [14] (Fig. 3). Various endoscopic instruments for ESD have been developed, including endoscopic knives, specific hemostatic forceps, and high-performance electrical surgical units, and understanding the features of each instrument is essential because proper selection and use contribute to successful and safe ESD [15]. Additionally, measures to adapt to various situations, such as the use of a transparent cap, the optimization of the dissection plane by repeated submucosal injection, and the control of air insufflations and suctions are also very important [16].

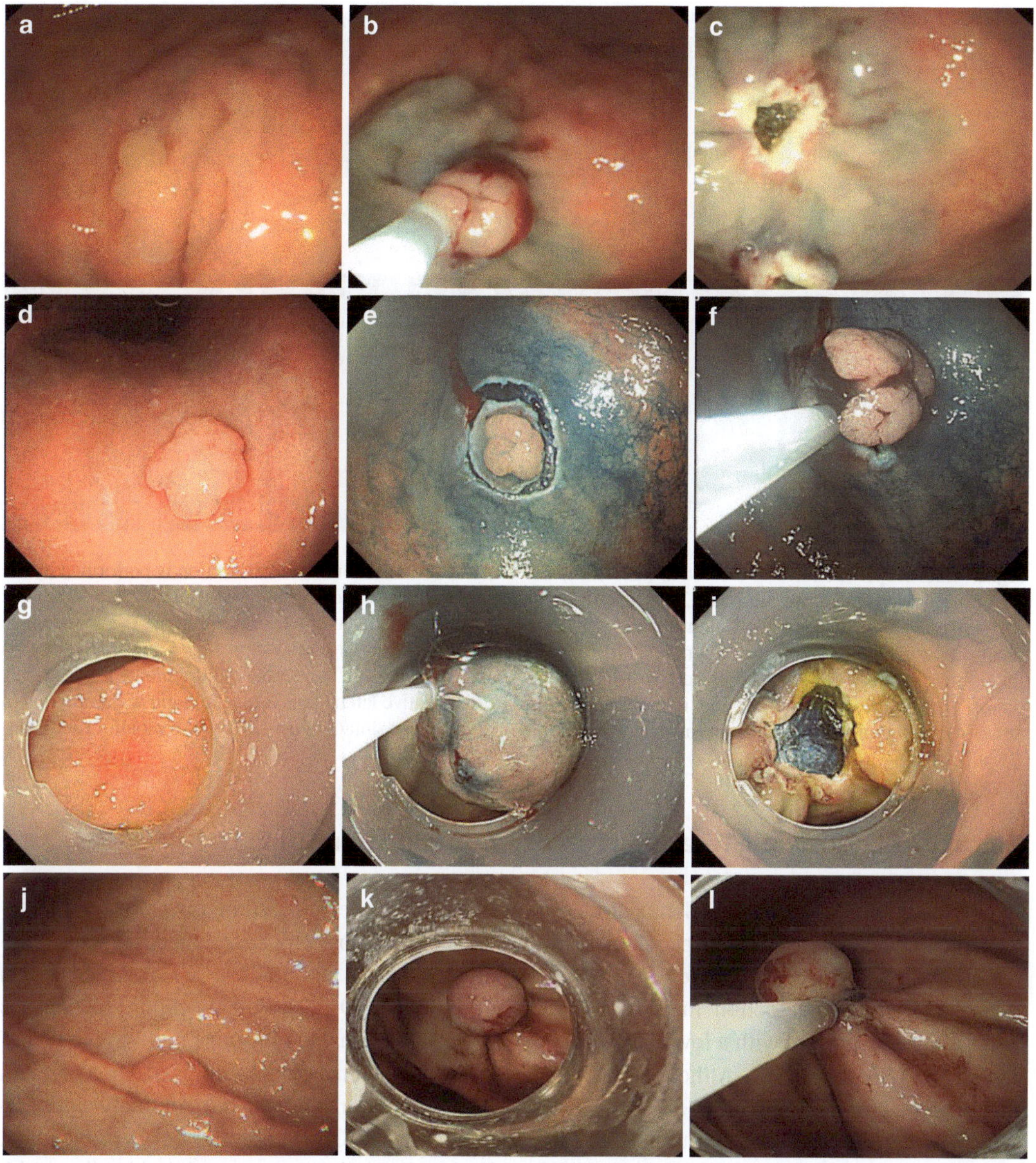

Fig. 2 Endoscopic mucosal resection (EMR). (**a**, **b**, **c**) Conventional injection-assisted EMR. (**d**, **e**, **f**) EMR after circumferential pre-cutting (EMR-P). (**g**, **h**, **i**) EMR using transparent plastic cap (EMR-C). (**j**, **k**, **l**) EMR using a ligation device (EMR-L)

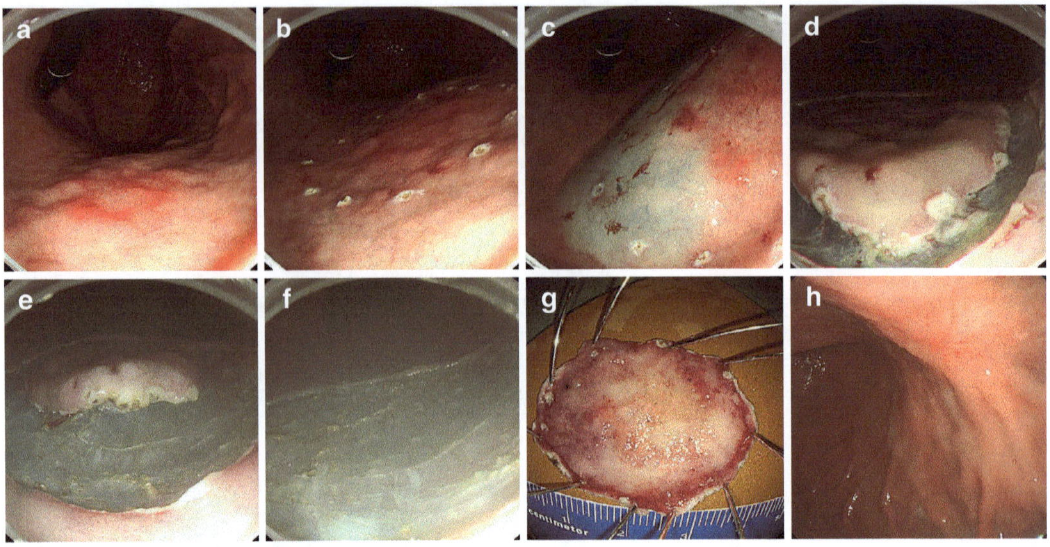

Fig. 3 Endoscopic submucosal dissection (ESD). (**a**) On the posterior wall side of the midbody, 2 cm type IIc + IIa early gastric cancer is seen. (**b**) Circumferential markings are places around the lesion at least 5 mm apart from the tumor margins. (**c**) Submucosal injection using saline mixed with diluted epinephrine and indigo carmine is done. (**d**) A circumferential incision is made outside of the markings. (**e**) Submucosal dissection is performed by the time the lesion is completely resected. (**f**) Artificial ulcer is observed after complete dissection. (**g**) Tissue specimen is fixed with pins on a plate. Final pathology is 2.2 cm × 2.0 cm moderately differentiated T1a cancer with negative lateral and vertical margin without lymphovascular invasion (**h**) Post-ESD scar 6 months after ESD

Efficacy of Endoscopic Treatment

In a recent meta-analysis, ESD demonstrated its superiority over EMR with respect to en bloc resection rates (OR 9.0), complete resection rates (OR 8.43), curative resection rates (OR 2.92), and was also associated with a lower risk of local recurrence (OR 0.18) [17]. Although ESD took longer procedure time (OR 1.12) and was associated with a greater risk of perforation (OR 2.55), the risk of bleeding was not significantly different between EMR and ESD. In studies in Japan and South Korea, ESD has shown en bloc resection rates of 95.3–99.2%, complete resection rates of 87.7–95.5% and curative resection rates of 81.7–84.1% [18]. En bloc resection rates and curative resection rates of ESD were 97.1–99.0% and 91.5–96.4% in absolute indications and 89.7–97.4% and 72.0–93.4% in expanded indications [19–21].

Complications of ESD

Bleeding is the most common major complication of ESD. Post-procedural bleeding rates ranging 1.3–11.9% and 50–70% are observed within 48 h after ESD [22]. Post-procedure bleeding is generally amenable to routine endoscopic hemostasis, and antisecretory drugs such as proton pump inhibitors, which are routinely administered after ESD to prevent delayed bleeding. Perforation is less common than bleeding, with rates reported between 1.5% and 9.6% [23]. Immediately recognized macroscopic perforations can be successfully treated with endoscopic clipping in most cases [24, 25]. Microperforations after ESD without endoscopically visible perforation can also usually be conservatively managed with fasting and broad-spectrum antibiotics [26]. However, in cases of unsuccessful endoscopic closure, signs of peritonitis, or delayed perforation, immediate surgical treatment is required. Stenosis events range from 0.7%–1.9%, and cardiac and pyloric resections are most common, with a frequency of 17% in the cardia and 7% in the pylorus [26]. Although data are limited, most patients were successfully treated with improvement in symptoms by endoscopic balloon dilation.

Post-procedural Management for non-Curative Resection

Curative resection is defined as a situation when the lesion which is resected en bloc, meets absolute and expanded indications with negative lateral and vertical margins, and does not show lymphovascular invasion in the final histology. Since non-curative resection (NCR) is associated with an increased risk of LNM and local recurrence, additional gastrectomy with regional lymph node dissection is usually recommended for these patients. However, the risk of LNM is variable depending on different predictive factors, and some patients with NCR are not eligible candidates or want to avoid further invasive surgery. Taking into account these issues, a low-risk NCR group for LNM, including lesions that were not resected en bloc or with a positive lateral margin, can be treated with redo-ESD, plasma argon coagulation, or close observation without additional surgery [27, 28]. Conversely, in cases with other NCR, an additional surgical resection is essential in view of the risk for LNM.

Long-Term Clinical Outcomes

Compared to surgery, although ESD does not generally compromise overall survival (OS) and disease-specific survival (DSS), it is associated with higher risks of recurrence [27–31]. In a recent meta-analysis, ESD was associated with a higher rate of local recurrence (OR 5.42), metachronous cancer (OR 10.84), and synchronous cancer (OR 6.59) than surgery, while OS (HR 0.92) and DSS (HR 0.73) showed no significant differences between the two groups [31]. Based on recent retrospective data, local recurrence rates have been documented to range from 0% to 1.8% in absolute indications and 0.6% to 7.0% in expanded indications [17]. In these same cohorts, there were no cases of LNM in absolute indications, while LNM rates ranged from 0% to 0.48% in expanded indications. In a prospective multicenter cohort study from Japan, ESD for expanded indications offered an OS of 97.0% [32]. In patients with EGCs fulfilling the criteria for curative resection, the 5-year DSS was 99.9% in both absolute and expanded indications, although the 5-year OS was 92.2% due to combined morbidities [33].

Surveillance

Since atrophic gastritis and intestinal metaplasia persist in the residual mucosa, a high incidence rate of metachronous cancers after ER has been reported, up to 6.9–13% [17]. For a strategy to reduce the incidence rate of metachronous cancers, *Helicobacter pylori* (*H. pylori*) eradication is recommended in *H. pylori*-positive patients [3, 28, 34–42]. However, as the risk of metachronous cancer may still persist after *H. pylori* eradication, more strict and careful endoscopic surveillance is needed. Recent Japanese and Korean guidelines recommend regular endoscopic surveillance every 6–12 months, and the ESGE guideline recommends the first endoscopic surveillance at 3–6 months, and regular endoscopic examination on a yearly basis thereafter [3, 28, 34]. In terms of detecting extra-gastric recurrence, precise standards for targeting subjects, examination tools, and the follow-up interval have not yet been established. In the Japanese guidelines, ultrasonography or abdominopelvic computed tomography is recommended at 6–12-month intervals for lesions meeting expanded indications while the Korean guideline suggests abdominopelvic computed tomography for lesions for both absolute and expanded indications [28, 34].

Conclusions

ER becomes the main procedure for the treatment of selected EGCs with a very low risk of LNM, and ESD is currently the preferred method. Compared to surgery, this preserves the entire stomach, improving the quality of life of patients, and many studies have reported favorable long-term results for patients receiving curative resection. However, even after achieving curative resection, endoscopists must pay careful attention during surveillance endoscopy due to a high incidence rate of metachronous gastric cancer.

References

1. Tada M, Murakami A, Karita M, Yanai H, Okita K. Endoscopic resection of early gastric cancer. Endoscopy. 1993;25(7):445–50.
2. Gotoda T, Kondo H, Ono H, Saito Y, Yamaguchi H, Saito D, et al. A new endoscopic mucosal resection procedure using an insulation-tipped electrosurgical knife for rectal flat lesions: report of two cases. Gastrointest Endosc. 1999;50(4):560–3.
3. Pimentel-Nunes P, Dinis-Ribeiro M, Ponchon T, Repici A, Vieth M, De Ceglie A, et al. Endoscopic submucosal dissection: European Society of Gastrointestinal Endoscopy (ESGE) guideline. Endoscopy. 2015;47(9):829–54.
4. Banks M, Graham D, Jansen M, Gotoda T, Coda S, Di Pietro M, et al. British Society of Gastroenterology guidelines on the diagnosis and management of patients at risk of gastric adenocarcinoma. Gut. 2019;68(9):1545–75.
5. Japanese Gastric Cancer Association. Japanese gastric cancer treatment guidelines 2014 (ver. 4). Gastric Cancer. 2017;20(1):1–19.
6. Gotoda T, Yanagisawa A, Sasako M, Ono H, Nakanishi Y, Shimoda T, et al. Incidence of lymph node metastasis from early gastric cancer: estimation with a large number of cases at two large centers. Gastric Cancer. 2000;3(4):219–25.
7. Kawahara Y, Takenaka R, Okada H, Kawano S, Inoue M, Tsuzuki T, et al. Novel chromoendoscopic method using an acetic acid-indigocarmine mixture for diagnostic accuracy in delineating the margin of early gastric cancers. Dig Endosc. 2009;21(1):14–9.
8. Asada-Hirayama I, Kodashima S, Sakaguchi Y, Ono S, Niimi K, Mochizuki S, et al. Magnifying endoscopy with narrow-band imaging is more accurate for determination of horizontal extent of early gastric cancers than chromoendoscopy. Endosc Int Open. 2016;4(6):E690–8.
9. Nagahama T, Yao K, Uedo N, Doyama H, Ueo T, Uchita K, et al. Delineation of the extent of early gastric cancer by magnifying narrow-band imaging and chromoendoscopy: a multicenter randomized controlled trial. Endoscopy. 2018;50(6):566–76.
10. Tsujii Y, Kato M, Inoue T, Yoshii S, Nagai K, Fujinaga T, et al. Integrated diagnostic strategy for the invasion depth of early gastric cancer by conventional endoscopy and EUS. Gastrointest Endosc. 2015;82(3):452–9.
11. Yoshida S, Tanaka S, Kunihiro K, Mitsuika Y, Hara M, Kitadai Y, et al. Diagnostic ability of high-frequency ultrasound probe sonography in staging early gastric cancer, especially for submucosal invasion. Abdom Imaging. 2005;30(5):518–23.
12. ASGE Technology Committee, Hwang JH, Konda V, Abu Dayyeh BK, Chauhan SS, Enestvedt BK, et al. Endoscopic mucosal resection. Gastrointest Endosc. 2015;82(2):215–26.
13. Min YW, Min BH, Lee JH, Kim JJ. Endoscopic treatment for early gastric cancer. World J Gastroenterol. 2014;20(16):4566–73.
14. Gotoda T. A large endoscopic resection by endoscopic submucosal dissection procedure for early gastric cancer. Clin Gastroenterol Hepatol. 2005;3(7 Suppl 1):S71–3.
15. Esaki M, Ihara E, Gotoda T. Endoscopic instruments and techniques in endoscopic submucosal dissection for early gastric cancer. Expert Rev Gastroenterol Hepatol. 2021;15(9):1009–20.
16. Lee WS, Cho JW, Kim YD, Kim JK, Jang BI. Technical issues and new devices of ESD of early gastric cancer. World J Gastroenterol. 2011;17(31):3585–90.
17. Tao M, Zhou X, Hu M, Pan J. Endoscopic submucosal dissection versus endoscopic mucosal resection for patients with early gastric cancer: a meta-analysis. BMJ Open. 2019;9(12):e025803.
18. Young E, Philpott H, Singh R. Endoscopic diagnosis and treatment of gastric dysplasia and early gastric cancer: current evidence and what the future may hold. World J Gastroenterol. 2021;27(31):5126–51.
19. Kang HJ, Kim DH, Jeon TY, Lee SH, Shin N, Chae SH, et al. Lymph node metastasis from intestinal-type early gastric cancer: experience in a single institution and reassessment of the extended criteria for endoscopic submucosal dissection. Gastrointest Endosc. 2010;72(3):508–15.
20. Choi MK, Kim GH, Park DY, Song GA, Kim DU, Ryu DY, et al. Long-term outcomes of endoscopic submucosal dissection for early gastric cancer: a single-center experience. Surg Endosc. 2013;27(11):4250–8.
21. Kosaka T, Endo M, Toya Y, Abiko Y, Kudara N, Inomata M, et al. Long-term outcomes of endoscopic submucosal dissection for early gastric cancer: a single-center retrospective study. Dig Endosc. 2014;26(2):183–91.
22. Lee BE, Kim GH, Song GA, Seo JH, Jeon HK, Baek DH, et al. Continuous infusion versus intermittent

dosing with pantoprazole for gastric endoscopic submucosal dissection. Gut Liver. 2019;13(1):40–7.
23. Arezzo A, Passera R, Marchese N, Galloro G, Manta R, Cirocchi R. Systematic review and metaanalysis of endoscopic submucosal dissection vs endoscopic mucosal resection for colorectal lesions. United European Gastroenterol J. 2016;4(1):18–29.
24. Minami S, Gotoda T, Ono H, Oda I, Hamanaka H. Complete endoscopic closure of gastric perforation induced by endoscopic resection of early gastric cancer using endoclips can prevent surgery (with video). Gastrointest Endosc. 2006;63(4):596–601.
25. Isomoto H, Nishiyama H, Yamaguchi N, Fukuda E, Ishii H, Ikeda K, et al. Clinicopathological factors associated with clinical outcomes of endoscopic submucosal dissection for colorectal epithelial neoplasms. Endoscopy. 2009;41(8):679–83.
26. Coda S, Oda I, Gotoda T, Yokoi C, Kikuchi T, Ono H. Risk factors for cardiac and pyloric stenosis after endoscopic submucosal dissection, and efficacy of endoscopic balloon dilation treatment. Endoscopy. 2009;41(5):421–42.
27. Hatta W, Gotoda T, Oyama T, Kawata N, Takahashi A, Yoshifuku Y, et al. A scoring system to stratify curability after endoscopic submucosal dissection for early gastric cancer: "eCura system". Am J Gastroenterol. 2017;112(6):874–81.
28. Ono H, Yao K, Fujishiro M, Oda I, Uedo N, Nimura S, et al. Guidelines for endoscopic submucosal dissection and endoscopic mucosal resection for early gastric cancer (second edition). Dig Endosc. 2021;33(1):4–20.
29. Shin DW, Hwang HY, Jeon SW. Comparison of endoscopic submucosal dissection and surgery for differentiated type early gastric cancer within the expanded criteria. Clin Endosc. 2017;50(2):170–8.
30. Fukunaga S, Nagami Y, Shiba M, Ominami M, Tanigawa T, Yamagami H, et al. Long-term prognosis of expanded-indication differentiated-type early gastric cancer treated with endoscopic submucosal dissection or surgery using propensity score analysis. Gastrointest Endosc. 2017;85(1):143–52.
31. Ryu SJ, Kim BW, Kim BG, Kim JH, Kim JS, Kim JI, et al. Endoscopic submucosal dissection versus surgical resection for early gastric cancer: a retrospective multicenter study on immediate and long-term outcome over 5 years. Surg Endosc. 2016;30(12):5283–9.
32. Liu Q, Ding L, Qiu X, Meng F. Updated evaluation of endoscopic submucosal dissection versus surgery for early gastric cancer: a systematic review and meta-analysis. Int J Surg. 2020;73:28–41.
33. Suzuki H, Oda I, Abe S, Sekiguchi M, Mori G, Nonaka S, et al. High rate of 5-year survival among patients with early gastric cancer undergoing curative endoscopic submucosal dissection. Gastric Cancer. 2016;19(1):198–205.
34. Fukase K, Kato M, Kikuchi S, Inoue K, Uemura N, Okamoto S, et al. Effect of eradication of helicobacter pylori on incidence of metachronous gastric carcinoma after endoscopic resection of early gastric cancer: an open-label, randomized controlled trial. Lancet. 2008;372(9636):392–7.
35. Choi IJ, Kook MC, Kim YI, Cho SJ, Lee JY, Kim CG, et al. Helicobacter pylori therapy for the prevention of metachronous gastric cancer. N Engl J Med. 2018;378(12):1085–95.
36. Choi JM, Kim SG, Choi J, Park JY, Oh S, Yang HJ, et al. Effects of helicobacter pylori eradication for metachronous gastric cancer prevention: a randomized controlled trial. Gastrointest Endosc. 2018;88(3):475–85.e2.
37. Xiao S, Li S, Zhou L, Jiang W, Liu J. Helicobacter pylori status and risks of metachronous recurrence after endoscopic resection of early gastric cancer: a systematic review and meta-analysis. J Gastroenterol. 2019;54(3):226–37.
38. Jung DH, Kim JH, Chung HS, Park JC, Shin SK, Lee SK, et al. Helicobacter pylori eradication on the prevention of metachronous lesions after endoscopic resection of gastric neoplasm: a meta-analysis. PLoS One. 2015;10(4):e0124725.
39. Chen HN, Wang Z, Li X, Zhou ZG. Helicobacter pylori eradication cannot reduce the risk of gastric cancer in patients with intestinal metaplasia and dysplasia: evidence from a meta-analysis. Gastric Cancer. 2016;19(1):166–75.
40. Yoon SB, Park JM, Lim CH, Cho YK, Choi MG. Effect of helicobacter pylori eradication on metachronous gastric cancer after endoscopic resection of gastric tumors: a meta-analysis. Helicobacter. 2014;19(4):243–8.
41. Bang CS, Baik GH, Shin IS, Kim JB, Suk KT, Yoon JH, et al. Helicobacter pylori eradication for prevention of metachronous recurrence after endoscopic resection of early gastric cancer. J Korean Med Sci. 2015;30(6):749–56.
42. Lee YC, Chiang TH, Chou CK, Tu YK, Liao WC, Wu MS, et al. Association between helicobacter pylori eradication and gastric cancer incidence: a systematic review and meta-analysis. Gastroenterology. 2016;150(5):1113–24.e5.

Surgical Treatment

Key Points

- Surgical treatment is a mainstay in the management of gastric cancer.
- The treatment algorithm for gastric cancer is well established.
- Gastric cancer surgery is composed of the resection of primary tumor, regional lymph node dissection, and reconstruction.
- For advanced gastric cancer, standard gastrectomy is recommended, and for early gastric cancer without suspicious lymph node metastasis, function-preserving gastrectomy can be applied.

Introduction

Surgical treatment represents the mainstay of gastric cancer management. Guidelines for surgical treatment have been established by the Japanese Gastric Cancer Association (JGCA) (Fig. 1) [1] and the Korean Gastric Cancer Association (KGCA) (Fig. 2) [2]. Indications for surgical treatment include patients with more advanced gastric cancer than the indications for endoscopic resection and patients with gastric cancer that can be resected without distant metastasis. The surgical approach for gastric cancer is diverse according to the location of the primary tumor and the status of disease progression.

Oh Kyoung Kwon is the lead author of this chapter.

H. J. Chun et al., *Gastrointestinal Cancer*, https://doi.org/10.1007/978-981-99-0815-8_7

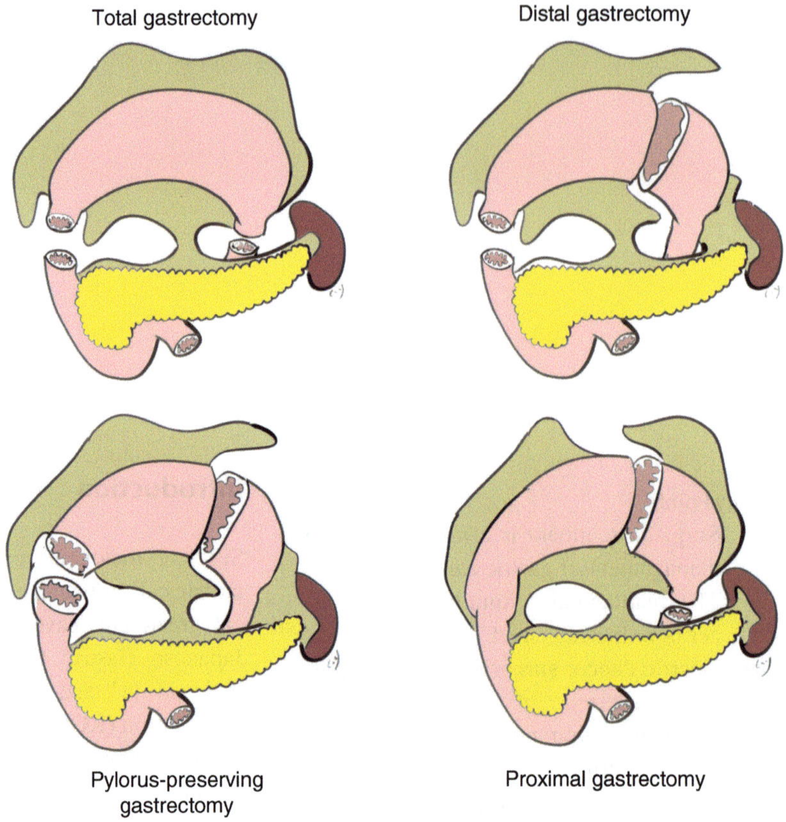

Fig. 1 Lymph node dissection in total gastrectomy, distal gastrectomy, pylorus-preserving gastrectomy, and proximal gastrectomy. (Adapted from Japanese Gastric Cancer Association [1])

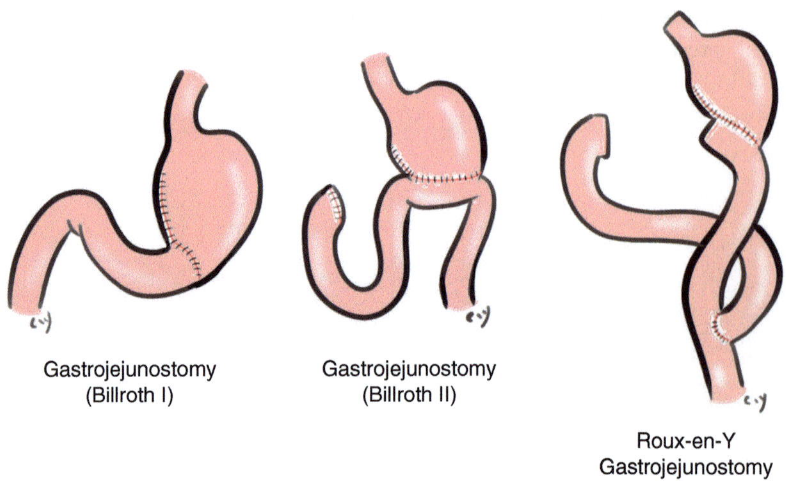

Fig. 2 Reconstructions after distal gastrectomy. (Adapted from UpToDate 2021)

Components in Surgical Treatment of Gastric Cancer

Resection of the Primary Tumor

Resection of the primary lesion is an essential surgical treatment for most solid cancers. The most important factor in determining the extent of resection of the stomach in gastric cancer is the location and gross type of the primary lesion. For advanced gastric cancer, distal gastrectomy and total gastrectomy are performed. In distal gastrectomy, it is recommended to secure 3–5 cm from the proximal margin of the lesion to the resection surface. Otherwise, absence of cancer cells in the resection surface should be checked through frozen section examination during surgery. When the location of the advanced gastric cancer or intramural cancerous infiltration from mid- or low-third gastric cancer is in the proximal part of the stomach, total gastrectomy should be performed. Furthermore, in linitis plastica (Borrmann type IV), total gastrectomy should be performed. For early gastric cancer without suspicion of lymph node metastasis clinically, in addition to the above mentioned two surgeries, pylorus-preserving gastrectomy, which can be performed for gastric cancer located in the middle of the stomach, and proximal gastrectomy for gastric cancer located in the proximal region of the stomach are also performed. In the case of direct infiltration to adjacent organs without distant metastasis, combined resection is recommended if resection is possible.

Dissection of Regional Lymph Nodes

Dissection of regional lymph nodes is essential in gastric cancer surgery not only to remove possible micro or macro-metastasis of gastric cancer, but also to assess exact pathological stage. Complete dissection of regional lymph node has contributed to improved survival of gastric cancer patients [3]. The recommended range of lymph node dissection is classified as D1, D1+, and D2 depending on the progression of gastric cancer while the composition of the lymph node groups to be resected depends on the extent of resection of the stomach [1] (Fig. 1).

Reconstruction of Gastrointestinal Integrity

After gastric resection, reconstruction of the gastrointestinal tract is necessary for continuity of the gastrointestinal tract for food intake and digestion. Reconstruction after gastrectomy depends on the extent of gastric resection. Gastroduodenostomy (Billroth I), gastrojejunostomy (Billroth II), and Roux-en-Y gastrojejunostomy are performed after distal gastrectomy (Fig. 2).

Roux-en-Y esophagojejunostomy is usually performed after total gastrectomy (Fig. 3).

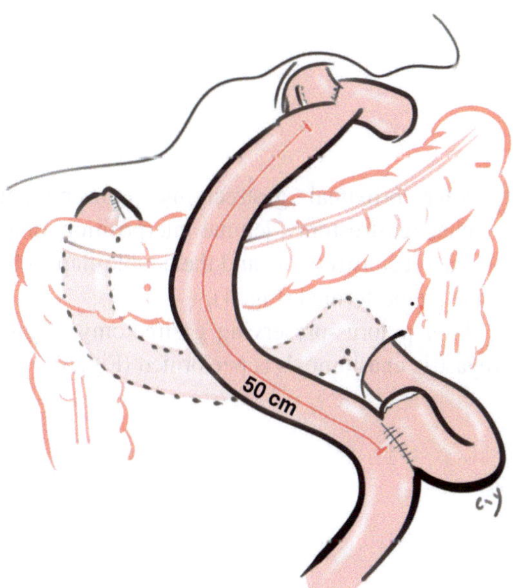

Fig. 3 Roux-en-Y esophagojejunostomy after total gastrectomy. (Adapted from Cho et al. [26])

Fig. 4 Reconstruction methods after proximal gastrectomy. (Adapted from park et al. [27], Nomura et al. [12], Nanobe et al. [28])

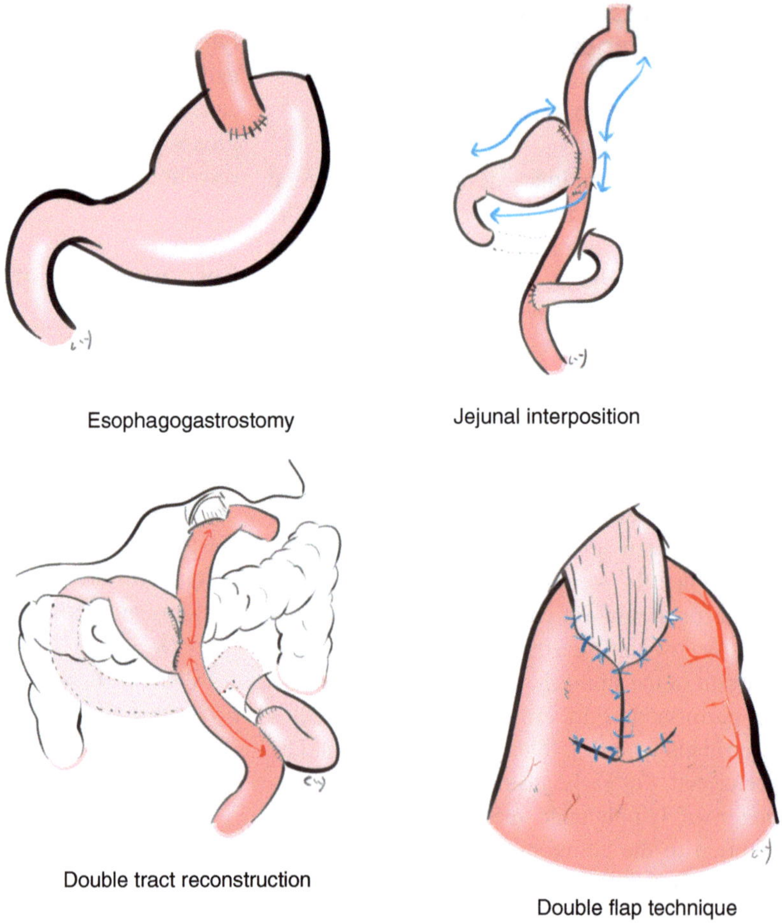

After proximal gastrectomy, conventional esophagogastrostomy, jejunal interposition, double tract reconstruction, and the double-flap technique are performed (Fig. 4).

After pylorus-preserving gastrectomy, a gastrogastric anastomosis is performed (Fig. 5).

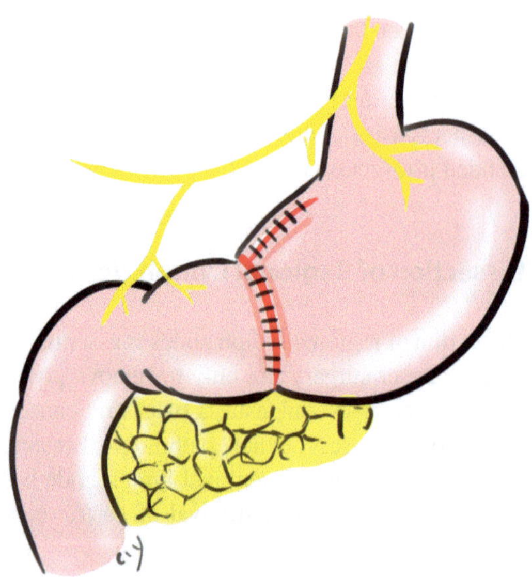

Fig. 5 Gastro-gastrostomy after pylorus-preserving gastrectomy. (Adapted from Sano et al. [29])

Surgical Treatment According to Disease Status

Surgical Treatment for Advanced Gastric Cancer

If the primary tumor has invaded the muscularis propria or beyond, it is classified as an advanced gastric cancer. Conversely, if gastric cancer is confined to the mucosa or submucosal layer (T1), regardless of metastasis to lymph nodes, it is classified as an early gastric cancer [4]. As a standard treatment for advanced gastric cancer, distal gastrectomy, which removes two-thirds of the distal part of the stomach, and total gastrectomy, which removes the entire stomach, are performed according to the location and gross type of the lesion [1]. For lymph node dissection, D2 is performed, and in some cases, further dissection is performed, such as paraaortic lymph node dissection. In case of gastric cancer with infiltration into adjacent organs, if complete resection is possible, concurrent resection is recommended. As for laparoscopic gastrectomy for advanced gastric cancer, it is not currently recommended in treatment guidelines as a first-line surgical approach in general practice. But recently published prospective clinical trials conducted in China and Korea demonstrated that laparoscopic distal gastrectomy for advanced gastric cancer is not inferior to open distal gastrectomy in terms of long-term survival [5, 6]. Therefore, it is likely that laparoscopic distal gastrectomy for advanced gastric cancer will soon be accepted as the standard treatment. A clinical study on the long-term survival outcome of laparoscopic total gastrectomy versus open total gastrectomy in patients with advanced gastric cancer is currently in progress [7].

Surgical Treatment for Early Gastric Cancer

The indication for surgical treatment in early gastric cancer with poor differentiation or deeper invasion is more/less than the indication for endoscopic resection and with a high-risk of lymph node metastasis. In addition, in the pathological results after endoscopic resection, cancers with a high-risk of lymph node metastasis or residual tumors that cannot be further resected are targeted [1]. The type of surgery in early gastric cancer is determined by the location of the tumor as in advanced gastric cancer, but the type of surgery according to the resection range is more diverse than in advanced gastric cancer. If the tumor is in the lower part of the stomach, distal gastrectomy is usually performed. If the tumor is in the middle of the stomach, distal gastrectomy or pylorus-preserving gastrectomy can be performed. When the tumor is in the upper part of the stomach, total gastrectomy or proximal gastrectomy can be performed. Among them, pylorus-preserving gastrectomy and proximal gastrectomy are classified as function-preserving gastrectomy [8]. Pylorus-preserving gastrectomy effectively reduces dumping syndrome and reflux of bile and pancreatic juice by preserving a part of the antrum, including the pylorus and the vagus nerve. Furthermore, pylorus-preserving gastrectomy significantly reduces the incidence of cholelithiasis occurring in the gallbladder by preserving the hepatic branch of the vagus nerve [9, 10]. However, delayed gastric emptying caused by poor pyloric relaxation was pointed out as a disadvantage [9]. Proximal gastrectomy was performed in the past, but conventional esophagogastric anastomosis has been rarely performed due to the high incidence of anastomosis-related complications such as reflux esophagitis and anastomotic stenosis [11]. Recently, anastomosis methods to prevent reflux have been introduced, and proximal gastrectomy has been increasingly performed. Mechanisms used to prevent reflux include reduction of reflux by interposition of an isoperistaltic jejunum that contracts downwards between the esophagus and the stomach (double tract reconstruction and jejunal interposition) [12–15], and valvuloplasty, which creates a valve that can prevent reflux during an esophagogastrostomy (double flap technique) [16–18]. However, there is still no conclusion on which of these two mechanisms is superior. Laparoscopic gastrectomy for early gastric cancer has been widely practiced. Through many clinical trials, laparoscopic gastrectomy for early gastric cancer showed a similar or lower incidence of postoperative complications compared to open gastrectomy [7, 19, 20]. There was a report indicating that the quality of life after surgery was better in the laparoscopic group [21], but there was no significant difference in long-term survival compared to open surgery [20, 22]. Currently, total gastrectomy, pylorus-preserving gastrectomy, and proximal gastrectomy are all performed laparoscopically.

Complications Associated with Surgery

Morbidity and Mortality Rates in Recent Studies

Recently published data of clinical trials from Korea and Japan have revealed a mortality rate less than 1%, and morbidity rate between 10% and 20% [7, 19, 23–25].

Surgery-Related Major Complications

Bleeding

Postoperative bleeding occurs in about 1% of patients. Early postoperative bleeding usually occurs as intraluminal or intraperitoneal bleeding. Most bleeding events can be controlled with conservative treatment, but in case of massive or continuous intraperitoneal bleeding, surgical hemostasis or embolization through angiography should be considered. In luminal bleeding endoscopic coagulation, epinephrine injection or clipping is needed if bleeding is refractory to conservative treatment. Late bleeding may occur 1 or 2 weeks after operation and this type of bleeding has a potential vascular origin such as erosion of vascular wall or rupture of pseudoaneurysm caused by abscess, anastomotic leakage, or pancreatic leakage. Therefore, careful monitoring and prompt surgical or angiographic intervention should be considered.

Anastomotic Leakage

There are various types of anastomoses in gastrectomy. Once anastomotic leakage occurs, intraluminal bowel contents, containing a large quantity of microbes and irritable chemicals, flow into the peritoneal cavity, resulting in localized abscess, wound disruption, severe peritonitis, and sepsis. Sometimes outcome is fatal, so early detection and treatment is essential for management of anastomotic leakage. Treatment for anastomotic leakage consists of effective peritoneal drainage, prevention of additional outflow of bowel contents through effective intraluminal decompression, and promotion of the closure of the opening.

Intraabdominal Abscess

Risk factors for intraabdominal abscess formation include malnutrition, diabetes, poor liver function, extended lymph node dissection, combined resection of other organs, and longer operation time. Causes of intraabdominal abscess are intraoperative contamination, spillage of intraluminal contents, pancreatic leakage, and anastomotic leakage. Treatment for intraabdominal abscess is percutaneous drainage or open surgical drainage when there are multiple abscesses or when percutaneous drainage is not feasible.

Pancreatic Leakage and Fistula Formation

Pancreatic injury and leakage may occur without resection of pancreatic parenchyma because pancreas can be injured during peripancreatic lymph node dissection and stripping of pancreatic capsule. Pancreatic juice containing trypsin can cause secondary injury to adjacent structures and secondary anastomosis leakage or intraabdominal bleeding may occur. Diagnosis can be made with high amylase level in the drained fluid. Administration of somatostatin analogue and effective drainage is recommended.

Conclusion

Surgical treatment of gastric cancer still occupies an important part of gastric cancer treatment and is performed as an adjuvant treatment for incomplete endoscopic resection, and also represents a form of conversion surgery for advanced gastric cancer patients who show good response to systemic chemotherapy. The target of gastric cancer surgery is local gastric cancer that can be resected without residual cancers that are gastric cancers beyond the scope of endoscopic resection. Gastric cancer surgery consists of resection of the primary lesion, lymph node resection, and reconstruction of the gastrointestinal tract. The extent of gastric resection is determined based on the location, degree of progression, and gross type of gastric cancer, and the extent of lymph node resection is determined according to the degree of gastric cancer and the extent of gastric resection, and various reconstruction methods can be applied according to the extent of gastric resection. It is reported that minimally invasive surgery in gastric cancer reduces pain and complications associated with surgery and has advantages in health-related quality of life in the early postoperative period. Currently, minimally invasive surgery is increasingly being applied in gastric cancer, which is a trend that will increasingly be applied to all gastric cancer surgeries, including advanced gastric cancer.

References

1. Japanese Gastric Cancer Association. Japanese gastric cancer treatment guidelines 2018 (5th edition). Gastric Cancer. 2021;24(1):1–21.
2. Guideline Committee of the Korean Gastric Cancer Association DWG, Review P. Korean practice guideline for gastric Cancer 2018: an evidence-based, multi-disciplinary approach. J Gastric Cancer. 2019;19(1):1–48.
3. Symeonidis D, Diamantis A, Bompou E, Tepetes K. Current role of lymphadenectomy in gastric cancer surgery. J BUON. 2019;24(5):1761–7.
4. Japanese Gastric Cancer A. Japanese classification of gastric carcinoma: 3rd English edition. Gastric Cancer. 2011;14(2):101–12.
5. Wong J. Effect of laparoscopic vs. open distal gastrectomy on 3-year disease free survival in patients with locally advanced gastric cancer: commentary on the class-01 randomized clinical trial. Transl. Gastroenterol Hepatol. 2019;4:78.
6. Hyung WJ, Yang HK, Park YK, Lee HJ, An JY, Kim W, et al. Long-term outcomes of laparoscopic distal gastrectomy for locally advanced gastric Cancer: the KLASS-02-RCT randomized clinical trial. J Clin Oncol. 2020;38(28):3304–13.
7. Hyung WJ, Yang HK, Han SU, Lee YJ, Park JM, Kim JJ, et al. A feasibility study of laparoscopic total gastrectomy for clinical stage I gastric cancer: a prospective multi-center phase II clinical trial, KLASS 03. Gastric Cancer. 2019;22(1):214–22.
8. Hiki N, Nunobe S, Kubota T, Jiang X. Function-preserving gastrectomy for early gastric cancer. Ann Surg Oncol. 2013;20(8):2683–92.
9. Suh YS, Han DS, Kong SH, Kwon S, Shin CI, Kim WH, et al. Laparoscopy-assisted pylorus-preserving gastrectomy is better than laparoscopy-assisted distal gastrectomy for middle-third early gastric cancer. Ann Surg. 2014;259(3):485–93.
10. Hosoda K, Yamashita K, Sakuramoto S, Katada N, Moriya H, Mieno H, et al. Postoperative quality of life after laparoscopy-assisted pylorus-preserving gastrectomy compared with laparoscopy-assisted distal gastrectomy: A cross-sectional postal questionnaire survey. Am J Surg. 2017;213(4):763–70.
11. Wang S, Lin S, Wang H, Yang J, Yu P, Zhao Q, et al. Reconstruction methods after radical proximal gastrectomy: A systematic review. Medicine (Baltimore). 2018;97(11):e0121.
12. Nomura E, Lee SW, Kawai M, Yamazaki M, Nabeshima K, Nakamura K, et al. Functional outcomes by reconstruction technique following laparoscopic proximal gastrectomy for gastric cancer: double tract versus jejunal interposition. World J Surg Oncol. 2014;12:20.
13. Takiguchi N, Takahashi M, Ikeda M, Inagawa S, Ueda S, Nobuoka T, et al. Long-term quality-of-life comparison of total gastrectomy and proximal gastrectomy by postgastrectomy syndrome assessment scale (PGSAS-45): a nationwide multi-institutional study. Gastric Cancer. 2015;18(2):407–16.
14. Ohashi M, Morita S, Fukagawa T, Oda I, Kushima R, Katai H. Functional advantages of proximal gastrectomy with jejunal interposition over total gastrectomy with roux-en-Y esophagojejunostomy for early gastric cancer. World J Surg. 2015;39(11):2726–33.
15. Jung DH, Lee Y, Kim DW, Park YS, Ahn SH, Park DJ, et al. Laparoscopic proximal gastrectomy with double tract reconstruction is superior to laparoscopic total gastrectomy for proximal early gastric cancer. Surg Endosc. 2017;31(10):3961–9.
16. Hayami M, Hiki N, Nunobe S, Mine S, Ohashi M, Kumagai K, et al. Clinical outcomes and evaluation of laparoscopic proximal gastrectomy with double-flap technique for early gastric cancer in the upper third of the stomach. Ann Surg Oncol. 2017;24(6):1635–42.
17. Tsumura T, Kuroda S, Nishizaki M, Kikuchi S, Kakiuchi Y, Takata N, et al. Short-term and long-

term comparisons of laparoscopy-assisted proximal gastrectomy with esophagogastrostomy by the double-flap technique and laparoscopy-assisted total gastrectomy for proximal gastric cancer. PLoS One. 2020;15(11):e0242223.

18. Saze Z, Kase K, Nakano H, Yamauchi N, Kaneta A, Watanabe Y, et al. Functional benefits of the double flap technique after proximal gastrectomy for gastric cancer. BMC Surg. 2021;21(1):392.
19. Kim W, Kim HH, Han SU, Kim MC, Hyung WJ, Ryu SW, et al. Decreased morbidity of laparoscopic distal gastrectomy compared with open distal gastrectomy for stage I gastric cancer: short-term outcomes from a multicenter randomized controlled trial (KLASS-01). Ann Surg. 2016;263(1):28–35.
20. Katai H, Mizusawa J, Katayama H, Morita S, Yamada T, Bando E, et al. Survival outcomes after laparoscopy-assisted distal gastrectomy versus open distal gastrectomy with nodal dissection for clinical stage IA or IB gastric cancer (JCOG0912): a multicentre, non-inferiority, phase 3 randomised controlled trial. Lancet Gastroenterol Hepatol. 2020;5(2):142–51.
21. Kim YW, Yoon HM, Yun YH, Nam BH, Eom BW, Baik YH, et al. Long-term outcomes of laparoscopy-assisted distal gastrectomy for early gastric cancer: result of a randomized controlled trial (COACT 0301). Surg Endosc. 2013;27(11):4267–76.
22. Kim HH, Han SU, Kim MC, Kim W, Lee HJ, Ryu SW, et al. Effect of laparoscopic distal gastrectomy vs open distal gastrectomy on long-term survival among patients with stage I gastric Cancer: the KLASS-01 randomized clinical trial. JAMA Oncol. 2019;5(4):506–13.
23. Katai H, Mizusawa J, Katayama H, Takagi M, Yoshikawa T, Fukagawa T, et al. Short-term surgical outcomes from a phase III study of laparoscopy-assisted versus open distal gastrectomy with nodal dissection for clinical stage IA/IB gastric cancer: Japan Clinical Oncology Group Study JCOG0912. Gastric Cancer. 2017;20(4):699–708.
24. Kim HH, Hyung WJ, Cho GS, Kim MC, Han SU, Kim W, et al. Morbidity and mortality of laparoscopic gastrectomy versus open gastrectomy for gastric cancer: an interim report--a phase III multicenter, prospective, randomized Trial (KLASS Trial). Ann Surg 2010;251(3):417–420.
25. Fujitani K, Yang HK, Kurokawa Y, Park DJ, Tsujinaka T, Park BJ, et al. Randomized controlled trial comparing gastrectomy plus chemotherapy with chemotherapy alone in advanced gastric cancer with a single non-curable factor: Japan Clinical Oncology Group Study JCOG 0705 and Korea Gastric Cancer Association Study KGCA01. Jpn J Clin Oncol. 2008;38(7):504–6.
26. Cho MH, Son T, Kim HI, Noh SH, Choi S, Seo WJ, et al. Similar hematologic and nutritional outcomes after proximal gastrectomy with double-tract reconstruction in comparison to total gastrectomy for early upper gastric cancer. Surg Endosc. 2019;33(6):1757–68.
27. Park DJ, Park YS, Ahn SH, Kim HH. Laparoscopic proximal gastrectomy as a surgical treatment for upper third early gastric cancer. Korean J Gastroenterol. 2017;70(3):134–40.
28. Souya N, Masaru H, Naoki H. Morphological and functional reconstruction of the esophago-gastric junction with a double-flap technique after laparoscopic proximal gastrectomy. Ann Laparosc Endosc Surg. 2017;2:25.
29. Sano T, Hollowood A. Early gastric cancer: diagnosis and less invasive treatments. Scand J Surg. 2006;95(4):249–55.

Adjuvant Chemotherapy

Key Points

- Postoperative chemotherapy is recommended for patients who have undergone primary D2 lymph node dissection, especially in Asian countries.
- Perioperative chemotherapy is also a recommended standard of care for patients with resectable gastric cancer.
- The addition of postoperative radiotherapy to postoperative treatment is currently not recommended and should be reserved for patients who received less than a D2 lymph node dissection.

Introduction

In recent decades, substantial evidence has been accumulated on the use of adjuvant treatment for patients with locoregional gastric cancer. However, standard treatment varies between countries or regions around the world due to surgical procedure, tumor heterogeneity, historical/epidemiological background, and clinical setting, despite several phase III clinical trials of adjuvant combined modality therapy have shown beneficial effects of adjuvant treatment [1]. In particular, D2 gastrectomy is essential and minimally invasive surgery is also being explored increasingly around the world [2]. In East Asian countries, postoperative chemotherapy is recommended for patients who have undergone primary dissection of D2 lymph nodes [3, 4], perioperative chemotherapy is the preferred approach to resectable gastric cancer in Europe [5, 6], and postoperative chemoradiation has been accepted as standard therapy in the United States for patients who received less than a D2 lymph node dissection [7]. Therefore, this chapter will summarize previous studies and discuss current treatment options for adjuvant treatment of gastric cancer.

Postoperative Chemotherapy

Current evidence is based on the results of two landmark Asian trials. The first trial, the CLASSIC trial, conducted in South Korea, established the benefit of adjuvant capecitabine and oxaliplatin (XELOX) in patients who undergo gastrectomy with D2 lymph node dissection [3]. This trial was performed in South Korea, China, and Taiwan, and randomized 1035 patients, who underwent D2 gastrectomy for stages II–IIIB gastric cancer, to receive adjuvant XELOX for 6 months or observation alone. After a preplanned interim analysis at 34 months of median follow-up, the study reached its primary end point, strengthening the role of adjuvant chemotherapy in this setting. Significantly improved disease-free survival (DFS) was observed in the chemotherapy group versus the surgery-only group (74 versus 59%; HR: 0.56; 95% CI, 0.44–

Byung Woog Kang is the lead author of this chapter.

H. J. Chun et al., *Gastrointestinal Cancer*, https://doi.org/10.1007/978-981-99-0815-8_8

0.72) despite the relatively high incidence of grade 3 or higher toxicities in the chemotherapy arm (56 versus 6%). The results were confirmed after 5 years of follow-up (9% improvement in the 5-year overall survival [OS] and 15% in DFS) [8].

In Japan, postoperative chemotherapy with S-1, an oral prodrug of 5-fluorouracil (5-FU), for 1 year confirmed an improvement in OS in comparison to D2 surgery alone in pathological stage II/III gastric cancer [4]. In this phase III trial (ACTS-GC), 1059 patients with pathological stage II/III gastric cancer, according to the 13th edition of the Japanese Classification of Gastric Carcinoma (JCGC), were randomized to either a surgery-alone arm or surgery with S-1 arm, between 2001 and 2004. The improved 5-year OS of the surgery with the S-1 group was confirmed by the 5-year follow-up results (71.7 versus 61.1%; HR, 0.67; 95% CI, 0.54–0.83) [9]. However, subgroup analysis indicated that the relative risk reduction for survival was not significant in patients with stage IIIB tumors, suggesting the insufficiency of the treatment intensity for patients with more advanced diseases [1]. Another question raised was whether the duration of adjuvant S-1 treatment in patients with stage II can be reduced. The possible feasibility of shorter S-1 duration was then evaluated in JCOG1104 [10]. The study was terminated at the first interim analysis with an HR for the 6-month group versus the 12-month group of 2.52 (95% CI, 1.11–5.77), which met the predefined criteria for early termination. Plus, since direct comparison between capecitabine-based and S-1-based regimens was limited, which regimen is better for pathological stage II/III gastric cancer is yet to be established [11]. Therefore, adjuvant treatment with 6 months XELOX or 1 year S-1 is considered the standard of care in Asian patients with stage II/III resectable gastric cancer after D2 surgery. However, this approach is less preferred in western countries and the benefits of postoperative chemotherapy following a D0/1 lymph node dissection have not been documented in randomized clinical trials [12].

More recently, the Japan Clinical Cancer Research Organization (JACCRO) GC-07 randomized 915 Japanese patients with stage III gastric cancer to receive adjuvant S-1 alone or in association with docetaxel [13]. At the second planned interim analysis, the 3-year relapse-free survival (RFS) of the S-1 plus docetaxel arm was significantly superior to that of the control arm (65.9 vs 49.6%; HR, 0.63; 95% CI, 0.40–0.99), but the combination arm showed higher adverse events. Based on these results, S-1 plus docetaxel after D2 gastrectomy can be considered a new standard of care for patients with stage III gastric cancer. Table 1 summarizes the pivotal trials of adjuvant chemotherapy for gastric cancer.

Table 1 Pivotal trials of adjuvant chemotherapy for gastric cancer

Study name	Phase	Treatment arms	Number (n)	Primary endpoints	HR	95% CI	*P* value
ACTS-GC [3]	III	Surgery/S-1 Surgery	529 530	OS	0.68	0.52–0.87	0.003
CLASSIC [4]	III	Surgery/XELOX Surgery	520 515	3-year DFS	0.56	0.44–0.72	<0.0001
MAGIC [5]	III	Surgery/perioperative ECF Surgery	250 253	OS	0.75	0.60–0.93	0.009
FLOT4-AIO [6]	III	Surgery/perioperative FLOT Surgery/perioperative ECF/ECX	356 360	OS	0.77	0.63–0.94	0.012
JACCRO GC-07 [13]	III	Surgery/S-1/docetaxel Surgery/S-1	454 459	3-year RFS	0.63	0.40–0.99	<0.001
INT-0116 [7]	III	Surgery Surgery/5-FU/LV/radiotherapy	275 281	RFS	1.52	1.23–1.86	<0.001
ARTIST [20]	III	Surgery/XP/XRT/XP Surgery/XP	230 228	DFS	0.74	0.52–1.05	0.0922

HR hazard ratio, *CI* confidence interval, *OS* overall survival, *XELOX* capecitabine plus oxaliplatin, *DFS* disease-free survival, *ECF* epirubicin, cisplatin, plus 5-fluorouracil, *FLOT* 5-fluorouracil, leucovorin, oxaliplatin, plus docetaxel, *ECX* epirubicin, cisplatin, plus capecitabine, *RFS* relapse-free survival, *5-FU* 5-fluorouracil, *LV* leucovorin, *XP* capecitabine plus cisplatin, *XRT* capecitabine plus radiotherapy

Perioperative Chemotherapy

Perioperative chemotherapy can have several advantages, including the eradication of micrometastatic disease, downstaging of the tumor, and increased chance for curative resection, but a potential limitation is that compliance may be relatively low and non-responders miss their opportunity for curative resection [2]. This strategy in the perioperative setting has mainly been applied in Europe. The United Kingdom Medical Research Council's MAGIC trial was a landmark phase III study that established the survival benefit of perioperative chemotherapy plus surgery versus surgery alone in patients with resectable gastric, esophagogastric junction, or lower esophageal adenocarcinoma [6]. This study randomized 503 patients to receive surgery alone or six cycles of perioperative ECF chemotherapy (epirubicin, cisplatin, and 5-FU) in addition to surgery. Patients treated with perioperative chemotherapy had an improved 5-year progression-free survival (PFS) and OS, with an increase from 23% to 36% for OS (HR, 0.66; 95% CI, 0.53–0.81). This encouraging result then led to a phase III trial (FLOT4-AIO) that compared perioperative 5-FU, leucovorin, oxaliplatin, and docetaxel (FLOT) with ECF in patients with resectable gastric cancer [5]. This randomized controlled phase III German trial enrolled 716 patients with cT2–4/cN-any/cM0 or cT-any/cN+/cM0 to receive FLOT or ECF. The study met its primary end point of OS, and all secondary end points, including PFS, complete resection rate, surgical morbidity and mortality, and toxicity, were also better in the experimental arm with FLOT. In particular, perioperative FLOT resulted in superior OS compared with ECF (50 versus 35 months; HR: 0.77; 95% CI, 0.63–0.94). The rate of R0 resections was significantly higher in the FLOT arm (84% vs 77%) and the completion rates of the planned chemotherapy in the preoperative and postoperative periods were 91% and 37% in the control arm, respectively, and 90% and 50% in the FLOT arm, respectively. Furthermore, FLOT was comparable in toxicity to ECF, even if the rates of grade 3 and 4 neutropenia and infection were higher. Therefore, FLOT is now the recommended standard of care for patients with locally advanced gastric cancer who can tolerate a perioperative three drug combination regimen [14].

Recently, in the PRODIGY trial in South Korea, a novel regimen with docetaxel/oxaliplatin/S-1 (DOS) was compared with postoperative S-1 [15]. The addition of preoperative DOS to D2 gastrectomy and postoperative adjuvant S1 chemotherapy led to significant tumor downstaging and improved PFS with acceptable safety. Another trial conducted in China (RESOLVE) compared the efficacy and safety of perioperative chemotherapy with oxaliplatin plus S-1 (SOX) [16]. The results showed that perioperative SOX improved 3-year DFS compared to postoperative XELOX and adjuvant SOX was not inferior to adjuvant XELOX. As a result, these findings suggest that the perioperative option is effective and can also be considered as a treatment approach for Asian patients with resectable gastric cancer.

Postoperative Chemoradiotherapy

Local treatment, including radiotherapy, can be applied as an adjuvant strategy to reduce the probability of local recurrence for resected gastric cancer [17]. However, the role of adjuvant chemoradiotherapy remains unclear. The landmark INT-0116 trial investigated the effectiveness of surgery followed by postoperative chemotherapy plus chemoradiotherapy on survival in patients with resectable gastric or esophagogastric junction cancer [7]. The study randomized 556 patients to receive adjuvant CRT with 5-FU/leucovorin followed by 4500 cGy radiotherapy at 180 cGy per day. The majority of patients had T3/4 tumors (69%) and node-positive disease (85%). Patients treated with chemoradiotherapy had significantly better OS (HR, 1.35; 95% CI, 1.09–1.66) and RFS (HR, 1.52; 95% CI, 1.23–1–86) than those in the surgery-only group, and the survival benefit was confirmed at the 10-year follow-up [18]. However, the study was limited by the finding that only 10% of the patients underwent D2 node dissection. The dosing and schedule of chemotherapy were also associated with high rates of grade 3 and 4 toxicities, and 17% of the patients receiving chemoradiotherapy discontinued treatment.

The ARTIST trial was conducted in South Korea to assess the impact of adjuvant chemoradiotherapy in patients who had undergone a D2 lymph node dissection [19]. This study randomized 458 patients to receive six cycles of adjuvant capecitabine plus cisplatin (XP) versus XP plus radiotherapy (XP/XRT/XP). The results confirmed that postoperative chemoradiotherapy did not significantly reduce recurrence rates after D2 dissection compared to postoperative chemotherapy (3-year DFS, 78.2 versus 74.2%). In the updated analysis with 7-year follow-up, no statistically significant differences were observed for DFS and OS [20]. Interestingly, considering the population of patients with node-positive involvement (396/458, 86%), there was a statistically significant prolongation of DFS in a subgroup of patients with positive nodes (77.5 versus 72.3%). Subsequently, the phase III ARTIST II trial was conducted to determine the role of chemoradiotherapy in patients with node-positive tumors. The results did not show benefit for postoperative chemoradiotherapy in these patients following D2 dissection (3-year DFS, 78% versus 73%) [21]. Taken together, although these studies suggest that adjuvant chemoradiotherapy may play a role in patients with suboptimal surgery or lymph node positive disease, there are limited data to recommend routine use of chemoradiotherapy for resected gastric cancer.

Conclusion

Despite the gap between regions, multimodal treatment represents the mainstay of cure for resectable gastric cancer. In Eastern countries, 5-FU-based chemotherapy or in association with oxaliplatin/docetaxel can be considered as an adjuvant postoperative treatment. In Western countries, the FLOT regimen was recently shown to be effective in the perioperative chemotherapy setting. In addition, novel regimens, such as DOS or SOX, would seem to be beneficial and tolerable for Asian patients and can be an option for these patients. Although these treatment strategies provide improved treatment outcomes in patients with resectable gastric cancer, the benefit is still disappointing. Consequently, additional trials are needed to identify the best treatment strategy and refine the benefits of adjuvant treatment, and more evidence is required to improve the management of gastric cancer.

References

1. Shimizu D, Kanda M, Kodera Y, Sakamoto J. Cutting-edge evidence of adjuvant treatments for gastric cancer. Expert Rev Gastroenterol Hepatol. 2018;12(11):1109–22.
2. Smyth EC, Nilsson M, Grabsch HI, van Grieken NCT, Lordick F. Gastric cancer. Lancet. 2020;396(10251):635–48.
3. Bang Y-J, Kim Y-W, Yang H-K, Chung HC, Park Y-K, Lee KH, et al. Adjuvant capecitabine and oxaliplatin for gastric cancer after D2 gastrectomy (CLASSIC): a phase 3 open-label, randomised controlled trial. Lancet. 2012;379(9813):315–21.
4. Sakuramoto S, Sasako M, Yamaguchi T, Kinoshita T, Fujii M, Nashimoto A, et al. Adjuvant chemotherapy for gastric cancer with S-1, an Oral fluoropyrimidine. N Engl J Med. 2007;357(18):1810–20.
5. Al-Batran S-E, Homann N, Pauligk C, Goetze TO, Meiler J, Kasper S, et al. Perioperative chemotherapy with fluorouracil plus leucovorin, oxaliplatin, and docetaxel versus fluorouracil or capecitabine plus cisplatin and epirubicin for locally advanced, resectable gastric or gastro-oesophageal junction adenocarcinoma (FLOT4): a randomised, phase 2/3 trial. Lancet. 2019;393(10184):1948–57.
6. Cunningham D, Allum WH, Stenning SP, Thompson JN, Van de Velde CJH, Nicolson M, et al. Perioperative chemotherapy versus surgery alone for resectable gastroesophageal cancer. N Engl J Med. 2006;355(1):11–20.
7. Macdonald JS, Smalley SR, Benedetti J, Hundahl SA, Estes NC, Stemmermann GN, et al. Chemoradiotherapy after surgery compared with surgery alone for adenocarcinoma of the stomach or gastroesophageal junction. N Engl J Med. 2001;345(10):725–30.
8. Noh SH, Park SR, Yang H-K, Chung HC, Chung I-J, Kim S-W, et al. Adjuvant capecitabine plus oxaliplatin for gastric cancer after D2 gastrectomy (CLASSIC): 5-year follow-up of an open-label, randomised phase 3 trial. Lancet Oncol. 2014;15(12):1389–96.
9. Sasako M, Sakuramoto S, Katai H, Kinoshita T, Furukawa H, Yamaguchi T, et al. Five-year outcomes of a randomized phase III trial comparing adjuvant chemotherapy with S-1 versus surgery alone in stage II or III gastric cancer. J Clin Oncol. 2011;29(33):4387–93.

10. Yoshikawa T, Terashima M, Mizusawa J, Nunobe S, Nishida Y, Yamada T, et al. Four courses versus eight courses of adjuvant S-1 for patients with stage II gastric cancer (JCOG1104 [OPAS-1]): an open-label, phase 3, non-inferiority, randomised trial. Lancet Gastroenterol Hepatol. 2019;4(3):208–16.
11. Pelcovits A, Almhanna K. Locoregional gastric cancer: a narrative review of multidisciplinary management. Ann Transl Med. 2020;8(17):1108.
12. Petrillo A, Smyth EC. Multimodality treatment for localized gastric cancer: state of the art and new insights. Curr Opin Oncol. 2020;32(4):347–55.
13. Yoshida K, Kodera Y, Kochi M, Ichikawa W, Kakeji Y, Sano T, et al. Addition of docetaxel to oral fluoropyrimidine improves efficacy in patients with stage III gastric cancer: interim analysis of JACCRO GC-07, a randomized controlled trial. J Clin Oncol. 2019;37(15):1296–304.
14. Wagner AD, Lordick F, Grabsch HI, Terashima M, Terada M, Yoshikawa T, et al. Multidisciplinary management of stage II-III gastric and gastro-oesophageal junction cancer. Eur J Cancer. 2020;124:67–76.
15. Kang Y-K, Yook JH, Park Y-K, Lee JS, Kim Y-W, Kim JY, et al. PRODIGY: a phase III study of neoadjuvant docetaxel, oxaliplatin, and S-1 plus surgery and adjuvant S-1 versus surgery and adjuvant S-1 for resectable advanced gastric cancer. J Clin Oncol. 2021;39(26):2903–13.
16. Zhang X, Liang H, Li Z, Xue Y, Wang Y, Zhou Z, et al. Perioperative or postoperative adjuvant oxaliplatin with S-1 versus adjuvant oxaliplatin with capecitabine in patients with locally advanced gastric or gastro-oesophageal junction adenocarcinoma undergoing D2 gastrectomy (RESOLVE): an open-label, superiority and non-inferiority, phase 3 randomised controlled trial. Lancet Oncol. 2021;22(8):1081–92.
17. Joshi SS, Badgwell BD. Current treatment and recent progress in gastric cancer. CA Cancer J Clin. 2021;71(3):264–79.
18. Smalley SR, Benedetti JK, Haller DG, Hundahl SA, Estes NC, Ajani JA, et al. Updated analysis of SWOG-directed intergroup study 0116: a phase III trial of adjuvant radiochemotherapy versus observation after curative gastric cancer resection. J Clin Oncol. 2012;30(19):2327–33.
19. Lee J, Lim DH, Kim S, Park SH, Park JO, Park YS, et al. Phase III trial comparing capecitabine plus cisplatin versus capecitabine plus cisplatin with concurrent capecitabine radiotherapy in completely resected gastric cancer with D2 lymph node dissection: the ARTIST trial. J Clin Oncol. 2012;30(3):268–73.
20. Park SH, Sohn TS, Lee J, Lim DH, Hong ME, Kim K-M, et al. Phase III trial to compare adjuvant chemotherapy with capecitabine and cisplatin versus concurrent chemoradiotherapy in gastric cancer: final report of the adjuvant chemoradiotherapy in stomach tumors trial, including survival and subset analyses. J Clin Oncol. 2015;33(28):3130–6.
21. Park SH, Lim DH, Sohn TS, Lee J, Zang DY, Kim ST, et al. A randomized phase III trial comparing adjuvant single-agent S1, S-1 with oxaliplatin, and postoperative chemoradiation with S-1 and oxaliplatin in patients with node-positive gastric cancer after D2 resection: the ARTIST 2 trial☆. Ann Oncol. 2021;32(3):368–74.

Palliative Chemotherapy in Advanced or Metastatic Gastric Cancer. IX-1. Overview and Cytotoxic Agents

Key Points

- Palliative chemotherapy can significantly improve the quality of life and survival of patients as compared to best supportive care in advanced or metastatic gastric cancer.
- Doublet or triplet platinum/fluoropyrimidine combination is the mainstay of chemotherapy in advanced or metastatic gastric cancer.
- In patients with HER2 overexpression/amplification, trastuzumab + cytotoxic agents could be the first choice in advanced or metastatic gastric cancer.
- Combination therapy of ramucirumab + paclitaxel may be useful in patients who worsen after using oxaliplatin as first-line therapy.
- Combination therapy with docetaxel has the disadvantage of high toxicity, but has a strong anticancer effect, so it can be considered in patients with a good performance status.

Introduction

Gastric cancer is one of the most common malignancies worldwide. Gastric cancer is often diagnosed at an advanced stage, except in Korea and Japan, and the prognosis of advanced gastric cancer is very poor. Due to national cancer screening programs, advanced gastric cancer is on the decline, especially in East Asia, but remains the leading cause of death elsewhere. For inoperable, advanced, or metastatic gastric cancer, palliative chemotherapy is the last treatment option. Compared to the best supportive care, palliative chemotherapy can significantly improve patient's quality of life and survival [1]. This chapter will review the chemotherapy regimens currently available in these clinical settings.

First-Line Treatment

Doublet or Triplet Platinum/Fluoropyrimidine Combination

The ESMO guidelines recommended doublet or triplet platinum/fluoropyrimidine combination for patients with advanced gastric cancer [2]. For many years, infusion 5-fluorouracil (5-FU) has been used as a basic therapy for the treatment of gastric cancer. In a meta-analysis, combination chemotherapy showed a modest survival benefit over single-agent chemotherapy [3]. The combination that has long been considered as the primary treatment for advanced gastric cancer is the platinum derivative cisplatin + 5-FU combination. In a phase 3 randomized controlled trial in Japan, the combination of cisplatin + 5-FU was found to be superior to 5-FU monotherapy [4].

Sun Hyung Kang is the lead author of this chapter.

H. J. Chun et al., *Gastrointestinal Cancer*, https://doi.org/10.1007/978-981-99-0815-8_9

Continuous infusion of 5-FU has the inconvenience of requiring hospitalization, so there have been attempts to replace it with oral 5-FU drugs. Kang et al., conducted a phase 3 study to compare the effects of oral 5-FU, capecitabine, and infusion 5-FU [5]. Each drug was used in combination with cisplatin, and the study demonstrated that capecitabine could replace 5-FU infusion because there was no difference in progression-free survival (PFS) between the two groups. Furthermore, in a meta-analysis, capecitabine showed better overall survival (OS) than 5-FU [6]. S-1 is another oral 5-FU formulation. S-1 is a combination of tegafur with two enzyme inhibitors: 5-chloro-2,4-dihydroxypyridine (CDHP), a reversible inhibitor of dihydropyrimidine dehydrogenase, and potassium oxonate (Oxo). CDHP improves the anticancer activity of tegafur by increasing its half-life, and Oxo reduces the gastrointestinal toxicity of tegafur [7]. Because the activity of CYP 2A6, which converts tegafur to 5-FU, is high in Caucasians, S-1 showed a high effect in Caucasians, but has the disadvantage of increasing its toxicity [8].

Because cisplatin has nephrotoxicity and ototoxicity, its use is limited in elderly patients or patients with impaired renal or cardiac function. Therefore, attempts have been made to replace cisplatin with other types of platinum derivatives. AI-Batran et al., conducted a comparative study between oxaliplatin and cisplatin [9]. Oxaliplatin and cisplatin were used in combination with 5-FU and leucovorin, respectively. OS was not statistically significant in this study, but the oxaliplatin group showed better PFS. Furthermore, the oxaliplatin group showed better tolerability, and in a subgroup analysis comparing elderly patients over 65 years of age, the oxaliplatin group showed a better response rate and OS. Currently, the FOLFOX regimen is widely used as primary anticancer therapy in Korea.

Irinotecan is another alternative to platinum derivatives. In a phase 3 study, irinotecan showed no significance difference in time to progression and OS compared to cisplatin, but tolerability was better [10]. Another phase 2 study showed similar results [11]. The FOLFIRI regimen, like the FOLFOX regimen, can be used as a first-line anticancer therapy.

Trastuzumab + Cytotoxic Agents

Approximately 20% of gastric cancers are characterized by the overexpression or/and amplification of the HER2 gene. HER2 overexpression is more common in the intestinal type than in the diffuse type, and more common in cancer of the gastroesophageal junction than in distal cancer. The HER2 gene is involved in cancer cell proliferation, apoptosis, adhesion, migration, and differentiation [12]. Trastuzumab is a monoclonal antibody against the HER2 receptor and has been shown to be effective in breast cancer [13]. The effectiveness of trastuzumab in gastric cancer was demonstrated in the ToGA trial, a large study involving a total of 584 patients in 12 countries [14]. In the ToGA trial, trastuzumab + cisplatin + 5-FU group showed better OS and PFS than cisplatin + 5-FU group (OS: 13.8 months vs. 11.1 months, PFS: 6.7 months vs. 5.5 months). In terms of quality of life, trastuzumab combination therapy showed superior results compared to chemotherapy alone [15].

Comparison of Treatment Outcomes between Regimens

Doublet or triplet platinum/fluoropyrimidine combination regimens do not differ significantly in overall therapeutic outcome. In a phase 2 study in Korea, four doublet regimens were performed: S-1 and cisplatin (SP); oxaliplatin and 5-FU (FOLFOX); docetaxel and 5-FU (DF) and paclitaxel and 5-FU (PF) did not differ in OS, but SP showed the most favorable results in PFS [16]. To date, no studies have directly compared trastuzumab combination chemotherapy with other regimens. The regimen can be selected considering the policy of the oncologist or institution and the clinical characteristics of each patient.

Second Line and beyond

Taxane-Based Chemotherapy

Taxanes are a type of drug that block cell growth by stopping mitosis (cell division). In the V-325 study, docetaxel + cisplatin + 5-FU triplet (DCF arm) showed better OS and PFS than the combination of cisplatin + 5-FU (CF arm) [17]. However, the difference in OS between the two groups was only 0.6 months (9.2 months vs. 8.6 months), which was statistically significant, but did not show a substantial difference. In terms of toxicity, the DCF arm showed significantly higher toxicity than the CF arm, so it was difficult to apply to patients in poor disease status. To reduce the toxicity of docetaxel, a recent Japanese study conducted a study by increasing the dose of docetaxel [18]. Although it was a small study in which only 16 patients were enrolled, the disease control rate was 100%, the overall response rate was 78%, and the median survival was 19.6 months, showing an excellent treatment effect. If toxicity can be overcome, good treatment results can be expected with anticancer therapy with docetaxel.

Ramucirumab + Paclitaxel

Ramucirumab is an Ig1 monoclonal antibody and an antagonist of the VEGF receptor 2, blocking the binding of VEGF A, C, and D. Because angiogenesis plays an important role in cancer progression, drugs that inhibit it have been tried in several carcinomas. In the REGARD trial, ramucirumab monotherapy showed an increased median survival (5.2 vs. 3.8 months, hazard ratio [HR] = 0.776) and PFS (2.1 months vs. 1.3 months, HR = 0.483) compared to placebo [19]. The efficacy of ramucirumab + cytotoxic agent was confirmed by the RAINBOW trial [20]. The RAINBOW trial compared combination chemotherapy with ramucirumab (8 mg/kg, every 15 days) plus weekly paclitaxel (80 mg/m^2, on days 1, 8, and 15) with paclitaxel monotherapy. Patients treated with ramucirumab combination chemotherapy showed significant improvements in median OS (9.6 months vs. 7.4 months, HR = 0.807), PFS (4.4 months vs. 2.9 months, HR = 0.635, $p < 0.0001$), and response rate (28% vs. 54%, $p = 0.0001$) [20]. It is currently widely used as a second-line rescue therapy in patients who worsen after receiving FOLFOX treatment.

Other Regimens

Because the difference in therapeutic efficacy between regimens in advanced or metastatic gastric cancer is not clear, a definitive treatment of choice has not been established. Therefore, secondary therapy can be performed sequentially according to the condition of each patient or the policy of the medical institution or oncologist, and use of a drug not used in the previous line of treatment. Epirubicin, an anthracycline, has been proven effective in the MAGIC trial and is widely used in European countries, but its use is gradually decreasing in the Eastern countries, including Korea [21].

Conclusion

Table 1 summarizes various regimens of palliative chemotherapy in gastric cancer.

Table 1 Various regimens of palliative chemotherapy in gastric cancer

Regimen	Control	No. of patients	OS (months, regimen vs. control)
Oxaliplatin + 5-FU + leucovorin [9]	Cisplatin + 5-FU + leucovorin	220	10.7 vs. 8.8
Trastuzumab + cisplatin + 5-FU [14]	Cisplatin + 5-FU or capeitabine	594	13.8 vs. 11.1
Docetaxel + cisplatin + 5-FU [17]	Cisplatin + 5FU	445	9.2 vs. 8.6
Ramucirumab + paclitaxel [20]	Paclitaxel	665	9.6 vs. 7.4

5-FU 5-fluorouracil

In patients diagnosed with inoperable, advanced, or metastatic gastric cancer, HER2 gene expression should first be assessed. If the bioptic tissue is positive for HER2 gene expression, combined chemotherapy with trastuzumab + cisplatin + 5-FU can be attempted first. If HER2 gene expression is negative, palliative chemotherapy such as FOLFOX, FOLFIRI, cisplatin + 5FU, or capecitabine + 5-FU can be attempted. In principle, drugs not included in previous regimens should be used to treat patients who worsen after first-line chemotherapy. Combination therapy of ramucirumab + paclitaxel may be useful in patients who worsen after using FOLFOX as first-line therapy. Combination therapy with docetaxel has the disadvantage of high toxicity, but has a strong anticancer effect, so it can be considered in patients with a good performance status.

References

1. Wagner AD, Grothe W, Haerting J, Kleber G, Grothey A, Fleig WE. Chemotherapy in advanced gastric cancer: a systemic review and meta-analysis based on aggregate data. J Clin Oncol. 2006;24:2903–9.
2. Smyth EC, Verheij M, Allum W, Cunningham D, Cervantes A, Arnold D. ESMO guidelines committee. Gastric cancer: ESMO clinical practice guidelines for diagnosis, treatment and follow-up. Ann Oncol. 2016;27:v38–49.
3. Wagner AD, Unverzagt S, Grothe W, Kleber G, Grothey A, Haerting J, et al. Chemotherapy for advanced gastric cancer. Cochrane Database Syst Rev. 2010;3:CD004064.
4. Ohtsu A, Shimada Y, Shirao K, Boku N, Hyodo I, Saito H, et al. Randomized phase III trial of fluorouracilalone versus fluorouracil plus cisplatin versus uracil and tegafur plus mitomycin in patients with unresectable, advanced gastric cancer: The Japan clinical oncology group study (JCOG9205). J Clin Oncol. 2003;21:54–9.
5. Kang YK, Kang WK, Shin DB, Chen J, Xiong J, Wang J, et al. Capecitabine/cisplatin versus 5-fluorouracil/cisplatin as first-line therapy in patients with advanced gastric cancer: a randomised phase III noninferiority trial. Ann Oncol. 2009;20(4):666–73.
6. Okines AFC, Norman AR, McCloud P, Kang YK, Cunningham D. Meta-analysis of the REAL-2 and ML17032 trials: evaluating capecitabine-based combination chemotherapy and infused 5-fluorouracil-based combination chemotherapy for the treatment of advanced oesophago-gastric cancer. Ann Oncol. 2009;20:1529–34.
7. Digklia A, Wagner AD. Advanced gastric cancer: current treatment landscape and future perspectives. World J Gastroenterol. 2016;22:2403–14.
8. Ajani JA, Rodriguez W, Bodoky G, Moiseyenko V, Lichinitser M, Gorbunova V, et al. Multicenter phase III comparison of cisplatin/S-1 with cisplatin/infusional fluorouracil in advanced gastric or gastroesophageal adenocarcinoma study: the FLAGS trial. J Clin Oncol. 2010;28:1547–53.
9. Al-Batran SE, Hartmann JT, Probst S, Schmalenberg H, Hollerbach S, Hofheinz R, et al. Phase III trial in metastatic gastroesophageal adenocarcinoma with fluorouracil, leucovorin plus either oxaliplatin or cisplatin: a study of the Arbeitsgemeinschaft Internistische Onkologie. J Clin Oncol. 2008;26:1435–42.
10. Dank M, Zaluski J, Barone C, Valvere V, Yalcin S, Peschel S, et al. Randomized phase III study comparing irinotecan combined with 5-fluorouracil and folinic acid to cisplatin combined with 5-fluorouracil in chemotherapy naive patients with advanced adenocarcinoma of the stomach or esophagogastric junction. Ann Oncol. 2008;19:1450–7.
11. Moehler M, Kanzler S, Geissler M, Raedle J, Ebert MP, Daum S, et al. A randomized multicenter phase II study comparing capecitabine with irinotecan or cisplatin in metastatic adenocarcinoma of the stomach or esophagogastric junction. Ann Oncol. 2010;21:71–7.
12. Wadhwa R, Song S, Lee JS, Yao Y, Wei Q, Ajani JA. Gastric cancer-molecular and clinical dimensions. Nat Rev Clin Oncol. 2013;10:643–55.
13. Genuino AJ, Chaikledkaew U, The DO, Reungwetwattana T, Thakkinstian A. Adjuvant trastuzumab regimen for HER2-positive early-stage breast cancer: a systematic review and meta-analysis. Expert Rev Clin Pharmacol. 2019;12:815–24.
14. Bang YJ, Van Custem E, Feyereislova A, Chung HC, Shen L, Sawaki A, et al. Trastuzumab in combination with chemotherapy versus chemotherapy alone for treatment of HER2-positive advanced gastric or gastro-oesophageal junction cancer (ToGA): a phase 3, open-label, randomised controlled trial. Lancet. 2010;376:687–97.
15. Satoh T, Bang YJ, Gotovkin EA, Hamamoto Y, Kang YK, Moiseyenko VM, et al. Quality of life in the trastuzumab for gastric cancer trial. Oncologist. 2014;19:712–9.
16. Kim C, Chon HJ, Kim JH, Jung MK, Nam CM, Kim HS, et al. Randomised phase II trial comparing four front-line doublets in Asian patients with metastatic gastric cancer. Eur J Cancer. 2019;112:20–8.
17. Van Cutsem E, Moiseyenko VM, Tjulandin S, Majlis A, Constenla M, Boni C, et al. Phase III study of docetaxel and cisplatin plus fluorouracil compared with cisplatin and fluorouracil as first-line therapy for advanced gastric cancer: a report of the V325 study group. J Clin Oncol. 2006;24:4991–7.

18. Sato Y, Sagawa T, Ohnuma H, Hirakawa M, Takahashi Y, Hamakuchi K, et al. A dose-escalation study of docetaxel, oxaliplatin, and S-1 (DOS) as a first-line therapy for patients with unresectable metastatic gastric cancer. Cancer Chemother Pharmacol. 2019;83:161–7.
19. Fuchs CS, Tomasek J, Yong CJ, Dumitru F, Passalacqua R, Goswami C, et al. Ramucirumab monotherapy for previously treated advanced gastric or gastro-oesophageal junction adenocarcinoma (REGARD): an international, randomised, multicentre, placebo-controlled, phase 3 trial. Lancet. 2014;383:31–9.
20. Wilke H, Muro K, Van Cutsem E, Oh SC, Bodoky G, Shimada Y, et al. Ramucirumab plus paclitaxel versus placebo plus paclitaxel in patients with previously treated advanced gastric or gastro-oesophageal junction adenocarcinoma (RAINBOW): a double-blind, randomised phase 3 trial. Lancet Oncol. 2014;15:1224–35.
21. Cunningham D, Allum WH, Stenning SP, Thompsom JN, De Velde C, Nicolson M, et al. Perioperative chemotherapy versus surgery alone for resectable gastroesophageal cancer. N Engl J Med. 2006;355:11–20.

Palliative Chemotherapy in Advanced or Metastatic Gastric Cancer. IX-2. Target Agents and Immunotherapy

Key Points

- Gastric cancer has recently been recognized as a very heterogeneous disease.
- The prognosis of advanced or metastatic advanced inoperable gastric cancer is unfavorable.
- Targeted therapy is currently being used as a standard treatment for advanced gastric cancer.
- Immune checkpoint inhibitors in first-line treatment for advanced and inoperable metastatic gastric cancer are promising.

Introduction

Globally, gastric cancer ranks sixth in incidence and second in cancer-related mortality [1]. It is a fatal malignant disease that accounts for two-thirds of all gastric cancer cases in East Asia, Eastern Europe, and South America. The rate of advanced gastric cancer is gradually decreasing, thanks to more frequent routine health checkups, but the prevalence of gastric cancer remains high with no significant change. For local gastric cancers without distant metastasis, treatment by endoscopic resection and surgery are the only approaches that can lead to a cure, if indicated. However, a large number of patients are still diagnosed with locally advanced gastric cancer or metastatic gastric cancer that cannot be surgically resected at the time of diagnosis, and chemotherapy is the primary standard treatment in these cases. In recent years, as the molecular genetic characteristics of gastric cancer have been revealed, targeted therapy and immunotherapy have been introduced into the treatment arena.

Targeted Agents

Recently, through various studies, molecular targets that are important for cancer cell survival and progression have been revealed, and relevant targeted therapeutics have been developed (Fig. 1). However, since these targeted therapies alone have limitations in the removal and inhibition of cancer cells, efforts are currently being made to overcome these limitations by combining them with chemotherapy. Although many studies have been conducted to date, it is still not clear whether the clinical effects of targeted therapies are significant, except for the findings from a few studies. The ToGA study was conducted in advanced or metastatic gastric cancer and esophageal-gastric junction cancer [2] and enrolled a total of 3807 patients. This was the first phase 3 clinical study to demonstrate the effectiveness of target treatment. Comparing capecitabine/cisplatin (XP) (or 5-fluorouracil/cisplatin (FP)) + trastuzumab therapy with XP (or FP) therapy in 548 patients with positive

Hee Seok Moon is the lead author of this chapter.

H. J. Chun et al., *Gastrointestinal Cancer*, https://doi.org/10.1007/978-981-99-0815-8_10

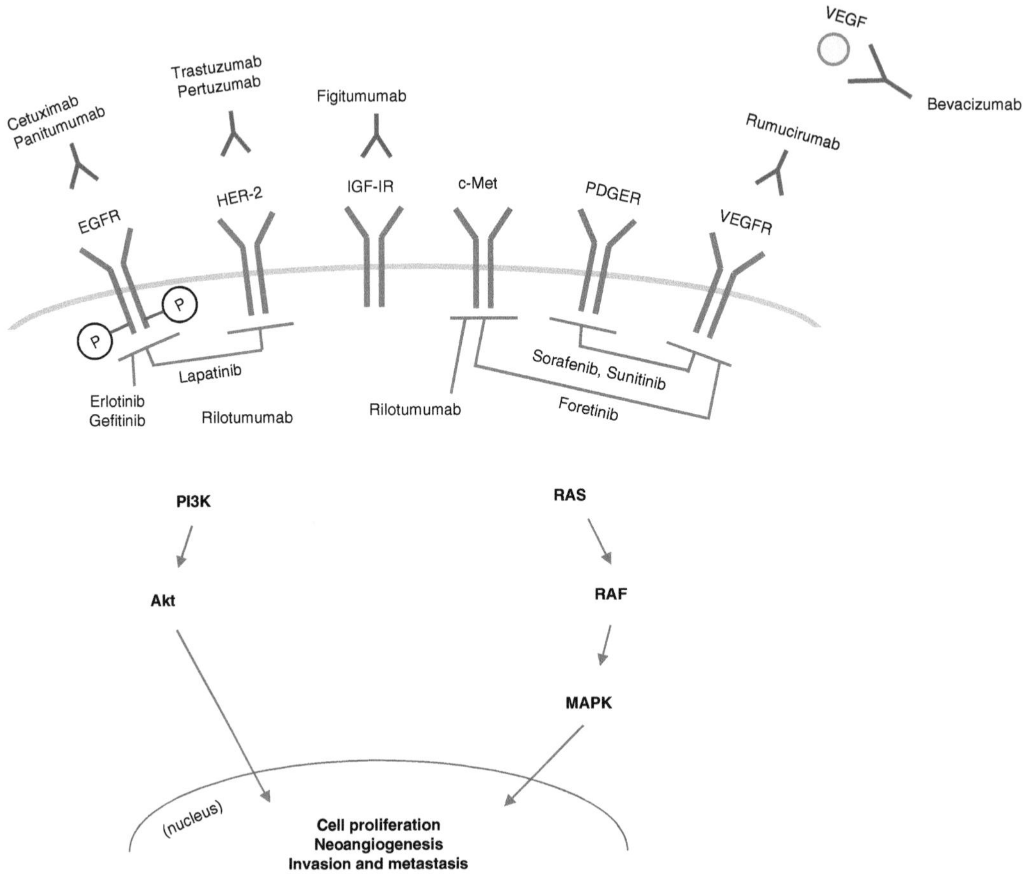

Fig. 1 Mechanism of molecular targeted therapy in gastric cancer

expression of Human epidermal factor receptor 2 (HER2) through immunohistochemistry (IHC) and FISH, the median overall survival (OS) was 13.8 months and 11.1 months (p = 0.0046), respectively, with median progression-free survival (PFS) of 6.7 months and 5.5 months (p = 0.0002), with tumor response rates of 47% and 35% (p = 0.0017), respectively. There was no increase in therapeutic toxicity. Based on the results of this study, combination therapy of chemotherapy based on fluoropyrimidine and platinum with trastuzumab was established as the first-line standard of care in patients with advanced or metastatic gastric cancer positive for HER2. Meanwhile, a study on advanced esophageal junction adenocarcinoma and gastric cancer using ramucirumab, a human IgG1 monoclonal antibody that inhibits Vascular endothelial growth factor receptor-2 (VEGFR-2), which is closely related to cancer cell proliferation and angiogenesis, has been reported. In the REGARD study, a multi-institutional Phase 3 clinical trial, the best conservative treatment and ramucirumab (8 mg/kg IV every 2 weeks) alone was compared and analyzed [3]. The ramucirumab group reported a statistically significant improvement in OS (5.2 vs 3.8 months, HR 0.78, 95% CI 0.60–0.998). In the RAINBOW study, 665 patients with metastatic gastric cancer and gastroesophageal junction cancer were compared with ramucirumab in combination with paclitaxel and placebo [4]. The mean OS rate was 9.6 vs 7.4 months (HR 0.807,

95% CI, 0.678–0.962), the combination treatment group receiving ramucirumab and paclitaxel reported a significant improvement. A phase 3 clinical study was completed in 273 gastric cancer patients using apatinib, another drug targeting VEGF-2, as third-line chemotherapy [5]. This study was conducted in a 2:1 randomization between apatinib and placebo. Apatinib was reported to be superior in terms of median OS: 6.5 versus 4.7 months (HR 0.71, 95% CI, 0.54–0.94; p = 0.0149). A new agent, trastuzumab deruxtecan, was introduced consisting of a conjugate of the HER2-directed antibody trastuzumab and a topoisomerase I inhibitor. Compared to existing trastuzumab, the drug-to-Ab ratio was 8 and it has shown excellent linker stability and bystander effects. In the DESTINY-Gastric 01 study, the survival rate and PFS were statistically higher than those of the control group. Thus, it has also been introduced as a treatment for gastric cancer [6].

Immune Checkpoint Inhibitors

Cancer cells are known to evade the immune response of the body by suppressing the function of tumor-specific T lymphocytes through changes in immune checkpoint function as an immune escape strategy. Immune checkpoint inhibitors (ICIs) function by using a monoclonal antibody targeting the cytotoxic T lymphocyte antigen (CTLA)-4, PD-1, or the PD-L1 ligand, which is the immune checkpoint at the final stage of the immune response, the stage of the activation of T cells. ICIs achieve an antitumor effect on cancer cells by enhancing suppressed tumor-specific T lymphocyte activation and inhibiting tumor growth (Fig. 2). Ipilimumab, a monoclonal antibody directed at CTLA-4, has demonstrated clinical efficacy in patients with advanced malignant melanoma, and was first approved as an ICI by the United States Food and Drug Administration (US FDA) in 2010 [7, 8]. Since then, another monoclonal antibody against CTLA-4, tremelimumab, has been developed. Pembrolizumab and nivolumab, which are fully humanized IgG4 PD-1 inhibitory monoclonal antibodies, and atezolizumab, durvalumab, and avelumab (a fully humanized anti-PD-L1 IgG1) targeting PD-L1, have been approved and are being used in clinical trials. In cohort 1 of the phase 2 study KEYNOTE-059, pembrolizumab was administered to 259 patients with gastric and gastroesophageal junction cancer as a third-line or subsequent treatment [9]. The response rate was 12% in all patients, 16% in patients positive for PD-L1, and 6% in patients negative for PD-L1. Based on this study, the US FDA approved pembrolizumab for patients with PD-L1-positive gastric cancer and gastroesophageal junction cancer. However, a phase III trial, comparing pembroli-

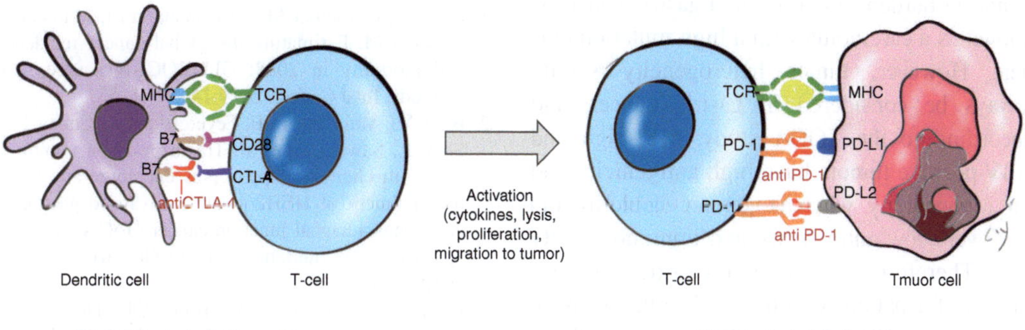

Fig. 2 Blocking CTLA-4 and PD-1. Abbreviations: *VEGFR* vascular endothelial growth factor receptor, *PDGFR* platelet-derived growth factor receptor, *IGF-1R* insulin-like growth factor 1 receptor, *FGFR* fibroblast growth factor receptor

zumab to paclitaxel as second-line treatment for advanced gastric cancer, has not met the primary endpoint to show the clinical efficacy of pembrolizumab monotherapy (OS: risk ratio = 0.82, 95% CI, 0.66–1.03; one-sided $p = 0.0421$) (PFS: risk ratio = 1.27, 95% CI, 1.03–1.57) [10]. A phase 3 clinical study on nivolumab was conducted for third-line and subsequent treatments in 493 patients with advanced gastric cancer. In this study, nivolumab and placebo were randomized 2:1 and the median survival rate was 5.3 months and 4.1 months, respectively (HR; 0.63%, 95% CI; 0.50–0.78, $p < 0.0001$) and the 1-year survival rates were reported to be 26.2% and 10.9%, respectively [11], leading to the establishment of standard options for a third-line treatment for advanced gastric cancer in the Japanese guideline. A recent meta-analysis of clinical trials with ICI (anti-PD1, anti-PD-L1, and anti-CTLA4) for advanced gastric cancer or esophago-gastric junction tumors in a total of 2003 patients from 9 clinical trials reported that the ORR of all ICI-treated patients, the anti-PD-1/PD-L1 subgroup, and the anti CTLA-4 subgroup were 9.9%, 12.0%, and 2.1%, respectively, and the disease control ratio was 33.3%, 34.7%, and 30.1%, respectively [12]. The median PFS of all ICI-treated patients, the anti-PD-1/PD-L1, and the anti-CTLA-4 subgroups were 1.6, 1.6, and 2.9 months, respectively. The median OS values of the three groups were 6.0, 5.4, and 7.7 months, respectively.

The effects of ICIs are correlated with the mutation burden of cancer, and gastric cancer is known as a carcinoma with a high mutation burden. However, tumor heterogeneity should always be considered in gastric cancer, and according to the TGCA study, MSI-high and EBV-positive tumors have high antigenicity and immunogenicity, whereas genome-stable tumors have very low antigenicity and immunogenicity [13]. Therefore, it is necessary to develop biomarkers for patient selection before the decision to recommend ICI therapy. Conversely, methods that increase the effects of immune modulation are being sought through the co-administration of existing cytotoxic anticancer drugs, targeted therapeutics, and immunotherapeutic agents with different mechanisms. Clinical research is being conducted, focusing on conservative and postoperative adjuvant treatment using ICIs, so it can be expected that the application of immunotherapy for gastric cancer will expand in the future.

Conclusion

Gastric cancer has recently been recognized as a very heterogeneous disease instead of disease of uniform nature. In the case of advanced or metastatic inoperable gastric cancer, the prognosis is unfavorable and the median survival period is known to be very poor, approximately 3–6 months without chemotherapy. Therefore, the superiority of chemotherapy compared to the best supportive treatment in terms of quality of life and life extension has already been confirmed through several studies. Recently, chemotherapy has been applied to the treatment of advanced gastric cancer and several targeted therapies and immunotherapy have recently also been introduced. However, the remarkable life extension achieved in advanced gastric cancer patients compared to other carcinomas is still low and is at a standstill. It is expected that these difficulties will be overcome as the molecular biological characteristics of gastric cancer become known in detail in the future.

References

1. Ferlay J, Colombet M, Soerjomataram I, Mathers C, Parkin DM. Estimating the global cancer incidence and mortality in 2018: GLOBOCAN sources and methods. Int J Cancer. 2019;144:1941–53.
2. Bang YJ, Van Cutsem E, Feyereislova A, Chung HC, Shen L, Sawaki A, et al. Trastuzumab in combination with chemotherapy versus chemotherapy alone for treatment of HER2-positive advanced gastric or gastro-oesophageal junction cancer (ToGA): a phase 3, open-label, randomised controlled trial. Lancet. 2010;376:687–97.
3. Fuchs CS, Tomasek J, Yong CJ, Dumitru F, Passalacqua R, Goswami C, et al. Ramucirumab monotherapy for previously treated advanced gastric or gastro-oesophageal junction adenocarcinoma (REGARD): an international, randomised, multicentre, placebo-controlled, phase 3 trial. Lancet. 2014;383:31–9.

4. Wilke H, Muro K, Van Cutsem E, Oh SC, Bodoky G, Shimada Y, et al. Ramucirumab plus paclitaxel versus placebo plus paclitaxel in patients with previously treated advanced gastric or gastro-oesophageal junction adenocarcinoma (RAINBOW): a double-blind, randomised phase 3 trial. Lancet Oncol. 2014;15:1224–35.
5. Li J, Qin S, Xu J, Xiong J, Wu C, Bai Y, et al. Randomized, double-blind, placebo-controlled phase III study of apatinib in patients with chemotherapy-refractory advanced gastric cancer or metastatic adenocarcinoma of the stomach or gastroesophageal junction. J Clin Oncol. 2016;34(13):1448–54.
6. Shitara K, Bang YJ, Iwasa S, Sugimoto N, Ryu MH, Sakai D, et al. Trastuzumab deruxtecan in previously treated HER2-positive gastric cancer. N Engl J Med. 2020;382:2419–30.
7. Robert C, Thomas L, Bondarenko I, O'Day S, Weber J, Garbe C, et al. Ipilimumab plus dacarbazine for previously untreated metastatic melanoma. N Engl J Med. 2011;364:2517–26.
8. Hodi FS, O'Day SJ, McDermott DF, Weber RW, Sosman JA, Haanen JB, et al. Improved survival with ipilimumab in patients with metastatic melanoma. N Engl J Med. 2010;363:711–23.
9. Fashoyin-Aje L, Donoghue M, Chen H, He K, Veeraraghavan J, Goldberg KB, et al. FDA approval summary: pembrolizumab for recurrent locally advanced or metastatic gastric or gastroesophageal junction adenocarcinoma expressing PD-L1. Oncologist. 2019;24:103–9.
10. Shitara K, Özgüroğlu M, Bang YJ, Di Bartolomeo M, Mandalà M, Ryu MH, et al. Pembrolizumab versus paclitaxel for previously treated, advanced gastric or gastro-oesophageal junction cancer (KEYNOTE-061): a randomised, open-label, controlled, phase 3 trial. Lancet. 2018;392:123–33.
11. Kang YK, Boku N, Satoh T, Ryu MH, Chao Y, Kato K, et al. Nivolumab in patients with advanced gastric or gastro-oesophageal junction cancer refractory to, or intolerant of, at least two previous chemotherapy regimens (ONO-4538-12, ATTRACTION-2): a randomised, double-blind, placebo-controlled, phase 3 trial. Lancet. 2017;390:2461–71.
12. Chen C, Zhang F. Efficacy and safety of immune checkpoint inhibitors in advanced gastric or gastroesophageal junction cancer: a systematic review and meta-analysis. Oncoimmunology. 2019;8:e1581547.
13. Bass AJ, Thorsson V, Shmulevich I, Reynolds SM, Miller M, Bernard B, et al. Comprehensive molecular characterization of gastric adenocarcinoma. Nature. 2014;513:202.

Primary Gastric Lymphoma: Extranodal Marginal B-Cell Lymphoma of Mucosa-Associated Lymphoid Tissue (MALT) Type

Key Points

- Gastric mucosa-associated lymphoid tissue (MALT) lymphomas are strongly associated with *Helicobacter pylori* (*H. pylori*) infection.
- Gastric MALT lymphoma involves genetic aberrations in the nuclear factor κB (NFκB) pathway, and 5 recurrent cytogenetic alterations have been described that converge on NFκB pathways.
- Eradication of *H. pylori* should be performed in all patients with gastric MALT lymphoma, regardless of stage.
- Eradication of *H. pylori* can induce complete regression in 75%–80% of patients.
- After eradication of *H. pylori,* serial endoscopies with multiple biopsies should be performed every 3 months, subsequently (every 6 months for 2 years), and long-term endoscopic and systemic follow-up is recommended.
- In the cases of persistent but stable residual disease or only histological relapse without distant dissemination and/or gross tumor, a watch-and-wait policy is recommended.
- Radiotherapy, chemotherapy, and anti-CD20 target therapy (rituximab) can be applied for *H. pylori* eradication-refractory gastric MALT lymphomas.
- Gastric MALT lymphoma can undergo aggressive diffuse large B-cell lymphoma and the risk of gastric adenocarcinoma increases.
- After complete remission, relapse mostly occurs within 5 years.

Introduction

Primary gastric lymphoma is the most common extranodal site of non-Hodgkin lymphoma [1] and represents 3–5% of gastric neoplastic lesions [2]. The most frequent histologic subtypes are extranodal marginal B-cell lymphoma of mucosa-associated lymphoid tissue (MALT) type and diffuse large B-cell lymphoma (DLBCL) [3]. The incidence of developing primary gastric lymphoma is 2–3 times higher in men than in women [4]. The incidence of MALT lymphoma increased significantly in patients over 40 years of age in a retrospective study [5]. Even if gastric MALT lymphomas are low-grade lesions and localized [6], they can rarely be transformed into high-

Su Youn Nam is the lead author of this chapter.

H. J. Chun et al., *Gastrointestinal Cancer*, https://doi.org/10.1007/978-981-99-0815-8_11

grade diffuse large B-cell lymphomas [7, 8]. Herein, the etiology, risk factors, diagnosis, treatment, and prognosis of gastric MALT lymphomas are summarized.

Etiology and Risk Factors

Gastric MALT lymphomas are strongly associated with *Helicobacter pylori* (*H. pylori*) infection [9]. Chronic *H. pylori* infection induces T-cell activation, B-cell proliferation, and migration of neutrophils to the gastric mucosa. Further proliferation of B cells is driven by the interaction of the CD40-CD40 ligand with reactive T cells and evolves into a monoclonal lymphoma [10–12]. Chronic proliferation of B cells and neutrophil-mediated release of reactive oxygen species induce additional oncogenic events that eventually make lymphoproliferation independent of antigenic stimulation.

Gastric MALT lymphoma involves genetic aberrations in the nuclear factor κB (NFκB) pathway [10] and 5 recurrent cytogenetic alterations have been identified, convergent on the NFκB pathway [13]. Recurrent translocations induce rearrangements of the genes encoding their encoded proteins: Mucosa-associated lymphoid tissue translocation protein 1 (*MALT1*), B-cell chronic lymphocytic leukemia/lymphoma protein 10 (*BCL10*), Immunoglobulin heavy chain (*IGH*), Immunoglobulin kappa light chain (*IGK*), Apoptosis inhibitor (*API2*), and Forkhead box P1 gene (*FOXP1*) (Table 1). The three most common translocations—t(11;18) (q21;q21), t(1;14) (p22;q32) and t(14;18) (q32;q21)—generate oncogenic fusion proteins that activate the NF-κB pathway [13]. The t(11;18) (q21;q21) produces the fusion of *API2* and *MALT1*. MALT1 activates NF-κB and is controlled by the *API2* promoter, which is itself stimulated by NF-κB [14, 15]. This fusion gene forms a positive feedback cycle that leads to the constitutive activation of NF-κB. The API2-MALT1 fusion protein induces constitutive activation of NF-κB through an alternative non-canonical pathway [16]. The presence of t(11;18) correlates with non-responsiveness to the eradication of *H. pylori* [14, 17]. The t(14;18) (q32;q21) produces the fusion of *IGH* with *MALT1* and induces the overexpression of *MALT1*, which activates NF-κB [14]. The t(1;14) (p22;q32) translocation results in the fusion of *BCL10* with the *IGH* gene enhancer region and produces juxtaposition of *BCL10* to *IGK*, which results in the overexpression of BCL10 [15]. The t(3;14) (p14;q32) fusion gene product includes *FOXP1* with the *IGH* enhancer, resulting in the overexpression of *FOXP1* [18]. *FOXP1* overexpression is an adverse prognostic factor [18, 19].

Table 1 Chromosomal translocations in MALT lymphomas

Translocation	Fusion protein	Role of fusion protein
t(11;18) (q21;q21)	API2-MALT1	Positive feedback cycle that leads to the constitutive activation of NF-κB Constitutive activation of NF-κB through an alternative non-canonical pathway No regression of lymphoma following *H. pylori* eradication
t(14;18) (q32;q21)	IGH-MALT1	Activates NF-κB Common in hepatic tumor
t(1;14) (p22;q32)	BCL10-IGH	Induces overexpression of BCL10 and activation of NF-κB
t(1;2) (p22;p12)	BCL10-IGK	Overexpression of BCL10
t(3;14) (p14;q32)	FOXP1-IGH	Overexpression of *FOXP1* Commonly found in thyroid tissue

API2 apoptosis inhibitor 2, *MALT1* mucosa-associated lymphoid tissue translocation protein 1, *BCL10* B-cell chronic lymphocytic leukemia/lymphoma protein 10, *IGH* immunoglobulin heavy chain, *IGK* immunoglobulin kappa light chain, *FOXP1* Forkhead box protein P1

Diagnosis

Patients with gastric MALT lymphoma present with the absence of symptoms or nonspecific symptoms. The diagnosis of gastric lymphoma is suggested by endoscopic findings and confirmed by histopathological examination; immunohistochemistry, flow cytometry, cytogenetics, and molecular biology [20].

Endoscopic Biopsy

Endoscopy with multiple biopsies is the gold standard for the diagnosis of gastric MALT lymphoma. Endoscopic findings of gastric MALT lymphoma present various features, usually multiple lesions including superficial erythema or erosion, multifocal atrophic gastritis-like lesion, nodular lesions, polypoid lesion, gastric ulcer, early gastric cancer-like lesion, or thickened gastric folds [21]. Endoscopic ultrasound (EUS) helps to determine the depth of invasion and perigastric nodes [14, 22, 23]. Superficial or diffuse EUS infiltrating lesions are observed in MALT lymphoma while mass-forming lesions are observed in DLBCL [24]. Endoscopists should obtain a large biopsy specimen as soon as possible for diagnostic evaluation. Magnified endoscopy for the evaluation of the distribution of abnormal vessels and microstructural pattern could be useful for both diagnosis and follow-up [25]. Compared to histopathology, the presence of abnormal vessels has both a sensitivity and a specificity of 86% while non-structural areas have a sensitivity of 77% and a specificity of 87% [25]. When EUS findings are characteristic, excisional biopsy can be replaced by ultrasound-guided core-needle biopsy [26]. When repeated biopsies show negative pathology in a suspicious lesion, endoscopic submucosal resection may provide even greater diagnostic capability.

Medical Imaging

Imaging studies are fundamental for the diagnosis and appropriate staging of lymphoma at presentation. A contrast-enhanced computed tomography (CT) scan of the abdomen, pelvis, and chest should be performed to evaluate distant disease [27]. For some patients, a neck CT may be required. Abdominal CT can detect locally advanced gastric MALT lymphoma, lymphadenopathy, local complications, and hepatosplenomegaly [27]. Abdominal CT scanning is less useful for the follow-up of localized gastric MALT lymphoma [28]. In patients with early-stage gastric MALT lymphoma in complete remission, recurrence may occur in 5.7% and is restricted to the mucosa, and thus undetectable on CT [28]. Therefore, serial endoscopy with multiple biopsies is mandatory for the follow-up of gastric MALT lymphoma. Positron emission tomography has limited diagnostic accuracy in the early stage of the disease [29].

Histopathology

Histopathological and immunohistochemical evaluations are fundamental for the diagnosis of MALT lymphoma. The diagnostic criterion for gastric MALT lymphoma is the presence of a variable number of lymphoepithelial lesions defined by invasion and destruction of the adjacent epithelium, as described by Wotherspoon (Table 2) [12, 30]. Immunohistochemistry is valuable in the differentiation between MALT lymphomas and other small-cell lymphomas, including follicular lymphoma, chronic lymphocytic leukemia/small lymphocytic lymphoma (CLL/SLL), and mantle-cell lymphoma (MCL) [31]. MALT lymphoma B-cells show positivity for the B-cell surface markers CD19, CD20, and CD22, and negativity for CD5 (unlike CLL/SLL), cyclin D1 (unlike MCL), and CD10 [31]. Polymerase chain reaction (PCR)-based analysis of IgH gene rearrangements is also helpful to distinguish MALT lymphoma from reactive proliferations.

MALT lymphoma can be divided into *H. pylori*-positive or *H. pylori*-negative. Most gastric MALT lymphoma are positive for *H. pylori* (>90%). *H. pylori*-negative MALT lymphoma has a higher frequency for t(11;18) (q21;q21) translocation compared to *H. pylori*-positive MALT lymphoma [32, 33]. The most common translocations are t(11;18) (q21;q21), t(14;18) (q32;q21), t(1;14)(p22;q32), and t(3;14) (p13;q32) (Table 1). Patients should be tested for *H. pylori*, detected by histological examination,

Table 2 Wotherspoon scoring system for Gastric MALT Lymphoma

Score	Diagnosis	Histological features
0	Normal	Scattered plasma cells in lamina propria. No lymphoid follicles
1	Chronic active gastritis	Small clusters of lymphocytes in lamina propria. No lymphoid follicle. No lymphoepithelial lesions
2	Chronic active gastritis with florid lymphoid follicle formation	Prominent lymphoid follicles with surrounding mantle zone and plasma cells. No lymphoepithelial lesions
3	Suspicious lymphoid infiltrate, probably reactive	Lymphoid follicles surrounded by small lymphocytes that infiltrate diffusely in lamina propria and occasionally into epithelium
4	Suspicious lymphoid infiltrate, probably lymphoma	Lymphoid follicles surrounded by marginal zone cells that infiltrate diffusely in lamina propria and into epithelium in small groups
5	MALT lymphoma	Presence of dense infiltrate of marginal zone cells in lamina propria with prominent lymphoepithelial lesions

rapid urease test, urea breath test, stool antigen test, or serology. Furthermore, fluorescence in situ hybridization (FISH) or PCR testing for t(11;18) should be performed. Bone marrow involvement is rarely reported in superficial gastric MALT lymphoma [34]. A recent study showed that bone marrow involvement was found in 4.3% of gastric MALT lymphomas [35]. But bone marrow involvement does not change treatment options or outcome in gastric MALT lymphoma confined to the stomach wall. Therefore, bone marrow biopsy and aspiration are not mandatory in superficial MALT lymphoma confined to the gastric wall.

Table 3 Work up for gastric MALT lymphoma

Exam	Note
EGD	Mandatory
EUS	Optional, to evaluate the regional lymph nodes and gastric wall infiltration
IHC	Mandatory, to evaluate helicobacter pylori status. Fecal antigen or breath test and serology studies are recommended when the results of histology are negative
FISH or PCR	Optional, to detect t(11;18) translocation
CT	Mandatory
Bone marrow biopsy	Optional
PET	Optional, limited value

Modified from Zucca et al. [36]

CT computed tomography, *EGD* esophagogastroduodenoscopy, *EUS* endoscopic ultrasound, *FISH* fluorescent in situ hybridization, *IHC* immunohistochemistry, *PCR* polymerase chain reaction, *PET* positron emission tomography

Staging

A staging for gastric MALT lymphoma includes 1) physical examination, 2) EUS is optional, 3) CT of the neck, chest, and abdomen to detect involvement of nodes above and below the diaphragm and other extranodal involvement not pertaining to the GI tract, 4) Positron emission tomography is not generally indicated as a staging procedure, especially in MALT lymphomas. 5) Bone marrow biopsy is not mandatory in gastric MALT lymphoma confined to the superficial gastric wall, but it should be performed according to stage and pathology [36] (Table 3).

The classic staging system of lymphoma is the Ann Arbor system. This system has intrinsic limitations in primary extranodal lymphomas of the gastrointestinal tract. The most popular staging system for primary gastrointestinal lymphomas is the Lugano staging system, a modification of the Ann Arbor staging system. It was developed to incorporate measures of depth of invasion and distant nodal involvement (Table 4) [37]. In stage I disease, the tumor is confined to the gastrointestinal tract. In stage II, the tumor extends into the abdomen and has nodal involvement. There is no stage III in the Lugano system. In stage IV, there is disseminated extranodal involvement or concomitant supradiaphragmatic nodal involvement. To overcome the shortcomings of various adaptations of the lymphoma staging system, the Paris staging System was proposed [38] (Table 4). The

Table 4 Lugano and Paris system for staging of gastrointestinal lymphomas

	Lugano staging system	Paris staging system	Tumor extension
Stage	Extent of disease		
Stage I	Confined to the gastrointestinal tract(single primary or multiple, non-contiguous)		
Stage I1	Tumor not exceeding the mucosa and submucosa	T1m N0 M0 T1sm N0 M0	Mucosa Submucosa
Stage I2	Tumor infiltrates into muscularis propria and/or subserosa and/or serosa	T2 N0 M0 T3 N0 M0	Muscularis propria Serosa
Stage II	Extending into abdomen		
• Stage II1	Local nodal involvement (paragastric nodes for gastric lymphoma or Para-intestinal nodes for intestinal lymphoma)	T1–3 N1 M0	Perigastric lymph nodes More distant regional nodes
• Stage II2	Distant nodal involvement (Para-aortic, Para-caval, pelvic, or inguinal nodes for most tumors; mesenteric nodes in the case of intestinal lymphoma)	T1–3 N2 M0	Invasion of adjacent structures with or without abdominal lymph nodes
• Stage IIE	Penetration of serosa to involve adjacent organs or tissues	T4 N0–2 M0	Invasion of adjacent structures with or without abdominal lymph nodes
Stage IV	Disseminated extranodal involvement or concomitant supra-diaphragmatic nodal involvement	T1–4 N3 M0 T1–4 N0–3 M1 T1–4 N0–3 M2	Extra-abdominal lymph nodes Distant (non-contiguous) GI sites involvement Non-GI sites involvement

Adapted from Rohatiner et al. [37] and Ruskoné-Fourmestraux et al. [38]

Paris staging system describes the depth of gastric wall involvement more accurately, a parameter that may predict the response to *H. pylori* eradication.

Treatment and Prognostic Factors

Initial Antibiotic Therapy in Gastric MALT Lymphoma

H. pylori eradication should be attempted in all patients with gastric marginal zone lymphomas (MZL), regardless of stage [36]. The anti-*H. pylori* regimen should be chosen based on the regional sensitivity of the microbes to antibiotics. The outcome of eradication therapy should be investigated by a urea breath test at least 4 weeks after the last administration of eradication therapy and at least 2 weeks after the withdrawal of the proton-pump inhibitor. When *H. pylori* eradication is not successful, second-line treatment should be attempted.

For early-stage gastric MALT lymphoma (I/II) with *H. pylori* infection, *H. pylori* eradication can induce complete regression in 75% of patients. For stage I disease, the cure rate is approximately 80% (most patients in stage IE1 and a smaller proportion of patients in stage IE2), while lymphomas in stage IIE and above are generally less responsive [14]. The length of time to obtain a remission varies from a few weeks to more than a year. In patients who acquire clinical and endoscopic remission after eradication of *H. pylori* but still have persistent microscopic lymphoma on histology, a watch-and-wait strategy is recommended for at least 12 months before starting another treatment [39]. Several studies have shown the frequent persistence of monoclonal B cells after histological regression [39, 40].

There are no clear predictive factors for the response to *H. pylori* eradication, and primary refractoriness is reported in 10–20% of low-grade gastric MALT lymphomas [41, 42]. There are 7% of non-responders among stage IE1 patients. Complete remissions are achieved in more than 98% of distal tumors, but only in 70% of proximal tumors [43]. Testing for resistance-associated genetic alterations such as t(11;18) could provide a helpful predictor of response to *H. pylori* eradication therapy [30, 44]. The presence of the t(11;18) translocation is a criterion for alternative therapies [45]. Approximately 20%–30% of patients do not respond to *H. pylori* eradication therapy or demonstrate relapse during follow-up. These patients should be reviewed to confirm MALT lymphoma and exclude more aggressive lymphomas [46].

The optimal treatment of *H. pylori*-negative and eradication-resistant *H. pylori*-positive gastric lymphomas has not been convincingly defined [39]. Even if regression of lymphoma after antibiotic treatment in *H. pylori*-negative gastric MZL is less likely, anti-Helicobacter therapy is still worthwhile because lymphoma occasionally responds to antibiotic therapy due to a false-negative test or infection by other Helicobacter species [39, 47]. In *H. pylori negative* cases, radiotherapy should be considered if no signs of lymphoma regression are observed at follow-up endoscopy 3 to 6 months after antibiotic therapy (Fig. 1). For advanced disease (stage IV), anti-*H. pylori* treatment is still effective as the first-line therapy and a watch-and-wait management is recommended if the lymphoma is asymptomatic. Chemotherapy can be considered in symptomatic lymphoma or patients with other treatment indications (Fig. 2).

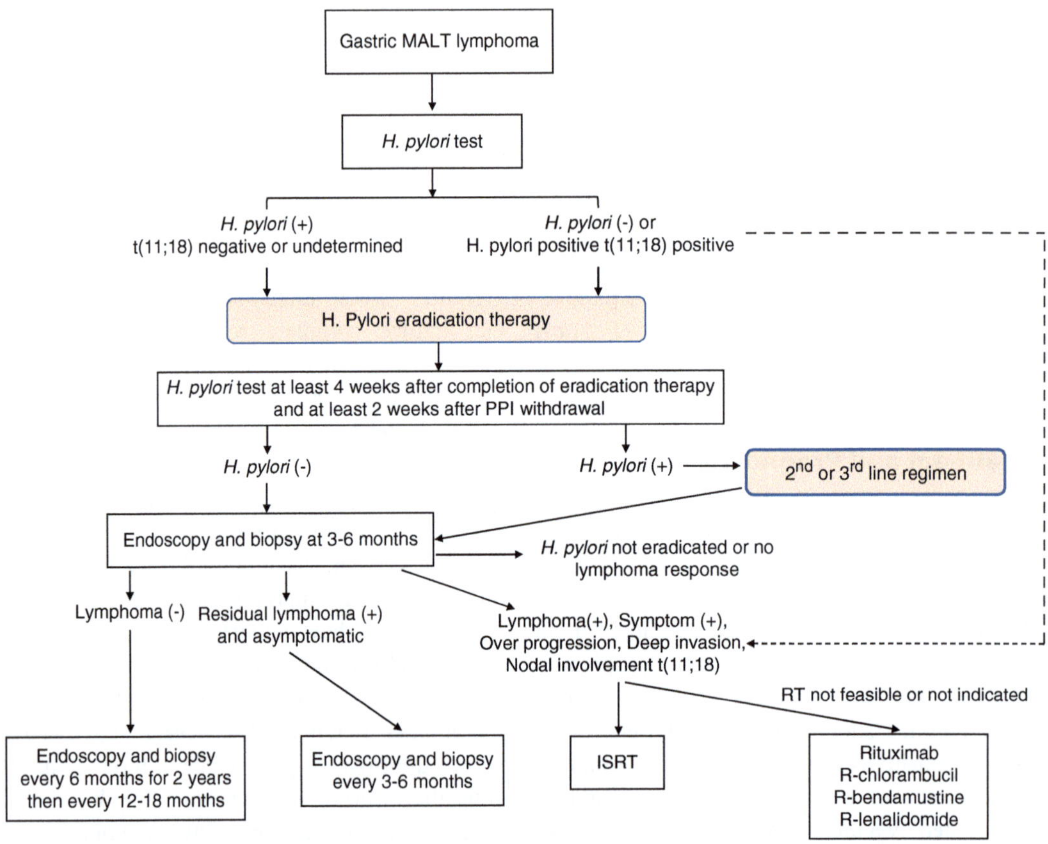

Fig. 1 Treatment algorithm for localized gastric MZL. (Modified from Zucca et al. [36]). *EGD* esophagogastroduodenoscopy, *ISRT* involved-site radiotherapy, *PPI* proton-pump inhibitor, *R* rituximab, *RT* radiotherapy

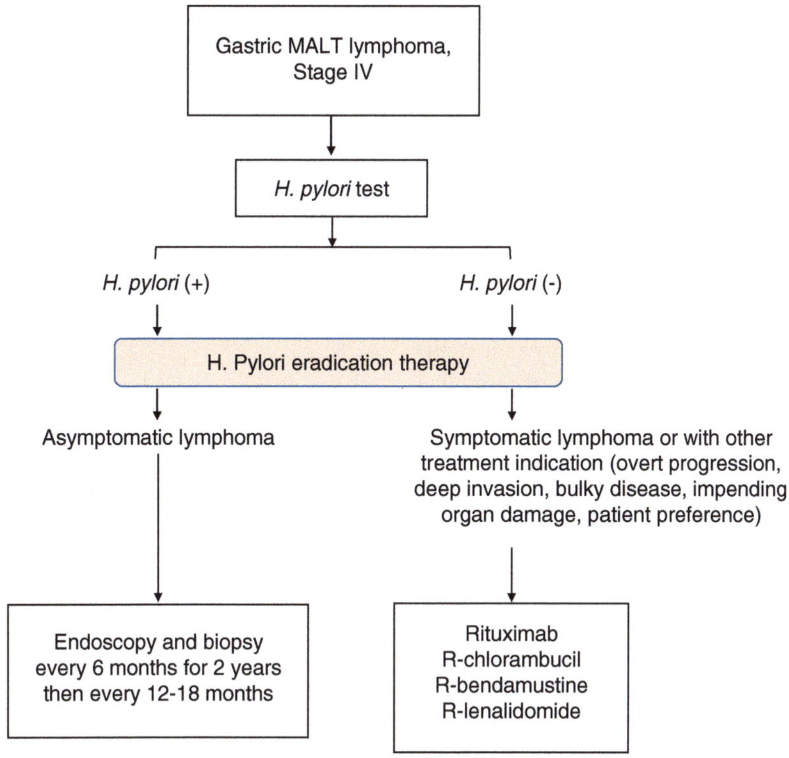

Fig. 2 Treatment algorithms for advanced gastric MZL. (Modified from Zucca et al. [36]). *EGD* esophagogastroduodenoscopy, *PPI* proton-pump inhibitor, *R* rituximab

Surgical Treatment

In gastric MALT lymphoma, surgical resection is not first-line therapy. A surgical resection can be curative in MALT lymphomas when the lymphoma coexists with a more aggressive carcinoma that is completely resected.

Radiotherapy

Radiotherapy has a high curative potential in *H. pylori*-negative patients or patients with non-response to eradication in *H. pylori*-positive patients. Approximately 80% of patients with eradication-refractory disease achieve complete remission with radiotherapy; a dose of 30–40 Gy in 15–20 fractions [48, 49].

Chemotherapy

H. pylori eradication-refractory gastric MALT lymphomas have high response rates to chemotherapy. Single drugs such as chlorambucil or cyclophosphamide may be used. Sometimes, a combination of chemotherapy drugs (cyclophosphamide, doxorubicin, vincristine, and prednisone) is used. Thalidomide is an immunomodulatory drug with anti-NF-κB activity, which has potential utility in MALT lymphomas [50]. Thalidomide salvage therapy in *H. pylori* eradication-refractory chemoresistant gastric MALT lymphomas shows an overall response rate (ORR) of 0% in patients with the API2-MALT1 transcript and 86% in patients without the transcript [50].

Target therapy with an anti-CD20 monoclonal antibody (rituximab) can induce complete remissions of MALT lymphoma [51, 52]. Rituximab has also been used in combination with immunochemotherapy and radiotherapy, with good results and tolerable side effects in MALT lymphoma [53, 54]. Radioimmunotherapy with 90Y-ibritumomab tiuxetan (an anti-CD20 monoclonal antibody containing a radioactive isotope) has been shown to induce high rates of complete remissions of up to 24 months in highly treated resistant patients, and furthermore, a tenfold reduction in the dose of radiotherapy potentially overcomes the local complications of radiotherapy [55, 56].

Response Evaluation and Follow-Up

Asymptomatic patients with disseminated gastric MZL are treated expectantly (watch-and-wait) with monitoring by physical examination, imaging, blood counts, and biochemistry every 3–6 months [36]. Periodic endoscopic biopsies are essential for gastric MZL to exclude either persistent disease or the appearance of gastric carcinoma, particularly in patients with persistent *H. pylori* infection. The interpretation of lymphoid infiltrates in post-treatment biopsies is difficult and there is no definition of histological remission. The Groupe d' Etude des Lymphomes de l' Adulte (GELA) scoring system is commonly used (Table 5) [57].

Following the eradication of *H. pylori*, serial endoscopies with multiple biopsies should be performed every 3 months to assess the disease response and recurrence, and subsequently (every 6 months for 2 years) to monitor lymphoma histological regression. Long-term endoscopic and systemic follow-up (clinical examination, blood counts every 12 months) is recommended.

Gastric MALT lymphoma has a limited tendency to distant spread and histological transformation. Transient histological relapses are occasionally observed in endoscopic follow-up biopsies, but they are usually self-limited, especially in the absence of *H. pylori* reinfection. They are considered relapse only if they are sustained and progressive. Therefore, in cases of persistent but stable residual disease or histological relapse alone (without distant dissemination and/or gross endoscopic tumor), a watch-and-wait policy is recommended [58, 59].

Table 5 GELA grading system proposed to define the histological response of gastric MZL after *Helicobacter pylori* eradication

Score	Histological characteristics
Complete histological remission (CR)	Normal or empty LP and/or fibrosis with absent or scattered plasma cells and small lymphoid cells in the LP, no LEL
Probable minimal residual disease (pMRD)	Empty LP and/or fibrosis with aggregates of lymphoid cells or lymphoid nodules in the LP/MM and/or SM, no LEL
Responding residual disease (rRD)	Focal empty LP and/or fibrosis with dense, diffuse, or nodular lymphoid infiltrate, extending around glands in the LP, focal LEL or absent
No change (NC)	Dense, diffuse, or nodular lymphoid infiltrate, LEL usually present

GELA Groupe d'Etude des Lymphomes de l'Adulte, *LEL* lymphoepithelial lesion, *LP* lamina propria, *MM* muscularis mucosa, *MZL* marginal zone B-cell lymphoma, *SM* submucosa
Adapted from Copie-Bergman et al. [57]

Although MALT lymphoma is a low-grade disease, transformation to large B cells rarely occurs and may undergo aggressive diffuse large B-cell lymphoma [60, 61]. Transformed MALT/DLBCL has a prognosis similar to de novo DLBCL [62]. The risk of gastric adenocarcinoma among patients with gastric MZLs is sixfold higher than in the general population [42, 63, 64], thus, long-term endoscopic follow-up is recommended. In addition, the risk of other non-Hodgkin lymphomas may also increase [64].

Gastric MALT lymphomas follow an indolent clinical course with prolonged OS (80% at 5 years) and disease-free survival; however, they showed a high recurrence rate, with most relapses within 5 years [58]. Second remissions can be achieved with retreatment, but the disease-free interval tends to decrease after subsequent remission [65]. Survival is inversely correlated with the stage at diagnosis; 5-year survival is 90%–95% for stage I, 75% for stage II, and 30% for stage IV [66].

Conclusion

Gastric MALT lymphomas are strongly associated with *H. pylori* infection and involve genetic aberrations in the NFκB pathway, and 5 recurrent cytogenetic alterations, converging on the NFB pathways, have been described. Eradication *of H. pylori* should be performed in all patients with gastric MALT lymphoma, regardless of stage, and it can induce complete regression in 75%–80% of patients. Following *H. pylori* eradication, serial endoscopies with multiple biopsies should be performed. In cases of persistent but stable residual disease or only histological relapse without distant dissemination and/or gross tumor, a watch-and-wait policy is recommended. Radiotherapy, chemotherapy, and anti-CD20 target therapy can be applied to *H. pylori* eradication-refractory gastric MALT lymphomas.

References

1. Ghimire P, Wu GY, Zhu L. Primary gastrointestinal lymphoma. World J Gastroenterol. 2011;17(6):697–707.
2. Gurney KA, Cartwright RA. Increasing incidence and descriptive epidemiology of extranodal non-Hodgkin lymphoma in parts of England and Wales. Hematol J. 2002;3(2):95–104.
3. Wang YG, Zhao LY, Liu CQ, Pan SC, Chen XL, Liu K, et al. Clinical characteristics and prognostic factors of primary gastric lymphoma. Medicine (Baltimore). 2016;95(31):e4250.
4. Juárez-Salcedo LM, Sokol L, Chavez JC, Dalia S. Primary gastric lymphoma, epidemiology, clinical diagnosis, and treatment. Cancer Control. 2018;25(1):107327481877825.
5. Ge Z, Liu Z, Hu X. Anatomic distribution, clinical features, and survival data of 87 cases primary gastrointestinal lymphoma. World J Surg Oncol. 2016;14(1):1–7.
6. Wang YG, Zhao LY, Liu CQ, Pan SC, Chen XL, Liu K, et al. Clinical characteristics and prognostic factors of primary gastric lymphoma: a retrospective study with 165 cases. Med (Baltimore). 2016;95:e4250.
7. Stathis A, Chini C, Bertoni F, Proserpio I, Capella C, Mazzucchelli L, et al. Long-term outcome following helicobacter pylori eradication in a retrospective study of 105 patients with localized gastric marginal zone B-cell lymphoma of MALT type. Ann Oncol. 2009;20:1086–93.
8. Fischbach W, Goebeler ME, Ruskone-Fourmestraux A, Wündisch T, Neubauer A, Raderer M, et al. Most patients with minimal histological residuals of gastric MALT lymphoma after successful eradication of helicobacter pylori can be managed safely by a watch and wait strategy: experience from a large international series. Gut. 2007;56:1685–7.
9. Hussell T, Isaacson PG, Crabtree JE, Spencer J. The response of cells from low-grade B-cell gastric lymphomas of mucosa-associated lymphoid tissue to helicobacter pylori. Lancet. 1993;342:571–4.
10. Sagaert X, Van Cutsem E, De Hertogh G, Geboes K, Tousseyn T. Gastric MALT lymphoma: a model of chronic inflammation-induced tumor development. Nat Rev. Gastroenterol Hepatol. 2010;7:336–46.
11. Zucca E, Bertoni F, Roggero E, Bosshard G, Cazzaniga G, Pedrinis E, et al. Molecular analysis of the progression from helicobacter pylori-associated chronic gastritis to mucosa-associated lymphoid-tissue lymphoma of the stomach. N Engl J Med. 1998;338:804–10.
12. Wotherspoon AC, Ortiz-Hidalgo C, Falzon MR, Isaacson PG. Helicobacter pylori-associated gastritis and primary B-cell gastric lymphoma. Lancet. 1991;338:1175.
13. Du MQ. MALT lymphoma: many roads lead to nuclear factor-κb activation. Histopathology. 2011;58:26–38.
14. Isaacson PG. Update on MALT lymphomas. Best Pract Res Clin Haematol. 2005;18:57–68.
15. Nakagawa M, Hosokawa Y, Yonezumi M, Izumiyama K, Suzuki R, Tsuzuki S, et al. MALT1 contains nuclear export signals and regulates cytoplasmic localization of BCL10. Blood. 2005;106:4210–6.
16. Rosebeck S, Madden L, Jin X, Gu S, Apel IJ, Appert A, et al. Cleavage of NIK by the API2-MALT1 fusion oncoprotein leads to noncanonical NF-kappaB activation. Science. 2011;331:468–72.
17. Dong G, Liu C, Ye H, Gong L, Zheng J, Li M, et al. BCL10 nuclear expression and t(11; 18)(q21; q21) indicate nonresponsiveness to helicobacter pylori eradication of Chinese primary gastric MALT lymphoma. Int J Hematol. 2008;88:516–23.
18. Streubel B, Vinatzer U, Lamprecht A, Raderer M, Chott A. T(3; 14)(p14.1; q32) involving IGH and FOXP1 is a novel recurrent chromosomal aberration in MALT lymphoma. Leukemia. 2005;19:652–8.
19. Sagaert X, de Paepe P, Libbrecht L, Vanhentenrijk V, Verhoef G, Thomas J, et al. Forkhead box protein P1 expression in mucosa associated lymphoid tissue lymphomas predicts poor prognosis and transformation to diffuse large B-cell lymphoma. J Clin Oncol. 2006;24:2490–7.
20. Owens SR, Smith LB. Molecular aspects of H. pylori-related MALT lymphoma. Patholog Res Int. 2011;2011:193149.
21. Fork FT, Haglund U, Högström H, Wehlin L. Primary gastric lymphoma versus gastric cancer. An endo-

scopic and radiographic study of differential diagnostic possibilities. Endoscopy. 1985;17:5.

22. Fujishima H, Misawa T, Maruoka A, Chijiiwa Y, Sakai K, Nawata H. Staging and follow-up of primary gastric lymphoma by endoscopic ultrasonography. Am J Gastroenterol. 1991;86:719.
23. Caletti G, Ferrari A, Brocchi E, Barbara L. Accuracy of endoscopic ultrasonography in the diagnosis and staging of gastric cancer and lymphoma. Surgery. 1993;113:14.
24. Suekane H, Iida M, Yao T, Matsumoto T, Masuda Y, Fujishima M. Endoscopic ultrasonography in primary gastric lymphoma: correlation with endoscopic and histologic findings. Gastrointest Endosc. 1993;39:139–45.
25. Ono S, Kato M, Ono Y, Nishida U, Yamamoto K, Shimizu Y, et al. Target biopsy using magnifying endoscopy in clinical management of gastric mucosa-associated lymphoid tissue lymphoma. J Gastroenterol Hepatol. 2011;26:1133–8.
26. Bahn YE, Lee SK, Kwon SY, Kim SP. Sonographic appearances of mucosa-associated lymphoid tissue lymphoma of the submandibular gland confirmed with sonographically guided core needle biopsy. J Clin Ultrasound. 2011;39:228–32.
27. Kim HJ, Ha HK, Kim HJ, Byeon JS, Kim MJ, Lee SS, et al. Gastrointestinal dissemination of mucosa-associated lymphoid tissue lymphoma: computed tomographic findings. J Comput Assist Tomogr. 2010;34:187–92.
28. Choi JY, Lee GH, Ahn JY, Kim MY, Lee JH, Choi KS, et al. The role of abdominal CT scan as follow-up after complete remission with successful helicobacter pylori eradication in patients with H. pylori-positive stage I(E1) gastric MALT lymphoma. Helicobacter. 2011;16:36–41.
29. Perry C, Herishanu Y, Metzer U, Bairey O, Ruchlemer R, Trejo L, et al. Diagnostic accuracy of PET/CT in patients with extranodal marginal zone MALT lymphoma. Eur J Haematol. 2007;79:205.
30. Dreyling M, Thieblemont C, Gallamini A, Arcaini L, Campo E, Hermine O, et al. ESMO consensus conferences: guidelines on malignant lymphoma. Part 2: marginal zone lymphoma, mantle cell lymphoma, peripheral T-cell lymphoma. Ann Oncol. 2013;24:857–77.
31. Eck M, Fischbach W. Gastric MALT-type lymphoma. Pathology, pathogenesis, diagnostics and therapy. Pathologe. [Article in German]. 2010;31:188–94.
32. Nakamura S, Matsumoto T, Nakamura S, Jo Y, Fujisawa K, Suekane H, et al. Chromosomal translocation t(11;18)(q21;q21) in gastrointestinal mucosa associated lymphoid tissue lymphoma. J Clin Pathol. 2003;56:36–42.
33. Novak U, Basso K, Pasqualucci L, Dalla-Favera R, Bhagat G. Genomic analysis of non-splenic marginal zone lymphomas (MZL) indicates similarities between nodal and extranodal MZL and supports their derivation from memory B-cells. Br J Haematol. 2011;155:362.
34. Park JY, Kim SG, Kim JS, Jung HC. Bone marrow involvement is rare in superficial gastric mucosa-associated lymphoid tissue lymphoma. Dig Liver Dis. 2016;48:81–6.
35. Choi SI, Kook MC, Hwang SH, Kim YI, Lee JY, Kim CG, et al. Prevalence and implications of bone marrow involvement in patients with gastric mucosa-associated lymphoid tissue lymphoma. Gut Liver. 2018;12(3):278–87.
36. Zucca E, Arcaini L, Buske C, Johnson PW, Ponzoni M, Raderer M, et al. Marginal zone lymphomas: ESMO clinical practice guidelines for diagnosis, treatment and follow-up. Ann Oncol. 2020;31(1):17–29.
37. Rohatiner A, d'Amore F, Coiffier B, Crowther D, Gospodarowicz M, Isaacson P, et al. Report on a workshop convened to discuss the pathological and staging classifications of gastrointestinal tract lymphoma. Ann Oncol. 1994;5(5):397–400.
38. Ruskoné-Fourmestraux A, Dragosics B, Morgner A, Wotherspoon A, De Jong D. Paris staging system for primary gastrointestinal lymphomas. Gut. 2003;52:912–3.
39. Ruskoné-Fourmestraux A, Fischbach W, Aleman BM, Boot H, Du MQ, Megraud F, et al. EGILS consensus report. Gastric extranodal marginal zone B-cell lymphoma of MALT. Gut. 2011;60:747–58.
40. Zucca E, Bertoni F. The spectrum of MALT lymphoma at different sites: biological and therapeutic relevance. Blood. 2016;127:2082–92.
41. Suzuki H, Saito Y, Hibi T. Helicobacter pylori and gastric mucosa-associated lymphoid tissue (MALT) lymphoma: updated review of clinical outcomes and the molecular pathogenesis. Gut Liver. 2009;3:81–7.
42. Ono S, Kato M, Takagi K, Kodaira J, Kubota K, Matsuno Y, et al. Long-term treatment of localized gastric marginal zone B-cell mucosa associated lymphoid tissue lymphoma including incidence of metachronous gastric cancer. J Gastroenterol Hepatol. 2010;25:804–9.
43. Kim SJ, Yang S, Min BH, Lee JH, Rhee PL, Rhee JC, et al. Helicobacter pylori eradication for stage I(E1) gastric mucosa-associated lymphoid tissue lymphoma: predictive factors of complete remission. Korean J Gastroenterol. 2010;55:94–9.
44. Yepes S, Torres MM, Saavedra C, Andrade R. Gastric mucosa-associated lymphoid tissue lymphomas and helicobacter pylori infection: a Colombian perspective. World J Gastroenterol. 2012;18:685–91.
45. Alpen B, Neubauer A, Dierlamm J, Marynen P, Thiede C, Bayerdörfer E, et al. Translocation t(11;18) absent in early gastric marginal zone B-cell lymphoma of MALT type responding to eradication of helicobacter pylori infection. Blood. 2000;95:4014–5.
46. Neubauer A, Thiede C, Morgner A, Alpen B, Ritter M, Neubauer B, et al. Cure of helicobacter pylori infection and duration of remission of low-grade gastric mucosa-associated lymphoid tissue lymphoma. J Natl Cancer Inst. 1997;89:1350–5.
47. Zullo A, Hassan C, Ridola L, Francesco VD, Rossi L, Tomao S, et al. Eradication therapy in helicobacter

pylori-negative, gastric low-grade mucosa-associated lymphoid tissue lymphoma patients: a systematic review. J Clin Gastroenterol. 2013;47:824–7.
48. Aleman BM, Haas RL, van der Maazen RW. Role of radiotherapy in the treatment of lymphomas of the gastrointestinal tract. Best Pract Res Clin Gastroenterol. 2010;24:27–34.
49. Deinbeck K, Geinitz H, Haller B, Fakhrian K. Radiotherapy in marginal zone lymphoma. Radiat Oncol. 2013;8:2.
50. Kuo SH, Cheng AL, Lin CW, Hsu CH, Wu MS, Yeh KH, et al. T(11; 18)(q21; q21) translocation as predictive marker for non-responsiveness to salvage thalidomide therapy in patients with marginal zone B-cell lymphoma with gastric involvement. Cancer Chemother Pharmacol. 2011;68:1387–95.
51. Tektonidou MG. MALT lymphoma of the lacrimal gland in the context of systemic lupus erythematosus: complete remission after treatment with rituximab. Lupus. 2010;19:1243–5.
52. Nakajima T, Yasufuku K, Sekine Y, Yoshida S, Yoshino I. Mucosa-associated lymphoid tissue lymphoma of the left mainstem bronchus. Ann Thorac Surg. 2011;91:1281–3.
53. Kang HJ, Kim WS, Kim SJ, Lee JJ, Yang DH, Kim JS, et al. Phase II trial of rituximab plus CVP combination chemotherapy for advanced stage marginal zone lymphoma as a first-line therapy: consortium for improving survival of lymphoma (CISL) study. Ann Hematol. 2012;91:543–51.
54. Zucca E, Conconi A, Laszlo D, López-Guillermo A, Bouabdallah R, Coiffier B, et al. Addition of rituximab to chlorambucil produces superior event-free survival in the treatment of patients with extranodal marginal-zone B-cell lymphoma: 5-year analysis of the IELSG-19 randomized study. J Clin Oncol. 2013;31:565–72.
55. Hoffmann M, Troch M, Eidherr H, Traub-Weidinger T, Jonak C, Muellauer L, et al. 90Y-ibritumomab tiuxetan (Zevalin) in heavily pretreated patients with mucosa associated lymphoid tissue lymphoma. Leuk Lymphoma. 2011;52:42–5.
56. Esmaeli B, McLaughlin P, Pro B, Samaniego F, Gayed I, Hagemeister F, et al. Prospective trial of targeted radioimmunotherapy with Y-90 ibritumomab tiuxetan (Zevalin) for front-line treatment of early-stage extranodal indolent ocular adnexal lymphoma. Ann Oncol. 2009;20:709–14.
57. Copie-Bergman C, Wotherspoon A.C, Capella C, Motta T, Pedrinis E, Pileri SA, et al. Gela histological scoring system for post-treatment biopsies of patients with gastric MALT lymphoma is feasible and reliable in routine practice. Br J Haematol. 2013; 160: 47–52.
58. Nakamura S, Sugiyama T, Matsumoto T, Iijima K, Ono S, Tajika M, et al. Long-term clinical outcome of gastric MALT lymphoma after eradication of helicobacter pylori: a multicentre cohort follow-up study of 420 patients in Japan. Gut. 2012;61:507–13.
59. Wundisch T, Thiede C, Morgner A, Dempfle A, Gunther A, Liu H, et al. Long-term follow-up of gastric MALT lymphoma after helicobacter pylori eradication. J Clin Oncol. 2005;23:8018–24.
60. Craig VJ, Cogliatti SB, Imig J, Renner C, Neuenschwander S, Rehrauer H, et al. Myc-mediated repression of microRNA-34a promotes high-grade transformation of B-cell lymphoma by dysregulation of FoxP1. Blood. 2011;117:6227–36.
61. Ferrucci PF, Zucca E. Primary gastric lymphoma pathogenesis and treatment: what has changed over the past 10 years? Br J Haematol. 2007;136:521–38.
62. Li X, Xia B, Guo S, Zhan Z, Zhang L, Zhao D, et al. A retrospective analysis of primary gastric diffuse large B-cell lymphoma with or without concomitant mucosa-associated lymphoid tissue (MALT) lymphoma components. Ann Hematol. 2013;92:807–15.
63. Capelle LG, de Vries AC, Looman CW, Casparie MK, Booot H, Meijer GA, et al. Gastric MALT lymphoma: epidemiology and high adenocarcinoma risk in a nation-wide study. Eur J Cancer. 2008;44:2470–6.
64. Wündisch T, Dieckhoff P, Greene B, Thiede C, Wilhelm C, Stolte M, et al. Second cancers and residual disease in patients treated for gastric mucosa-associated lymphoid tissue lymphoma by helicobacter pylori eradication and followed for 10 years. Gastroenterology. 2012;143:936–42; quiz e13-e14
65. Kirschbaum M, Frankel P, Popplewell L, Zain J, Delioukina M, Pullarkat V, et al. Phase II study of vorinostat for treatment of relapsed or refractory indolent non-Hodgkin's lymphoma and mantle cell lymphoma. J Clin Oncol. 2011;29:1198–203.
66. Oh SY, Kim WS, Lee DH, Kim SJ, Kim SH, Ryoo BY, et al. Phase II study of gemcitabine for treatment of patients with advanced stage marginal zone B-cell lymphoma: consortium for improving survival of lymphoma (CISL) trial. Invest New Drugs. 2010;28:171–7.

Part II

Gastroesophageal Junction and Esophageal Cancer

Epidemiology, Risk Factors, and Clinical Manifestation

Key Points

- Esophageal cancer is classified mainly as squamous cell carcinoma and adenocarcinoma.
- Squamous cell carcinoma arises in the middle and lower esophagus, with tobacco and alcohol use being the main risk factors.
- Adenocarcinoma occurs in the lower esophagus and gastroesophageal junction, with Barrett's esophagus and gastroesophageal reflux disease as the primary risk factors.
- Typical symptoms in patients with advanced esophageal cancer are progressive dysphagia and weight loss.

Introduction

Esophageal cancers are generally classified as squamous cell carcinoma (SCC) and adenocarcinoma (ADC). Both histopathological types have a similar clinical manifestation, but different characteristics, including tumor location and risk factors. For most of the twentieth century, SCC predominated; however, recently, the incidence of ADC arising from Barrett's esophagus (BE) has dramatically increased in Western countries. However, SCC is still the main histopathological type in most countries; and SCC, especially, comprises more than 90% of all cases of esophageal cancer in Eastern Asian countries, including Korea, Japan, and China. The epidemiology, risk factors, and clinical manifestation of SCC and ADC of the esophagus and gastroesophageal junction (GEJ) will be reviewed here.

Epidemiology

Esophageal cancer is the tenth most common cancer in the world and the sixth leading cause of cancer mortality [1]. A varied distribution of the histopathological type of esophageal cancer (SCC vs ADC) is present based on geographic location. SCC is predominant in the area known as the esophageal cancer belt, extending from northern Iran, through central Asia, to central China. In the past, SCC represented more than 90% of all esophageal cancers; however, for the last three decades, the frequency of ADC of the esophagus and GEJ has increased dramatically in Western countries and also in some Eastern countries [2]. Men are 3–4 times more likely to be diagnosed with esophageal cancer than women [3]. Esophageal cancer is frequently associated with synchronous or metachronous multiple carcinomas.

Gwang Ha Kim is the lead author of this chapter.

H. J. Chun et al., *Gastrointestinal Cancer*, https://doi.org/10.1007/978-981-99-0815-8_12

Risk Factors

The risk factors are also different according to the histopathological type (Table 1). Tobacco smoking and alcohol consumption are the main risk factors in more than 90% of patients with SCC [4]. Cigar and pipe smoking are also associated with an increased risk of SCC, but the magnitude of the risk is less with cigarettes [5, 6]. The type and amount of alcoholic beverages could affect the risk of SCC. Although hard liquor may have a higher risk than wine or beer, the cumulative amount of alcohol consumption is more important than the type of alcohol [7, 8]. Tobacco smokers have a fivefold risk of developing SCC as compared to non-smokers [9], and the relative risk of SCC increases in proportion to the amount of alcohol consumed, varying between 1.8 and 7.4 depending on the weekly volume ingested [10]. Concomitant use of tobacco and alcohol is associated with a multiplied risk of developing SCC [11]. Smoking and alcohol are also risk factors for other aerodigestive cancers (head and neck cancer and lung cancer) as a result of field cancerization. Thus, patients with head and neck cancer or lung cancer have an increased risk of synchronous and second esophageal cancer and vice versa compared with the age-matched general population [12]. The presence of pre-existing esophageal diseases such as achalasia, caustic injury, and radiation-induced strictures can increase the risk of SCC. In a population-based study that included 1062 patients with achalasia; about 6% of the patients developed esophageal SCC, and on average, cancer was detected 14 years after the diagnosis of achalasia [13]. In a retrospective study that included 2414 patients with SCC, 63 patients had a history of caustic esophageal injury and the average time to diagnosis of SCC was 41 years after ingestion [14]. High-temperature beverages and foods could increase the risk of SCC by producing thermal damage to the esophageal mucosa [15]. Yerba mate tea is also associated with an increased risk of SCC, in terms of both the temperature of the beverage and the amount consumed. Poor nutritional status and vitamin deficiencies due to inadequate intake of fruits and vegetables have also been reported as risk factors for SCC. Foods containing N-nitroso compounds have been shown to increase the level of SCC by inducing alkyl adducts in DNA. Toxin (e.g., aflatoxin)-producing fungi present in food sources within endemic areas might exert mutagenic potential by reducing nitrates to nitroso compounds [16]. Other dietary risk factors for SCC include red meat intake and deficiency of selenium, zinc, and folate [17–19]. Plummer-Vinson syndrome, which is characterized by iron deficiency anemia, esophageal webbing, and glossitis, has a one in ten-lifetime risk of developing esophageal SCC [20]. Several genetic factors have also been suggested as risk factors for SCC. Tylosis palmaris et plantaris, an autosomal dominant disorder characterized by hyperkeratosis and pitting of the palms and soles, is associated with an increased risk (a 40% to 95% lifetime risk) of SCC in the mid-to-lower esophagus [21]. Genome-wide association studies have suggested several single nucleotide polymorphisms, enzymes related to alcohol metabolism (alcohol dehydrogenase and

Table 1 Risk factors for esophageal cancers

	Squamous cell carcinoma	Adenocarcinoma
Age	60–70 years	50–60 years
Sex	Men > women	Men > women
Lifestyle	High alcohol consumption Cigarette smoking Hot tea Ingested carcinogens (nitrates, smoked opiates, fundal toxins) Low intake of fruits and vegetables Dietary deficiencies of selenium, molybdenum, zinc, and vitamin A	Cigarette smoking Obesity
Medical history	Past ingestion of lye Achalasia Radiation-induced strictures	Barrett's esophagus Gastroesophageal reflux disease
Others	Plummer-Vinson syndrome Tylosis palmaris et plantaris	

acetyl dehydrogenase), and loci present on phospholipase C and chromosome 20 as genetic susceptibility factors [22]. A relationship has been suggested between the human papilloma virus and the development of SCC in certain high-risk subpopulations, but the role of the virus remains unclear [23].

BE caused by persistent inflammation of the lower esophagus due to gastroesophageal reflux disease (GERD) is known to be an important risk factor for ADC of the esophagus and GEJ. Many studies have shown that GERD, high body mass index (BMI), and smoking are involved in the development of ADC [24–26]. A meta-analysis showed that weekly and daily GERD symptoms were associated with a fivefold and sevenfold increased risk of ADC, respectively [27]. Although GERD itself can directly lead to ADC, it progresses to ADC more commonly through a preneoplastic condition, such as BE.

BE is defined as columnar metaplasia that replaces the normal stratified squamous epithelium of the distal esophagus. In the United States, specialized intestinal metaplasia, including goblet cells, is required for the diagnosis of BE. Conversely, the presence of goblet cells is not necessary for the diagnosis of BE in other countries [28]. Patients with BE have a 30-fold increased risk of ADC as compared to the general population, but the absolute risk of developing ADC is low (estimated annual incidence, 0.12%) [29].

Tobacco smokers have a 2.1-fold risk of developing ADC as compared to non-smokers, and the risk increases with increasing total dose (pack-years of smoking) [30]. In contrast, no association between alcohol consumption and ADC has been documented, even at higher levels of consumption [31]. Obesity is associated with an increased risk for ADC of the esophagus and GEJ; the relative risks of ADC for BMI between 25 and 30 kg/m^2 and > 30 kg/m^2 are 1.7 and 2.3, respectively [32]. Race, sex, and age are also risk factors. Whites are affected five times more frequently than blacks, and men are eight times more likely to develop ADC than women [33]. Seventy percent of the patients are between 55 and 85 years of age, and more than 50% are older than 70 years [34]. In contrast, aspirin and non-steroidal anti-inflammatory drugs (NSAID), which inhibit cyclooxygenase, may play a protective role against the development of ADC, particularly in the presence of BE. NSAID use is associated with a significantly reduced risk of ADC of the esophagus (odds ratio [OR] 0.68; 95% confidence interval [CI], 0.56–0.82) and with a trend toward a reduced risk of ADC of the GEJ [35]. Increased frequency (daily or more) and duration of use (≥10 years) are associated with an approximately 40% reduction in both ADC of the esophagus (OR 0.56; 95% CI, 0.43–0.73) and GEJ (OR 0.63; 95% CI, 0.45–0.90) [35].

Clinical Manifestations

Esophageal cancers occur mainly in the lower third (75%) and middle third (25%) of the esophagus. Most patients with early esophageal cancer are asymptomatic, and those with advanced esophageal cancer typically present with progressive dysphagia (difficulty in swallowing from solids to liquids), odynophagia, and unintentional weight loss. Dysphagia usually occurs once the diameter of the esophageal lumen is less than 13 mm (reduction by approximately 70% of the luminal diameter), indicating a locally advanced stage. Weight loss is mainly caused by changes in diet to accommodate dysphagia and tumor-related anorexia can also be a contributing factor. Approximately 20% of patients also complain of odynophagia.

Regurgitation of saliva or food uncontaminated by gastric secretions may also occur. Hoarseness and/or cough can occur when the recurrent laryngeal nerve is invaded by the primary tumor or associated nodal metastases. Aspiration pneumonia is infrequent. Iron deficiency anemia due to chronic gastrointestinal blood loss from cancers is common [36]. However, patients seldom notice melena or hematemesis. Acute upper gastrointestinal bleeding caused by tumor invasion into the aorta or bronchial artery is rare. When patients complain of intractable coughing, especially after eating, or recurrent pneumonia, the formation of an esophageal-tracheal or esophageal-bronchial fistula by direct invasion of the tumor into the trachea or mainstem bronchus is suspected; this is a late complication of esophageal cancer. Some patients present symptoms or signs attributable to metastatic disease from the time of first diagnosis. The most common metastatic lesions are the liver, lungs, bones, and adrenal glands [37]. SCC frequently metastasizes to intrathoracic sites, while ADC frequently metastasizes to intraabdominal sites (liver, peritoneum). As with SCC of other organs, hypercalcemia can occur as a part of paraneoplastic syndromes (probably due to parathormone-related peptide secreted by tumor cells) in the absence of osseous metastases.

Conclusion

Esophageal cancers are classified as SCC and ADC. Although ADC has increased dramatically in Western countries, SCC remains the main histopathological type in most countries. SCC occurs primarily in the middle and lower esophagus, and tobacco and alcohol use are the main risk factors. Conversely, ADC occurs in the lower esophagus and GEJ, with BE and GERD as the primary risk factors. Typical symptoms in patients with advanced esophageal cancer are progressive dysphagia and weight loss, regardless of histopathological types.

References

1. Sung H, Ferlay J, Siegel RL, Laversanne M, Soerjomataram I, Jemal A, et al. Global cancer statistics 2020: GLOBOCAN estimates of incidence and mortality worldwide for 36 cancers in 185 countries. CA Cancer J Clin. 2021;71:209–49.
2. Thrift AP. The epidemic of oesophageal carcinoma: where are we now? Cancer Epidemiol. 2016;41:88–95.
3. Kurtom S, Kaplan BJ. Esophagus and gastrointestinal junction yumors. Surg Clin North Am. 2020;100:507–21.
4. Engel LS, Chow WH, Vaughan TL, Gammon MD, Risch HA, Stanford JL, et al. Population attributable risks of esophageal and gastric cancers. J Natl Cancer Inst. 2003;95:1404–13.
5. Iribarren C, Tekawa IS, Sidney S, Friedman GD. Effect of cigar smoking on the risk of cardiovascular disease, chronic obstructive pulmonary disease, and cancer in men. N Engl J Med. 1999;340:1773–80.
6. Randi G, Scotti L, Bosetti C, Talamini R, Negri E, Levi F, et al. Pipe smoking and cancers of the upper digestive tract. Int J Cancer. 2007;121:2049–51.
7. Tuyns AJ, Pequignot G, Abbatucci JS. Oesophageal cancer and alcohol consumption; importance of type of beverage. Int J Cancer. 1979;23:443–7.
8. Brown LM, Hoover R, Gridley G, Schoenberg JB, Greenberg RS, Silverman DT, et al. Drinking practices and risk of squamous-cell esophageal cancer among black and white men in the United States. Cancer Causes Control. 1997;8:605–9.
9. Domper Arnal MJ, Ferrandez Arenas A, Lanas AA. Esophageal cancer: risk factors, screening and endoscopic treatment in Western and eastern countries. World J Gastroenterol. 2015;21:7933–43.
10. Wheeler JB, Reed CE. Epidemiology of esophageal cancer. Surg Clin North Am. 2012;92:1077–87.
11. Steevens J, Schouten LJ, Goldbohm RA, van den Brandt PA. Alcohol consumption, cigarette smoking and risk of subtypes of oesophageal and gastric cancer: a prospective cohort study. Gut. 2010;59:39–48.
12. Prabhu A, Obi KO, Rubenstein JH. The synergistic effects of alcohol and tobacco consumption on the risk of esophageal squamous cell carcinoma: a meta-analysis. Am J Gastroenterol. 2014;109:822–7.
13. Sandler RS, Nyren O, Ekbom A, Eisen GM, Yuen J, Josefsson S. The risk of esophageal cancer in patients with achalasia. A population-based study. JAMA. 1995;274:1359–62.
14. Appelqvist P, Salmo M. Lye corrosion carcinoma of the esophagus: a review of 63 cases. Cancer. 1980;45:2655–8.
15. Islami F, Boffetta P, Ren JS, Pedoeim L, Khatib D, Kamangar F. High-temperature beverages and foods and esophageal cancer risk--a systematic review. Int J Cancer. 2009;125:491–524.
16. Chu FS, Li GY. Simultaneous occurrence of fumonisin B1 and other mycotoxins in moldy corn collected from the People's Republic of China in regions with high incidences of esophageal cancer. Appl Environ Microbiol. 1994;60:847–52.
17. Cross AJ, Freedman ND, Ren J, Ward MH, Hollenbeck AR, Schatzkin A, et al. Meat consumption and risk of esophageal and gastric cancer in a large prospective study. Am J Gastroenterol. 2011;106:432–42.
18. Mark SD, Qiao YL, Dawsey SM, Wu YP, Katki H, Gunter EW, et al. Prospective study of serum selenium levels and incident esophageal and gastric cancers. J Natl Cancer Inst. 2000;92:1753–63.
19. Abnet CC, Lai B, Qiao YL, Vogt S, Luo XM, Taylor PR, et al. Zinc concentration in esophageal biopsy specimens measured by x-ray fluorescence and esophageal cancer risk. J Natl Cancer Inst. 2005;97:301–6.

20. Enzinger PC, Mayer RJ. Esophageal cancer. N Engl J Med. 2003;349:2241–52.
21. Lindor NM, McMaster ML, Lindor CJ, Greene MH. Concise handbook of familial cancer susceptibility syndromes - second edition. J Natl Cancer Inst Monogr. 2008:1–93.
22. Zhang HZ, Jin GF, Shen HB. Epidemiologic differences in esophageal cancer between Asian and Western populations. Chin J Cancer. 2012;31:281–6.
23. Far AE, Aghakhani A, Hamkar R, Ramezani A, Pishbigar HF, Mirmomen S, et al. Frequency of human papillomavirus infection in oesophageal squamous cell carcinoma in Iranian patients. Scand J Infect Dis. 2007;39:58–62.
24. Yousef F, Cardwell C, Cantwell MM, Galway K, Johnston BT, Murray L. The incidence of esophageal cancer and high-grade dysplasia in Barrett's esophagus: a systematic review and meta-analysis. Am J Epidemiol. 2008;168:237–49.
25. Lagergren J, Bergstrom R, Lindgren A, Nyren O. Symptomatic gastroesophageal reflux as a risk factor for esophageal adenocarcinoma. N Engl J Med. 1999;340:825–31.
26. Kubo A, Corley DA. Body mass index and adenocarcinomas of the esophagus or gastric cardia: a systematic review and meta-analysis. Cancer Epidemiol Biomarkers Prev. 2006;15:872–8.
27. Rubenstein JH, Taylor JB. Meta-analysis: the association of oesophageal adenocarcinoma with symptoms of gastro-oesophageal reflux. Aliment Pharmacol Ther. 2010;32:1222–7.
28. Sampliner RE. Practice guidelines on the diagnosis, surveillance, and therapy of Barrett's esophagus. The Practice Parameters Committee of the American College of Gastroenterology. Am J Gastroenterol. 1998;93:1028–32.
29. Hvid-Jensen F, Pedersen L, Drewes AM, Sorensen HT, Funch-Jensen P. Incidence of adenocarcinoma among patients with Barrett's esophagus. N Engl J Med. 2011;365:1375–83.
30. Cook MB, Kamangar F, Whiteman DC, Freedman ND, Gammon MD, Bernstein L, et al. Cigarette smoking and adenocarcinomas of the esophagus and esophagogastric junction: a pooled analysis from the international BEACON consortium. J Natl Cancer Inst. 2010;102:1344–53.
31. Tramacere I, Pelucchi C, Bagnardi V, Rota M, Scotti L, Islami F, et al. A meta-analysis on alcohol drinking and esophageal and gastric cardia adenocarcinoma risk. Ann Oncol. 2012;23:287–97.
32. Turati F, Tramacere I, La Vecchia C, Negri E. A meta-analysis of body mass index and esophageal and gastric cardia adenocarcinoma. Ann Oncol. 2013;24:609–17.
33. El-Serag HB, Mason AC, Petersen N, Key CR. Epidemiological differences between adenocarcinoma of the oesophagus and adenocarcinoma of the gastric cardia in the USA. Gut. 2002;50:368–72.
34. Sweed MR, Edmonson D, Cohen SJ. Tumors of the esophagus, gastroesophageal junction, and stomach. Semin Oncol Nurs. 2009;25:61–75.
35. Liao LM, Vaughan TL, Corley DA, Cook MB, Casson AG, Kamangar F, et al. Nonsteroidal anti-inflammatory drug use reduces risk of adenocarcinomas of the esophagus and esophagogastric junction in a pooled analysis. Gastroenterology. 2012;142:442–52 e5; quiz e22–3
36. Schatz RA, Rockey DC. Gastrointestinal bleeding due to gastrointestinal tract malignancy: natural history, management, and outcomes. Dig Dis Sci. 2017;62:491–501.
37. Meltzer CC, Luketich JD, Friedman D, Charron M, Strollo D, Meehan M, et al. Whole-body FDG positron emission tomographic imaging for staging esophageal cancer comparison with computed tomography. Clin Nucl Med. 2000;25:882–7.

Diagnosis, Staging, and Prognosis

Key Points

- EUS is the best imaging modality to determine the depth of tumor invasion (cT) and the presence of regional lymph node metastasis (cN).
- CT is used to evaluate the invasion of adjacent structures and to detect regional and non-regional nodal metastasis and distant systemic metastases.
- PET-CT is particularly useful to identify distant and unusual metastases.
- Bronchoscopy is necessary for tumors at or above the carina to rule out T4 disease to the airways.
- The staging of esophageal cancer has evolved over the years, and AJCC-8 has made significant modifications to overcome the shortcomings of previous editions.
- Appropriate staging for esophageal cancer leads to better treatment and improved patient outcomes.
- Avoiding over-staging or under-staging in esophageal cancer is critical.

Introduction

Esophageal cancer is a fatal disease with low survival rates. Formal staging is required and is confirmed by a detailed examination of tumor thickness, nodal involvement, and presence of metastases that make up the TNM staging classification. Optimal staging and optimal treatment decisions based on stage, histologic type, and location of the disease are very important.

Diagnosis

The diagnosis of esophageal cancer is almost always made by endoscopic biopsy, which is necessary for an accurate diagnosis of squamous cell carcinoma (SCC) or adenocarcinoma (AC). However, it may present as a flat or subtle lesion in the early stage, so the initial endoscopist is often unaware of the presence of cancer. Additionally, a single biopsy may not be diagnostic. Therefore, multiple biopsies should be performed for suspicious lesions. During endoscopy, the location of the tumor relative to the incisors and the esophagogastric junction (EGJ), the length of the tumor, and the degree of obstruction of the tumor should be noted. The most proximal and circumferential extent of Barrett's esophagus should also be noted according to the Prague criteria [1]. Although there is no consensus on the maximum size for small tumors or nodules, an experienced endoscopist should perform endo-

Joon Hyun Cho is the lead author of this chapter.

H. J. Chun et al., *Gastrointestinal Cancer*, https://doi.org/10.1007/978-981-99-0815-8_13

scopic en bloc resection in cases of well- or moderately-differentiated histology at the initial biopsy specimen and no obvious submucosal involvement to provide a specimen that accurately assesses the depth of invasion [2]. Unfortunately, only limited cases are diagnosed at an early stage and are amenable to endoscopic therapy, and these are usually detected in screening tests rather than in the investigation of symptoms. Thus, most tumors are usually diagnosed as larger lesions in an advanced stage.

After esophageal cancer is diagnosed by endoscopy and biopsy, accurate staging is essential for appropriate treatment and to predict the prognosis. Further staging with contrast-enhanced computed tomography (CT) scanning of the chest and abdomen and positron emission tomography-CT (PET-CT) imaging should be performed to evaluate distant metastatic disease. In case of the absence of evidence of distant metastatic disease, an endoscopic ultrasound (EUS) should be performed to assess the status of T and regional lymph nodes. EUS with fine needle aspiration of suspicious nodes further increases the accuracy of this test [3]. Evaluation by PET-CT before EUS has several advantages. The PET-CT scan can demonstrate distant metastatic disease and eliminate the need for the patient to undergo EUS. The PET-CT scan may also identify a suspicious lymph node that can be specifically examined and sampled during the EUS procedure. EUS is superior to CT or PET-CT for the assessment of both T- and N-status. It is highly accurate for celiac nodal status, but slightly lower for other regional lymph nodes due to the difficulty of accessing the node without crossing the tumor. It is also important to remember that for more superficial tumors (T1a–T2), the accuracy of EUS is significantly diminished and endoscopic resection provides the most accurate staging information [3, 4]. Obstructive lesions may make EUS assessment impossible. In these cases, ballooning on radial EUS examination is associated with a risk of perforation. These risks should be weighed against the benefits of obtaining additional staging information. Most tumors with such tight stenoses are locally advanced and should probably be treated with multimodal therapy.

Locally advanced disease can include airway invasion. This becomes more relevant in more proximal esophageal cancers. Although EUS provides information on invasion of adjacent structures, bronchoscopy with visualization and biopsies should also be performed for proximal and middle-third esophageal tumors located in or above the carina with no evidence of metastatic disease to assess direct tracheal invasion (T4 disease). Signs of tracheal involvement include a widened carina, external compression, tumor infiltration, and fistulization. The last two signs contraindicate surgical resection [5]. Bronchoscopic gross appearance may not be accurate; in fact, a bulge of the posterior tracheobronchial wall or minimal mucosal changes (erythema, edema) do not confirm the cancer invasion of the wall. Therefore, biopsy plus brush cytology is recommended. In a study of patients with supracarinal cancer, endoluminal tumor mass, protrusion of the posterior tracheal wall, and signs of mucosal invasion were visible in 5.9%, 28.6%, and 4.1% of bronchoscopic examinations, respectively. However, in only 8.6% of 220 bronchoscopic examinations, cancer invasion was confirmed by biopsy or cytology. Bronchoscopy excluded 18.1% of potentially operable patients from surgery due to airway invasion, with an overall accuracy of 93.3% [6]. In addition, other recent studies have shown that endobronchial ultrasound is more accurate in assessing tracheobronchial invasion by esophageal cancer as compared to conventional bronchoscopy, CT, and EUS [7].

The assessment of Siewert type (Fig. 1) should also be included as part of the initial investigation in all patients with EGJ AC [8, 9]. Siewert type I tumors are defined as an AC of the lower esophagus with the tumor epicenter located 1 to 5 cm above the anatomic EGJ, which usually arises from an area with specialized intestinal metaplasia of the esophagus (i.e., Barrett's esophagus). Siewert type II tumors are defined as a true cardia carcinoma with the epicenter of the tumor located within 1 cm above and 2 cm below the anatomic EGJ, which arises from the cardiac epithelium or short segments with intestinal metaplasia in the EGJ. This entity is often referred to as 'junctional carcinoma'. Siewert type III tumors are defined as a subcardial carcinoma with the tumor epicenter located between 2 and 5 cm below the EGJ, which infiltrates the EGJ and the lower esopha-

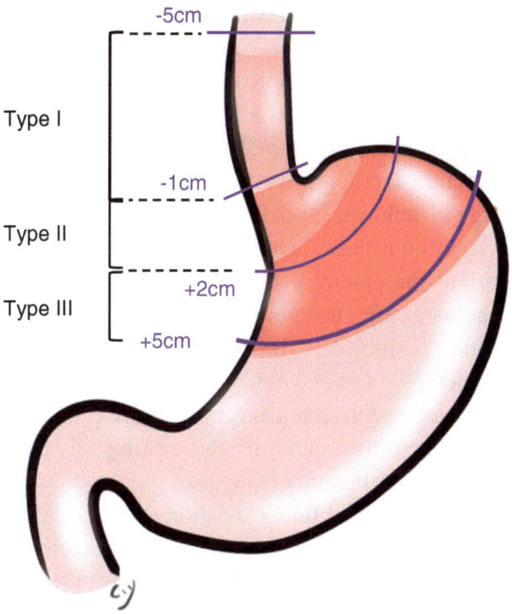

Fig. 1 Siewert classification for adenocarcinoma of the gastroesophageal junction. (Adapted from Shackelford's Surgery of the Alimentary Tract—Published December 31, Chevallay et al. [13])

gus from below. The American Joint Committee on Cancer (AJCC) criteria for distal esophageal and proximal gastric cancers have evolved over the years. In AJCC-7, tumors involving the EGJ and with epicenter <5 cm into the proximal stomach were staged as esophageal cancers, while in AJCC-8, this requirement has been reduced to <2 cm [10]. Thus, any tumor with an epicenter located ≥2 cm into the proximal stomach should now be classified as stomach cancer, even if it involves the EGJ [11]. Therefore, Siewert type I and II tumors should be treated according to the guidelines for esophageal and EGJ cancers while Siewert type III tumors are more appropriately managed according to the guidelines for gastric cancer.

Staging and Prognosis

The eighth Edition of the AJCC tumor node metastasis (TNM) staging system [11] acknowledges differences in the biology of AC and SCC by creating separate staging groups for the two histological types (Tables 1, 2, 3, and 4). Studies have shown that early-stage SCCs (pT1 or T2, N0) have a worse prognosis compared to AC. Therefore, SCC and AC are staged differently, specifically for stage I and stage II cancers. Furthermore, this is the first edition to separate

Table 1 Cancer staging categories for the esophagus and esophagogastric junction [12]

Definition of primary tumor (T)	
T category	
TX	Tumor cannot be assessed
T0	No evidence of primary tumor
Tis	High-grade dysplasia, defined as malignant cells confined to the epithelium by the basement membrane
T1	Tumor invades the lamina propria, muscularis mucosae, or submucosa
T1a	Tumor invades lamina propria, muscularis mucosa
T1b	Tumor invades submucosa
T2	Tumor invades muscularis propria
T3	Tumor invades adventitia
T4	Tumor invades adjacent structures
T4a	Tumor invades the pleura, pericardium, azygos vein, diaphragm, or peritoneum
T4b	Tumor invades other adjacent structures, such as the aorta, vertebral body, or airway
Definition of regional lymph nodes (N)	
N category	
NX	Regional lymph nodes cannot be assessed
N0	No regional lymph node metastasis
N1	Metastasis in one or two regional lymph nodes
N2	Metastasis in three to six regional lymph nodes
N3	Metastasis in seven or more regional lymph nodes
Definition of distant metastasis (M)	
M category	
M0	No distant metastasis
M1	Distant metastasis
Histologic grade (G)	
GX	Grade cannot be assessed
G1	Well differentiated
G2	Moderately differentiated
G3	Poorly differentiated, undifferentiated

(continued)

Table 1 (continued)

Location-applicable to squamous cell carcinoma only	
X	Location unknown
Upper	Cervical esophagus to lower border of azygos vein
Middle	Lower border of azygos vein to lower border of inferior pulmonary vein
Lower	Lower border of inferior pulmonary vein to stomach, including gastroesophageal junction
Note: Location is defined by the position of the epicenter of the tumor in the esophagus	

Table 2 Clinical stage groups (cTNM) for the esophagus and esophagogastric junction [12]

Stage	cT	cN	M
Squamous cell carcinoma			
0	Tis	N0	M0
I	T1	N0–1	M0
II	T2	N0–1	M0
	T3	N0	M0
III	T3	N1	M0
	T1–3	N2	M0
IVA	T4	N0–2	M0
	Any T	N3	M0
IVB	Any T	Any N	M1
Adenocarcinoma			
Stage	cT	cN	M
0	Tis	N0	M0
I	T1	N0	M0
IIA	T1	N1	M0
IIB	T2	N0	M0
III	T2	N1	M0
	T3	N0–1	M0
	T4a	N0–1	M0
IVA	T1-4a	N2	M0
	T4b	N0–2	M0
	Any T	N3	M0
IVB	Any T	Any N	M1

The cTNM is separate for AC and SCC, given the differences in epidemiology, pathogenesis, location, and outcomes of both subtypes. cTNM is based on imaging and biopsy specimens

stages into clinical (cTNM) (Table 2), pathologic (pTNM) (Table 3), and post-neoadjuvant (ypTNM) staging groups (Table 4) [12]. The inclusion of ypTNM is a response to an increasing proportion of operable patients who receive induction therapy prior to resection. Pathologic stage is included for patients who undergo resection without neoadjuvant therapy. ypTNM categorizes the extent of residual tumor in resected specimens after neoadjuvant treatment, where the prefix "y" indicates the use of neoadjuvant chemotherapy and/or radiation therapy. Unlike untreated esophageal cancers, both SCC and AC are staged the same in the setting of post-neoadjuvant therapy (Table 4).

Assessment of tumor location (Fig. 2) is conducted during esophagoscopy. Tumor location is defined as the location of the epicenter of the cancer relative to its distance from the incisors and is divided into four distinct anatomic regions. Clinically, the epicenter is determined from measurements at the upper and lower borders, which also provide the length of the cancer. Alternatively, the location of the tumor can be determined from CT of the chest [11]. The cervical esophagus begins at the hypopharynx and extends to the thoracic inlet, which is the level of the sternal notch. On endoscopy, this corresponds to approximately 15–20 cm from the incisors. The upper thoracic esophagus begins at the thoracic inlet and extends to the azygos vein, which is approximately 20–25 cm from the incisors. The middle thoracic esophagus begins at the lower border of the azygos vein and extends to the inferior pulmonary vein, which is approximately 25–30 cm from the incisors. The lower thoracic esophagus begins at the distal end of the lower border of the inferior pulmonary vein and extends to the GEJ and is usually more than 30 cm from the incisors. Tumor location affects the pathologic stage of SCC but not for AC, and only affects the outcome in patients with SCC with stage IIA and stage IIB disease (Table 3).

Histologic grade (G) reflects the biological activity of the tumor and is subcategorized as well differentiated (G1), moderately differentiated (G2), and poorly differentiated (G3). If G is undifferentiated, the tumor is considered G3. While histologic grade is considered prognosti-

Table 3 Pathologic stage groups (pTNM) for the esophagus and esophagogastric junction [12]

Stage	pT	pN	M	G	Location
Squamous cell carcinoma					
0	Tis	N0	M0	N/A	Any
IA	T1a	N0	M0	G1	Any
	T1a	N0	M0	GX	Any
IB	T1a	N0	M0	G2–3	Any
	T1b	N0	M0	G1–3	Any
	T1b	N0	M0	GX	Any
	T2	N0	M0	G1	Any
IIA	T2	N0	M0	G2–3	Any
	T2	N0	M0	GX	Any
	T3	N0	M0	G1–3	Lower
	T3	N0	M0	G1	Upper/middle
IIB	T3	N0	M0	G2–3	Upper/middle
	T3	N0	M0	GX	Upper/middle/lower
	T3	N0	M0	Any	Location X
	T1	N1	M0	Any	Any
IIIA	T1	N2	M0	Any	Any
	T2	N1	M0	Any	Any
IIIB	T2	N2	M0	Any	Any
	T3	N1–2	M0	Any	Any
	T4a	N0–1	M0	Any	Any
IVA	T4a	N2	M0	Any	Any
	T4b	N0–2	M0	Any	Any
	Any T	N3	M0	Any	Any
IVB	Any T	Any N	M1	Any	Any
Adenocarcinoma					
	pT	pN	M	G	
0	Tis	N0	M0	N/A	
IA	T1a	N0	M0	G1	
	T1a	N0	M0	GX	
IB	T1a	N0	M0	G2	
	T1b	N0	M0	G1–2	
	T1b	N0	M0	GX	
IC	T1	N0	M0	G3	
	T2	N0	M0	G1–2	
IIA	T2	N0	M0	G3	
	T2	N0	M0	GX	
IIB	T1	N1	M0	Any	
	T3	N0	M0	Any	
IIIA	T1	N2	M0	Any	
	T2	N1	M0	Any	
IIIB	T2	N2	M0	Any	
	T3	N1–2	M0	Any	
	T4a	N0–1	M0	Any	
IVA	T4a	N2	M0	Any	
	T4b	N0–2	M0	Any	
	Any T	N3	M0	Any	
IVB	Any T	Any N	M1	Any	

The pTNM is based on pathologic findings after esophagectomy. Differences in survival profiles make it necessary to separate stage groups for AC and SCC

Used with permission of the American Joint Committee on Cancer (AJCC), Chicago, Illinois. The original and primary source for this information is the AJCC Cancer Staging Manual, Eighth Edition (2017), published by Springer International Publishing [12]

Table 4 Postneoadjuvant therapy stage groups (ypTNM) for esophageal adenocarcinoma and squamous cell carcinoma [12]

Stage	ypT	ypN	M
I	T0–2	N0	M0
II	T3	N0	M0
IIIA	T0–2	N1	M0
IIIB	T3	N1	M0
	T0–3	N2	M0
	T4a	N0	M0
IVA	T4a	N1–2	M0
	T4a	NX	M0
	T4b	N0–2	M0
	Any T	N3	M0
IVB	Any T	Any N	M1

ypTNM is identical for both AC and SCC and is based on the pathologic review of the resected specimen in patients who have had neoadjuvant therapy

Used with permission of the American Joint Committee on Cancer (AJCC), Chicago, Illinois. The original and primary source for this information is the AJCC Cancer Staging Manual, Eighth Edition (2017), published by Springer International Publishing [12]

cally important and is included in pathologic staging for early-stage tumors for AC and SCC (Table 3), it is not included in clinical or post-neoadjuvant staging. In both histologies, the clinical and post-neoadjuvant staging include only the TNM classification without the use of tumor location or histologic grade.

The depth of invasion of the tumor defines the T-status (Fig. 3). High-grade dysplasia includes malignant cells confined to the epithelium by the basement membrane and is by definition non-invasive (Tis). T1a tumors invade the lamina propria or muscularis mucosa, and T1b tumors invade the submucosa. T2 tumors invade the muscularis propria, and T3 tumors invade the adventitia but not the surrounding structures. T4a tumors invade adjacent structures that are usually resectable (diaphragm, pleura, and pericardium). T4b tumors invade adjacent structures that are typically unresectable (trachea and aorta).

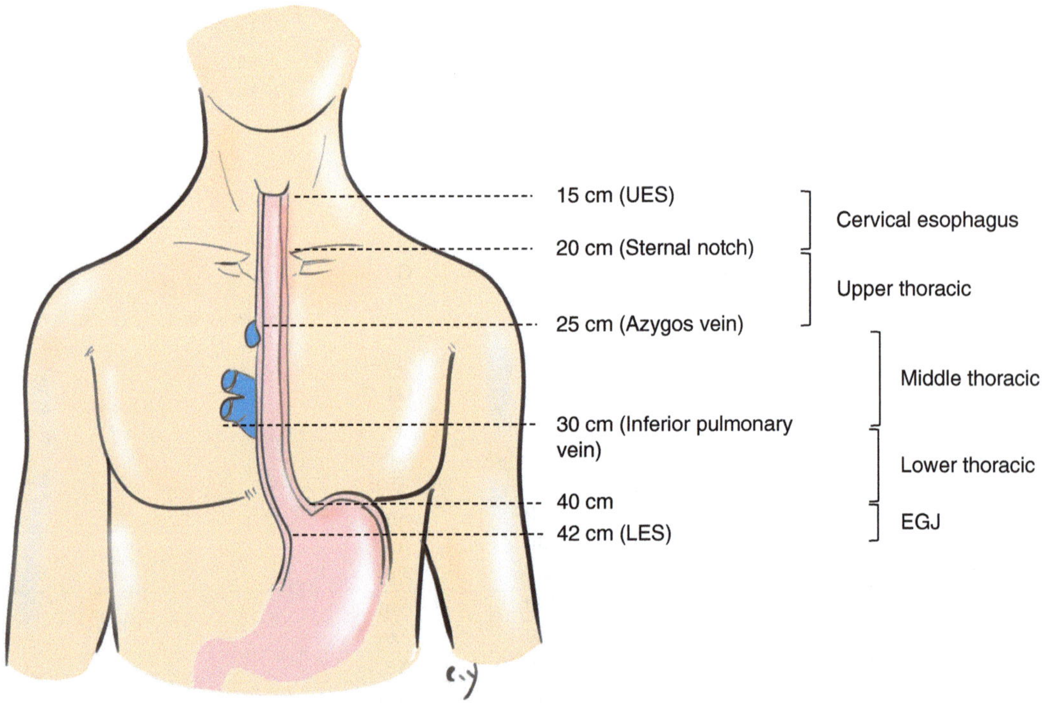

Fig. 2 Location of esophageal cancer based on endoscopic measurements from the incisors. The esophagus is divided into 4 distinct anatomic regions. The cervical esophagus extends from the upper esophageal sphincter to the suprasternal notch (15–20 cm from the incisors). The upper thoracic esophagus extends from the suprasternal notch to the lower border of the azygos vein (20–25 cm from the incisors). The midthoracic esophagus extends from the lower border of the azygos vein to the inferior pulmonary vein (25–30 cm from the incisors). The lower thoracic esophagus extends from the lower border of the inferior pulmonary vein to the gastroesophageal junction (30–40 cm from the incisors). (Adapted from Sabiston Textbook of Surgery. Published December 31, 2021. p1043, Betancourt-Cuellar et al. [14])

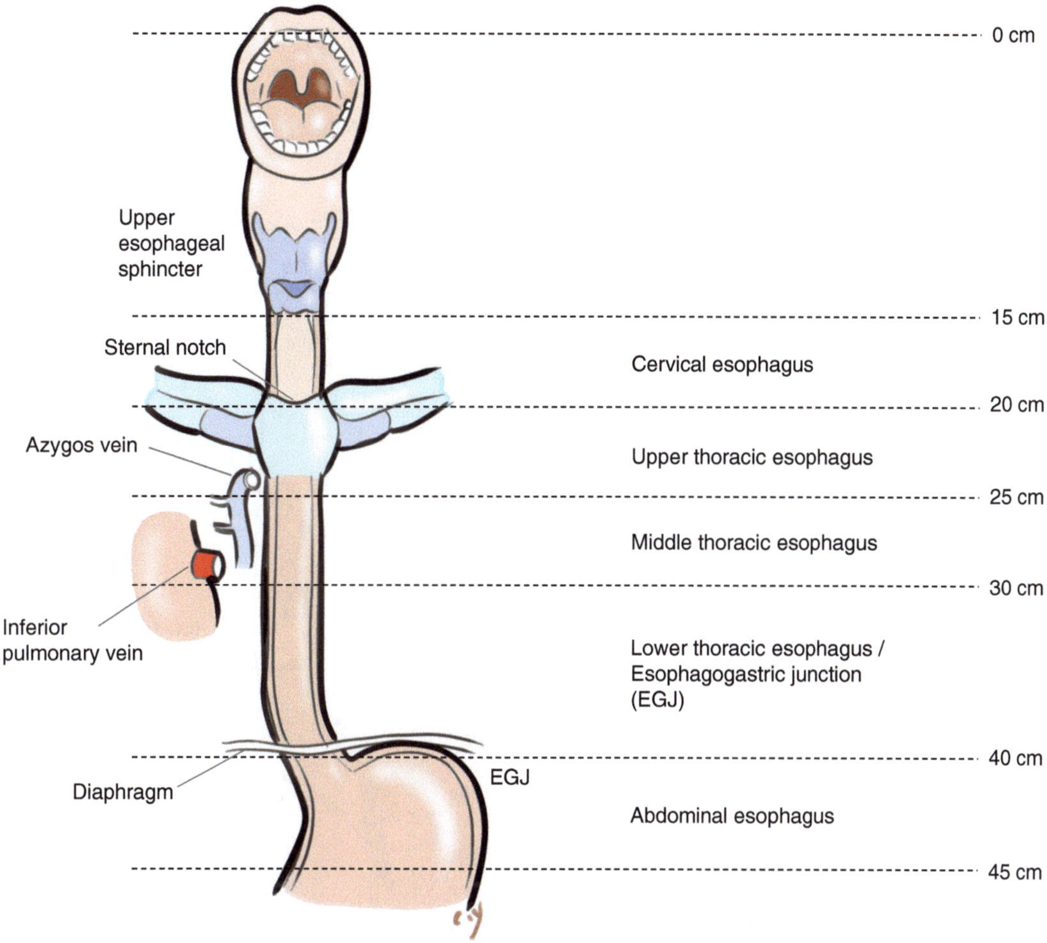

Fig. 2 (continued)

Nodal classification is based on the total number of regional lymph node metastases. The number of lymph nodes involved has been shown to have an influence on survival, and this is reflected in the subdivision of the N category into subcategories N1 (1–2 lymph nodes involved), N2 (3–6 lymph nodes involved), and N3 (>6 lymph nodes involved) (Fig. 3). The eighth Edition of the AJCC staging system introduces an esophagus-specific regional lymph node map for descriptive purposes [12]. Regional lymph nodes are defined as any periesophageal lymph node from the upper esophageal sphincter to the celiac axis. These include extrathoracic lymph nodes in the lower cervical periesophageal region, periesophageal intrathoracic lymph nodes, bilateral paratracheal and subcarinal nodes, diaphragmatic lymph nodes adjacent to the crura, paracardial lymph nodes, and upper abdominal lymph nodes (left gastric, common hepatic, splenic, and celiac lymph nodes). Lymph nodes outside these regions are considered distant metastatic diseases. Supraclavicular lymph nodes not located in the periesophageal region are considered M1 disease.

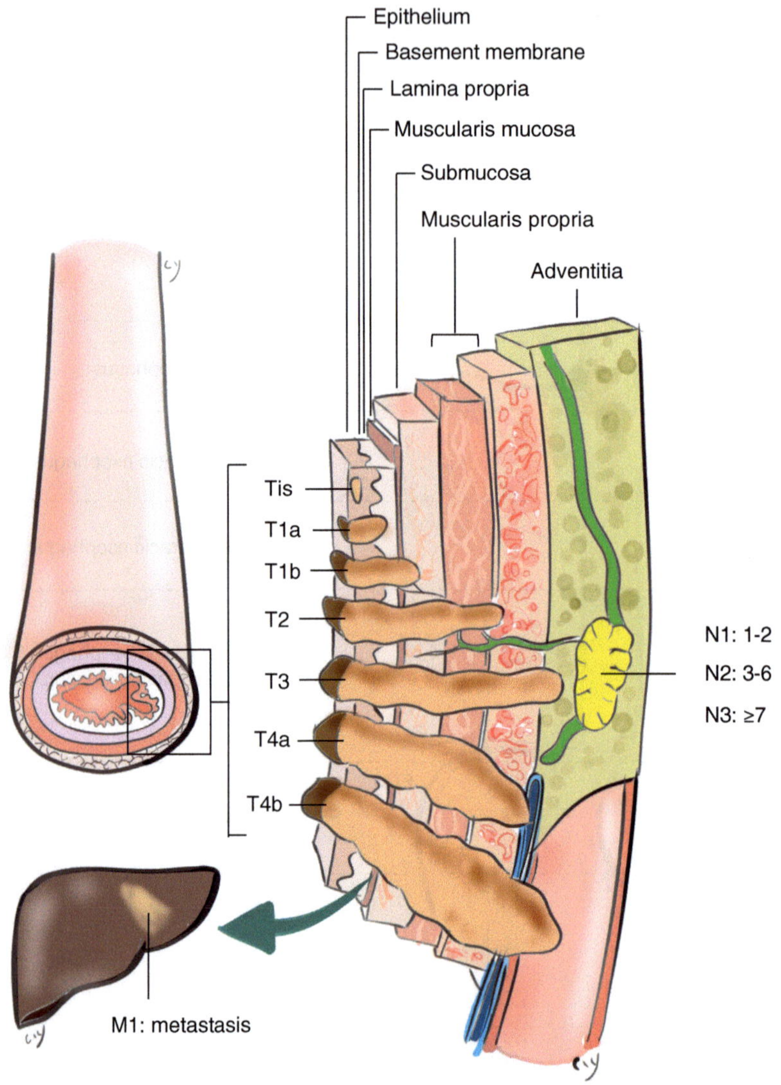

Fig. 3 TNM anatomic categories include the primary tumor (T), regional lymph node (N), and distant metastases (M). The T category provides information regarding the extension of tumor invasion into the esophageal wall. The N category represents regional lymph node involvement, and the M category represents metastasis to distant organ/s. (Adapted from Betancourt-Cuellar et al. [14], Sabiston Textbook of Surgery. Published December 31, 2021. p1044)

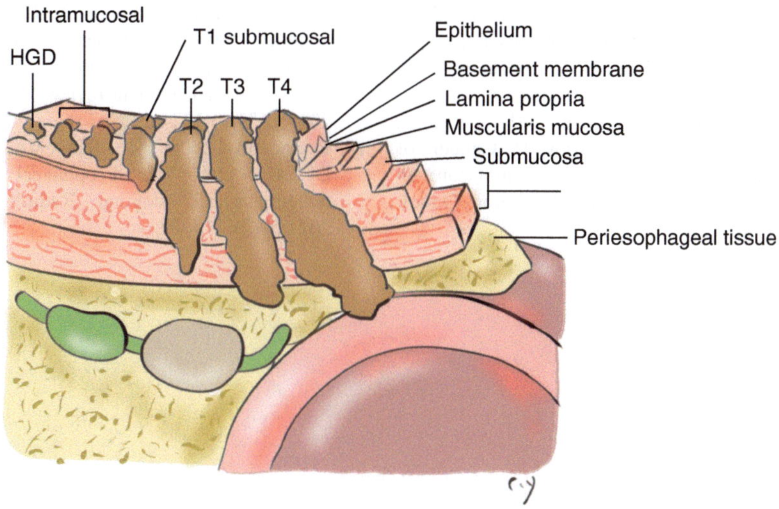

Fig. 3 (continued)

Conclusion

Esophageal cancer remains one of the tumors with the worst survival outcomes. Despite advances in multimodal therapy, survivor data did not improve. The treatment of esophageal cancer is stage-specific to ensure the best possible clinical outcomes. Accordingly, accurate pre-treatment staging is very important for appropriate treatment plans. Without accurate staging, patients are likely to be undertreated or over-treated, leading to decreased survival and quality of life.

References

1. Shaheen NJ, Falk GW, Iyer PG, Gerson LB. American College of Gastroenterology. ACG clinical guideline: diagnosis and management of Barrett's esophagus. Am J Gastroenterol. 2016;111(1):30–50.
2. Pimentel-Nunes P, Dinis-Ribeiro M, Ponchon T, Repici A, Vieth M, De Ceglie A, et al. Endoscopic submucosal dissection: European Society of Gastrointestinal Endoscopy (ESGE) Guideline. Endoscopy. 2015;47(9):829–54.
3. Esophageal and Esophagogastric Junction Cancers—Version 4.2021. National Comprehensive Cancer Network—Clinical Practice Guidelines in Oncology; 2021. www.nccn.org. Accessed Aug 2021.
4. Dhupar R, Rice RD, Correa AM, Weston BR, Bhutani MS, Maru DM, et al. Endoscopic ultrasound estimates for tumor depth at the gastroesophageal junction are inaccurate: implications for the liberal use of endoscopic resection. Ann Thorac Surg. 2015;100(5):1812–6.
5. Cheung HC, Siu KF, Wong J. A comparison of flexible and rigid endoscopy in evaluating esophageal cancer patients for surgery. World J Surg. 1988;12(1):117–22.
6. Riedel M, Stein HJ, Mounyam L, Lembeck R, Siewert JR. Extensive sampling improves preoperative bronchoscopic assessment of airway invasion by supracarinal esophageal cancer: a prospective study in 166 patients. Chest. 2001;119(6):1652–60.
7. Wakamatsu T, Tsushima K, Yasuo M, Yamazaki Y, Yoshikawa S, Koide N. Usefulness of preoperative endobronchial ultrasound for airway invasion around the trachea: esophageal cancer and thyroid cancer. Respiration. 2006;73(5):651–7.
8. Siewert JR, Stein HJ. Carcinoma of the gastroesophageal junction—classification, pathology and extent of resection. Dis Esophagus. 1996;9(3):173–82.
9. Siewert JR, Feith M, Werner M, Stein HJ. Adenocarcinoma of the esophagogastric junction: results of surgical therapy based on anatomical/topographic classification in 1002 consecutive patients. Ann Surg. 2000;232(3):353–61.
10. Inada M, Nishimura Y, Ishikawa K, Nakamatsu K, Wada Y, Uehara T, et al. Comparing the 7th and 8th editions of the American Joint Committee on Cancer/Union for International Cancer Control TNM staging system for esophageal squamous cell carcinoma treated by definitive radiotherapy. Esophagus. 2019;16(4):371–6.

11. Rice TW, Patil DT, Blackstone EH. 8th edition AJCC/UICC staging of cancers of the esophagus and esophagogastric junction: application to clinical practice. Ann Cardiothorac Surg. 2017;6(2):119–30.
12. Rice TW, Ishwaran H, Ferguson MK, Ferguson MK, Blackstone EH, Goldstraw P. Cancer of the esophagus and esophagogastric junction: an eighth edition staging primer. J Thorac Oncol. 2017;12(1):36–42.
13. Chevallay M, Bollschweiler E, Chandramohan SM, Schmidt T, Koch O, Demanzoni G, et al. Cancer of the gastroesophageal junction: a diagnosis, classification, and management review. Ann N Y Acad Sci. 2018;1434(1):132–8.
14. Betancourt-Cuellar SL, Benveniste MFK, Palacio DP, Hofstetter WL. Esophageal cancer: tumor-node-metastasis staging. Radiol Clin N Am. 2021;59(2):219–29.

Overview of Treatment

Key Points

- A multimodal approach is required for the treatment of esophageal and gastroesophageal junction cancers. This is particularly applicable to locally advanced esophageal cancer.
- Endoscopic submucosal dissection or endoscopic mucosal resection is the recommended treatment for small (≤3 cm) Tis and T1a esophageal squamous cell carcinoma (SCC) and adenocarcinoma.
- Preoperative chemoradiotherapy followed by surgery is widely accepted as the standard of care for locally advanced esophageal cancer in both SCC and adenocarcinoma.
- For the treatment of patients with metastatic esophageal cancer, large-scale studies using targeted therapy or immunotherapy are needed.

Introduction

Esophageal cancer is a devastating disease that not only causes progressive dysphagia, which reduces the quality of life of patients, but also has a low survival rate. Clinically, esophageal cancer can be divided into various stages (0–IVB) [1]; however, based on treatment, it can be classified as early disease, including superficial esophageal cancer, and locally advanced disease. Locally advanced disease can be further divided into resectable and unresectable disease. Several treatment options are available for early disease; however, as the disease progresses, treatment options become fewer and the disease becomes more difficult to treat.

Treatment of Superficial Esophageal Cancer

The Japan Esophageal Society classifies early and superficial esophageal cancer according to the depth of tumor invasion (Fig. 1). Early

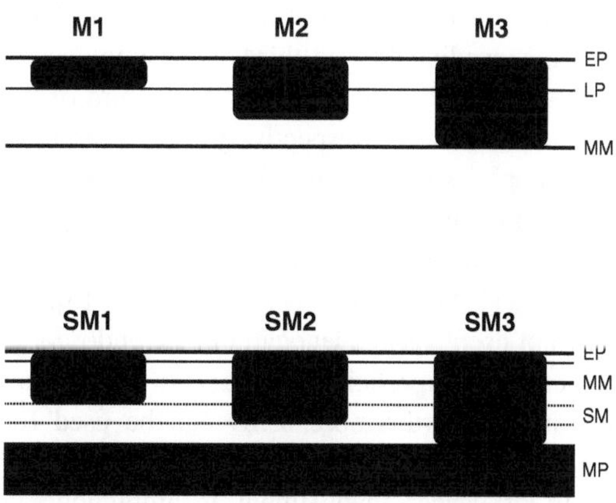

Fig. 1 Subclassification of depth of tumor invasion in superficial esophageal cancer. *EP* epithelium, *LP* lamina propria, *MM* muscularis mucosa, *SM* submucosa, *MP* muscularis propria

Sung Eun Kim is the lead author of this chapter.

H. J. Chun et al., *Gastrointestinal Cancer*, https://doi.org/10.1007/978-981-99-0815-8_14

esophageal cancer is defined as a tumor that invades the mucosa (T1a), irrespective of the presence or absence of lymph nodes or distant metastasis [2]. Superficial esophageal cancer is defined as a tumor that invades the mucosa (T1a) and submucosa (T1b), regardless of lymph node or distant metastasis [2]. The American Joint Committee on Cancer (AJCC) classifies clinical stage I esophageal squamous cell carcinoma (SCC) as T1N0-1 M0 and clinical stage I esophageal adenocarcinoma as T1N0M0 [3]. High-grade dysplasia or in situ carcinoma (Tis) is classified as mucosal cancer (T1a) [3]. Although there are minor differences in each definition, in terms of treatment, esophageal cancer cases confined to the mucosa or submucosa (T1) can be considered as an early disease.

Endoscopic Resection

Endoscopic resection can be a curative treatment for superficial esophageal cancer when the risk of lymph node metastasis is minimal. In a study evaluating 2418 Japanese patients, the incidence of lymph node metastasis in M1 (intraepithelial tumors), M2 (tumors invading the lamina propria), and M3 (tumors in contiguity with or invading the muscularis mucosa) cases was 0%, 3%, and 12.2%, respectively [4]. Moreover, 26.5%, 35.8%, and 45.9% cases were SM1 (tumors invading the upper third of the submucosa), SM2 (tumors invading the mid-third of the submucosa), and SM3 (tumors invading the lower third of the submucosa) cases, respectively [4]. Therefore, endoscopic submucosal dissection (ESD) or endoscopic mucosal resection is the most appropriate treatment for small (≤3 cm) Tis and T1a esophageal SCC and adenocarcinoma [5]. In cases of esophageal adenocarcinoma, endoscopic resection of superficial T1b cancers may be an option [5]. Furthermore, ESD can be used for diagnostic and therapeutic purposes when the depth of cancer involvement is ambiguous in cases of superficial esophageal cancer [6].

Ablation Therapy with/without Endoscopic Resection

Ablation therapy is a minimally invasive procedure that destroys abnormal tissue. There are various ablation methods, such as radiofrequency ablation (RFA), cryoablation, and photodynamic therapy. Among them, RFA has recently been used for the treatment of superficial esophageal SCC and esophageal adenocarcinoma originating from Barrett's esophagus [5].

Regarding esophageal adenocarcinoma (i.e., Barrett's adenocarcinoma). RFA for the remaining Barrett's esophagus after endoscopic resection of visible lesions may be more effective than either treatment alone [7]. Some guidelines recommend combination therapy (endoscopic resection with RFA) when endoscopically resected specimens are confirmed to be high-grade dysplasia or intramucosal cancer [7–10].

RFA has been recommended for flat, early SCC in several studies, and M1/2 T1a lesions are considered suitable for RFA [11]. However, it is difficult to differentiate the depth of cancer invasion by endoscopy alone, and there is a continual risk of lymph node metastasis. Thus, the Japanese guidelines do not recommend RFA for clinical T1a esophageal cancer [12].

Esophagectomy

Esophagectomy has long been the initial treatment for localized esophageal cancer. However, the mortality rate after esophagectomy is 2–5% [13] and several studies have not reported significant differences in oncological outcomes comparing esophagectomy and endoscopic resection for T1 esophageal cancer, including esophageal SCC and adenocarcinoma [14, 15]. Therefore, although esophagectomy can be performed for all T1 esophageal cancers, it is more appropriate for T1b lesions [5].

Treatment of Locally Advanced Esophageal Cancer

Resectable locally advanced esophageal cancer refers to T2-4N0 or TanyN1–3. Of these, clinical T2N0 (cT2N0) esophageal cancer can be distinguished from the other stages of esophageal cancer.

Clinical T2N0 Esophageal Cancer

T2 disease defines tumors that invade the muscularis propria of the esophagus. Although tumors are located on the esophageal wall, they are associated with an increased risk of lymphatic metastasis. The role of neoadjuvant chemoradiotherapy (CRT) before esophagectomy in patients with cT2N0 disease is controversial. Recent large-scale studies and a systematic review have failed to show oncological benefits of neoadjuvant therapy in cT2N0 disease in terms of long-term survival and reduced recurrence risk [16–18]. Esophagectomy is generally preferred for patients with cT2N0 esophageal cancer [5]. However, neoadjuvant therapy is appropriate for patients with cT2N0 disease and one or more risk factors for lymphatic metastasis, including the presence of lymphovascular invasion, poorly differentiated carcinoma, or tumors sized >3 cm [5].

Locally Advanced Resectable Esophageal Cancer

Treatment options for locally advanced esophageal cancer are limited. However, it is necessary to use a multimodal approach that considers the individual conditions of patients with esophageal cancer.

In both SCC and esophageal adenocarcinoma, preoperative CRT followed by surgery have shown survival benefits in patients with locally advanced cancer, and R0 resection rates should also be higher than those of surgery alone [19–21]. Currently, surgery after preoperative CRT is widely considered the gold standard for locally advanced esophageal cancer [5, 22].

Several studies have compared the efficacy of preoperative chemotherapy followed by surgery alone. Preoperative chemotherapy has shown better overall effects than surgery alone; however, more significant effects have been observed in patients with esophageal adenocarcinoma than in patients with SCC [23, 24].

Cervical Esophageal Cancer

Esophagectomy is not recommended for the treatment of cervical esophageal cancer due to the risk of major complications, including high mortality and morbidity rates and poor quality of life [25]. Therefore, definitive CRT is recommended for patients with cervical esophageal cancer [5].

Unresectable Locally Advanced Esophageal Cancer

Unresectable locally advanced esophageal cancer refers to T4b disease, indicating invasion of the tumor into other adjacent structures, such as the aorta, vertebral body, trachea, heart, and great vessels, or the presence of a tracheoesophageal fistula [3]. Definitive CRT is recommended for the treatment of patients with T4b esophageal cancer without distant metastasis [5]. Induction chemotherapy followed by definitive CRT may also be considered in some patients [6].

Treatment of Metastatic Esophageal Cancer

If esophageal cancer has metastasized, targeted therapy or immune checkpoint inhibitors may be additional treatment options. In terms of targeted therapy, the addition of trastuzumab, a monoclonal HER2/neu (tyrosine kinase receptor) antibody, increased overall survival (OS) compared to chemotherapy alone in the ToGA trial [26].

Furthermore, apatinib, a vascular endothelial growth factor receptor-2 tyrosine kinase inhibitor, has been shown to improve OS in patients with gastroesophageal junction (GEJ) adenocarcinoma refractory to chemotherapy (at least two lines) [27].

Several well-designed studies have reported that nivolumab and pembrolizumab, anti-PD-1 antibodies, improve oncological outcomes in patients with GEJ adenocarcinoma refractory to chemotherapy [28, 29]. Nivolumab and pembrolizumab have also demonstrated promising activity in patients with refractory esophageal SCC to chemotherapy [30, 31].

Conclusion

Treatment of esophageal cancer is challenging. However, the multimodal approach has been instrumental in advancing the treatment of esophageal cancer (Table 1). Many researchers are conducting large-scale studies to improve the results of esophageal cancer treatment. Therefore, more advanced treatment methods are expected to be proposed based on the results of their studies. Furthermore, as the role of targeted therapy and immune checkpoint inhibitors is elucidated, treatment of patients with metastatic esophageal cancer will be further developed.

Table 1 Treatment options for gastroesophageal junction and esophageal cancers

TNM classification	Treatment options
pTis	Endoscopic treatments
	• ESD or EMR
	• Ablation
	• ESD or EMR followed by ablation
	or esophagectomy
pT1a	Endoscopic treatments
	• ESD or EMR
	• ESD or EMR followed by ablation
	or esophagectomy
cT1bN0–cT2N0 (low-risk; <3 cm, well differentiated)	Esophagectomy[a]
cT2N0(high-risk; ≥ 3 cm, LVI (+), poorly differentiated) or cT1b–cT4a, Nany	Non-cervical esophagus Preoperative chemoradiation followed by esophagectomy Cervical esophagus Definitive chemoradiation
cT4b	Definitive chemoradiation or
	Chemotherapy

ESD endoscopic submucosal dissection, *EMR* endoscopic mucosal resection, *LVI* lymphovascular invasion

[a] Endoscopic resection or endoscopic resection followed by ablation can be considered in superficial pT1b esophageal adenocarcinoma patients

References

1. Rice TW, Ishwaran H, Blackstone EH, Hofstetter WL, Kelsen DP, Apperson-Hansen C, et al. Recommendations for clinical staging (cTNM) of cancer of the esophagus and esophagogastric junction for the eighth edition AJCC/UICC staging manuals. Dis Esophagus. 2016;29:913–9.
2. Japan ES. Japanese classification of esophageal cancer, 11th ed.: part I. Esophagus. 2017;14:1–36.
3. Rice TW, Kelsen DP, Blackstone EH, et al. Esophagus and esophagogastric juction. In: Amin MB, Edge SB, Greene FL, et al., editors. AJCC cancer staging manual. 8th ed. New York: Springer; 2017. p. 185–202.
4. Kodama M, Kakegawa T. Treatment of superficial cancer of the esophagus: a summary of responses to a questionnaire on superficial cancer of the esophagus in Japan. Surgery. 1998;123:432–9.
5. National Comprehensive Cancer Network. Esophageal and esophagogastric junction cancers (version 4.2021). 2021. https://www.nccn.org/professionals/physician_gls/pdf/esophageal.pdf.
6. Cilbir E, Yalcin S. Esophageal and gastroesophageal junction tumors. In: Yalcin S, Philip P, editors. Textbook of gastrointestinal oncology. New York: Springer; 2019. p. 55–71.
7. 2018 surveillance of Barrett's oesophagus: ablative therapy (NICE guideline CG106). London; 2018.
8. Sharma P, Shaheen NJ, Katzka D, Bergman J. AGA clinical practice update on endoscopic treatment of Barrett's esophagus with dysplasia and/or early cancer: expert review. Gastroenterology. 2020;158:760–9.
9. Weusten B, Bisschops R, Coron E, Dinis-Ribeiro M, Dumonceau JM, Esteban JM, et al. Endoscopic management of Barrett's esophagus: European Society of Gastrointestinal Endoscopy (ESGE) Position Statement. Endoscopy. 2017;49:191–8.
10. Shaheen NJ, Falk GW, Iyer PG, Gerson LB, American College of G. ACG clinical guideline: diagnosis and management of Barrett's esophagus. Am J Gastroenterol. 2016;111:30–50.
11. Lei S, Mulmi Shrestha S, Shi R. Radiofrequency ablation for early superficial flat esophageal squamous cell neoplasia: a comprehensive review. Gastroenterol Res Pract. 2020;2020:4152453.

12. Ishihara R, Arima M, Iizuka T, Oyama T, Katada C, Kato M, et al. Endoscopic submucosal dissection/endoscopic mucosal resection guidelines for esophageal cancer. Dig Endosc. 2020;32:452–93.
13. Schieman C, Wigle DA, Deschamps C, Nichols Iii FC, Cassivi SD, Shen KR, et al. Patterns of operative mortality following esophagectomy. Dis Esophagus. 2012;25:645–51.
14. Das A, Singh V, Fleischer DE, Sharma VK. A comparison of endoscopic treatment and surgery in early esophageal cancer: an analysis of surveillance epidemiology and end results data. Am J Gastroenterol. 2008;103:1340–5.
15. Prasad GA, Wu TT, Wigle DA, Buttar NS, Wongkeesong LM, Dunagan KT, et al. Endoscopic and surgical treatment of mucosal (T1a) esophageal adenocarcinoma in Barrett's esophagus. Gastroenterology. 2009;137:815–23.
16. Mota FC, Cecconello I, Takeda FR, Tustumi F, Sallum RAA, Bernardo WM. Neoadjuvant therapy or upfront surgery? A systematic review and meta-analysis of T2N0 esophageal cancer treatment options. Int J Surg. 2018;54:176–81.
17. Hardacker TJ, Ceppa D, Okereke I, Rieger KM, Jalal SI, LeBlanc JK, et al. Treatment of clinical T2N0M0 esophageal cancer. Ann Surg Oncol. 2014;21:3739–43.
18. Esophageal Cancer Study Group Participating C. Predictors of staging accuracy, pathologic nodal involvement, and overall survival for cT2N0 carcinoma of the esophagus. J Thorac Cardiovasc Surg. 2019;157(1264–72):e6.
19. Walsh TN, Noonan N, Hollywood D, Kelly A, Keeling N, Hennessy TP. A comparison of multimodal therapy and surgery for esophageal adenocarcinoma. N Engl J Med. 1996;335:462–7.
20. Graham AJ, Shrive FM, Ghali WA, Manns BJ, Grondin SC, Finley RJ, et al. Defining the optimal treatment of locally advanced esophageal cancer: a systematic review and decision analysis. Ann Thorac Surg. 2007;83:1257–64.
21. Shapiro J, van Lanschot JJB, Hulshof M, van Hagen P, van Berge Henegouwen MI, Wijnhoven BPL, et al. Neoadjuvant chemoradiotherapy plus surgery versus surgery alone for oesophageal or junctional cancer (CROSS): long-term results of a randomised controlled trial. Lancet Oncol. 2015;16:1090–8.
22. Shah MA, Kennedy EB, Catenacci DV, Deighton DC, Goodman KA, Malhotra NK, et al. Treatment of locally advanced esophageal carcinoma: ASCO guideline. J Clin Oncol. 2020;38:2677–94.
23. Allum WH, Stenning SP, Bancewicz J, Clark PI, Langley RE. Long-term results of a randomized trial of surgery with or without preoperative chemotherapy in esophageal cancer. J Clin Oncol. 2009;27:5062–7.
24. Medical Research Council Oesophageal Cancer Working G. Surgical resection with or without preoperative chemotherapy in oesophageal cancer: a randomised controlled trial. Lancet. 2002;359:1727–33.
25. Hoeben A, Polak J, Van De Voorde L, Hoebers F, Grabsch HI, de Vos-Geelen J. Cervical esophageal cancer: a gap in cancer knowledge. Ann Oncol. 2016;27:1664–74.
26. Bang YJ, Van Cutsem E, Feyereislova A, Chung HC, Shen L, Sawaki A, et al. Trastuzumab in combination with chemotherapy versus chemotherapy alone for treatment of HER2-positive advanced gastric or gastro-oesophageal junction cancer (ToGA): a phase 3, open-label, randomised controlled trial. Lancet. 2010;376:687–97.
27. Li J, Qin S, Xu J, Xiong J, Wu C, Bai Y, et al. Randomized, double-blind, placebo-controlled phase III trial of apatinib in patients with chemotherapy-refractory advanced or metastatic adenocarcinoma of the stomach or gastroesophageal junction. J Clin Oncol. 2016;34:1448–54.
28. Kang YK, Boku N, Satoh T, Ryu MH, Chao Y, Kato K, et al. Nivolumab in patients with advanced gastric or gastro-oesophageal junction cancer refractory to, or intolerant of, at least two previous chemotherapy regimens (ONO-4538-12, ATTRACTION-2): a randomised, double-blind, placebo-controlled, phase 3 trial. Lancet. 2017;390:2461–71.
29. Fuchs CS, Doi T, Jang RW, Muro K, Satoh T, Machado M, et al. Safety and efficacy of pembrolizumab monotherapy in patients with previously treated advanced gastric and gastroesophageal junction cancer: phase 2 clinical KEYNOTE-059 trial. JAMA Oncol. 2018;4:e180013.
30. Kudo T, Hamamoto Y, Kato K, Ura T, Kojima T, Tsushima T, et al. Nivolumab treatment for oesophageal squamous-cell carcinoma: an open-label, multicentre, phase 2 trial. Lancet Oncol. 2017;18:631–9.
31. Doi T, Piha-Paul SA, Jalal SI, Saraf S, Lunceford J, Koshiji M, et al. Safety and antitumor activity of the anti-programmed death-1 antibody pembrolizumab in patients with advanced esophageal carcinoma. J Clin Oncol. 2018;36:61–7.

Endoscopic Treatment

Key Points

- Endoscopic resection, including endoscopic mucosal resection and endoscopic submucosal dissection, is a feasible alternative to surgical resection for superficial esophageal cancer based on favorable results in suitable indications.
- Endoscopic resection for superficial esophageal cancer is usually associated with a low-risk of morbidity and mortality compared to surgery.
- The endoscopist should consider adverse events such as bleeding, perforation, and stricture during and after endoscopic resection.
- In superficial esophageal cancers less than 10–20 mm in size, endoscopic mucosal resection can be applied instead of endoscopic submucosal dissection.

Introduction

Esophageal cancer is a gastrointestinal cancer with an extremely poor prognosis despite advances in diagnostic and treatment methods. This is because esophageal cancer is often diagnosed in an advanced stage, and lymph node metastasis is common. The standard treatment for esophageal cancer is surgical resection; however, the morbidity and mortality rate following the intervention is high and restoring the patient's quality of life after surgery is prolonged. With these limitations of surgery, endoscopic treatment is performed for radical resection of specific superficial esophageal cancers with no possibility of lymph node metastasis. In this review, the indications, treatment modality, and outcomes of endoscopic treatment for superficial esophageal cancer are summarized.

Ji Yong Ahn is the lead author of this chapter.

Indications of Endoscopic Resection

Superficial esophageal cancer is defined as cancer localized to the mucosa and submucosa regardless of lymph node metastasis. The absence of distant metastasis and low-risk of lymph node metastasis are indications for endoscopic treatment. Although endoscopic resection of superficial esophageal cancer can preserve the esophagus, it is important to carefully select the patients who will receive the procedure, as there is still the possibility of lymph node metastasis. Therefore, the most important factor to consider when deciding on the treatment plan is to estimate the possibility of lymph node metastasis before the procedure. To evaluate clinical staging before making a treatment plan, examinations such as esophagogastroduodenoscopy, endoscopic ultrasound, computed tomography, and positron emission tomography are needed.

H. J. Chun et al., *Gastrointestinal Cancer*, https://doi.org/10.1007/978-981-99-0815-8_15

Risk factors for lymph node metastasis include the size of the lesion, endoscopic findings, lymphatic invasion, and depth of invasion. Of these, the depth of tumor invasion is closely associated with the possibility of lymph node metastasis [1–3]. Previous studies examining surgical reports of superficial esophageal cancer have revealed that the rates of lymph node metastasis were 0–5.6% when tumor invasion is limited to the intraepithelial layer or lamina propria layer. However, in cases of invasion of the muscularis mucosa or submucosal invasion of less than 200 μm, the rates of lymph node metastasis increase to 9.0–27.0% and 15.0–53.1%, respectively [2, 4, 5]. Considering this evidence, the absolute indication for endoscopic resection in superficial esophageal cancer can be defined as intraepithelial or lamina propria invasion tumor [6, 7]. Therefore, the depth of invasion of superficial esophageal cancer must be accurately determined using esophagogastroduodenoscopy, endoscopic ultrasound, and magnifying endoscopy with narrow-band imaging before performing the endoscopic resection [8–11].

In the guidelines of the European Society for Gastrointestinal Endoscopy (ESGE) and the Japan Esophageal Society (JES), superficial esophageal cancer without lymph node metastasis and invasion into the lamina propria layer is presented as absolute indications for endoscopic resection [6, 7]. However, Korean studies report that there was no significant difference in long-term survival between patients with superficial esophageal cancer without obvious submucosal invasion who underwent endoscopic resection and those who received esophagectomy; the postoperative complication rate was significantly higher in operated patients [12]. A Chinese study also reported no significant differences in survival rates between patients with superficial esophageal cancer who underwent endoscopic resection and those who underwent surgical resection [13]. In addition, despite the high morbidity rate and a 1–2% mortality rate that can occur after surgery, endoscopic resection can be performed as an alternative treatment option when the patient's conditions are poor or when the patient refuses surgery [14–16]. Thus, according to the guidelines of the ESGE and JES, endoscopic resection can be performed in superficial esophageal cancer with M3 or SM1 invasion as relative indication because the risk of lymph node metastasis is low if there is no vascular or lymphatic invasion [6, 7].

In a similar opinion, the Korean clinical practice guidelines recommend endoscopic resection for superficial esophageal cancer without distant or lymph node metastasis, excluding those with obvious submucosal invasion [17] and the National Comprehensive Cancer Network (NCCN) guidelines also recommend endoscopic resection for superficial esophageal cancer located in the mucosa and esophagectomy in the presence of submucosal invasion [18].

Therefore, if the pathological examination subsequent to the complete resection of the superficial esophageal cancer shows that the depth of infiltration does not exceed the layer of the muscularis mucosa and there is no vascular or lymphatic invasion, careful follow-up with close monitoring can be performed instead of additional surgery.

Methods of Endoscopic Resection

Endoscopic submucosal dissection (ESD), endoscopic mucosal resection (EMR), argon plasma coagulation, and photodynamic therapy are the types of endoscopic treatment. EMR or ESD is recommended for complete resection of the lesion and pathological examination of the tissue after resection. Esophageal EMR began in Japan as a treatment for superficial esophageal cancer in the late 1980s and has since spread worldwide. However, because the EMR allows only a narrow area to be resected in a single procedure, it is not easy to resect tumors larger than 1–2 cm in size and it is difficult to obtain accurate pathological information. Furthermore, the curative resection rate is low, and the local recurrence rate is high compared to ESD [19–21]. With instrumental and technical improvement of endoscopic treatments, ESD is considered the first therapeutic option compared to EMR because it can remove larger tumors (Fig. 1) or even lesions that completely surround the esophageal lumen [19, 20] (Fig. 2).

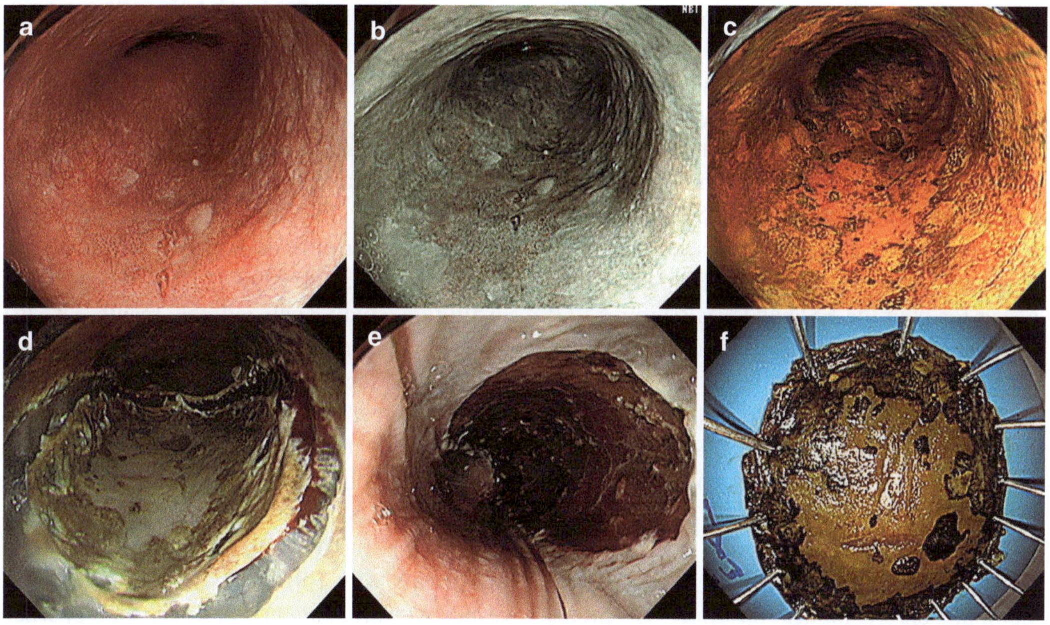

Fig. 1 Endoscopic submucosal dissection of superficial esophageal cancer. (**a**) Conventional white light endoscopy shows a flat lesion with coarsening of the mucosa and surface granularity in the middle esophagus. (**b**) Non-magnifying endoscopy with narrow-band imaging of the corresponding lesion. (**c**) Chromoendoscopy with iodine staining demarcates the lesion from the non-neoplastic area. (**d**) Circumferential mucosal precutting after submucosal injection. (**e**) Artificial ulcer after submucosal dissection. (**f**) En bloc resection by endoscopic submucosal dissection and iodine staining

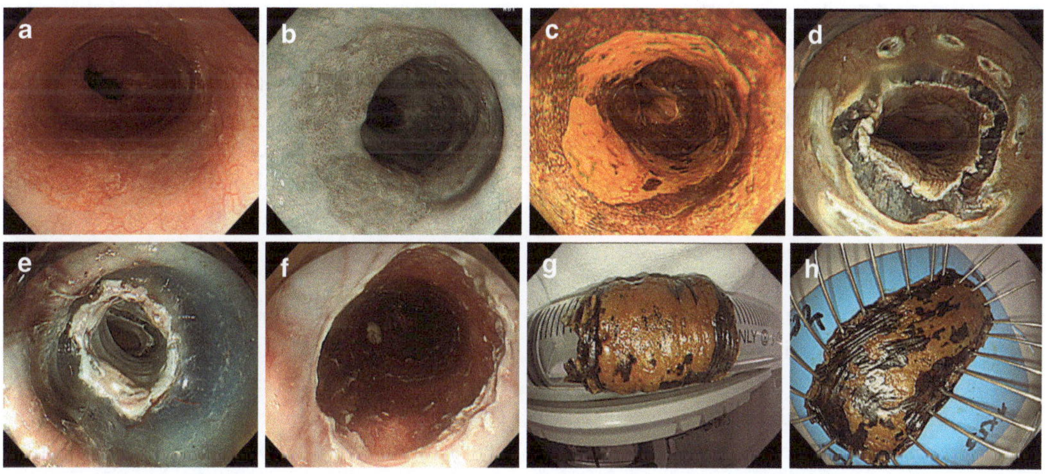

Fig. 2 Endoscopic circumferential submucosal dissection of superficial esophageal neoplasm. (**a**) Conventional white light endoscopy shows a flat lesion that affects the entire circumference of the lower esophagus. (**b**) Non-magnifying endoscopy with narrow-band imaging of the corresponding lesion. (**c**) Chromoendoscopy with iodine staining demarcates the circumferential lesion from the nonneoplastic area. (**d**) Circumferential mucosal precutting after submucosal injection. (**e**) Circumferential submucosal dissection. (**f**) Artificial ulcer after submucosal dissection. (**g**) En bloc resection by endoscopic circumferential submucosal dissection. (**h**) Resected specimen after iodine staining

A recent meta-analysis of 20 studies revealed that patients receiving ESD had a significantly higher en bloc resection rate, curative resection rate, and R0 resection rate compared to EMR, regardless of the size of the lesion [22]. However, when tumor size was ≤10 mm, there was no significant difference between the ESD and EMR in en bloc resection and curative resection, and the R0 resection rate was similar for lesions ≤20 mm in size for both the ESD and EMR groups [22]. The procedure time was longer in ESD compared to EMR of any size, and the risk of perforation was also higher in the ESD group [22]. Therefore, for better treatment results, ESD is a better method than EMR for endoscopic resection of superficial esophageal cancer [6, 7, 19].

However, ESD is technically difficult and a more time-consuming procedure than EMR; in addition, the complication rate is higher. Therefore, the potential of EMR in treating small tumors (≤10–20 mm sized tumor) should not be underestimated, as it achieves good en bloc, curative resection, and R0 resection rates with fewer complications [22].

Outcomes of Endoscopic Resection

The outcomes of endoscopic resection treatment in superficial esophageal cancer are excellent. After an average of 50 months of follow-up of 402 patients following endoscopic resection, the 5-year survival rate was 90.5% if the tumor was confined to the intraepithelial layer or the lamina propria layer. However, the survival rate was lower, 71.1% and 70.8%, respectively, when the tumor invaded muscularis mucosa layer or submucosa layer [23].

The survival rate and the risk of metastasis are closely related to the depth of tumor invasion, especially in mucosal cancer, and the risk of metastasis is significantly higher when the vascular or lymphatic invasion is present. Other studies have reported that the en bloc resection rate and the complete resection rate of ESD in 373 superficial esophageal cancers were 96.7% and 84.5%, respectively, and a 5-year disease-free survival rate was 84.8% after curative resection [24].

In previous studies, the en bloc resection and the curative resection rate of endoscopic resection were reported to range from 80.3%–97.2% and 81.8%–91.7%, respectively, and the frequency of recurrence or deaths related to esophageal cancer was very low [21, 25–27]. A single institution study analyzed the results of 261 ESD lesions subjected to en bloc resection and complete resection; the rates were 93.9% and 89.7%, respectively, and the 5-year disease-specific survival (DSS) rate was 100% during a median 35-month follow-up period [26]. Studies comparing ESD and surgical treatment also showed that the overall survival and DSS rates of patients with ESD were 93.9% and 92.8%, respectively, for patients receiving surgery when compared to 120 pairs of patients using propensity score matching [12]. In a recent meta-analysis of clinical outcomes between the ESD and the surgery group, the 5-year survival rate (86.4% and 81.8%, respectively) and the DSS rate (97.5% and 94.1%, respectively) were similar, but ESD was associated with fewer adverse events [28]. The rates of complications related to treatment were significantly higher in the surgery group (55.5%) than in the endoscopic treatment group (18.5%). Therefore, endoscopic resection for superficial esophageal cancer showed similar clinical outcomes compared to surgery and allowed patients to preserve quality of life [21, 25, 26].

Complications of endoscopic treatment include bleeding, perforation, and stenosis. Endoscopic resection of esophageal disease is technically difficult because the esophagus has a narrow and curved lumen and is influenced by the heartbeat or breathing of the patient. In addition, the risk of perforation is higher as compared to the stomach because the esophageal wall is relatively thin and there is no serosa in the esophagus. In addition to these anatomical factors, the experience and proficiency of the endoscopist also influence the occurrence of complications, so it is desirable for an experienced endoscopist to perform the procedure under general anesthesia [24]. Bleeding associated with the procedure has been reported in 0–5.6% and perforation in 4–9.3% cases, and most events could be successfully treated with endoscopic hemostasis or closure [12, 24–26, 29].

Endoscopists should consider prevention and management of stricture after endoscopic treatment in superficial esophageal cancer (Fig. 3). After endoscopic treatment, stricture occurs in 5.4–13.9% cases, especially if mucosal defects after resection account for more than 75% of the circumference. The risk of stricture is very high, so additional treatments are needed to prevent stricture [12, 24–26, 29]. Balloon dilatation can be performed as a treatment after stricture occurs; however, repetitive procedures are usually required [30, 31]. A method of temporary insertion and removal of the esophageal stent can also be used [32]. In patients who are expected to present stricture after the procedure, local steroids can be injected into the submucosal layer immediately after the procedure, or oral steroids can be used to reduce the incidence of stricture [33–35]. A total of 12 network meta-analysis studies including 513 patients showed that steroid injection or oral steroid can reduce the risk of stricture and the number of balloon dilation treatments compared to the control group [36]. However, the prevention and treatment methods for stricture have not yet been standardized and attempts at novel approaches as well as studies comparing the effects of current methods are still needed (Fig. 4).

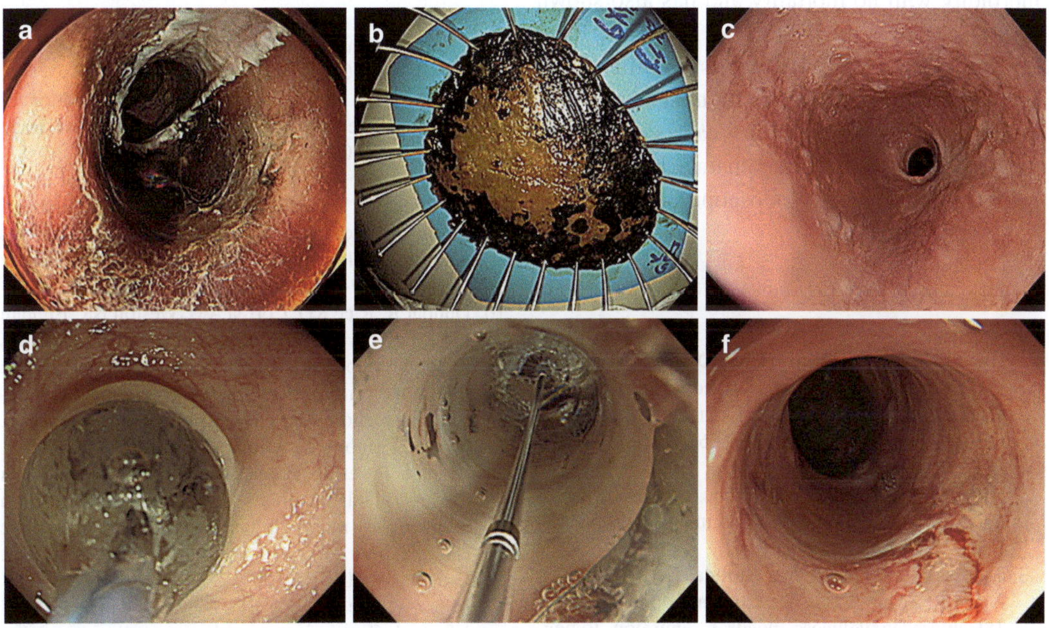

Fig. 3 Esophageal ballooning for stricture after endoscopic submucosal dissection. (**a**) Esophageal ulcer immediately after endoscopic submucosal dissection affecting approximately 90% of the lumen. (**b**) En bloc resection by endoscopic submucosal dissection and iodine staining. (**c**) Luminal stricture at the site of the ESD scar. (**d**) Endoscopic balloon dilation at the stricture site. (**e**) Direct endoscopic visualization. (**f**) Dilated stricture site after endoscopic ballooning

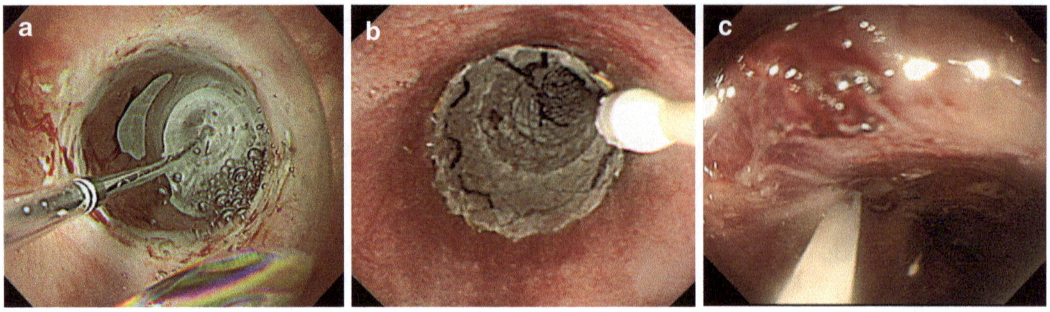

Fig. 4 Various methods for treating or preventing esophageal stricture after submucosal dissection. (**a**) Endoscopic balloon dilatation. (**b**) Temporary endoscopic insertion of a stent. (**c**) Steroid injection into the esophageal ulcer immediately after endoscopic submucosal dissection

Conclusions

Endoscopic resection for superficial esophageal cancer is usually associated with a low risk of morbidity with no mortality and has also shown favorable long-term outcomes. However, there remains a long-term risk of metastasis after endoscopic resection and complications such as perforation, bleeding, and stricture can occur, which vary according to the tumor characteristics, treatment modality, and the endoscopist experience.

References

1. Huh CW, Jung DH, Kim JH, Ma DW, Youn YH, Park H. Clinical implication of endoscopic gross appearance in superficial esophageal squamous carcinoma: revisited. Surg Endosc. 2018;32:367–75.
2. Choi JY, Park YS, Jung HY, Ahn JY, Kim MY, Lee JH, et al. Feasibility of endoscopic resection in superficial esophageal squamous carcinoma. Gastrointest Endosc. 2011;73(881–9):9.e1–2.
3. Tsurusaki M, Okada M, Kuroda H, Matsuki M, Ishii K, Murakami T. Clinical application of 18F-fluorodeoxyglucose positron emission tomography for assessment and evaluation after therapy for malignant hepatic tumor. J Gastroenterol. 2014;49:46–56.
4. Akutsu Y, Uesato M, Shuto K, Kono T, Hoshino I, Horibe D, et al. The overall prevalence of metastasis in T1 esophageal squamous cell carcinoma: a retrospective analysis of 295 patients. Ann Surg. 2013;257:1032–8.
5. Kim DU, Lee JH, Min BH, Shim SG, Chang DK, Kim YH, et al. Risk factors of lymph node metastasis in T1 esophageal squamous cell carcinoma. J Gastroenterol Hepatol. 2008;23:619–25.
6. Anonymous. Japanese classification of esophageal cancer, 11th edition: part I. Esophagus. 2017;14:1–36.
7. Pimentel-Nunes P, Dinis-Ribeiro M, Ponchon T, Repici A, Vieth M, De Ceglie A, et al. Endoscopic submucosal dissection: European Society of Gastrointestinal Endoscopy (ESGE) Guideline. Endoscopy. 2015;47:829–54.
8. Anonymous. Update on the Paris classification of superficial neoplastic lesions in the digestive tract. Endoscopy. 2005;37:570–8.
9. Lee WC, Lee TH, Jang JY, Lee JS, Cho JY, Lee JS, et al. Staging accuracy of endoscopic ultrasound performed by nonexpert endosonographers in patients with resectable esophageal squamous cell carcinoma: is it possible? Dis Esophagus. 2015;28:574–8.
10. Dhupar R, Rice RD, Correa AM, Weston BR, Bhutani MS, Maru DM, et al. Endoscopic ultrasound estimates for tumor depth at the gastroesophageal junction are inaccurate: implications for the Liberal use of endoscopic resection. Ann Thorac Surg. 2015;100:1812–6.
11. Oyama T, Inoue H, Arima M, Momma K, Omori T, Ishihara R, et al. Prediction of the invasion depth of superficial squamous cell carcinoma based on microvessel morphology: magnifying endoscopic classification of the Japan esophageal society. Esophagus. 2017;14:105–12.
12. Min YW, Lee H, Song BG, Min BH, Kim HK, Choi YS, et al. Comparison of endoscopic submucosal dissection and surgery for superficial esophageal squamous cell carcinoma: a propensity score-matched analysis. Gastrointest Endosc. 2018;88:624–33.
13. Zhang Y, Ding H, Chen T, Zhang X, Chen WF, Li Q, et al. Outcomes of endoscopic submucosal dissection vs esophagectomy for T1 esophageal squamous cell carcinoma in a real-world cohort. Clin Gastroenterol Hepatol. 2019;17:73–81.e3.
14. Chang AC, Ji H, Birkmeyer NJ, Orringer MB, Birkmeyer JD. Outcomes after transhiatal and trans-

thoracic esophagectomy for cancer. Ann Thorac Surg. 2008;85:424–9.
15. Ra J, Paulson EC, Kucharczuk J, Armstrong K, Wirtalla C, Rapaport-Kelz R, et al. Postoperative mortality after esophagectomy for cancer: development of a preoperative risk prediction model. Ann Surg Oncol. 2008;15:1577–84.
16. Connors RC, Reuben BC, Neumayer LA, Bull DA. Comparing outcomes after transthoracic and transhiatal esophagectomy: a 5-year prospective cohort of 17,395 patients. J Am Coll Surg. 2007;205:735–40.
17. Park CH, Yang DH, Kim JW, Kim JH, Kim JH, Min YW, et al. Clinical practice guideline for endoscopic resection of early gastrointestinal cancer. Clin Endosc. 2020;53:142–66.
18. Ajani JA, D'Amico TA, Almhanna K, Bentrem DJ, Besh S, Chao J, et al. Esophageal and esophagogastric junction cancers, version 1.2015. J Natl Compr Cancer Netw. 2015;13:194–227.
19. Takahashi H, Arimura Y, Masao H, Okahara S, Tanuma T, Kodaira J, et al. Endoscopic submucosal dissection is superior to conventional endoscopic resection as a curative treatment for early squamous cell carcinoma of the esophagus (with video). Gastrointest Endosc. 2010;72:255–64, 64.e1–2
20. Ishihara R, Iishi H, Uedo N, Takeuchi Y, Yamamoto S, Yamada T, et al. Comparison of EMR and endoscopic submucosal dissection for en bloc resection of early esophageal cancers in Japan. Gastrointest Endosc. 2008;68:1066–72.
21. Kim DH, Jung HY, Gong EJ, Choi JY, Ahn JY, Kim MY, et al. Endoscopic and oncologic outcomes of endoscopic resection for superficial esophageal neoplasm. Gut Liver. 2015;9:470–7.
22. Han C, Sun Y. Efficacy and safety of endoscopic submucosal dissection versus endoscopic mucosal resection for superficial esophageal carcinoma: a systematic review and meta-analysis. Dis Esophagus. 2021;34:doaa081.
23. Yamashina T, Ishihara R, Nagai K, Matsuura N, Matsui F, Ito T, et al. Long-term outcome and metastatic risk after endoscopic resection of superficial esophageal squamous cell carcinoma. Am J Gastroenterol. 2013;108:544–51.
24. Tsujii Y, Nishida T, Nishiyama O, Yamamoto K, Kawai N, Yamaguchi S, et al. Clinical outcomes of endoscopic submucosal dissection for superficial esophageal neoplasms: a multicenter retrospective cohort study. Endoscopy. 2015;47:775–83.
25. Park JS, Youn YH, Park JJ, Kim JH, Park H. Clinical outcomes of endoscopic submucosal dissection for superficial esophageal squamous neoplasms. Clin Endosc. 2016;49:168–75.
26. Park HC, Kim DH, Gong EJ, Na HK, Ahn JY, Lee JH, et al. Ten-year experience of esophageal endoscopic submucosal dissection of superficial esophageal neoplasms in a single center. Korean J Intern Med. 2016;31:1064–72.
27. Hsu MH, Wang WL, Chen TH, Tai CM, Wang HP, Lee CT. Long-term outcomes of endoscopic submucosal dissection for superficial esophageal squamous cell carcinoma in Taiwan. BMC Gastroenterol. 2021;21:308.
28. Yeh JH, Huang RY, Lee CT, Lin CW, Hsu MH, Wu TC, et al. Long-term outcomes of endoscopic submucosal dissection and comparison to surgery for superficial esophageal squamous cancer: a systematic review and meta-analysis. Ther Adv Gastroenterol. 2020;13:1756284820964316.
29. Joo DC, Kim GH, Park DY, Jhi JH, Song GA. Long-term outcome after endoscopic submucosal dissection in patients with superficial esophageal squamous cell carcinoma: a single-center study. Gut Liver. 2014;8:612–8.
30. Lian JJ, Ma LL, Hu JW, Chen SY, Qin WZ, Xu MD, et al. Endoscopic balloon dilatation for benign esophageal stricture after endoscopic submucosal dissection for early esophageal neoplasms. J Dig Dis. 2014;15:224–9.
31. Ezoe Y, Muto M, Horimatsu T, Morita S, Miyamoto S, Mochizuki S, et al. Efficacy of preventive endoscopic balloon dilation for esophageal stricture after endoscopic resection. J Clin Gastroenterol. 2011;45:222–7.
32. Wen J, Lu Z, Yang Y, Liu Q, Yang J, Wang S, et al. Preventing stricture formation by covered esophageal stent placement after endoscopic submucosal dissection for early esophageal cancer. Dig Dis Sci. 2014;59:658–63.
33. Isomoto H, Yamaguchi N, Nakayama T, Hayashi T, Nishiyama H, Ohnita K, et al. Management of esophageal stricture after complete circular endoscopic submucosal dissection for superficial esophageal squamous cell carcinoma. BMC Gastroenterol. 2011;11:46.
34. Hashimoto S, Kobayashi M, Takeuchi M, Sato Y, Narisawa R, Aoyagi Y. The efficacy of endoscopic triamcinolone injection for the prevention of esophageal stricture after endoscopic submucosal dissection. Gastrointest Endosc. 2011;74:1389–93.
35. Kataoka M, Anzai S, Shirasaki T, Ikemiyagi H, Fujii T, Mabuchi K, et al. Efficacy of short period, low dose oral prednisolone for the prevention of stricture after circumferential endoscopic submucosal dissection (ESD) for esophageal cancer. Endosc Int Open. 2015;3:E113–7.
36. Wang W, Ma Z. Steroid administration is effective to prevent strictures after endoscopic esophageal submucosal dissection: a network meta-analysis. Medicine (Baltimore). 2015;94:e1664.

Surgical Resection and Perioperative Chemotherapy

> **Key Points**
> - Surgery alone in resectable esophageal cancer is invasive and associated with a high incidence of morbidity and mortality.
> - Preoperative chemoradiotherapy followed by surgery results in an optimal outcome while managing locally advanced esophageal cancer.
> - A complete pathological response to preoperative chemoradiotherapy is the important factor to obtain a survival benefit.
> - Postoperative management is based on surgical margin, nodal status, differentiation grade, and previous treatment.

Introduction

In general, patients with locally advanced esophageal cancer (cT1N+ and cT2-4aN0-3) are potential candidates for surgical resection. However, esophagectomy is a particularly complicated surgical procedure and is associated with high perioperative morbidity and mortality. A recent review of the Surveillance, Epidemiology, and End Result (SEER) database demonstrated that esophagectomy mortality increased from 8.9% at the 30-day follow-up to 15.8% at 90 days [1]. In addition, unsatisfactory treatment results are achieved due to the high rate of local and systemic recurrence and postoperative complications. In fact, the 5-year survival rate of surgery alone in locally advanced esophageal cancer is reported to be less than 20–30% [2]. Therefore, there is a worldwide consensus that surgery alone should no longer be the standard of care for the treatment of esophageal cancer. In esophageal cancer, many studies have been conducted evaluating the efficacy of chemotherapy (CT) and radiotherapy (RT) as preoperative or postoperative therapy to improve the long-term survival following surgical resection by improving the control of micrometastases and the resection rate through tumor downsizing. This review summarizes recent progress in the multidisciplinary treatment of locally advanced esophageal cancer.

Preoperative Chemotherapy and Chemoradiotherapy

Outcome of Preoperative Chemotherapy and Radiotherapy

In locally advanced esophageal cancer, several studies have been conducted in an attempt to increase the effectiveness of surgical treatment through preoperative CT and RT because the effects of surgery alone do not meet expectations.

Young Sin Cho is the lead author of this chapter.

H. J. Chun et al., *Gastrointestinal Cancer*, https://doi.org/10.1007/978-981-99-0815-8_16

In a meta-analysis comparing a surgery-alone group and a preoperative RT group, preoperative RT was found to lower the risk of death by 11% compared to surgery alone but did not show a statistically significant improvement in the survival rate [3]. A meta-analysis of preoperative CT in 2122 patients with esophageal cancer showed that the preoperative CT group achieved a significant survival benefit compared to the surgery-alone group (hazard ratio [HR] = 0.88; 95% confidence interval [CI], 0.80–0.96, $p = 0.003$) [4]. In another meta-analysis, preoperative CT showed a survival benefit when compared to surgery alone, especially when tumors were limited to adenocarcinoma (HR = 0.83, 95% CI, 0.71–0.95, $p = 0.01$). However, when the target group was limited to squamous cell carcinoma, preoperative chemotherapy did not show a significant reduction in mortality compared to the surgery-alone group (HR = 0.92; 95% CI, 0.81–1.04, $p = 0.18$) [5]. In a meta-analysis of perioperative CT and surgery alone, perioperative CT overall survival (OS) (HR, 0.73; 95% CI, 0.61–0.88), disease-free survival (HR, 0.65; 95% CI, 0.48–0.89), and progression-free survival (PFS) (HR, 0.66; 95% CI, 0.53–0.81) showed a significant effect [6].

Outcome of Preoperative Chemoradiotherapy

Under the theoretical background of CT reducing cancer mass and increasing the therapeutic effect of RT, studies have attempted a combination treatment using concurrent chemoradiotherapy (CRT) and surgery. The CROSS trial [7, 8] was a landmark trial comparing preoperative CRT with surgery alone. In this study, preoperative CRT was associated with improved OS, pathological complete response (pCR), R0 resection (no cancer at the resection margin), and PFS compared to surgery alone in patients with locally advanced esophageal cancer (Table 1). In the NEOCRTEC5010 trial [9] that enrolled patients with squamous cell carcinoma of the esophagus, the preoperative CRT group had a higher rate of R0 resection (98.4% vs. 91.2%; $p = 0.002$), a better median OS (100.1 vs 66.5 months; $p = 0.03$), and a prolonged disease-free survival (100.1 vs. 41.7 months; $p = 0.001$) compared to the surgery-alone group. In a recent network meta-analysis [10], preoperative CRT reported a HR of 0.75 compared to surgery alone and additionally reported that preoperative CRT was more effective in OS than preoperative CT (Table 2).

Table 1 Summary of the CROSS trial assessing the role of preoperative chemoradiotherapy in esophageal cancer

Parameter	Preoperative chemoradiotherapy	Surgery alone	*P*-value
Subjects, *n*	178	188	>0.05
Adenocarcinoma/squamous carcinoma, *n*	134/41	141/43	
Complete resection (R0), %	92	69	<0.001
Postoperative complications, *n*	46	44	
Pulmonary	22	30	
Anastomotic leakage			
Death (in hospital/30 days)	4/2	4/3	
Median OS, months	49.4	24	0.003
DFS (5 years), %	44	27	<0.001
OS (5 years), %	47	33	<0.05

DFS disease-free survival; *OS* overall survival
Adapted from van Hagen et al. [7]

Table 2 Network meta-analysis of preoperative therapy for locally advanced, resectable esophageal cancer

Parameter	Preoperative CT vs. surgery alone	Preoperative RT vs. surgery alone	Preoperative CRT vs. surgery alone	Preoperative CRT vs. surgery alone
Overall survival	HR 0.91 (95% CR 0.81–1.03)	HR 0.93 (95% CR 0.80–1.07)	HR 0.75 (95% CR 0.67–0.85)	HR 0.83 (95% CR 0.70–0.96)
Postoperative mortality	RR 0.93 (95% CR 0.68–1.26)	RR 1.14 (95% CR 0.76–1.72)	RR 1.46 (95% CR 1.00–2.14)	RR 1.58 (95% CR 1.00–2.49)
Locoregional recurrence	RR 0.80 (95% CR 0.64–1.00)	RR 0.39 (95% CR 0.08–1.98)	RR 0.57 (95% CR 0.45–0.72)	RR 0.72 (95% CR 0.54–0.95)
Distant metastases	RR 1.00 (95% CR 0.82–1.22)	RR 0.98 (95% CR 0.36–2.70)	RR 0.91 (95% CR 0.77–1.06)	RR 0.90 (95% CR 0.71–1.14)
Locoregional and distant metastases	RR 1.07 (95% CR 0.77–1.50)	RR 0.98 (95% CR 0.06–15.68)	RR 0.67 (95% CR 0.43–1.03)	RR 0.62 (95% CR 0.37–1.05)

CR credible region; *CT* chemotherapy; *CRT* chemoradiotherapy; *CR* credible region; *HR* hazard ratio; *RR* risk ratio; *RT* radiotherapy
Adapted from van Chan et al. [10]

Table 3 Network meta-analysis of preoperative therapy for locally advanced, resectable esophageal cancer

Guidelines	Statement	Level of evidence and grade of recommendation
ESMO [11]	Patients with locally advanced SCC benefit from preoperative chemotherapy or, most likely to a greater extent, from preoperative CRT, with higher rates of complete tumor resection and better local tumor control and survival	I/A
NCCN [12]	Preoperative CRT is the preferred approach for localized adenocarcinoma of the thoracic esophagus or EGJ. Perioperative chemotherapy is an alternative option for distal esophagus and EGJ	2/A
ASCO [6]	Preoperative CRT or perioperative CT should be offered to patients with locally advanced esophageal adenocarcinoma. Preoperative CRT or CRT without surgery should be offered to patients with locally advanced esophageal squamous cell carcinoma	Moderate/strong

SCC squamous cell carcinoma; *CRT* chemoradiotherapy; *EGJ* esophagogastric junction; *CT* chemotherapy

Therefore, the main guidelines for esophageal cancer recommend preoperative CRT as the preferred approach for locally advanced esophageal cancer (Table 3) [6, 11, 12].

Pathological Response of Preoperative Chemoradiotherapy

In previous studies, the rate of pCR to preoperative CRT was reported to be 15–43% (Table 4) [7, 13–23]. Burmeister et al. [17] showed that pCR was more common in patients with esophageal squamous cell carcinoma than in adenocarcinoma. In general, it is reported that confirmed pCR after preoperative CRT was associated with the survival rate of patients with esophageal cancer. In a study by Saeki et al. [23], the pathological effectiveness of preoperative CRT was classified into grades 0–1 (ineffective and lightly effective), grade 2 (moderately effective), and grade 3 (markedly effective), and the 5-year survival rate was 36.9%, 53.8%, and 100%, respectively. Hsu et al. [24] reported that nonresponders to preoperative CRT had no benefit and worse outcomes compared to those who underwent primary resection for locally advanced esophageal cancer. Therefore, it is necessary to identify predictors of pathological response after preoperative CRT in locally advanced esophageal cancer. In previous studies, older age, smoking, and tumor length exceeding 3 cm were reported as predictors of pCR [25]. In addition, biochemical and molecular markers such as the neutrophil-to-lymphocyte ratio and *TP53* mutation status have been reported as predictive factors in the evaluation of treatment response to preoperative CRT [26].

Table 4 Pathological efficacy of preoperative chemoradiotherapy

Author	Year	Histology	Number of patients	pCR (%)
Bosset et al. [13]	1997	SCC	Preoperative CRT 143/ surgery 139	26
Urba et al. [14]	2001	AC 75%/SCC 25%	Preoperative CRT 50/ surgery 50	28
Heise et al. [15]	2001	SCC	Preoperative CRT 33/ surgery 170	33
Lee et al. [16]	2004	SCC	Preoperative CRT 51/ surgery 50	43
Burmeister et al. [17]	2005	AC 62%/SCC 37%	Preoperative CRT 128/ surgery 128	16
Natsugoe et al. [18]	2006	SCC	Preoperative CRT 22/ surgery 23	15
Tepper et al. [19]	2008	AC 75%/SCC 25%	Preoperative CRT 30/ surgery 26	40
Cao et al. [20]	2009	SCC	Preoperative CRT 118/ surgery 118	22.3
Van Hagen et al. [7]	2012	AC 75%/SCC 23%	Preoperative CRT 178/ surgery 188	29
Chen et al. [21]	2012	SCC	Preoperative CRT 57/ surgery 14	37
Fujiwara et al. [22]	2013	SCC	Preoperative CRT 52/ surgery 36	30.8
Saeki et al. [23]	2013	SCC	Preoperative CRT 76/ surgery 921	21.1

SCC squamous cell carcinoma; *AC* adenocarcinoma; *pCR* pathological complete response; *CRT* chemoradiotherapy

Ideal Timing for Surgery

Although preoperative CT or CRT shows an effective outcome in locally advanced esophageal cancer, the ideal time between preoperative CT or CRT and surgery has not yet been established. However, optimal surgery timing is important because early surgery has a higher risk of side effects and late surgery increases the risk of cancer progression. In landmark preoperative CT trials, the preoperative interval was performed 2–6 weeks after CT [27, 28]. In the case of preoperative CRT, an interval of 4–6 weeks was recommended in the CROSS trial [7]. However, there is an opinion that a longer interval after CT increases the chance of a pCR and lowers the risk of postoperative complications due to fibrosis after RT. Therefore, in the Enhanced Recovery After Surgery (ERAS) guidelines [29], the recommended optimal time for surgery after preoperative CT is 3–6 weeks after CT completion. Furthermore, the optimal time for surgery after preoperative CRT is 6–10 weeks after the completion of RT.

Perioperative Chemotherapy/ Chemoradiotherapy

Surgical Approach

Esophageal surgery should be considered for all medically fit patients with resectable esophageal cancer (>5 cm from the cricopharyngeus). R0 resection is important for the prognosis of esophageal cancer. Presently, esophagectomy is performed using a thoracoabdominal or transhiatal approach using an open or minimally invasive technique. Minimally invasive esophagectomy has a lower perioperative complication rate and lower in-hospital mortality than open esophagectomy [30]. The Siewert tumor type should be

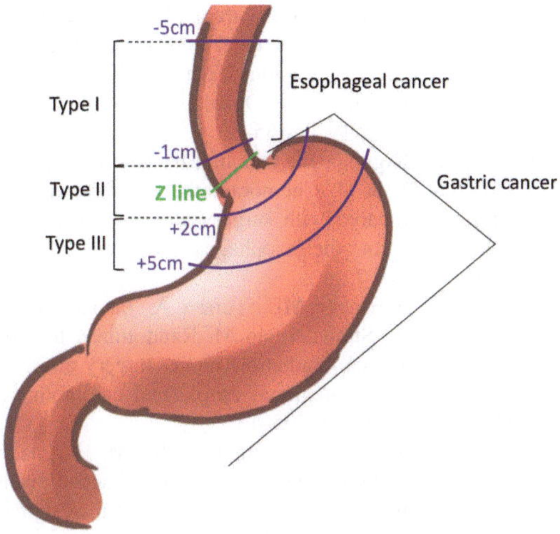

Fig. 1 Siewert classification esophagogastric junction tumor (EGJ). **Type I**: adenocarcinoma of the distal esophagus (epicenter of lesion 1–5 cm above the EGJ). **Type II**: adenocarcinoma of the cardia (epicenter of lesion up to 1 cm above and 2 cm below the EGJ). **Type III**: sub-cardial-type adenocarcinoma (epicenter of lesion 2–5 cm below the EGJ). (Adapted from Siewert et al. [31])

assessed in all patients with adenocarcinoma involving the gastroesophageal junction [31] (Fig. 1). The Siewert classification has implications for lymph node spread and is the most widely used classification [32]. Prognosis has been shown to differ according to the frequency of esophagectomy, and the overall mortality rate was lower in higher volume center than in low volume center (HR, 0.82; 95% CI 0.75–0.90) [33]. Patients who have undergone esophagectomy often have certain survival problems, including decreased quality of life (QoL), eating disorders, and malnutrition, and poor long-term survival. A population-based cohort study found that surgery can have a strong negative effect on several health-related QoL measures such as reflux, dysphagia, and eating disorders up to 10 years after surgery [34].

Postoperative Management

Postoperative management is based on surgical margin, nodal status, differentiation grade, and previous treatment, but to date there is insufficient evidence on the efficacy of postoperative CT. The National Comprehensive Cancer Network recommends their management by classifying tumors into squamous cell carcinoma and adenocarcinoma [12]. In squamous cell carcinoma, CRT or palliative management is considered for R1 (microscopic residual cancer) or R2 (macroscopic residual cancer) resection, and surveillance is recommended for R0 resection. Nivolumab may be considered if there is residual cancer in patients undergoing preoperative CRT [35]. In adenocarcinoma, surveillance is recommended for patients with R0 and negative nodal status, but CRT is recommended as an alternative option for patients with pT3–4 or pT2 with high-risk features (i.e., poorly differentiated or higher-grade cancer, lymphovascular invasion, perineural invasion, or age < 50 years). CT or CRT is recommended for patients with R0 resection and negative nodal status. In patients with R1 or R2 resection, CRT or palliative management is recommended depending on the patient's condition. All patients who underwent R0 resection and received preoperative therapy can be monitored until disease progression, regardless of the status of the nodule. Because perioperative CT showed an improvement in PFS and OS over surgery alone [36], perioperative CT is recommended for patients with completely resected, nodular-negative, or nodular-positive disease. Postoperative CRT is not recommended for patients with node-positive disease after R0 resection. Patients with R1 or R2 resection should be treated with CRT, if not received preoperatively. Alternatively, patients with R1 resection can be observed until disease progression or may be considered for re-resection. Palliative care is an alternative option for patients with R2 resection.

Conclusion

Although esophageal resection is a cornerstone of curative treatment for patients with locally advanced esophageal cancer, perioperative therapy has been introduced to compensate for its high morbidity and mortality. In the future, it will be necessary to confirm the results of clinical trials using appropriate strategies based on the histological type and stage.

References

1. Walters DM, McMurry TL, Isbell JM, Stukenborg GJ, Kozower BD. Understanding mortality as a quality indicator after esophagectomy. Ann Thorac Surg. 2014;98:506–11; discussion 11–2.
2. Rice TW, Rusch VW, Apperson-Hansen C, Allen MS, Chen LQ, Hunter JG, et al. Worldwide esophageal cancer collaboration. Dis Esophagus. 2009;22:1–8.
3. Arnott SJ, Duncan W, Gignoux M, Hansen HS, Launois B, Nygaard K, et al. Preoperative radiotherapy for esophageal carcinoma. Cochrane Database Syst Rev. 2005;2005:Cd001799.
4. Kidane B, Coughlin S, Vogt K, Malthaner R. Preoperative chemotherapy for resectable thoracic esophageal cancer. Cochrane Database Syst Rev. 2015;2015:Cd001556.
5. Sjoquist KM, Burmeister BH, Smithers BM, Zalcberg JR, Simes RJ, Barbour A, et al. Survival after neoadjuvant chemotherapy or chemoradiotherapy for resectable oesophageal carcinoma: an updated meta-analysis. Lancet Oncol. 2011;12:681–92.
6. Shah MA, Kennedy EB, Catenacci DV, Deighton DC, Goodman KA, Malhotra NK, et al. Treatment of locally advanced esophageal carcinoma: ASCO guideline. J Clin Oncol. 2020;38:2677–94.
7. van Hagen P, Hulshof MC, van Lanschot JJ, Steyerberg EW, van Berge Henegouwen MI, Wijnhoven BP, et al. Preoperative chemoradiotherapy for esophageal or junctional cancer. N Engl J Med. 2012;366:2074–84.
8. Shapiro J, van Lanschot JJB, Hulshof M, van Hagen P, van Berge Henegouwen MI, Wijnhoven BPL, et al. Neoadjuvant chemoradiotherapy plus surgery versus surgery alone for oesophageal or junctional cancer (CROSS): long-term results of a randomised controlled trial. Lancet Oncol. 2015;16:1090–8.
9. Yang H, Liu H, Chen Y, Zhu C, Fang W, Yu Z, et al. Neoadjuvant chemoradiotherapy followed by surgery versus surgery alone for locally advanced squamous cell carcinoma of the esophagus (NEOCRTEC5010): a phase III multicenter, randomized, open-label clinical trial. J Clin Oncol. 2018;36:2796–803.
10. Chan KKW, Saluja R, Delos Santos K, Lien K, Shah K, Cramarossa G, et al. Neoadjuvant treatments for locally advanced, resectable esophageal cancer: a network meta-analysis. Int J Cancer. 2018;143:430–7.
11. Lordick F, Mariette C, Haustermans K, Obermannová R, Arnold D. Oesophageal cancer: ESMO Clinical Practice Guidelines for diagnosis, treatment and follow-up. Ann Oncol. 2016;27:v50–v7.
12. Ajani JA, D'Amico TA, Bentrem DJ, Chao J, Corvera C, Das P, et al. Esophageal and Esophagogastric Junction Cancers, Version 2.2019, NCCN Clinical Practice Guidelines in Oncology. J Natl Compr Cancer Netw. 2019;17:855–83.
13. Bosset JF, Gignoux M, Triboulet JP, Tiret E, Mantion G, Elias D, et al. Chemoradiotherapy followed by surgery compared with surgery alone in squamous-cell cancer of the esophagus. N Engl J Med. 1997;337:161–7.
14. Urba SG, Orringer MB, Turrisi A, Iannettoni M, Forastiere A, Strawderman M. Randomized trial of preoperative chemoradiation versus surgery alone in patients with locoregional esophageal carcinoma. J Clin Oncol. 2001;19:305–13.
15. Heise JW, Heep H, Frieling T, Sarbia M, Hartmann KA, Röher HD. Expense and benefit of neoadjuvant treatment in squamous cell carcinoma of the esophagus. BMC Cancer. 2001;1:20.
16. Lee JL, Park SI, Kim SB, Jung HY, Lee GH, Kim JH, et al. A single institutional phase III trial of preoperative chemotherapy with hyperfractionation radiotherapy plus surgery versus surgery alone for resectable esophageal squamous cell carcinoma. Ann Oncol. 2004;15:947–54.
17. Burmeister BH, Smithers BM, Gebski V, Fitzgerald L, Simes RJ, Devitt P, et al. Surgery alone versus chemoradiotherapy followed by surgery for resectable cancer of the oesophagus: a randomised controlled phase III trial. Lancet Oncol. 2005;6:659–68.
18. Natsugoe S, Okumura H, Matsumoto M, Uchikado Y, Setoyama T, Yokomakura N, et al. Randomized controlled study on preoperative chemoradiotherapy followed by surgery versus surgery alone for esophageal squamous cell cancer in a single institution. Dis Esophagus. 2006;19:468–72.
19. Tepper J, Krasna MJ, Niedzwiecki D, Hollis D, Reed CE, Goldberg R, et al. Phase III trial of trimodality therapy with cisplatin, fluorouracil, radiotherapy, and surgery compared with surgery alone for esophageal cancer: CALGB 9781. J Clin Oncol. 2008;26:1086–92.
20. Cao XF, He XT, Ji L, Xiao J, Lv J. Effects of neoadjuvant radiochemotherapy on pathological staging and prognosis for locally advanced esophageal squamous cell carcinoma. Dis Esophagus. 2009;22:477–81.
21. Chen WH, Chao YK, Chang HK, Tseng CK, Wu YC, Liu YH, et al. Long-term outcomes following neoadjuvant chemoradiotherapy in patients with clinical T2N0 esophageal squamous cell carcinoma. Dis Esophagus. 2012;25:250–5.
22. Fujiwara Y, Yoshikawa R, Kamikonya N, Nakayama T, Kitani K, Tsujie M, et al. Neoadjuvant chemoradiotherapy followed by esophagectomy vs. surgery alone in the treatment of resectable esophageal squamous cell carcinoma. Mol Clin Oncol. 2013;1:773–9.
23. Saeki H, Morita M, Nakashima Y, Sonoda H, Hashimoto K, Egashira A, et al. Neoadjuvant chemoradiotherapy for clinical stage II-III esopha-

geal squamous cell carcinoma. Anticancer Res. 2011;31:3073–7.
24. Hsu PK, Chien LI, Huang CS, Hsieh CC, Wu YC, Hsu WH, et al. Comparison of survival among neoadjuvant chemoradiation responders, non-responders and patients receiving primary resection for locally advanced oesophageal squamous cell carcinoma: does neoadjuvant chemoradiation benefit all? Interact Cardiovasc Thorac Surg. 2013;17:460–6.
25. Huang RW, Chao YK, Wen YW, Chang HK, Tseng CK, Chan SC, et al. Predictors of pathological complete response to neoadjuvant chemoradiotherapy for esophageal squamous cell carcinoma. World J Surg Oncol. 2014;12:170.
26. Li Y, Liu J, Cai XW, Li HX, Cheng Y, Dong XH, et al. Biomarkers for the prediction of esophageal cancer neoadjuvant chemoradiotherapy response: a systemic review. Crit Rev Oncol Hematol. 2021;167:103466.
27. Cunningham D, Allum WH, Stenning SP, Thompson JN, Van de Velde CJ, Nicolson M, et al. Perioperative chemotherapy versus surgery alone for resectable gastroesophageal cancer. N Engl J Med. 2006;355:11–20.
28. Kelsen DP, Ginsberg R, Pajak TF, Sheahan DG, Gunderson L, Mortimer J, et al. Chemotherapy followed by surgery compared with surgery alone for localized esophageal cancer. N Engl J Med. 1998;339:1979–84.
29. Low DE, Allum W, De Manzoni G, Ferri L, Immanuel A, Kuppusamy M, et al. Guidelines for perioperative care in esophagectomy: enhanced recovery after surgery (ERAS(®)) society recommendations. World J Surg. 2019;43:299–330.
30. Yibulayin W, Abulizi S, Lv H, Sun W. Minimally invasive oesophagectomy versus open esophagectomy for resectable esophageal cancer: a meta-analysis. World J Surg Oncol. 2016;14:304.
31. Siewert JR, Stein HJ. Classification of adenocarcinoma of the oesophagogastric junction. Br J Surg. 1998;85:1457–9.
32. Zhang S, Orita H, Fukunaga T. Current surgical treatment of esophagogastric junction adenocarcinoma. World J Gastrointest Oncol. 2019;11:567–78.
33. Brusselaers N, Mattsson F, Lagergren J. Hospital and surgeon volume in relation to long-term survival after oesophagectomy: systematic review and meta-analysis. Gut. 2014;63:1393–400.
34. Schandl A, Lagergren J, Johar A, Lagergren P. Health-related quality of life 10 years after oesophageal cancer surgery. Eur J Cancer. 2016;69:43–50.
35. Kelly RJ, Ajani JA, Kuzdzal J, Zander T, Van Cutsem E, Piessen G, et al. Adjuvant nivolumab in resected esophageal or gastroesophageal junction cancer. N Engl J Med. 2021;384:1191–203.
36. Ychou M, Boige V, Pignon JP, Conroy T, Bouché O, Lebreton G, et al. Perioperative chemotherapy compared with surgery alone for resectable gastroesophageal adenocarcinoma: an FNCLCC and FFCD multicenter phase III trial. J Clin Oncol. 2011;29:1715–21.

Definitive Chemoradiotherapy

Key Points

- Chemotherapy and radiotherapy are synergistic in the treatment of esophageal cancer.
- Concurrent chemoradiotherapy or a combination of chemotherapy and radiotherapy provides at least equivalent oncological outcomes to surgery in resectable/locally advanced esophageal cancer.
- Definitive chemoradiotherapy and trimodality treatment have both been considered equivalent in overall survival, as well as progression-free survival. However, local disease control is better with trimodality treatment. Surgery-related complications and mortality compromise the benefits.
- Additional esophagectomy after chemoradiation may improve survival in patients achieving a chemoradiation response and in surgically fit conditions.
- New targeted agents and immune therapeutic agents are under investigation and will contribute to the treatment of esophageal cancer.

Introduction

Radiotherapy has been used as a substitute for surgery or to alleviate symptoms in patients who are unfit to undergo surgical treatment. However, the clinical outcomes of radiation therapy alone are unsatisfactory and are not recommended as an option for first-line treatment. When radiotherapy and chemotherapy are combined, the local cure rate and survival rate improve greatly, and several clinical studies have been published showing clinical outcomes close to those of surgery. Chemoradiotherapy (CRT) is used in lieu of surgery in patients with locally advanced esophageal cancer when the patient's general condition indicates the patient is unfit to receive surgery, and CRT also has been proven to play a role in increasing the complete resection rate and improving the survival. Nowadays, multidisciplinary treatment with surgery after chemoradiation is being established as standard treatment.

Radiotherapy exerts a lethal effect on cells by inducing DNA damage through a direct or indirect route. DNA damage can take many forms, but DNA double-strand break is the most biologically important. Radiation can break a double strand by directly irradiating ionizing particles to DNA. But the direct irradiation on water molecules, which occupy 80–90% of the cell and gen-

Dae Young Cheung is the lead author of this chapter.

H. J. Chun et al., *Gastrointestinal Cancer*, https://doi.org/10.1007/978-981-99-0815-8_17

erate DNA-damaging reactive oxygen species in response to irradiation, is the main mechanism. The mechanism by which chemotherapeutic agents increase the radiation lethality of cancer cells is not fully understood. The sensitization mechanism of cancer cells to radiation is hypothesized to include synergistic killing, reducing accelerated repopulation, cell cycle arrest in the radiosensitive phase, enhancement of radiation injury, and inhibition of DNA damage repair. Based on these theories, clinical studies on combination CRT have been conducted [1]. By confirming the combined effect of cisplatin and radiation treatment for non-small cell lung cancer, the role of chemotherapy as a radiosensitizer was firmly established [2].

Combination of Chemotherapy and Radiotherapy

The results of early monotherapy strategies for esophageal cancer were very poor. The long-term survival rate of radiotherapy alone was less than 10%, and even when a dose of 50 Gy or more was used, local control and distant failure rates reached 66%.

When chemotherapy was added to radiotherapy (CRT), the response rate improved. Single-center studies were the first to be conducted, and the results were reported. In a Japanese study in which bleomycin was combined with radiotherapy, the response rate was 69% [3]. When cisplatin and 5-fluorouracil (5-FU) were combined with radiotherapy with a total dose of 30 Gy, the median survival was 9.8 months, and the 2-year survival rate was 20% [4]. When the radiation dose was increased to 50 Gy, the median survival improved to 19 months, and the 2-year survival rate also improved to 36%. Even when 5-FU and mitomycin were combined with 60 Gy dose of radiotherapy, the median survival was 18 months, and 3-year survival was 29%. In particular, oncological outcomes differed according to stage of esophageal cancer, and the 3-year survival rate for stage I patients was 73% [5].

In 1992, the results of the RTOG85–01 of Radiation Therapy Oncology Group study, a representative randomized multicenter clinical study comparing definitive CRT (dCRT) and radiotherapy alone, were published [6]. In this study, 121 patients were randomized and each group received 64 Gy of radiotherapy alone or two cycles of 5-FU/cisplatin chemotherapy and 50 Gy of concurrent radiotherapy, followed by two cycles of 5-FU/cisplatin chemotherapy. The median survival duration of patients in dCRT group was 14.1 months, which was significantly better than the 9.3 months achieved by the radiotherapy alone group. The 5-year survival rate was 26% in the case of dCRT patients, but there were no survivors in the case of radiotherapy alone.

A phase 3 study by the Eastern Oncology Cooperative Group published in 1998 compared the effects of 60 Gy dose of radiotherapy with or without concurrent 5-FU and mitomycin C chemotherapy [7]. As a result of the study, the median survival duration and the 2-year survival rate of patients treated with dCRT were 14.8 months and 27%, which were significant improvement from those of 9.2 months and 12% of patients treated with radiotherapy alone ($p = 0.04$). In particular, tumor stage was analyzed as the only factor with significant differences in survival between patients in the same treatment group. Conversely, severe acute toxicity occurred in 44% of patients who received dCRT, and life-threatening toxicity occurred in 20% of patients. This was significantly different from the frequency of acute severe or life-threatening toxicity of 25% and 3%, respectively, of patients who received radiotherapy alone.

Based on the results of this series of studies, CRT has been established as the standard of care for locally advanced esophageal cancer. It should be noted that acute toxicity must be tolerated in return for benefits such as improved local control, decreased distant failure, and longer overall survival (OS), which can be obtained by adding chemotherapy to radiotherapy.

Definitive Chemoradiotherapy Versus Primary Surgery for Resectable Disease

Early-stage esophageal cancer can be cured with primary surgery. Considering clinical efficacy and safety, dCRT for early-stage esophageal cancer may be considered instead of primary surgery. Mottori et al. conducted a comparative study of esophagectomy and CRT in clinical T1bN0M0 esophageal cancer [8, 9]. Although there was an issue with stage underestimation, the results were quite clear. There were no significant differences in OS between the surgery group and the CRT group. Progression-free survival (PFS) was better in the primary surgery group, and the incidence of distant recurrence was similar. Surgery showed better local control, but the benefit did not include improved survival of the patients.

Teoh et al. from China reported the findings of a small randomized controlled trial [10]. All enrolled patients were in resectable disease stage and were assigned either to surgery or CRT (50–60 Gy with two cycles of cisplatin and 5-FU). Overall, the 5-year survival favored CRT, but the difference did not reach statistical significance (surgery 29.4% and CRT 50%, $p = 0.147$). The 5-year disease-free survival also showed a trend toward significance favoring CRT ($P = 0.068$). In the surgery group, postoperative mortality reached 6.8%.

In conclusion, surgery can provide better local control and probably improves recurrence-free survival; however, surgery-related mortality compromises the marginal benefit. Distant metastasis can occur beyond surgery and local treatment. Even for resectable esophageal cancer, dCRT is equivalent to surgery.

Radiation Dose Escalation in Concurrent Chemoradiotherapy

Clinical studies have also been conducted on whether radiation dose escalation can further improve the clinical effects of CRT combination therapy. The Intergroup (INT) 0123 trial, which was conducted with the expectation of reducing local failure and increasing survival rate, was a phase 3 clinical trial based on the previous design of the RTOG85-01 study stratified. However, the study was stopped because it was judged to have a low probability of a significant gain in the interim analysis. As a result, the median survival of the high-dose group was 13 months, which was shorter than that of the low-dose group, which was 18.1 months. Treatment-related toxicity was disproportionately higher in the high-dose group. As a result of this study, 50.4 Gy was established as the standard dose for combined treatment. To date, it is not clear whether radiation doses greater than 50 Gy may provide additional benefit to oncological outcomes.

Altered Fractionation in Chemoradiation

Instead of dose escalation, studies were also conducted on whether altered fractionation schemes are feasible and effective as a treatment strategy for esophageal cancer. This concept is based on the experience of head and neck cancer and lung cancer applied to esophageal cancer.

The Cleveland Clinic study published in 1997 was a phase 2 study that enrolled 74 patients. In the study, two courses of 5-FU and cisplatin chemotherapy were performed, and accelerated fractionation radiation (1.5 Gy twice daily to 45 Gy) was performed from the first day of each course [11]. Finally, 93% of the participating patients underwent surgery, and 27% showed no residual pathological evidence of tumor. However, 18% of the patients died during treatment, and most of the patients experienced preoperative toxicity.

A phase 2 clinical study at the Massachusetts General Hospital published in 2004 investigated the effects of fractionation radiation in 46 patients with stage T2-3N0-1M0 [12]. Two cycles of chemotherapy consisting of cisplatin, 5-FU, and paclitaxel were administered, and 58.5 Gy of radiation was divided into 34 fractions and administered bid as qd or as a booster dose. Finally, surgery was performed in 87% of the patients, and 45% of the patients who underwent the operation had a pathological complete response (pT0N0). The median survival time was 34 months, and the 5-year survival rate was 37%. Although the results of the study are encouraging, the fact that treatment-related toxicity increased to a significant level is another consideration for future studies.

Need for Surgery on Chemoradiotherapy: dCRT vs. Trimodality Therapy

Curative surgery serves as the most effective and meaningful treatment for various solid cancers, and the same is true for esophageal cancer. However, due to the anatomical and structural characteristics of the esophagus, radical surgery is difficult, and the risk of complications is very high. Therefore, the debate over whether adding surgical treatment to CRT, which is accepted as the standard treatment for esophageal cancer, would be beneficial in terms of oncological outcomes is still under consideration. This is because the balance between efforts to improve the disease control of esophageal cancer and effort to reduce the treatment-related mortality and morbidity is important.

For comparative evaluation of dCRT and neoadjuvant chemoradiation and surgery, i.e., trimodality therapy, two European studies are cited as representative. In a study conducted in France, a total of 259 patients with T3N0-1M0 thoracic esophageal cancer were enrolled [13]. The patients received two cycles of 5-FU and cisplatin and conventional (46 Gy in 4.5 weeks) or split course (15 Gy, days 1–5 and 22–26) concomitant radiotherapy. Patients with a response and no contraindication to either treatment were randomly assigned to surgery or continuation of chemoradiation (three cycles of FU/cisplatin and up to 20 Gy radiotherapy). The 2-year survival rate was 34% in the trimodality group versus 40% in the cCRT group (HR 0.90; adjusted $P = 0.44$). The median survival time was 17.7 months and 19.3 months, respectively. The 3-month mortality rate was 9.3% in the surgery group compared to 0.8% in the dCRT group. Therefore, the authors concluded that in patients who respond to chemoradiation, there is no benefit in adding surgery after chemoradiation compared to the continuation of additional chemoradiation.

At approximately the same time, a German study enrolled 172 patients with locally advanced squamous cell carcinoma of the esophagus [14]. Patients were randomly allocated to either induction chemotherapy followed by CRT (40 Gy) followed by surgery or the same induction chemotherapy followed by CRT (at least 65 Gy) without surgery. After 6 years of follow-up, OS was equivalent between the two treatment groups. However, treatment-related mortality was significantly increased in the surgery group than in the CRT group (12.8% vs. 3.5%, respectively; $p = 0.03$). The authors found that tumor response to induction chemotherapy could predict favorable outcomes in these high-risk patients, regardless of the treatment group. Two phase 3 studies reported very similar results; the reason both treatment strategies had the same OS was that surgery-related mortality and morbidity compromised the outcome gain obtained with multimodality treatment. Therefore, if the risk of surgery could be reduced and suitable patients for surgery may be selected, it can be expected that trimodality treatment will have a more favorable result.

Recent studies adopting the propensity score-matching approach report results that differ from the present opinions. A 2018 study by Barbetta et al. enrolled stage II and III patients and analyzed the results after propensity score-matching [15]. The results showed that the median OS and disease-free survival were 3.1 and 1.8 years for trimodality versus 2.3 and 1.0 years for dCRT, respectively. Surgery was independently associated with improved OS (hazard ratio [HR], 0.57; 95% confidence interval [CI], 0.34–0.97; $p = 0.039$) and disease-free survival (HR, 0.51; 95% CI, 0.32–0.83; $p = 0.007$). In a recent meta-analysis including this study, neoadjuvant CRT with surgery had superior OS compared to dCRT, HR was 0.55 (95% CI 0.49–0.62), and complications and toxicity induced by the two treatment strategies were similar [16].

If esophageal cancer patients are equally suitable for both dCRT and neoadjuvant CRT with surgery, the results of both treatment strategies are likely to be equally effective. However, the patients encountered in real-world practice are more likely to be relatively better suited to a specific treatment. Therefore, it is not easy to ignore these factors and perform randomization and treatment. Considering the existence of residual and inherent confounding in prospective randomized studies as well as in all retrospective cohort studies to date, the results of previous studies should be accepted. Toxicity is a very important factor to consider in the decision and implementation of a treatment strategy. Due to the intrinsic nature of treatment, surgery has a high risk of immediate adverse events and treatment-related death, while dCRT is likely to suffer late toxicity. Radiation dose also has an effect, so if dose escalation is used, it has beneficial effects on PFS, but OS can be reduced. This can be explained by the increased risk of toxicity to the heart, lung, and esophagus under the influence of an increase in dose.

Induction Chemotherapy Ahead of CRT

As a variant of dCRT, induction chemotherapy prior to CRT may be beneficial in improving local control and inhibiting distant metastases. A study by Stahl et al. [14] also used the design of CRT with or without surgery after induction chemotherapy. The study by Ajani et al. was designed and performed to assess the feasibility of induction chemotherapy in addition to CRT to improve the rate of curative resection, local control, and survival [17]. Thirty-eight patients with locally advanced esophageal cancer were enrolled. Ninety-five percent of patients achieved R0 resection following surgery, and the pathologic complete response could be confirmed at 30%. However, other similar studies have reported that the overall benefit is offset by an increase in toxicity associated with induction chemotherapy. Therefore, the use of induction chemotherapy is still limited.

Targeting Agents

Due to the advancements in the understanding of tumorigenesis and the accumulated findings involving signaling cascades related to tumor cell growth and differentiation, new systemic therapies have been introduced into the clinical field. Agents specifically targeting cellular growth, protein receptors, and downstream signaling pathways are also showing promising results in the field of tumor therapy.

Epidermal growth factor receptor (EGFR, ErbB-1) is overexpressed in approximately 90% of esophageal cancers and is associated with a poor prognosis. Cetuximab, a monoclonal (IgG1) antibody against the extracellular domain of EGFR, has been reported to have a synergistic effect when combined with radiotherapy for head and neck cancer [18]. As a result of the study adding cetuximab to radiation, the median survival duration increased from 29.3 to 49.0 months. Notably, there was no increase in toxicity with the addition of cetuximab. However, so far, the effect of cetuximab on esophageal cancer is still unclear. A recent meta-analysis of ten studies was reported and included patients with locally advanced resectable esophageal cancer and metastatic disease [19]. In the study results, for these patients with localized esophageal cancer, cetuximab could not significantly improve response rate, OS, or PFS. However, for patients with metastatic disease, the addition of cetuximab significantly increased response rate (OR = 3.34; 95%CI, 1.90–5.88), disease control rate (OR = 2.92; 95% CI,1.49–5.71), and OS at 2 years (OR = 2.78; 95% CI,1.20–6.46).

HER-2 (ErbB2) is another member of the ErbB receptor family. Overexpression of HER-2 has been shown in esophageal cancers and is known to be associated with increased tumor invasiveness, lymph node metastasis, and chemoresistance. Trastuzumab is a humanized IgG1 antibody against the HER-2 receptor. The addition of trastuzumab to first-line chemotherapy has been shown to improve OS in patients with HER-2-positive metastatic gastric cancer and is also effective in gastroesophageal junction and esophageal adenocarcinoma. Furthermore, pembrolizumab, an inhibitor of the PD-1 immune checkpoint, has shown a beneficial impact for HER-2-positive metastatic esophagogastric cancer (gastric, esophageal, or gastroesophageal junction) when combined with trastuzumab and conventional chemotherapy. However, more investigation and evidence is needed for esophageal squamous cell cancer.

Bevacizumab is an antibody against vascular endothelial growth factor (VEGF) which is known to have apoptotic effects and be involved in cancer angiogenesis. However, in clinical trials to date, the combination of bevacizumab with cisplatin and 5-FU chemotherapy did not appear to improve resection rate or OS compared to previous regimens [20].

Conclusion

Chemotherapy and radiotherapy are synergistic in the treatment of esophageal cancer. Concurrent chemoradiotherapy or a combination of chemotherapy and radiation therapy provides at least equivalent oncological outcomes to surgery in locally advanced resectable esophageal cancer. Definitive CRT and trimodality treatment have both been considered equivalent in terms of OS as well as PFS. However, local disease control is better with trimodality treatment. Surgery-related complications and mortality compromise the benefits. Additional esophagectomy after chemoradiation may improve survival in patients with chemoradiation response and in surgically fit conditions. New target agents and immune therapeutic agents are under investigation and will likely participate in the treatment of esophageal cancer in the future.

References

1. Mohiuddin JJ, Jethwa KR, Grandhi N, Breen WG, Wang X, Anvari A, et al. Multi-institutional comparison of intensity modulated photon versus proton radiation therapy in the management of squamous cell carcinoma of the anus. Adv Radiat Oncol. 2021;6:100744.
2. Schaake-Koning C, van den Bogaert W, Dalesio O, Festen J, Hoogenhout J, van Houtte P, et al. Effects of concomitant cisplatin and radiotherapy on inoperable non-small-cell lung cancer. N Engl J Med. 1992;326:524–30.
3. Fujimake M, Soga J, Kawaguchi M, Maeda M, Sasaki K. Role of preoperative administration of bleomycin and radiation in the treatment of esophageal cancer. Jpn J Surg. 1975;5:48–55.
4. Herskovic A, Leichman L, Lattin P, Han I, Ahmad K, Leichman G, et al. Chemo/radiation with and without surgery in the thoracic esophagus: the Wayne State experience. Int J Radiat Oncol Biol Phys. 1988;15:655–62.
5. Coia LR, Engstrom PF, Paul AR, Stafford PM, Hanks GE. Long-term results of infusional 5-FU, mitomycin-C and radiation as primary management of esophageal carcinoma. Int J Radiat Oncol Biol Phys. 1991;20:29–36.
6. Herskovic A, Martz K, Al-Sarraf M, Leichman L, Brindle J, Vaitkevicius V, et al. Combined chemotherapy and radiotherapy compared with radiotherapy alone in patients with cancer of the esophagus. N Engl J Med. 1992;326:1593–8.
7. Smith TJ, Ryan LM, Douglass HO Jr, Haller DG, Dayal Y, Kirkwood J, et al. Combined chemoradiotherapy vs. radiotherapy alone for early stage squamous cell carcinoma of the esophagus: a study of the Eastern Cooperative Oncology Group. Int J Radiat Oncol Biol Phys. 1998;42:269–76.
8. Motoori M, Yano M, Ishihara R, Yamamoto S, Kawaguchi Y, Tanaka K, et al. Comparison between radical esophagectomy and definitive chemoradiotherapy in patients with clinical T1bN0M0 esophageal cancer. Ann Surg Oncol. 2012;19:2135–41.
9. Stahl M, Budach W. Definitive chemoradiotherapy. J Thorac Dis. 2017;9:S792–s8.
10. Teoh AY, Chiu PW, Yeung WK, Liu SY, Wong SK, Ng EK. Long-term survival outcomes after definitive chemoradiation versus surgery in patients with resectable squamous carcinoma of the esophagus: results from a randomized controlled trial. Ann Oncol. 2013;24:165–71.
11. Adelstein DJ, Rice TW, Becker M, Larto MA, Kirby TJ, Koka A, et al. Use of concurrent chemotherapy, accelerated fractionation radiation, and surgery for patients with esophageal carcinoma. Cancer. 1997;80:1011–20.
12. Choi N, Park SD, Lynch T, Wright C, Ancukiewicz M, Wain J, et al. Twice-daily radiotherapy as concurrent boost technique during two chemotherapy cycles in neoadjuvant chemoradiotherapy for resectable esophageal carcinoma: mature results of phase II study. Int J Radiat Oncol Biol Phys. 2004;60:111–22.
13. Bedenne L, Michel P, Bouché O, Milan C, Mariette C, Conroy T, et al. Chemoradiation followed by surgery compared with chemoradiation alone in squamous cancer of the esophagus: FFCD 9102. J Clin Oncol. 2007;25:1160–8.

14. Stahl M, Stuschke M, Lehmann N, Meyer HJ, Walz MK, Seeber S, et al. Chemoradiation with and without surgery in patients with locally advanced squamous cell carcinoma of the esophagus. J Clin Oncol. 2005;23:2310–7.
15. Barbetta A, Hsu M, Tan KS, Stefanova D, Herman K, Adusumilli PS, et al. Definitive chemoradiotherapy versus neoadjuvant chemoradiotherapy followed by surgery for stage II to III esophageal squamous cell carcinoma. J Thorac Cardiovasc Surg. 2018;155:2710–21.e3.
16. Chow R, Murdy K, Vaska M, Lee SL. Definitive chemoradiotherapy versus neoadjuvant chemoradiotherapy and esophagectomy for the treatment of esophageal and gastroesophageal carcinoma—a systematic review and meta-analysis. Radiother Oncol. 2021;165:37–43.
17. Ajani JA, Komaki R, Putnam JB, Walsh G, Nesbitt J, Pisters PW, et al. A three-step strategy of induction chemotherapy then chemoradiation followed by surgery in patients with potentially resectable carcinoma of the esophagus or gastroesophageal junction. Cancer. 2001;92:279–86.
18. Bonner JA, Harari PM, Giralt J, Azarnia N, Shin DM, Cohen RB, et al. Radiotherapy plus cetuximab for squamous-cell carcinoma of the head and neck. N Engl J Med. 2006;354:567–78.
19. Huang ZH, Ma XW, Zhang J, Li X, Lai NL, Zhang SX. Cetuximab for esophageal cancer: an updated meta-analysis of randomized controlled trials. BMC Cancer. 2018;18:1170.
20. Idelevich E, Kashtan H, Klein Y, Buevich V, Baruch NB, Dinerman M, et al. Prospective phase II study of neoadjuvant therapy with cisplatin, 5-fluorouracil, and bevacizumab for locally advanced resectable esophageal cancer. Onkologie. 2012;35:427–31.

Palliative Chemotherapy: CTx Regimen (First-Line, Second-Line, Targeted Therapies, and Immunotherapy)

Key Points

- Although recurrent/metastatic esophageal cancer has an extremely poor prognosis, palliative chemotherapy helps improve survival and quality of life.
- For palliative therapy for recurrent/metastatic esophageal cancer, fluoropyrimidine-/platinum-containing combination chemotherapy is the choice for first-line treatment over single-agent chemotherapy.
- Docetaxel- and irinotecan-based chemotherapies are standard options for second-line chemotherapy.
- Recently, targeted therapy and immunotherapy have been implemented to overcome the low response rate of conventional chemotherapy, and the survival rate has improved.
- In the future, targeted/immune treatment will be planned based on HER2 positivity and PD-L1 expression level in patients with recurrent/metastatic esophageal cancer prior to treatment.

Introduction

About 40% of esophageal cancers have metastasized to distant lymph nodes or other organs at the time of diagnosis [1]. Recurrence is also experienced in 21–39% of patients who achieve complete pathological remission through multidisciplinary treatment of advanced esophageal cancer. Although recurrent/metastatic esophageal cancer has an extremely poor prognosis (<5% in 5-year survival rate) [1], a meta-analysis of the Cochrane review published in 2017 confirmed that palliative chemotherapy was more effective than best supportive care in improving overall survival (OS) and quality of life and for alleviating symptoms such as dysphagia [2]. In recent years, more treatment options have emerged as a result of research on new targeted drugs and immunotherapy [3, 4]. In this chapter, palliative combination chemotherapy, which is widely used for metastatic or recurrent advanced esophageal cancer, is discussed, and the therapeutic effects of recently implemented targeted chemotherapy and immunotherapy are summarized (Tables 1 and 2).

Kyoungwon Jung is the lead author of this chapter.

H. J. Chun et al., *Gastrointestinal Cancer*, https://doi.org/10.1007/978-981-99-0815-8_18

Table 1 Pivotal trials of targeted therapy for recurrent/metastatic esophageal cancer

Study name	Phase	Cell of origin	Treatment arms	Minimum previous lines	Number (*n*)	ORR	PFS (months)	mOS (months)
HER2								
ToGA [30]	3	GA: 478 (81.8%) EGJA: 106 (18.2%)	Trastuzumab + chemotherapy Chemotherapy alone	NA	294 290	47%[a] 35%	6.7[a] 5.5	13.8[a] 11.1
JACOB [31]	3	GA: 572 (73.3%) EGJA: 208 (26.7%)	Pertuzumab + trastuzumab + chemotherapy Placebo + trastuzumab + chemotherapy	Naive	388 392	NA	8.5[a] 7.0	17.5 14.2
TRIO-013/LOGiC [32]	3	EAC: 20 (4.1%) EGJA: 43 (8.8%) GA: 424 (87.1%)	Lapatinib + capecitabine + oxaliplatin Placebo + capecitabine + oxaliplatin	Naive	249 238	53%[a] 39%	6.0[a] 5.4	12.2 10.5
VEGF								
REGARD [35]	3	GA: 265 (74.6%) EGJA: 90 (25.4%)	Ramucirumab Placebo	1	238 117	NA 6-month survival 41.8% 31.6%	2.1[a] 1.3	5.2[a] 3.8
RAINBOW [36]	3	GA: 528 (79.4%) EGJA: 137 (20.6%)	Ramucirumab + paclitaxel Placebo + paclitaxel	1	330 335	NA 6-month survival 72% 57%	4.4[a] 2.9	9.6[a] 7.4

NA not available; *ORR* overall response rate; *PFS* progression-free survival; *mOS* median overall survival; *GA* gastric adenocarcinoma; *EGJA* esophagogastric junction adenocarcinoma; EAC esophageal adenocarcinoma

[a] Difference is statistically significant

Table 2 Pivotal trials of immunotherapy for recurrent/metastatic esophageal cancer

Study name	Phase	Cell of origin	Treatment arms	Minimum previous lines	Number (*n*)	ORR	PFS (months)	mOS (months)
Pembrolizumab								
KEYNOTE-180 [45]	2	ESCC: 63 (52.1%) EA: 40 (33.1%) EGJA: 18 (14.9%) [PD-L1 positive (CPS ≥10) 58 (47.9%)]	Single arm, pembrolizumab	2	121	9.9%	2.0	5.8
KEYNOTE-181 [46]	3	ESCC: 401 (63.9%) EA: 227 (36.1%) [PD-L1 positive (CPS ≥10) 222 (35.4%)]	Pembrolizumab Chemotherapy	1	314 314	13.1% 6.7%	2.1 3.4	7.1 7.1 (PD-L1 positive [CPS ≥10]: 9.3[a] vs. 6.7)
KEYNOTE-590 [49]	3	ESCC: 548 (73.2%) EAC: 110 (14.7%) EGJA: 91 (12.1%) [PD-L1 positive (CPS ≥10) 383 (51.1%)]	Pembrolizumab + 5-FU/cisplatin Placebo + 5-FU/cisplatin	Naive	373 376	45.0%[a] 29.3%	6.3[a] 5.8	12.4[a] 9.8 (PD-L1 positive [CPS ≥10]: 13.5[a] vs. 9.4)
Pembrolizumab + trastuzumab [51]	2	EAC: 14 (38%) EGJA: 12 (32%) GA: 11 (30%)	Single arm, pembrolizumab + trastuzumab	Naive	37	NA # PFR 26% on 6 months	13.0	27.3
Nivolumab								
ATTRACTION-2 [47]	3	EGJA 42 (8.5%) GA 407 (82.6%) NA 44 (8.9%)	Nivolumab Placebo	2	493 330 163	11.2% 0%	1.61[a] 1.45	5.26[a] 4.14 (PD-L1 expression ≥1% 5.22 vs. 3.83)
ATTRACTION-3 [48]	3	ESCC 419 (100%)	Nivolumab Chemotherapy	1	419 210 209	19% 22%	1.7 3.4	10.9[a] 8.4
CheckMate 649 [50]	3	EAC: 211 (13.3%) EGJA: 260 (16.4%) GA: 1110 (70.2%)	Nivolumab + chemotherapy Chemotherapy alone	Naive	1581 789 792	58% 46%	7.7[a] 6.9	13.8[a] 11.6 (PD-L1 positive [CPS ≥5]: 14.4[a] vs. 11.1)

NA not available; *ORR* overall response rate; *PFS* progression-free survival; *mOS* median overall survival; *GA* gastric adenocarcinoma; *EGJA* esophagogastric junction adenocarcinoma; *EAC* esophageal adenocarcinoma; *ESCC* esophageal squamous cell carcinoma; *5-FU* 5-fluorouracil; *PD-L1* programmed cell death 1 ligand-1; *PFR* progression-free response; *CPS* combined positive score

[a] Difference is statistically significant

First-Line Chemotherapy

Similar to other metastatic cancers, systemic chemotherapy is the first-line treatment for metastatic and recurrent esophageal cancer. As a first-line treatment for esophageal cancer, chemotherapy has the advantage of inhibiting tumor growth and preventing distant metastasis. Various single-drug chemotherapeutic agents such as bleomycin, cisplatin, 5-fluorouracil (5-FU), methotrexate, methyl-GAG, mitomycin-C, and vindesine have been shown to be effective in the treatment of esophageal cancer, but the overall response rate was less than 20% [5]. Among these, the single agents most commonly used are 5-FU and cisplatin, which have a response rate of 6–15% and a median OS of 3–7 months [6, 7]. Other agents, such as paclitaxel, docetaxel, and irinotecan, have also shown single-agent efficacy with similar response rates [8–10].

Combination chemotherapy, which uses multiple known effective chemotherapy drugs together, has been developed to improve the low response rate and survival of monotherapy. The combination of cisplatin with 5-FU resulted in higher response rates and median OS compared to monotherapy. In a phase 2 study including 92 patients with advanced or metastatic squamous cell esophageal cancer published by Bleiberg et al., the response rate increased by 35% in the cisplatin and 5-FU combination therapy group and by 19% in the cisplatin-alone group. The median survival time was 33 weeks, showing a survival gain of approximately 5 weeks in combination therapy [11]. However, hematological and nonhematological toxicity increased in the combination therapy group, so additional studies were conducted to reduce toxicity. In a phase 3 study conducted by Al-Batran et al. involving 220 patients with metastatic gastroesophageal junction adenocarcinoma, they compared the 5-FU and cisplatin combination and the 5-FU and oxaliplatin combination. Most adverse events such as anemia, vomiting, alopecia, fatigue, renal toxicity, thromboembolic events, and serious adverse events were significantly lower in the oxaliplatin-treated group, and only peripheral neuropathy was less in the cisplatin group. Although there were no significant differences in median survival between the two groups, the response rate was higher in the oxaliplatin group in patients over 65 years of age, and progression-free survival (PFS) of 6 months and 3.1 months was more prolonged in the oxaliplatin group [12]. In the study by Ajani et al. based on S-1, an oral analog of 5-FU, 1053 patients with advanced gastric/gastroesophageal junction adenocarcinoma participated in the study. When the cisplatin/S-1 group and the cisplatin/5-FU group were compared, there were no significant differences in median survival values between the two groups, but statistically significant safety advantages were observed for the cisplatin/S-1 group, which was confirmed to be safer than 5-FU [13]. In a phase 2 study conducted by Lee et al. involving 94 patients with recurrent or metastatic esophageal squamous cell carcinoma, they were divided into the capecitabine and cisplatin combined group and the capecitabine and paclitaxel combined group, respectively. The response rate and median survival were 57% and 10.5 months in the cisplatin group and 58% and 13.2 months in the paclitaxel group, respectively. Although neutropenia and thrombocytopenia were more common in the cisplatin group, and neuropathy and alopecia were more common in the paclitaxel group, the two groups showed similar efficacy in the quality-of-life analysis. These results indicated that both regimens were effective and well tolerated as first-line treatment in patients with metastatic esophageal squamous cell carcinoma [14].

After the fluoropyrimidine/platinum combination became the most standard treatment among palliative chemotherapies, studies were conducted on other third-line agents to further improve the effect of response to treatment. Cisplatin/5-FU plus epirubicin combination therapy in patients with advanced gastroesophageal cancer had an overall response rate of 45% and a median survival of 8.9 months [15]. The REAL-2 study, a large study by Cunningham et al., confirmed that capecitabine and oxaliplatin were as effective as 5-FU and cisplatin, respectively, in combination therapy with epirubicin in patients with previously untreated esophageal cancer [16]. A V325 phase 3 study was conducted in which docetaxel was added to the basic combination therapy, cisplatin/5-FU. Although only 22% had gastroesophageal junction cancer, an increase in treatment response and OS was confirmed in the docetaxel group [17]. However, in a network meta-analysis that comprehensively analyzed combined chemotherapy, it was confirmed that this triplet therapy showed clinically significant anticancer drug-related toxicity compared to fluoropyrimidine/platinum and had limitations due to inconsistent clinical treatment response effects [18].

Second-Line Chemotherapy

Second-line chemotherapy is usually performed when treatment failure is confirmed in the treatment response evaluation during first-line chemotherapy. Approximately 40–50% of patients are well tolerant of first-line chemotherapy toxicity and are medically eligible for additional chemotherapy. In this setting, mainly taxane-based and irinotecan-based chemotherapies are considered standard options for second-line treatment [19].

The drug most studied among second-line treatments is docetaxel, which showed a median survival and duration of 4–8.3 months in a nonrandomized monotherapy study [20]. When combination therapy containing docetaxel and platinum was administered, the survival period was approximately 5–9 months [20]. However, most studies were directed at patients with histologically confirmed adenocarcinoma or gastric or gastroesophageal junction cancers. As a study that included squamous cell carcinoma limited to the esophagus as the main study population, Muro et al. conducted a phase 2 study on docetaxel monotherapy in 49 patients, and 94% had squamous cell carcinoma [9]. The response rate to chemotherapy was 20%, and among the patients who showed a response to treatment, six patients who had previously received chemotherapy were identified, and the median survival period was confirmed to be 8.1 months [9]. In a study conducted by Jin et al. on the combination therapy of docetaxel and nedaplatin, a response rate of 37.1% and a median survival of 5.9 months were confirmed [21]. Regarding the results of these nonrandomized studies, Ford et al. confirmed in a randomized study that docetaxel improved the OS rate of 1.6 months in recurrent gastroesophageal adenocarcinoma [22]. More recently, a non-inferiority study using nanoparticle albumin-binding (nab)-paclitaxel confirmed the therapeutic effects [23].

A drug that has been extensively studied, in addition to taxane, is irinotecan. A study by Burkart et al. showed a partial remission rate of 15% and disease stabilization in 23% of patients with weekly single-agent irinotecan [24]. Considering the 29–29.6% treatment response rate achieved by the irinotecan/5-FU combination therapy, it was confirmed that it could be considered as a second-line chemotherapy regimen for failed recurrent/metastatic esophageal cancer [25, 26]. Based on the results of a previous study, the results of the ESWN 01 trial comparing irinotecan/S-1 with S-1 monotherapy were recently reported in 123 patients with previously treated recurrent/metastatic esophageal cancer. Compared to the S-1 monotherapy group, patients who received irinotecan combination therapy showed a significant response rate of 24.6% versus 9.7%, and PFS also increased to 3.8 months compared to 1.7 months, confirming that irinotecan was also effective as combination therapy [27]. Recently, the therapeutic effect of a new drug TAS-102 (a combination of trifluridine [nucleoside analog] and tipiracil [thymidine phosphorylase inhibitor] in metastatic gastroesophageal/gastric adenocarcinoma pretreated with multiple chemotherapy) (TAGS trial) was reported [28]. Of note, the NCCN guidelines mention TAS-102 as a third-line treatment for selected patients with minimal symptoms and minimal disease due to the hematologic toxicity of neutropenia despite an increase in OS.

Targeted Therapy

Targeting HER2

The human epidermal growth factor receptor type 2 (HER2) gene is an oncogene encoding a transmembrane receptor protein with intracellular tyrosine kinase activity. This protein plays a key role in the activation of signaling pathways that regulate cell proliferation and was reported to be overexpressed in about 22% of patients undergoing esophageal cancer surgery [29]. The therapeutic effect of trastuzumab, a monoclonal antibody that targets HER2 and induces antibody-dependent cytotoxicity, was confirmed through the ToGA trial. In this study, patients who received trastuzumab plus chemotherapy had a higher median OS (13.8 vs. 11.1 months) and a higher objective response rate (47% vs. 35%) [30]. These results have made it the standard chemotherapy regimen for patients with advanced gastric/gastroesophageal junction HER2-positive adenocarcinoma. Since then, studies with pertuzumab, a recombinant monoclonal antibody against the extracellular domain II of the HER2 protein, which is required for heterodimerization of HER2 with other HER receptors, and lapatinib, a small-molecule inhibitor of EGFR type 1 and HER2, also have shown an increased survival rate [31, 32].

Targeting VEGF

Angiogenesis, or the formation of new blood vessels, is an important process necessary for the proliferation and growth of cancer. Vascular endothelial growth factor (VEGF) is one of the major proangiogenic factors involved in tumor angiogenesis, and it is known that the level of VEGF increases in many malignant tumors, including esophageal cancer [33, 34]. Therefore, blocking the VEGF pathway has been an important target in the development of esophageal cancer therapeutics. Ramucirumab is a monoclonal antibody that binds to VEGFR2 and inhibits receptor activation. In previously treated patients with advanced gastric/gastroesophageal junction adenocarcinoma, patients receiving ramucirumab improved PFS and OS compared to patients receiving best supportive care (REGARD trial) [35]. In the phase 3 RAINBOW trial of patients previously treated with chemotherapy containing fluoropyrimidine/platinum, when ramucirumab was administered weekly in combination with paclitaxel, OS (9.6 versus 7.4 months) was improved compared to patients treated with paclitaxel alone [36]. Other studies have investigated VEGF target-related agents such as bevacizumab, apatinib, sorafenib, regorafenib, and sunitinib [37–41]; however, their clinical usefulness is still limited because it does not significantly affect the overall response rate or the improvement in survival rate, and the results of large-scale clinical studies are lacking.

Immunotherapy

As cancer progresses and metastasizes, malignant cells evolve to evade surveillance by the innate immune system. A major mechanism of this immune evasion involves the expression of one or more molecules on the cell surface, effectively limiting T cell activation [42]. The best known and most studied immune checkpoints are those that are expressed on the surface of tumor cells, such as the programmed cell death 1 ligand-1 (PD-L1) and the cytotoxic T lymphocyte-associated antigen-4 (CTLA-4) [43]. These can act as inhibitory signal by binding to receptors on immune cells and suppressing immune cell function.

Immunotherapy Trials

PD-1 inhibitors are considered effective targeting drugs to address cancer cell evasion of T cells. Common PD-1 inhibitors, such as pembrolizumab (humanized IgG4 kappa monoclonal antibody), can bind to PD-1 in T cells, which prevents PD-1 from binding to PD-L1 in tumor cells and subsequently stops T cell suppression, eventually allowing T cells to exert their apoptotic effects on cancer cells [44].

In the phase 2 KEYNOTE-180 clinical study, the objective response rate was 9.9% after pembrolizumab monotherapy in patients with esophageal adenocarcinoma and esophageal squamous cell carcinoma [45]. A subgroup analysis showed that pembrolizumab treatment was more effective in patients with PD-L1-positive esophageal squamous cell carcinoma [45]. Based on these results, the KEYNOTE-181 study, a randomized controlled study of the pembrolizumab group and the standard chemotherapy group, was also published [46]. This study included 628 patients with advanced/metastatic esophageal cancer who progressed after one previous therapy. Although OS was not significantly different between the two groups at 7.1 months, OS in patients with combined positive score (CPS) ≥ 10 was prolonged in the pembrolizumab group compared to the chemotherapy group (9.3 vs. 6.7 months, HR 0.69; $p = 0.0074$) [46]. Based on these results, the US Food and Drug Administration has now approved pembrolizumab as a second-line treatment option for patients with advanced esophageal squamous cell carcinoma positive for PD-L1.

Nivolumab, a fully human IgG4 monoclonal antibody targeting PD-1, has a high affinity for PD-1 and can inhibit the binding of PD-L1/PD-L2 to PD-1. In the phase 3 ATTRACTION-2 trial in patients with advanced gastric/gastroesophageal junction adenocarcinoma who had previously received two or more chemotherapy regimens, the overall 1-year survival rate of patients treated with nivolumab was improved compared to placebo, regardless of PD-L1 expression (26.2% vs. 10.9%) [47]. Subsequently, an additional study called the phase 3 ATTRACTION-3 trial was conducted [48]. In patients with unresectable advanced or recurrent esophageal squamous cell carcinoma who had failed previous chemotherapy, OS improved with nivolumab compared to chemotherapy (docetaxel or paclitaxel) (10.5 vs. 8.0 months), and the rate of adverse events was lower in the nivolumab group (18% vs. 63%) [48]. Through these results, not only the therapeutic efficacy but also safety was confirmed.

Immunotherapy with Chemotherapy Combination

In the KEYNOTE-590 study with 749 patients with esophageal cancer, after stratifying the conventional chemotherapy-alone group and the pembrolizumab plus chemotherapy group, a comparison of the 2-year survival rate (28% vs. 16%) and the median survival rate (12.4 vs. 9.8 months) of the combination group pembrolizumab improved compared to the chemotherapy-alone group [49].

In the CheckMate 649 study of 1581 untreated patients with HER2-negative gastric/gastroesophageal/esophageal adenocarcinoma, the nivolumab plus chemotherapy group improved OS by 29% compared to the chemotherapy-alone group. This study showed the potential of nivolumab as a first-line treatment for previously untreated advanced esophageal adenocarcinoma [50].

In addition to the combination of immunotherapy with conventional chemotherapy, treatment with the combination of immunotherapy with targeted therapy is also being attempted. In a phase 2 study of 37 patients with HER2-positive esophageal/gastric/gastroesophageal junction cancer, 70% of the patients showed no progression at 6 months with the combination of pembrolizumab and trastuzumab, suggesting that various combination therapies for HER2-positive cancer should be investigated in the future [51].

Summary and Conclusions

Palliative chemotherapy helps to improve survival and quality of life despite the poor prognosis of recurrent/metastatic esophageal cancer. Combination chemotherapy containing fluoropyrimidine/platinum is the standard palliative initial chemotherapy rather than single-agent chemotherapy. However, recently, the importance of targeted and immunotherapeutic agents has increased due to the low response rate or disease progression during combination chemotherapy. Since the effectiveness of targeted and immunotherapeutic drugs has been proven in many studies, it will be important to check HER2 positivity and PD-L1 expression levels before treatment in patients with recurrent/metastatic esophageal cancer.

References

1. Rustgi AK, El-Serag HB. Esophageal carcinoma. N Engl J Med. 2014;371:2499–509.
2. Janmaat VT, Steyerberg EW, van der Gaast A, Mathijssen RH, Bruno MJ, Peppelenbosch MP, et al. Palliative chemotherapy and targeted therapies for esophageal and gastroesophageal junction cancer. Cochrane Database Syst Rev. 2017;11:Cd004063.
3. Yang YM, Hong P, Xu WW, He QY, Li B. Advances in targeted therapy for esophageal cancer. Signal Transduct Target Ther. 2020;5:229.
4. Zhao Q, Yu J, Meng X. A good start of immunotherapy in esophageal cancer. Cancer Med. 2019;8:4519–26.
5. Grünberger B, Raderer M, Schmidinger M, Hejna M. Palliative chemotherapy for recurrent and metastatic esophageal cancer. Anticancer Res. 2007;27:2705–14.
6. Ezdinli EZ, Gelber R, Desai DV, Falkson G, Moertel CG, Hahn RG. Chemotherapy of advanced esophageal carcinoma: Eastern Cooperative Oncology Group experience. Cancer. 1980;46:2149–53.
7. Kantarjian H, Ajani JA, Karlin DA. Cis-diaminodichloroplatinum (II) chemotherapy for advanced adenocarcinoma of the upper gastrointestinal tract. Oncology. 1985;42:69–71.
8. Ilson DH, Wadleigh RG, Leichman LP, Kelsen DP. Paclitaxel given by a weekly 1-h infusion in advanced esophageal cancer. Ann Oncol. 2007;18:898–902.
9. Muro K, Hamaguchi T, Ohtsu A, Boku N, Chin K, Hyodo I, et al. A phase II study of single-agent docetaxel in patients with metastatic esophageal cancer. Ann Oncol. 2004;15:955–9.
10. Enzinger PC, Kulke MH, Clark JW, Ryan DP, Kim H, Earle CC, et al. A phase II trial of irinotecan in patients with previously untreated advanced esophageal and gastric adenocarcinoma. Dig Dis Sci. 2005;50:2218–23.
11. Bleiberg H, Conroy T, Paillot B, Lacave AJ, Blijham G, Jacob JH, et al. Randomised phase II study of cisplatin and 5-fluorouracil (5-FU) versus cisplatin alone in advanced squamous cell oesophageal cancer. Eur J Cancer. 1997;33:1216–20.
12. Al-Batran SE, Hartmann JT, Probst S, Schmalenberg H, Hollerbach S, Hofheinz R, et al. Phase III trial in metastatic gastroesophageal adenocarcinoma with fluorouracil, leucovorin plus either oxaliplatin or cisplatin: a study of the Arbeitsgemeinschaft Internistische Onkologie. J Clin Oncol. 2008;26:1435–42.
13. Ajani JA, Buyse M, Lichinitser M, Gorbunova V, Bodoky G, Douillard JY, et al. Combination of cisplatin/S-1 in the treatment of patients with advanced gastric or gastroesophageal adenocarcinoma: results of noninferiority and safety analyses compared with cisplatin/5-fluorouracil in the First-Line Advanced Gastric Cancer Study. Eur J Cancer. 2013;49:3616–24.
14. Lee SJ, Kim S, Kim M, Lee J, Park YH, Im YH, et al. Capecitabine in combination with either cisplatin or weekly paclitaxel as a first-line treatment for metastatic esophageal squamous cell carcinoma: a randomized phase II study. BMC Cancer. 2015;15:693.
15. Webb A, Cunningham D, Scarffe JH, Harper P, Norman A, Joffe JK, et al. Randomized trial comparing epirubicin, cisplatin, and fluorouracil versus fluorouracil, doxorubicin, and methotrexate in advanced esophagogastric cancer. J Clin Oncol. 1997;15:261–7.
16. Cunningham D, Starling N, Rao S, Iveson T, Nicolson M, Coxon F, et al. Capecitabine and oxaliplatin for advanced esophagogastric cancer. N Engl J Med. 2008;358:36–46.
17. Van Cutsem E, Moiseyenko VM, Tjulandin S, Majlis A, Constenla M, Boni C, et al. Phase III study of docetaxel and cisplatin plus fluorouracil compared with cisplatin and fluorouracil as first-line therapy for advanced gastric cancer: a report of the V325 Study Group. J Clin Oncol. 2006;24:4991–7.
18. Ter Veer E, Haj Mohammad N, van Valkenhoef G, Ngai LL, Mali RMA, Anderegg MC, et al. The efficacy and safety of first-line chemotherapy in advanced esophagogastric cancer: a network meta-analysis. J Natl Cancer Inst 2016;108.
19. Thallinger CM, Raderer M, Hejna M. Esophageal cancer: a critical evaluation of systemic second-line therapy. J Clin Oncol. 2011;29:4709–14.
20. Ford H, Gounaris I. Docetaxel and its potential in the treatment of refractory esophagogastric adenocarcinoma. Ther Adv Gastroenterol. 2015;8:189–205.
21. Jin J, Xu X, Wang F, Yan G, Liu J, Lu W, et al. Second-line combination chemotherapy with docetaxel and nedaplatin for Cisplatin-pretreated refractory metastatic/recurrent esophageal squamous cell carcinoma. J Thorac Oncol. 2009;4:1017–21.
22. Ford HE, Marshall A, Bridgewater JA, Janowitz T, Coxon FY, Wadsley J, et al. Docetaxel versus active symptom control for refractory oesophagogastric adenocarcinoma (COUGAR-02): an open-label, phase 3 randomised controlled trial. Lancet Oncol. 2014;15:78–86.
23. Shitara K, Takashima A, Fujitani K, Koeda K, Hara H, Nakayama N, et al. Nab-paclitaxel versus solvent-based paclitaxel in patients with previously treated advanced gastric cancer (ABSOLUTE): an open-label, randomised, non-inferiority, phase 3 trial. Lancet Gastroenterol Hepatol. 2017;2:277–87.
24. Burkart C, Bokemeyer C, Klump B, Pereira P, Teichmann R, Hartmann JT. A phase II trial of weekly irinotecan in cisplatin-refractory esophageal cancer. Anticancer Res. 2007;27:2845–8.
25. Wang X, Wang X, Huang J. Irinotecan plus fluorouracil-based regimen as second or third-line

chemotherapy for recurrent or metastatic esophageal squamous cell carcinoma. Thorac Cancer. 2016;7:246–50.

26. Assersohn L, Brown G, Cunningham D, Ward C, Oates J, Waters JS, et al. Phase II study of irinotecan and 5-fluorouracil/leucovorin in patients with primary refractory or relapsed advanced oesophageal and gastric carcinoma. Ann Oncol. 2004;15:64–9.
27. Huang J, Xu B, Liu Y, Huang J, Lu P, Ba Y, et al. Irinotecan plus S-1 versus S-1 in patients with previously treated recurrent or metastatic esophageal cancer (ESWN 01): a prospective randomized, multicenter, open-labeled phase 3 trial. Cancer Commun (Lond). 2019;39:16.
28. Shitara K, Doi T, Dvorkin M, Mansoor W, Arkenau HT, Prokharau A, et al. Trifluridine/tipiracil versus placebo in patients with heavily pretreated metastatic gastric cancer (TAGS): a randomised, double-blind, placebo-controlled, phase 3 trial. Lancet Oncol. 2018;19:1437–48.
29. Chan DS, Twine CP, Lewis WG. Systematic review and meta-analysis of the influence of HER2 expression and amplification in operable oesophageal cancer. J Gastrointest Surg. 2012;16:1821–9.
30. Bang YJ, Van Cutsem E, Feyereislova A, Chung HC, Shen L, Sawaki A, et al. Trastuzumab in combination with chemotherapy versus chemotherapy alone for treatment of HER2-positive advanced gastric or gastro-oesophageal junction cancer (ToGA): a phase 3, open-label, randomised controlled trial. Lancet. 2010;376:687–97.
31. Tabernero J, Hoff PM, Shen L, Ohtsu A, Shah MA, Cheng K, et al. Pertuzumab plus trastuzumab and chemotherapy for HER2-positive metastatic gastric or gastro-oesophageal junction cancer (JACOB): final analysis of a double-blind, randomised, placebo-controlled phase 3 study. Lancet Oncol. 2018;19:1372–84.
32. Hecht JR, Bang YJ, Qin SK, Chung HC, Xu JM, Park JO, et al. Lapatinib in combination with capecitabine plus oxaliplatin in human epidermal growth factor receptor 2-positive advanced or metastatic gastric, esophageal, or gastroesophageal adenocarcinoma TRIO-013/LOGiC—a randomized phase III trial. J Clin Oncol. 2016;34:443–51.
33. Carmeliet P. VEGF as a key mediator of angiogenesis in cancer. Oncology. 2005;69(Suppl 3):4–10.
34. Xu WW, Li B, Cheung AL. The potential of targeted antiangiogenesis therapies in the treatment of esophageal cancer. Gastrointest Cancer Targets Therapy. 2015;5:79–88.
35. Fuchs CS, Tomasek J, Yong CJ, Dumitru F, Passalacqua R, Goswami C, et al. Ramucirumab monotherapy for previously treated advanced gastric or gastro-oesophageal junction adenocarcinoma (REGARD): an international, randomised, multicentre, placebo-controlled, phase 3 trial. Lancet. 2014;383:31–9.
36. Wilke H, Muro K, Van Cutsem E, Oh SC, Bodoky G, Shimada Y, et al. Ramucirumab plus paclitaxel versus placebo plus paclitaxel in patients with previously treated advanced gastric or gastro-oesophageal junction adenocarcinoma (RAINBOW): a double-blind, randomised phase 3 trial. Lancet Oncol. 2014;15:1224–35.
37. Ohtsu A, Shah MA, Van Cutsem E, Rha SY, Sawaki A, Park SR, et al. Bevacizumab in combination with chemotherapy as first-line therapy in advanced gastric cancer: a randomized, double-blind, placebo-controlled phase III study. J Clin Oncol. 2011;29:3968–76.
38. Li J, Qin S, Xu J, Xiong J, Wu C, Bai Y, et al. Randomized, double-blind, placebo-controlled phase III trial of apatinib in patients with chemotherapy-refractory advanced or metastatic adenocarcinoma of the stomach or gastroesophageal junction. J Clin Oncol. 2016;34:1448–54.
39. Janjigian YY, Vakiani E, Ku GY, Herrera JM, Tang LH, Bouvier N, et al. Phase II trial of sorafenib in patients with chemotherapy refractory metastatic esophageal and gastroesophageal (GE) junction cancer. PLoS One. 2015;10:e0134731.
40. Wu C, Mikhail S, Wei L, Timmers C, Tahiri S, Neal A, et al. A phase II and pharmacodynamic study of sunitinib in relapsed/refractory oesophageal and gastro-oesophageal cancers. Br J Cancer. 2015;113:220–5.
41. Moy RH, Dos Santos FG, Jonsson P, Chou JF, Basunia A, Ku GY, et al. Regorafenib in combination with first-line chemotherapy for metastatic esophagogastric cancer. Oncologist. 2020;25:e68–74.
42. Pardoll DM. The blockade of immune checkpoints in cancer immunotherapy. Nat Rev Cancer. 2012;12:252–64.
43. Drake CG, Lipson EJ, Brahmer JR. Breathing new life into immunotherapy: review of melanoma, lung and kidney cancer. Nat Rev Clin Oncol. 2014;11:24–37.
44. Yamamoto S, Kato K. Pembrolizumab for the treatment of esophageal cancer. Expert Opin Biol Ther. 2020;20:1143–50.
45. Shah MA, Kojima T, Hochhauser D, Enzinger P, Raimbourg J, Hollebecque A, et al. Efficacy and safety of pembrolizumab for heavily pretreated patients with advanced, metastatic adenocarcinoma or squamous cell carcinoma of the esophagus: the phase 2 KEYNOTE-180 study. JAMA Oncol. 2019;5:546–50.
46. Kojima T, Shah MA, Muro K, Francois E, Adenis A, Hsu CH, et al. Randomized phase III KEYNOTE-181 study of pembrolizumab versus chemotherapy in advanced esophageal cancer. J Clin Oncol. 2020;38:4138–48.
47. Kang YK, Boku N, Satoh T, Ryu MH, Chao Y, Kato K, et al. Nivolumab in patients with advanced gastric or gastro-oesophageal junction cancer refractory to, or intolerant of, at least two previous chemotherapy regimens (ONO-4538-12, ATTRACTION-2): a randomised, double-blind, placebo-controlled, phase 3 trial. Lancet. 2017;390:2461–71.
48. Kato K, Cho BC, Takahashi M, Okada M, Lin CY, Chin K, et al. Nivolumab versus chemotherapy in patients with advanced oesophageal squamous cell

carcinoma refractory or intolerant to previous chemotherapy (ATTRACTION-3): a multicentre, randomised, open-label, phase 3 trial. Lancet Oncol. 2019;20:1506–17.

49. Sun JM, Shen L, Shah MA, Enzinger P, Adenis A, Doi T, et al. Pembrolizumab plus chemotherapy versus chemotherapy alone for first-line treatment of advanced oesophageal cancer (KEYNOTE-590): a randomised, placebo-controlled, phase 3 study. Lancet. 2021;398:759–71.
50. Janjigian YY, Shitara K, Moehler M, Garrido M, Salman P, Shen L, et al. First-line nivolumab plus chemotherapy versus chemotherapy alone for advanced gastric, gastro-oesophageal junction, and oesophageal adenocarcinoma (CheckMate 649): a randomised, open-label, phase 3 trial. Lancet. 2021;398:27–40.
51. Janjigian YY, Maron SB, Chatila WK, Millang B, Chavan SS, Alterman C, et al. First-line pembrolizumab and trastuzumab in HER2-positive oesophageal, gastric, or gastro-oesophageal junction cancer: an open-label, single-arm, phase 2 trial. Lancet Oncol. 2020;21:821–31.

Part III

Small Bowel Cancer

Epidemiology and Prevention. I-1. Epidemiology and Risk Factors

Key Points

- Although small bowel cancer is a rare disease, its incidence has increased slowly in recent years.
- The segment of small bowel cancer that is the most frequently involved is the duodenum, followed by the jejunum and ileum.
- The median age at diagnosis is approximately 60 years, with a higher incidence rate in men than in women.
- Several lifestyle and dietary factors, including alcohol consumption, red meat, salted and smoked foods, and refined sugar, are associated with an increased risk of small bowel cancer.
- The risk of small bowel cancer increases in several familial cancer syndromes, including Lynch syndrome, familial adenomatous polyposis, and Peutz-Jeghers syndrome.
- The risk of small bowel cancer is higher in the context of long-standing inflammations, including Crohn's disease and celiac disease.

Introduction

The small bowel represents 75% of the length and 90% of the absorptive surface of the gastrointestinal system [1]. Despite its major role in digestion, the small intestine is a rare location for the development of neoplasms. Small bowel cancers include several histologic subtypes, such as adenocarcinoma, neuroendocrine tumor, lymphoma, and sarcoma. Due to the heterogeneity and scarcity of small bowel cancers, epidemiological literature regarding small bowel cancers has been very limited. In recent years, population-based studies have reported the epidemiology of small bowel cancer, and the incidence is gradual increasing. Although the cause of this increasing trend in small bowel cancer has not yet been elucidated, the recent development of diagnostic tools for the small intestine is believed to be one of the reasons. Small bowel cancer is primarily at increased risk in patients with underlying diseases known to be at high risk of small bowel cancer, including Lynch syndrome, familial adenomatous polyposis, Peutz-Jeghers syndrome, and Crohn's disease. Furthermore, lifestyle-related factors have been reported to be related to an increased risk of small bowel cancer in patients without those underlying diseases.

Jae Jun Park is the lead author of this chapter.

H. J. Chun et al., *Gastrointestinal Cancer*, https://doi.org/10.1007/978-981-99-0815-8_19

Epidemiology

Cancers of the small bowel are rare. According to recent epidemiological data from the United States, the approximate incidence of small bowel cancer is 2.3 per 100,000 in 2019 [2]. Meanwhile, according to the annual report of cancer statistics in Korea, the age-adjusted incidence rate of small bowel malignant neoplasm is 1.0 per 100,000 people in 2018 [3]. Although the small intestine constitutes three-quarters of the digestive tract, small bowel malignancies account for only 3% of all gastrointestinal tract neoplasms [4–7]. Historically, adenocarcinoma had been the dominant histological type of small bowel malignancy, followed by neuroendocrine cancer, lymphoma, and sarcoma [6, 7]; however, neuroendocrine carcinoma became the dominant type in recent years [8]. Presently, in all cases of small bowel cancer diagnosis, neuroendocrine tumors account for 39–40%, and small bowel adenocarcinomas for 31–40% [9]. The overall incidence of small bowel cancer has gradually increased since the early 1990s. The segment most frequently affected is the duodenum with 55–82% of cases, followed by the jejunum (11–25%) and the ileum (7–17%) [10]. Cancer in the small bowel is more common in men than in women (male-to-female ratio of 1.5:1) [11]. Regarding the mean age of diagnosis, the age at diagnosis of adenocarcinoma of the small intestine and neuroendocrine tumors is 67–68 years, which is older than the mean age of 60–62 years at diagnosis of lymphoma and sarcoma [12, 13].

Risk Factors

Dietary and Lifestyle Factors

Several case-control studies have reported that dietary factors including alcohol consumption, red meat, salted and smoked foods, and refined sugar are associated with an increased risk of small bowel cancer [14–17]. Meanwhile, no consistent results have been reported regarding the risk of small intestine cancer in smokers, and some studies address the increased risk but not in other studies [16, 18, 19]. Studies on the relationship between obesity and small bowel cancer also yielded inconsistent results [14, 19, 20]. Conversely, the consumption of fiber, fruits, vegetables, and fish is associated with a reduced risk of small bowel adenocarcinoma [21].

Hereditary Cancer Syndromes

In several familial cancer syndromes involving specific inherited genetic abnormalities, the risk of small bowel cancer has been reported to increase.

Lynch syndrome (hereditary nonpolyposis colorectal cancer) is an autosomal dominant genetic condition involving a germline mutation of the DNA mismatch repair gene and is related to increased risk of many types of cancer, particularly colon cancers. Furthermore, there is an increased risk of small bowel cancer in Lynch patients: the cumulative lifetime risk of small bowel adenocarcinoma is around 1% [22]. In a nationwide French study, the most common site of small bowel adenocarcinoma is the duodenum (61%) in Lynch syndrome, while the jejunal and ileal locations were reported in 30% and 9% of cases, respectively [23]. Lynch syndrome accounts for approximately 5–10% of small bowel adenocarcinoma [24, 25].

Familial adenomatous polyposis is an inherited condition caused by a defect in the adenomatous polyposis coli gene. Familial adenomatous polyposis causes hundreds to thousands of precancerous colorectal adenomatous polyps if left untreated, eventually developing colorectal cancer at an average age of 39 years. Moreover, adenomatous polyps frequently occur in the duodenum in addition to the colon in patients with familial adenomatous polyposis. Specifically, duodenal adenomas are present in 80% of patients with FAP and can develop into adenocarcinoma in 4% of cases. Familial adenomatous polyposis is present in approximately 2% of small bowel adenocarcinomas [23]. In patients with familial adenomatous polyposis, small bowel adenocarcinoma has been reported to occur mainly in the duodenum (83%) or the jejunum (16%) [23].

Peutz-Jeghers syndrome is an autosomal dominant disorder caused by the STK11 suppressor gene mutation. Peutz-Jeghers syndrome is characterized by multiple polyps of hamartoma in the gastrointestinal tract and, more importantly, is also associated with an increased risk of cancer in several organs, including the breast, colon, pancreas, stomach, testicles, ovaries, lung, cervix, etc. In addition, Peutz-Jeghers syndrome has been associated with an increased risk of adenocarcinoma of the small intestine [26]. The estimated cumulative risk of small bowel adenocarcinoma in Peutz-Jeghers syndrome is 13% [26], and it is thought to be responsible for less than 1% of small bowel adenocarcinoma [23].

Chronic Inflammation

Long-standing inflammation has been suggested as the etiology of cancer in several types of cancers. Crohn's disease induces chronic inflammation in the gastrointestinal tract, and the distal ileum is the site most frequently affected. It is known that the risk of small bowel adenocarcinoma is correlated with the duration and location of the inflammatory damage in Crohn's disease. The odds ratio in Crohn's disease for the risk of small bowel cancer is 9.8 in a pooled analysis involving nine studies [27]. The cumulative risk is estimated to be around 0.2% after 10 years and 2.2% after 25 years of Crohn's disease diagnosis [28]. In a nationwide French study, Crohn's disease was involved in approximately 9% of small bowel adenocarcinomas, mostly in the ileum [23]. Celiac disease is a disorder of the small bowel characterized by chronic mucosal inflammation, leading to atrophy of the intestinal villi, malabsorption, and various clinical manifestations. Celiac disease increases the relative risk of small bowel adenocarcinoma from 10 to 30 compared to the general population [29, 30]. Celiac disease is associated with small bowel adenocarcinoma in approximately 2% of cases; the main location is in the jejunum [23].

Cystic Fibrosis

Cystic fibrosis is an inherited condition that causes sticky mucus to build up in the lungs and digestive system, resulting in lung infections and difficulty in digesting food. The risk of small bowel cancer is known to increase in cystic fibrosis patients, with a standardized pooled incidence ratio of 18.9 in meta-analysis reports [31].

Conclusion

Although small bowel cancer is a rare disease, the incidence has slowly increased in recent years. Several dietary and lifestyle factors are associated with an increased risk of small bowel cancers. Additionally, the risk of small bowel cancer increases in the setting of familial cancer syndromes involving specific inherited genetic abnormalities and long-standing inflammation involving the small intestine, and a small bowel evaluation may be needed in these high-risk patients.

References

1. Schottenfeld D, Beebe-Dimmer JL, Vigneau FD. The epidemiology and pathogenesis of neoplasia in the small intestine. Ann Epidemiol. 2009;19:58–69.
2. Hase K, Ueno H, Kuranaga N, Utsunomiya K, Kanabe S, Mochizuki H. Intraperitoneal exfoliated cancer cells in patients with colorectal cancer. Dis Colon Rectum. 1998;41:1134–40.
3. Yamamoto S, Akasu T, Fujita S, Moriya Y. Long-term prognostic value of conventional peritoneal cytology after curative resection for colorectal carcinoma. Jpn J Clin Oncol. 2003;33:33–7.
4. Siegel RL, Miller KD, Fuchs HE, Jemal A. Cancer Statistics, 2021. CA Cancer J Clin. 2021;71:7–33.
5. DeSesso JM, Jacobson CF. Anatomical and physiological parameters affecting gastrointestinal absorption in humans and rats. Food Chem Toxicol. 2001;39:209–28.
6. Severson RK, Schenk M, Gurney JG, Weiss LK, Demers RY. Increasing incidence of adenocarcinomas and carcinoid tumors of the small intestine in adults. Cancer Epidemiol Biomark Prev. 1996;5:81–4.
7. Bilimoria KY, Bentrem DJ, Wayne JD, Ko CY, Bennett CL, Talamonti MS. Small bowel cancer in the United States: changes in epidemiology, treatment, and survival over the last 20 years. Ann Surg. 2009;249:63–71.
8. Pan SY, Morrison H. Epidemiology of cancer of the small intestine. World J Gastrointest Oncol. 2011;3:33–42.
9. Pedersen KS, Raghav K, Overman MJ. Small bowel adenocarcinoma: etiology, presentation, and

molecular alterations. J Natl Compr Cancer Netw. 2019;17:1135–41.
10. Aparicio T, Zaanan A, Svrcek M, Laurent-Puig P, Carrere N, Manfredi S, et al. Small bowel adenocarcinoma: epidemiology, risk factors, diagnosis and treatment. Dig Liver Dis. 2014;46:97–104.
11. Haselkorn T, Whittemore AS, Lilienfeld DE. Incidence of small bowel cancer in the United States and worldwide: geographic, temporal, and racial differences. Cancer Causes Control. 2005;16:781–7.
12. Hatzaras I, Palesty JA, Abir F, Sullivan P, Kozol RA, Dudrick SJ, et al. Small-bowel tumors: epidemiologic and clinical characteristics of 1260 cases from the connecticut tumor registry. Arch Surg. 2007;142:229–35.
13. Lepage C, Bouvier AM, Manfredi S, Dancourt V, Faivre J. Incidence and management of primary malignant small bowel cancers: a well-defined French population study. Am J Gastroenterol. 2006;101:2826–32.
14. Chow WH, Linet MS, McLaughlin JK, Hsing AW, Chien HT, Blot WJ. Risk factors for small intestine cancer. Cancer Causes Control. 1993;4:163–9.
15. Neugut AI, Jacobson JS, Suh S, Mukherjee R, Arber N. The epidemiology of cancer of the small bowel. Cancer Epidemiol Biomark Prev. 1998;7:243–51.
16. Wu AH, Yu MC, Mack TM. Smoking, alcohol use, dietary factors and risk of small intestinal adenocarcinoma. Int J Cancer. 1997;70:512–7.
17. Cross AJ, Leitzmann MF, Subar AF, Thompson FE, Hollenbeck AR, Schatzkin A. A prospective study of meat and fat intake in relation to small intestinal cancer. Cancer Res. 2008;68:9274–9.
18. Chen CC, Neugut AI, Rotterdam H. Risk factors for adenocarcinomas and malignant carcinoids of the small intestine: preliminary findings. Cancer Epidemiol Biomark Prev. 1994;3:205–7.
19. Negri E, Bosetti C, La Vecchia C, Fioretti F, Conti E, Franceschi S. Risk factors for adenocarcinoma of the small intestine. Int J Cancer. 1999;82:171–4.
20. Bjørge T, Tretli S, Engeland A. Height and body mass index in relation to cancer of the small intestine in two million Norwegian men and women. Br J Cancer. 2005;93:807–10.
21. Bennett CM, Coleman HG, Veal PG, Cantwell MM, Lau CC, Murray LJ. Lifestyle factors and small intestine adenocarcinoma risk: a systematic review and meta-analysis. Cancer Epidemiol. 2015;39:265–73.
22. Bonadona V, Bonaïti B, Olschwang S, Grandjouan S, Huiart L, Longy M, et al. Cancer risks associated with germline mutations in MLH1, MSH2, and MSH6 genes in Lynch syndrome. JAMA. 2011;305:2304–10.
23. Aparicio T, Henriques J, Manfredi S, Tougeron D, Bouché O, Pezet D, et al. Small bowel adenocarcinoma: results from a nationwide prospective ARCAD-NADEGE cohort study of 347 patients. Int J Cancer. 2020;147:967–77.
24. Rodriguez-Bigas MA, Vasen HF, Lynch HT, Watson P, Myrhøj T, Järvinen HJ, et al. Characteristics of small bowel carcinoma in hereditary nonpolyposis colorectal carcinoma. International Collaborative Group on HNPCC. Cancer. 1998;83:240–4.
25. Zhang MQ, Chen ZM, Wang HL. Immunohistochemical investigation of tumorigenic pathways in small intestinal adenocarcinoma: a comparison with colorectal adenocarcinoma. Mod Pathol. 2006;19:573–80.
26. Giardiello FM, Brensinger JD, Tersmette AC, Goodman SN, Petersen GM, Booker SV, et al. Very high risk of cancer in familial Peutz-Jeghers syndrome. Gastroenterology. 2000;119:1447–53.
27. Wan Q, Zhao R, Xia L, Wu Y, Zhou Y, Wang Y, et al. Inflammatory bowel disease and risk of gastric, small bowel and colorectal cancer: a meta-analysis of 26 observational studies. J Cancer Res Clin Oncol. 2021;147:1077–87.
28. Palascak-Juif V, Bouvier AM, Cosnes J, Flourié B, Bouché O, Cadiot G, et al. Small bowel adenocarcinoma in patients with Crohn's disease compared with small bowel adenocarcinoma de novo. Inflamm Bowel Dis. 2005;11:828–32.
29. Askling J, Linet M, Gridley G, Halstensen TS, Ekström K, Ekbom A. Cancer incidence in a population-based cohort of individuals hospitalized with celiac disease or dermatitis herpetiformis. Gastroenterology. 2002;123:1428–35.
30. Green PH, Fleischauer AT, Bhagat G, Goyal R, Jabri B, Neugut AI. Risk of malignancy in patients with celiac disease. Am J Med. 2003;115:191–5.
31. Yamada A, Komaki Y, Komaki F, Micic D, Zullow S, Sakuraba A. Risk of gastrointestinal cancers in patients with cystic fibrosis: a systematic review and meta-analysis. Lancet Oncol. 2018;19:758–67.

Epidemiology and Prevention. I-2. Pathological and Molecular Characteristics

Key Points

Small intestinal adenocarcinoma

- Nearly identical to colorectal carcinoma.
- Arises from adenomas or dysplasia (Crohn's disease).
- Duodenal tumors may have an intestinal, gastric, or pancreaticobiliary phenotype.

Ampullary adenocarcinoma

- Most are gland-forming (tubular adenocarcinoma).
- Approximately 60% show intestinal or biliary phenotypes, while 40% have a mixed phenotype.

Small Intestinal neuroendocrine tumor

- Nested or trabecular pattern of homogeneous cells with ample cytoplasm.
- Well-differentiated tumors have few mitoses and bland nuclei.
- Poorly differentiated tumors have a high mitotic count (Ki-67 index >20%) with necrosis.

Introduction

Small intestinal adenocarcinomas are rare, with a much lower prevalence than adenocarcinomas in any other part of the gastrointestinal tract. However, several studies have shown an increasing incidence of duodenal adenocarcinomas [1, 2]. Most duodenal cancers arise in the ampullary region and are broadly divided into intestinal and pancreaticobiliary types based on histomorphology and immunohistochemical characteristics [3]. In this chapter, the histology and molecular pathology of malignant epithelial tumors and neuroendocrine tumors will be described, and, due to limited space, mesenchymal tumors and hematolymphoid malignancy will be excluded.

Non-ampullary Adenocarcinoma

Definition

Non-ampullary adenocarcinoma is a malignant epithelial neoplasm of the small bowel with glandular differentiation.

Histopathology

Small intestinal adenocarcinomas are similar to their counterparts in the colorectum but show a

Sung Hak Lee is the lead author of this chapter.

H. J. Chun et al., *Gastrointestinal Cancer*, https://doi.org/10.1007/978-981-99-0815-8_20

higher proportion of poorly differentiated histology with glandular, squamous, and undifferentiated components [4]. Therefore, the histological subclassification of small bowel adenocarcinoma includes adenocarcinoma (not otherwise characterized), mucinous adenocarcinoma, poorly cohesive cell carcinoma (with or without signet-ring cells), medullary carcinoma, adenosquamous carcinoma, squamous cell carcinoma, and undifferentiated carcinoma (Figs. 1, 2, 3, and 4).

Despite morphological similarities with colorectal cancers, small intestinal carcinomas show different immunohistochemical profiles of cytokeratin 7/20, with 50% positive for cytokeratin 7 and 40% positive for cytokeratin 20 [5]. Furthermore, duodenal adenocarcinomas, unlike distal small intestine adenocarcinomas, often have an immunophenotype closer to that of gastric or pancreatobiliary cancers, with positive for immunohistochemical markers of the upper gastrointestinal tract (cytokeratin 7, EMA, MUC5AC, and MUC6) in half of the tumors [6, 7].

Molecular Pathology

The molecular data for small intestinal adenocarcinoma are limited. However, most small bowel adenocarcinomas arise from adenomas, and several studies suggest that an adenoma-carcinoma sequence with molecular genetics may be similar to those that arise in colorectal carcinogenesis [8].

The mutational landscape of small intestinal adenocarcinoma is summarized in Box 1.

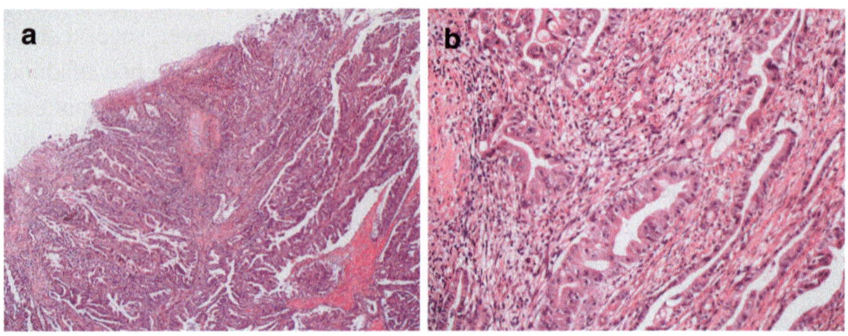

Fig. 1 Duodenal adenocarcinoma. (**a**) Moderately differentiated malignant glands are shown. (**b**) High-power view

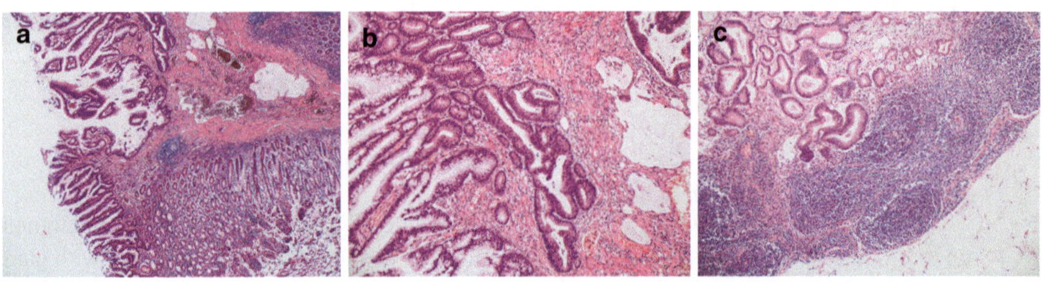

Fig. 2 Duodenal adenocarcinoma. (**a**) Villous adenoma adjacent to invasive cancer is shown (left down). (**b**) Well-differentiated, invasive adenocarcinoma component is visible, high-power view. (**c**) Metastatic tumors in the regional lymph node

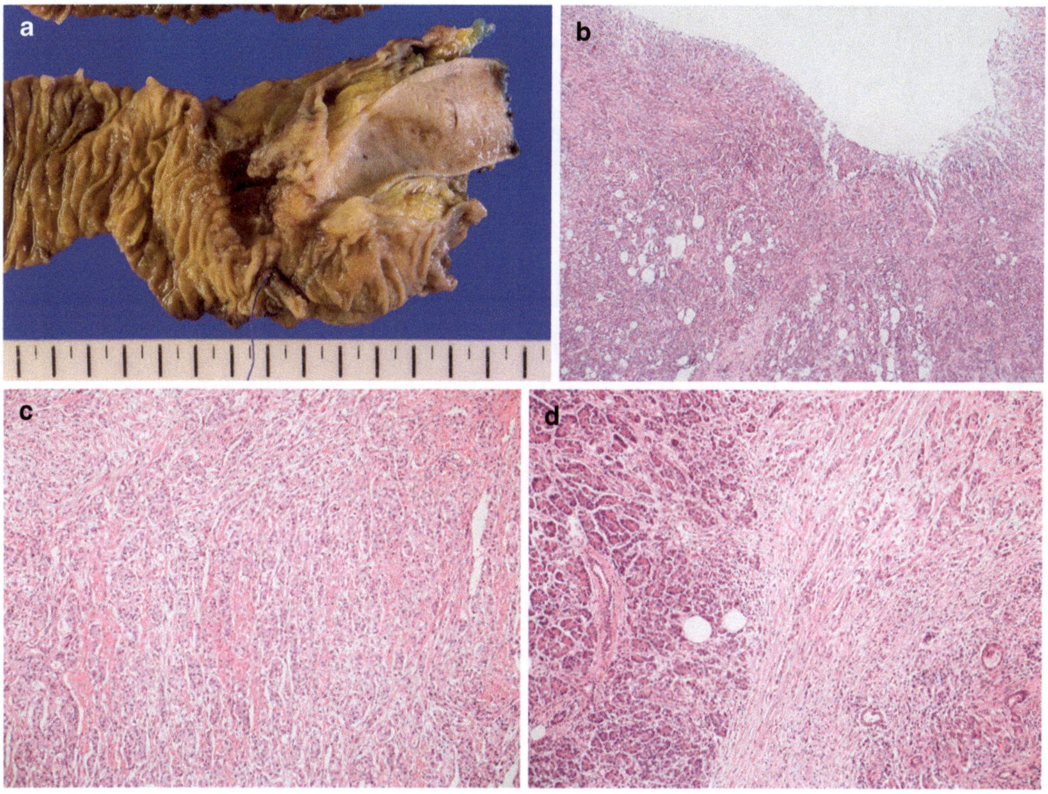

Fig. 3 Duodenal adenocarcinoma. (**a**) Deep ulcerative mass encircling the lumen is shown adjacent ampulla of Vater. (**b**) Poorly differentiated adenocarcinoma, low-power view. (**c**) High-power view. (**d**) Neoplastic cells infiltrating pancreatic tissue with desmoplastic reaction

Box 1 Molecular Alterations Identified in Small Intestinal Adenocarcinoma [3]

- *TP53* mutations
- Loss of E-cadherin and mutation of *CTNNB1* with nuclear localization
- *SMAD4*/*KRAS* mutations and activation of the RAS/RAF/MAPK pathway
- *IDH1, CDH1, KIT, FGFR2, FLT3, NPM1, PTEN. MET, AKT1, RET, ERBB2, NOTCH1*, and *ERBB4* mutations

Microsatellite instability (MSI) is reported in 5–35% of small bowel adenocarcinomas and is associated with a better prognostic outcome [6, 9]. SMARC gene alterations are reported in undifferentiated carcinomas with rhabdoid features [10]. There is a strong correlation between distal small intestinal adenocarcinoma and Crohn's disease, with an absolute risk of 2.2% at 25 years [11].

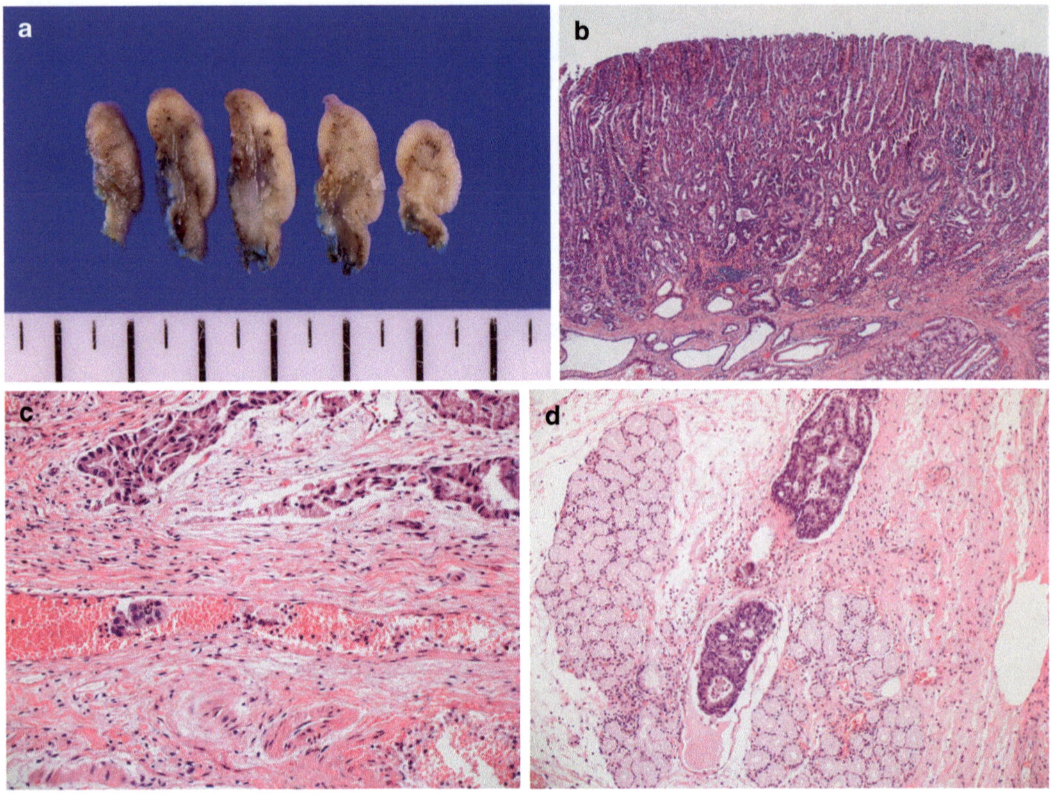

Fig. 4 Duodenal adenocarcinoma. (**a**) Cut section showing an ill-defined tumor invading submucosa. (**b**) Moderately differentiated adenocarcinoma, low-power view. (**c**) Infiltrating malignant glands with vascular invasion. (**d**) Lymphatic invasion

Ampullary Adenocarcinoma

Definition

Ampullary adenocarcinoma is a gland-forming malignant epithelial tumor of the small bowel, which originates in the ampulla of Vater.

Histopathology

Histomorphologically, ampullary adenocarcinomas have been broadly classified as intestinal (50–80%) or pancreatobiliary (15–20%) phenotypes [12, 13].

Immunohistochemically, intestinal subtypes are positive staining for CK20, CDX2, or MUC2, while the pancreatobiliary subtype was defined as positive for MUC1 and negative for CDX2 and MUC2 [14].

Intestinal-Type Adenocarcinoma

This tubule-forming adenocarcinoma is the most common malignant epithelial tumor of the ampulla and is morphologically similar to colonic adenocarcinomas [15]. The glands consist predominantly of tall columnar cells with elongated, pseudo-stratified nuclei. Scattered goblet, Paneth, and neuroendocrine cells may be detected in some carcinomas [16]. A considerable proportion is related to intestinal-type adenomas [17] (Fig. 5).

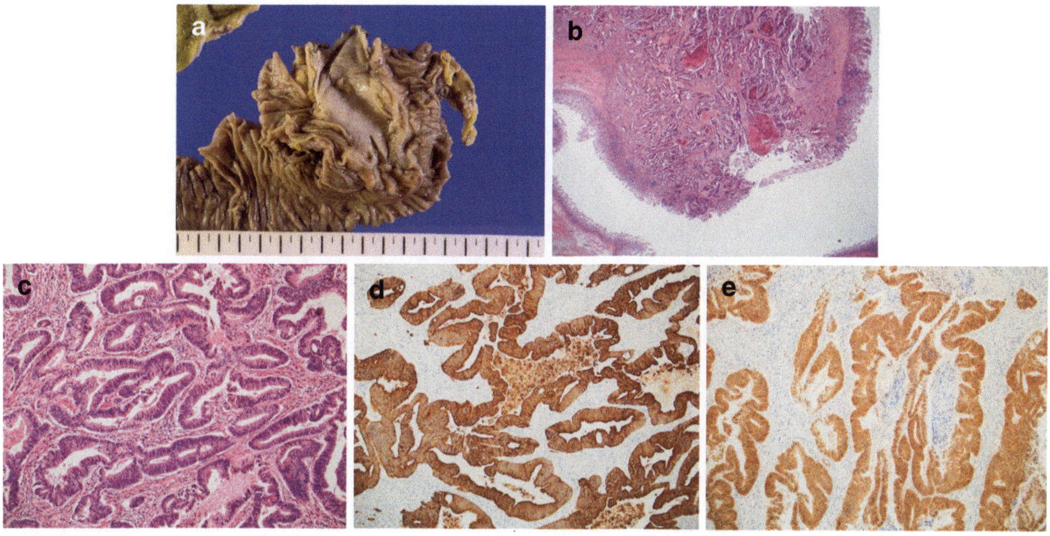

Fig. 5 Intestinal-type adenocarcinoma. (**a**) Protruding mass at the ampulla of Vater, luminal view. (**b**) Low-power view. (**c**) Neoplastic glands are made up of columnar cells with an intestinal phenotype. (**d**) Cytokeratin 20 immunoreactivity. (**e**) CDX2 immunoreactivity

Pancreatobiliary-Type or Gastric-Type Adenocarcinoma

This tubular adenocarcinoma is composed of relatively small glandular structures, which are similar to adenocarcinomas of the pancreatic ductal, gallbladder, and extrahepatic biliary tract, with a desmoplastic stroma. The glandular epithelium usually shows a single layer of cuboidal to low columnar cells, without considerable nuclear pseudostratification [15, 18] (Fig. 6).

Mucinous Adenocarcinoma

A tumor is defined as mucinous adenocarcinoma if >50% of the tumor areas are composed of extracellular mucin pools containing overt malignant epithelial cells, including signet-ring cells. Mucinous adenocarcinoma is proportionally more common in the duodenum. Mucinous adenocarcinomas account for approximately 10% of ampullary carcinoma [13] (Fig. 7).

Poorly Cohesive Cell Carcinoma

This subtype, which is relatively uncommon in the small bowel, is composed of tumor cells that are isolated or arranged in small aggregates without well-formed glandular units. Poorly cohesive cell carcinoma is usually diagnosed at an advanced stage and has a poorer prognosis than conventional adenocarcinomas [3].

Medullary Carcinoma

This type of tumor, which constitutes 3% of ampullary cancers, is characterized by malignant cells with vesicular nuclei, prominent nucleoli, and abundant eosinophilic cytoplasm with syncytial growth pattern and prominent infiltration of inflammatory cells. Medullary carcinomas can occur in the small intestine, especially in the duodenum and ampulla [6]. Like colonic medullary carcinomas, they are associated with a good prognosis despite their large size [3].

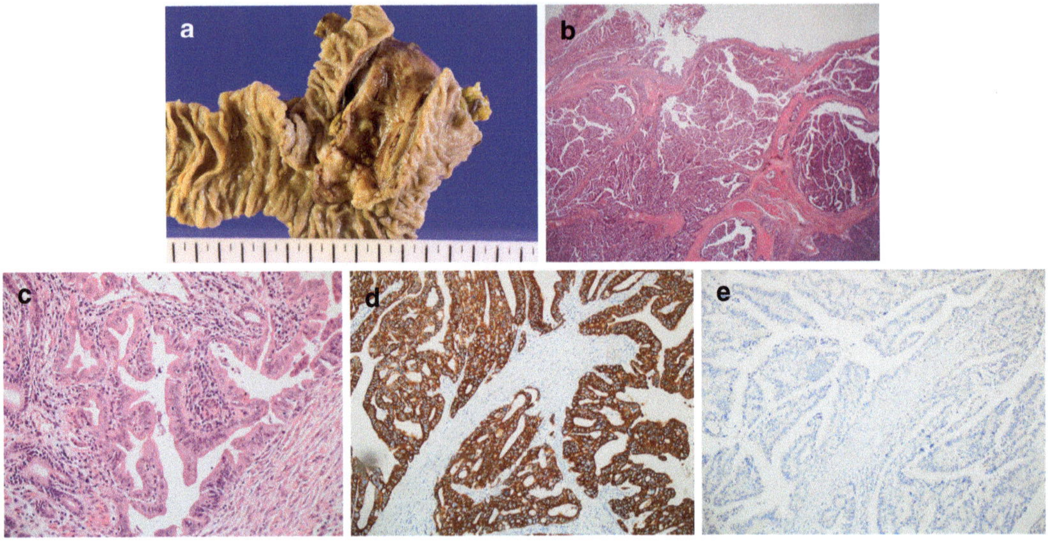

Fig. 6 Pancreatobiliary-type adenocarcinoma. (**a**) Protruding mass that circumferentially constricts the intra-ampullary duct, luminal view. (**b**) Low-power histological view. (**c**) Neoplastic glands are made up of a single layer of cuboidal or columnar cells without pseudostratification. (**d**) Cytokeratin 7 immunoreactivity. (**e**) No immunoreaction for CDX2 antibody

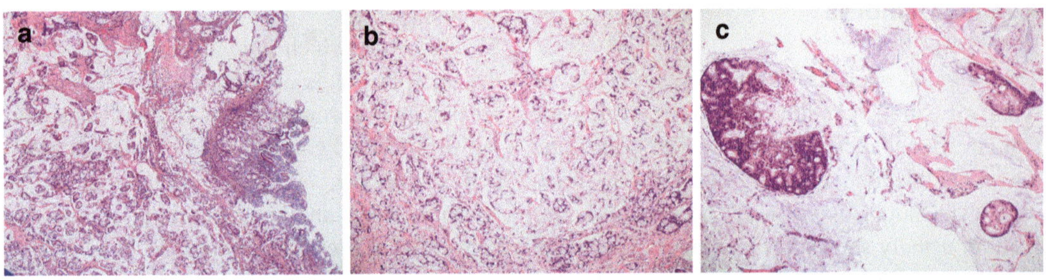

Fig. 7 Mucinous adenocarcinoma. (**a**) Malignant epithelial cell clumps within pools of extracellular mucin. (**b**) Nests of signet-ring cells floating in extracellular mucous. (**c**) Malignant glands are visible in extracellular mucinous pools

Adenosquamous Carcinoma

This rare subtype accounts for 1% of all ampullary carcinomas and has features of both adenocarcinoma and squamous cell carcinoma, similar to those seen elsewhere in the gastrointestinal tract [19].

High-Grade Neuroendocrine Carcinoma and Mixed Carcinomas

Both small-cell and large-cell neuroendocrine carcinoma (NEC) can arise from the small intestine, particularly in the ampulla [20, 21]. Usually, the solid and organoid patterns are observed in small-cell and large-cell NECs, respectively.

Undifferentiated Carcinoma

These tumors lack histological, immunohistochemical, and molecular evidence of differentiation toward the abovementioned epithelial tumors. Undifferentiated carcinoma with osteoclast-like giant cells similar to those reported in the pancreas occasionally arises in the small intestine, especially in the ampulla or duodenum [22].

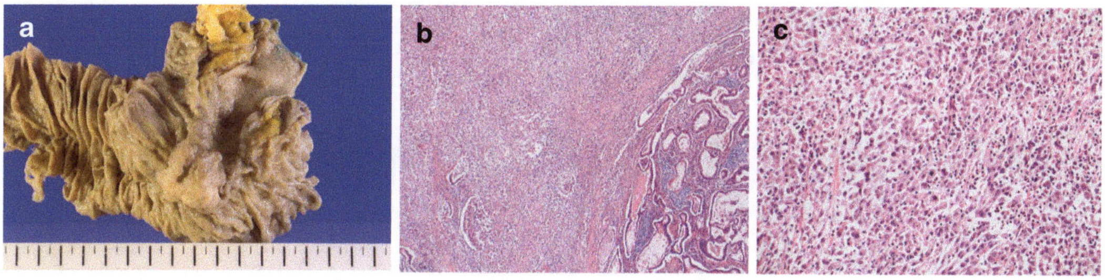

Fig. 8 Undifferentiated carcinoma. (**a**) Exophytic mass is seen in the ampullary area. (**b**) A minor glandular component is seen in most undifferentiated gastric carcinomas that are sufficiently sampled. (**c**) Rhabdoid differentiation

A small subgroup of undifferentiated carcinoma is characterized by a partially undifferentiated histomorphology and sarcomatous features such as spindle cell or rhabdoid components [10]. In general, patients have a poor outcome [3] (Fig. 8).

Molecular Pathology

Mutations in the *TP53* gene have been recorded in 59–94% of ampullary adenocarcinomas and appear to be a late event in cancer development [23, 24]. The KRAS mutation at codon 12 (and rarely codon 13) has been identified in 13–75% of ampullary adenocarcinomas and is a predictor of shorter recurrence-free survival [23, 25]. In addition, APC and β-catenin mutations have been reported in ampullary adenocarcinomas, with a lower frequency than in colorectal cancers [24]. Patients with familial adenomatous polyposis show a significantly increased risk of developing ampullary adenocarcinoma with a lifetime incidence of up to 12% [26]. MSI due to defective DNA mismatch repair has been identified in approximately 15% of ampullary carcinomas [3].

Small Intestinal and Ampullary Neuroendocrine Neoplasms

Definition

Neuroendocrine neoplasms (NENs) of the small intestine and ampulla are epithelial tumors with neuroendocrine differentiation, including well-differentiated neuroendocrine tumors (NETs) and poorly differentiated neuroendocrine carcinomas (NECs). Mixed neuroendocrine non-neuroendocrine neoplasms (MiNENs) show an exocrine component and a neuroendocrine component (typically NEC), each constituting >30% of the tumor.

Histopathology

Small intestinal NETs are composed of tumor cells with round to oval nuclei having finely granular chromatin. G-cell NETs (duodenal location) are typically arranged in trabecular pattern. D-cell NETs (ampullary location) have tubular or glandular pattern and may contain psammoma bodies. EC-cell NETs (jejunoileal location) are composed of tumor cell nests with peripheral palisading [3] (Fig. 9).

Poorly differentiated NECs are high-grade carcinomas with pleomorphic tumor cells and may show large-cell or small-cell patterns (Figs. 10 and 11).

Grading

NETs and NECs are graded on the basis of tumor differentiation and proliferative activity as assessed by mitotic rate and the Ki-67 proliferation index [27]. Small intestinal and ampullary NENs are graded using the same system for other gastrointestinal and pancreatic NENs (Table 1).

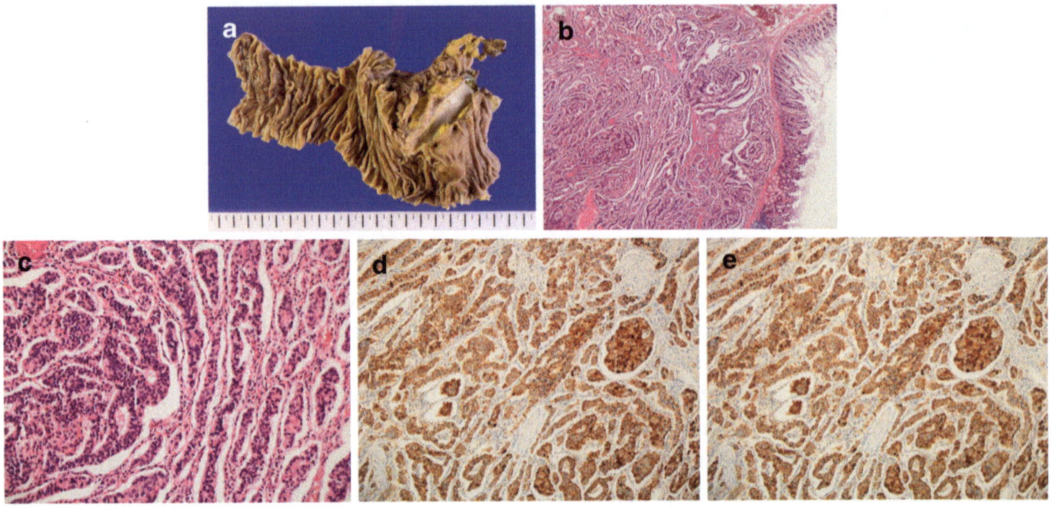

Fig. 9 Duodenal neuroendocrine tumor (NET). (**a**) Note the protruding mucosal nodule with central erosion (lower right side). (**b**) Tubuloglandular differentiation is shown, low-power view. (**c**) G1 NET showing packets of neuroendocrine cells separated by fibrovascular tissue. (**d**) Immunolabeling for synaptophysin. (**e**) Immunolabeling for chromogranin

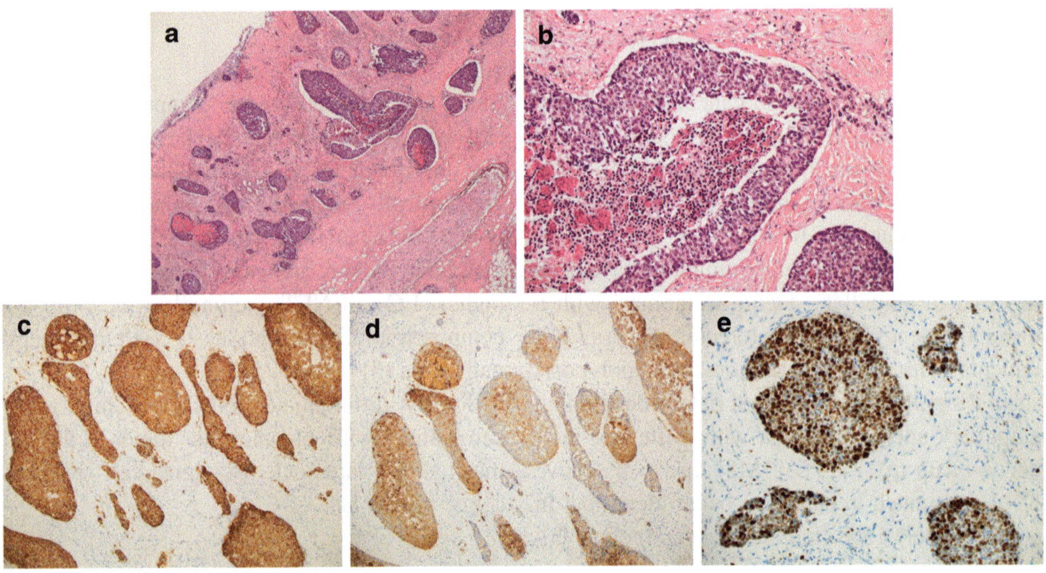

Fig. 10 Small intestinal neuroendocrine carcinoma, large-cell type. (**a**) Low-power histology. (**b**) Solid sheets of poorly differentiated tumor cells with central necrosis are seen. (**c**) Immunoreactivity for synaptophysin. (**d**) Immunoreactivity for chromogranin. (**e**) Ki-67 proliferative index of approximately 70%

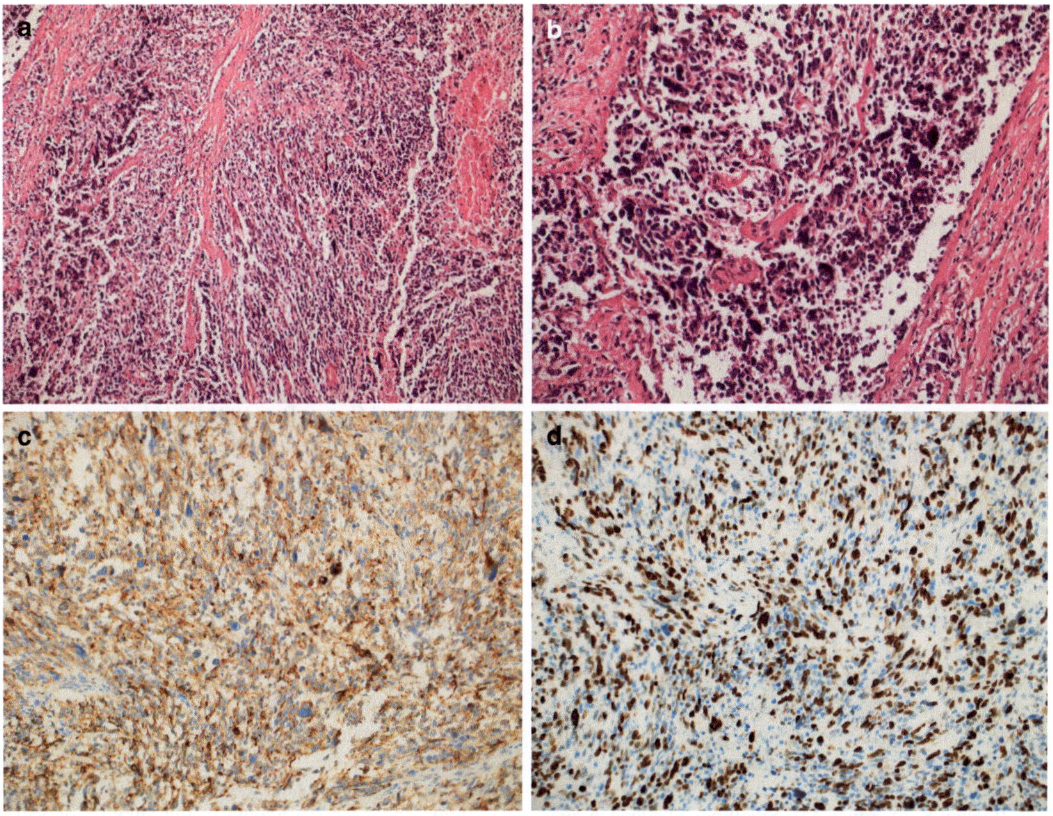

Fig. 11 Small intestinal neuroendocrine carcinoma, small-cell type. (**a**) Round to oval blue cells with minimal cytoplasm, low-power view. (**b**) Nuclear molding and smudging are shown. (**c**) Immunolabeling for synaptophysin. (**d**) Ki-67 proliferative index of approximately 70%

Table 1 Classification and grading criteria for NENs of the gastrointestinal tract and hepatobiliary systems

Terminology	Differentiation	Grade	Mitotic rate (mitoses/2 mm^2)	Ki-67 index
NET, G1	Well differentiated	Low	<2	<3%
NET, G2		Intermediate	2–20	3–20%
NET, G3		High	>20	>20%
NEC, small-cell type (SCNEC)	Poorly differentiated	High	>20	>20%
NEC, large-cell type (LCNEC)			>20	>20%
MiNEN	Well or poorly differentiated	Variable	Variable	Variable

Adapted from Klimstra et al. [3]

Molecular Pathology

Small intestine NETs have a complex genomic landscape, including frequent large-scale chromosomal abnormalities with a high rate of epigenetic changes [28, 29]. About 60–90% of jejunoileal NETs show deletion of chromosome 18 [30]. In addition, chromosome 14 gain is typically seen in advanced tumors and metastatic lesions, and therefore it may be a poor prognostic factor [31]. For epigenetic dysregulation, substantial portions of ileal NETs are the CpG island methylator phenotype [32].

Conclusion

Neoplasms of the small bowel in general are rare. The small intestinal and ampullary carcinomas have heterogeneous histopathology, with broad categories of intestinal and pancreatobiliary or gastric types. NETs are classified as G1, G2, or G3 based on proliferative activity. NECs are considered high grade by definition. The molecular characterization of small intestinal adenocarcinoma suggests that an adenoma-carcinoma sequence with molecular genetics may be similar to those arising in colorectal carcinogenesis. Identification of clinically relevant genomic alterations is encouraging in a population with limited treatment options and a poor prognosis.

References

1. Qubaiah O, Devesa SS, Platz CE, Huycke MM, Dores GM. Small intestinal cancer: a population-based study of incidence and survival patterns in the United States, 1992 to 2006. Cancer Epidemiol Biomark Prev. 2010;19:1908–18.
2. Raghav K, Overman MJ. Small bowel adenocarcinomas—existing evidence and evolving paradigms. Nat Rev Clin Oncol. 2013;10:534–44.
3. Klimstra D, Kloppell G, La Rosa S, Rindi G. WHO classification of tumours: digestive system tumours. Lyon, France: International Agency for Research on Cancer; 2019.
4. Maguire A, Sheahan K. Primary small bowel adenomas and adenocarcinomas-recent advances. Virchows Arch. 2018;473:265–73.
5. Lee MJ, Lee HS, Kim WH, Choi Y, Yang M. Expression of mucins and cytokeratins in primary carcinomas of the digestive system. Mod Pathol. 2003;16:403–10.
6. Xue Y, Vanoli A, Balci S, Reid MM, Saka B, Bagci P, et al. Non-ampullary-duodenal carcinomas: clinicopathologic analysis of 47 cases and comparison with ampullary and pancreatic adenocarcinomas. Mod Pathol. 2017;30:255–66.
7. Ushiku T, Arnason T, Fukayama M, Lauwers GY. Extra-ampullary duodenal adenocarcinoma. Am J Surg Pathol. 2014;38:1484–93.
8. Delaunoit T, Neczyporenko F, Limburg PJ, Erlichman C. Pathogenesis and risk factors of small bowel adenocarcinoma: a colorectal cancer sibling? Am J Gastroenterol. 2005;100:703–10.
9. Potter DD, Murray JA, Donohue JH, Burgart LJ, Nagorney DM, van Heerden JA, et al. The role of defective mismatch repair in small bowel adenocarcinoma in celiac disease. Cancer Res. 2004;64:7073–7.
10. Agaimy A, Daum O, Markl B, Lichtmannegger I, Michal M, Hartmann A. SWI/SNF complex-deficient undifferentiated/rhabdoid carcinomas of the gastrointestinal tract: a series of 13 cases highlighting mutually exclusive loss of SMARCA4 and SMARCA2 and frequent co-inactivation of SMARCB1 and SMARCA2. Am J Surg Pathol. 2016;40:544–53.
11. von Roon AC, Reese G, Teare J, Constantinides V, Darzi AW, Tekkis PP. The risk of cancer in patients with Crohn's disease. Dis Colon Rectum. 2007;50:839–55.
12. Kimura W, Futakawa N, Yamagata S, Wada Y, Kuroda A, Muto T, et al. Different clinicopathologic findings in two histologic types of carcinoma of papilla of Vater. Jpn J Cancer Res. 1994;85:161–6.
13. Albores-Saavedra J. Tumors of the gallbladder, extrahepatic bile ducts, and ampulla of Vater. Atlas of tumor pathology. J Clin Pathol. 2000;27:259–316.
14. Ang DC, Shia J, Tang LH, Katabi N, Klimstra DS. The utility of immunohistochemistry in subtyping adenocarcinoma of the ampulla of vater. Am J Surg Pathol. 2014;38:1371–9.
15. Reid MD, Balci S, Ohike N, Xue Y, Kim GE, Tajiri T, et al. Ampullary carcinoma is often of mixed or hybrid histologic type: an analysis of reproducibility and clinical relevance of classification as pancreatobiliary versus intestinal in 232 cases. Mod Pathol. 2016;29:1575–85.
16. Ferrell LD, Beckstead JH. Paneth-like cells in an adenoma and adenocarcinoma in the ampulla of Vater. Arch Pathol Lab Med. 1991;115:956–8.
17. Witteman BJ, Janssens AR, Terpstra JL, Eulderink F, Welvaart K, Lamers CB. Villous tumors of the duodenum. Presentation of five cases. Hepato-Gastroenterology. 1991;38:550–3.
18. Adsay V, Mino-Kenudson M, Furukawa T, Basturk O, Zamboni G, Marchegiani G, et al. Pathologic evaluation and reporting of intraductal papillary mucinous neoplasms of the pancreas and other tumoral intraepithelial neoplasms of pancreatobiliary tract: recommendations of verona consensus meeting. Ann Surg. 2016;263:162–77.
19. Yang SJ, Ooyang CH, Wang SY, Liu YY, Kuo IM, Liao CH, et al. Adenosquamous carcinoma of the ampulla of Vater—a rare disease at unusual location. World J Surg Oncol. 2013;11:124.
20. Sugawara G, Yamaguchi A, Isogai M, Watanabe Y, Kaneoka Y, Suzuki M. Small cell neuroendocrine carcinoma of the ampulla of Vater with foci of squamous differentiation: a case report. J Hepato-Biliary-Pancreat Surg. 2004;11:56–60.
21. Nassar H, Albores-Saavedra J, Klimstra DS. High-grade neuroendocrine carcinoma of the ampulla of vater: a clinicopathologic and immunohistochemical analysis of 14 cases. Am J Surg Pathol. 2005;29:588–94.
22. Kawamoto Y, Ome Y, Terada K, Hashida K, Kawamoto K, Ito T. Undifferentiated carcinoma with osteoclast-like giant cells of the ampullary region:

short term survival after pancreaticoduodenectomy. Int J Surg Case Rep. 2016;24:199–202.
23. Rashid A, Ueki T, Gao YT, Houlihan PS, Wallace C, Wang BS, et al. K-ras mutation, p53 overexpression, and microsatellite instability in biliary tract cancers: a population-based study in China. Clin Cancer Res. 2002;8:3156–63.
24. Bosman FT, Carneiro F, Hruban RH, Theise ND. WHO classification of tumours of the digestive system. World Health Organization; 2010.
25. Kwon MJ, Kim JW, Jung JP, Cho JW, Nam ES, Cho SJ, et al. Low incidence of KRAS, BRAF, and PIK3CA mutations in adenocarcinomas of the ampulla of Vater and their prognostic value. Hum Pathol. 2016;50:90–100.
26. Offerhaus GJ, Giardiello FM, Krush AJ, Booker SV, Tersmette AC, Kelley NC, et al. The risk of upper gastrointestinal cancer in familial adenomatous polyposis. Gastroenterology. 1992;102:1980–2.
27. van Velthuysen ML, Groen EJ, van der Noort V, van de Pol A, Tesselaar ME, Korse CM. Grading of neuroendocrine neoplasms: mitoses and Ki-67 are both essential. Neuroendocrinology. 2014;100:221–7.
28. Nilsson O. Profiling of ileal carcinoids. Neuroendocrinology. 2013;97:7–18.
29. Stalberg P, Westin G, Thirlwell C. Genetics and epigenetics in small intestinal neuroendocrine tumours. J Intern Med. 2016;280:584–94.
30. Wang GG, Yao JC, Worah S, White JA, Luna R, Wu TT, et al. Comparison of genetic alterations in neuroendocrine tumors: frequent loss of chromosome 18 in ileal carcinoid tumors. Mod Pathol. 2005;18:1079–87.
31. Andersson E, Sward C, Stenman G, Ahlman H, Nilsson O. High-resolution genomic profiling reveals gain of chromosome 14 as a predictor of poor outcome in ileal carcinoids. Endocr Relat Cancer. 2009;16:953–66.
32. How-Kit A, Dejeux E, Dousset B, Renault V, Baudry M, Terris B, et al. DNA methylation profiles distinguish different subtypes of gastroenteropancreatic neuroendocrine tumors. Epigenomics. 2015;7:1245–58.

Staging and Treatment. II-1. Staging and Prognosis

Key Points

- Small bowel cancer (adenocarcinoma) is a rare malignancy.
- Diagnostic methods include radiographic (computed tomography scan, small bowel series, enteroclysis) or endoscopic (wireless capsule endoscopy, push enteroscopy, double-balloon endoscopy).
- Small bowel cancer is more often diagnosed at advanced stages, suggesting the difficulty of early detection.
- As prognosis is closely related to the extent of the disease for small bowel cancers, early detection and treatment can contribute to a favorable outcome.

Introduction

The diagnosis of small bowel cancer is often established late in the course of the disease because these are generally rare conditions and the symptoms are nonspecific. Early diagnosis requires a high index of suspicion.

Hyun Seok Lee is the lead author of this chapter.

Diagnostic Evaluation

Patients with small bowel cancer require a complete staging workup, including biopsy (if appropriate), pathologic tissue review, complete blood count (CBC), serum electrolytes, liver function tests, carcinoembryonic antigen (CEA), carbohydrate antigen 19-9 (CA 19-9), and imaging studies. There is no single method that is best for imaging the small intestine in a patient with suspected small bowel cancer. The diagnostic options include radiographic (computed tomography [CT] scan, small bowel series, enteroclysis) or endoscopic (wireless capsule endoscopy, push enteroscopy, double-balloon endoscopy).

Radiographic Imaging

Multiple radiographic investigations are available for patients suspected of having a small bowel tumor.

Computed Tomography Scanning and Magnetic Resonance Imaging

Contrast-enhanced CT of the abdomen and pelvis is often obtained when evaluating vague or indeterminate abdominal complaints [1]. In addition to detecting the primary cancer, CT scans are of

H. J. Chun et al., *Gastrointestinal Cancer*, https://doi.org/10.1007/978-981-99-0815-8_21

critical importance for the appropriate evaluation of extraintestinal spread to distant sites and involvement of regional lymph nodes [2]. A chest CT (with or without IV contrast) is recommended for the initial workup and staging and to assess metastatic disease to the lungs. Magnetic resonance imaging (MRI) of the abdomen and pelvis is an alternative for cross-sectional imaging where there is a contraindication to CT. Magnetic resonance cholangiopancreatography (MRCP) may be required in the initial workup of duodenal malignancies to further determine the tumor site of origin, particularly in the presence of biliary obstruction.

CT enterography involves the administration of a large volume of an attenuation-neutral enteric contrast media (often low-concentration barium or water) to the gastrointestinal system via oral intake, which results in distension of the small bowel lumen with a contrast agent that does not interfere with the ability to visualize the lumen and the bowel wall with CT. Although not as widely available as CT enterography, MR enterography is emerging as an accurate technique for the diagnosis and exclusion of a small bowel neoplasm [3]. CT or magnetic resonance enterography may be considered when conventional CT or magnetic resonance with contrast has failed to discern a tumor [4, 5].

Positron Emission Tomography/ Computed Tomography

Positron emission tomography/computed tomography (PET/CT) may be useful for the initial diagnosis of small bowel cancer and staging. PET/CT allows the detection of primary lesion of small bowel cancers [6], although the sensitivity compared to other imaging methods has not been systematically studied. The ability of PET/CT to detect local and distant metastatic disease has not been formally evaluated. PET/CT may be useful as an adjunct to other imaging modalities such as CT or MR for nondiagnostic conventional imaging.

Endoscopy

Esophagogastroduodenoscopy (EGD) can reach only the proximal duodenum. It may be adequate if a proximal tumor of the small intestine is suspected. Endoscopic ultrasound (EUS) is useful for pretherapeutic staging of proximal small bowel cancers and may be used to discern duodenal lesions from ampullary, biliary, or pancreatic primaries [7]. Wireless video capsule endoscopy (VCE) and double-balloon enteroscopy (DBE) may be useful in certain circumstances, although they are not required for routine staging. VCE provides a noninvasive means of visualizing the entire small bowel. Although VCE allows for a more detailed examination of the entire small bowel mucosa and may result in the diagnosis of small bowel cancer when other imaging modalities have failed to reveal a primary lesion, it is not the preferred method for initial evaluation due to its inability to biopsy tissue for histopathological analysis [8, 9]. VCE is contraindicated for these conditions in the case of a small bowel obstruction or stricture [10].

Enteroscopy refers to the passage of a special enteroscope beyond the Treitz ligament using push, intraoperative, or DBE techniques [11]. The main advantage of enteroscopy compared to VCE is the ability to obtain tissue samples and perform therapeutic interventions. Enteroscopy can be complementary to VCE by allowing tissue sampling of lesions identified during VCE. However, the procedure is invasive and can be technically challenging (hence not always successful in visualizing the entire small bowel), and the required expertise and equipment are not always available.

Staging and Prognosis

As prognosis is closely linked to disease extent for small bowel cancers, early detection and treatment can contribute to a favorable outcome [12]. The staging of small bowel cancer is based on the tumor, node, metastasis (TNM) system of the American Joint Committee on Cancer (AJCC) (Tables 1 and 2) [13].

Table 1 Definitions for T, N, M staging

T category	Primary tumor (T)
TX	Primary tumor cannot be assessed
T0	No evidence of primary tumor
Tis	High-grade dysplasia/carcinoma in situ
T1	Tumor invades the lamina propria or submucosa
T1a	Tumor invades the lamina propria
T1b	Tumor invades the submucosa
T2	Tumor invades the muscularis propria
T3	Tumor invades the muscularis propria into the subserosa, or extends into nonperitonealized perimuscular tissue (mesentery or retroperitoneum) without serosal penetration*
T4	Tumor perforates the visceral peritoneum or directly invades other organs or structures (e.g., other loops of the small intestine, mesentery of adjacent loops of the bowel, and abdominal wall by means of serosa; for duodenum only, invasion of pancreas or bile duct)
N category	**Regional lymph nodes (N)**
NX	Regional lymph nodes cannot be assessed
N0	No regional lymph node metastasis
N1	Metastasis in one or two regional lymph nodes
N2	Metastasis in three or more regional lymph nodes
M category	**Distant metastasis (M)**
M0	No distant metastasis
M1	Distant metastasis present

Adapted from AJCC Cancer Staging Manual, 8th Ed. [13]

Table 2 AJCC prognostic stage groups

T	N	M	Prognostic stage group
Tis	N0	M0	0
T1–2	N0	M0	I
T3	N0	M0	IIA
T4	N0	M0	IIB
Any T	N1	M0	IIIA
Any T	N2	M0	IIIB
Any T	Any N	M1	IV

AJCC American Joint Committee on Cancer
Adapted from AJCC Cancer Staging Manual, 8th Ed. [13]

Conclusion

Small bowel cancer is a rare malignancy, with a rising incidence in recent decades. Small bowel cancer is often diagnosed in advanced stages, suggesting the difficulty of detecting these cancers. Although curative therapy involves surgical resection, most small bowel cancers arise in the duodenum and are associated with a poorer prognosis.

References

1. Laurent F, Raynaud M, Biset JM, Boisserie-Lacroix M, Grelet P, Drouillard J. Diagnosis and categorization of small bowel neoplasms: role of computed tomography. Gastrointest Radiol. 1991;16:115–9.
2. Horton KM, Fishman EK. Multidetector-row computed tomography and 3-dimensional computed tomography imaging of small bowel neoplasms: current concept in diagnosis. J Comput Assist Tomogr. 2004;28:106–16.
3. Masselli G, Di Tola M, Casciani E, Polettini E, Laghi F, Monti R, et al. Diagnosis of small-bowel diseases: prospective comparison of multi-detector row CT enterography with MR enterography. Radiology. 2016;279:420–31.
4. Soyer P, Aout M, Hoeffel C, Vicaut E, Placé V, Boudiaf M. Helical CT-enteroclysis in the detection of small-bowel tumours: a meta-analysis. Eur Radiol. 2013;23:388–99.
5. Masselli G, Casciani E, Polettini E, Laghi F, Gualdi G. Magnetic resonance imaging of small bowel neoplasms. Cancer Imaging. 2013;13:92–9.
6. Cronin CG, Scott J, Kambadakone A, Catalano OA, Sahani D, Blake MA, et al. Utility of positron emission tomography/CT in the evaluation of small bowel pathology. Br J Radiol. 2012;85:1211–21.
7. Nylund K, Ødegaard S, Hausken T, Folvik G, Lied GA, Viola I, et al. Sonography of the small intestine. World J Gastroenterol. 2009;15:1319–30.
8. Bailey AA, Debinski HS, Appleyard MN, Remedios ML, Hooper JE, Walsh AJ, et al. Diagnosis and outcome of small bowel tumors found by capsule endoscopy: a three-center Australian experience. Am J Gastroenterol. 2006;101:2237–43.
9. Cheung DY, Lee IS, Chang DK, Kim JO, Cheon JH, Jang BI, et al. Capsule endoscopy in small bowel

tumors: a multicenter Korean study. J Gastroenterol Hepatol. 2010;25:1079–86.
10. Hara AK, Leighton JA, Sharma VK, Heigh RI, Fleischer DE. Imaging of small bowel disease: comparison of capsule endoscopy, standard endoscopy, barium examination, and CT. Radiographics. 2005;25:697–711; discussion 711–8.
11. Fry LC, Bellutti M, Neumann H, Malfertheiner P, Mönkemüller K. Incidence of bleeding lesions within reach of conventional upper and lower endoscopes in patients undergoing double-balloon enteroscopy for obscure gastrointestinal bleeding. Aliment Pharmacol Ther. 2009;29:342–9.
12. North JH, Pack MS. Malignant tumors of the small intestine: a review of 144 cases. Am Surg. 2000;66:46–51.
13. Small Intestine. In: Amin MB editor, AJCC cancer staging manual, 8th ed. Chicago: AJCC; 2017. p. 221.

Staging and Treatment. II-2. Overview of Treatment

Key Points

- Surgery is the standard treatment for resectable small bowel adenocarcinoma, while cytotoxic chemotherapy, targeted therapy, or an immune checkpoint inhibitor could be considered in unresectable disease status. The efficacy of neoadjuvant or adjuvant systemic therapy in small bowel cancer has not yet been clearly determined.
- Complete resection without lymphadenectomy is the standard treatment for localized GIST due to rare metastasis to the regional lymph node. Adjuvant imatinib is recommended in intermediate- or high-risk malignant potential behavior. Unresectable GIST should be considered as medical therapy, including imatinib or sunitinib.
- Complete resection with regional lymphadenectomy is the standard treatment for localized neuroendocrine disease due to its indolent but metastatic potential. For patients with unresectable disease status and/or symptomatic carcinoid syndrome, somatostatin analogs, such as octreotide and lanreotide, which act as agonists of inhibitory somatostatin receptors, are the first-line medical therapy.

Introduction

Small bowel cancer is a very rare disease that accounts for approximately 3% of gastrointestinal cancers; however, the incidence rate has been steadily increasing recently, unlike other cancers of the gastrointestinal tract [1]. The most common cancers of the small bowel include adenocarcinoma, gastrointestinal stromal tumor, neuroendocrine tumor, and lymphoma. Since these small intestine cancers show different pathophysiological characteristics, a different therapeutic approach is required according to each histological type [2]. Due to the inherent limitations of the low incidence of small bowel cancers, research is limited to small treatment-related studies, and most are retrospective studies, and no clinical trials have been reported to date. In this chapter, we will provide an overview of treatment for small bowel cancers according to the histological subtypes.

Stage I–III. Adenocarcinoma

Endoscopic resection could be considered for stage I Tis and T1aN0 small bowel adenocarcinoma (SBA) with a high success rate in an experienced unit, although there has been no comparative trial with surgery to date [3].

Soo-Young Na is the lead author of this chapter.

H. J. Chun et al., *Gastrointestinal Cancer*, https://doi.org/10.1007/978-981-99-0815-8_22

However, surgery may be considered if endoscopic resection is not feasible due to difficult tumor location, large size, or deep invasion. The standard treatment of choice for SBA is curative surgical resection. For local SBA, of T1bN0 or T2N0 stage I to stage III, surgical resection with removal of the regional lymph nodes is recommended [4]. The type and extent of resection used to treat localized SBA depends on the location of the primary tumor. The SBA of the first and second portions of the duodenum may require pancreaticoduodenectomy (Whipple procedure) or segmental duodenal resection. A retrospective study of duodenal SBA of 1611 patients showed similar 5-year overall survival (odds ratio, 1.11; 95% confidential interval, 0.97–1.27) after controlling for confounding factors between radical resection (865 patients) and segmental resection groups (746 patients) [5]. For SBA of the third and fourth portions of the duodenum, jejunum, or proximal ileum, segmentectomy with resection of the mesentery and regional lymph nodes is preferred [6]. If the SBA is located in the terminal ileum, terminal ileal resection with right hemicolectomy is preferred [6]. Unfortunately, many SBA present at an advanced stage at diagnosis; therefore, 25–60% of patients are not feasible for surgery, and 15–25% of patients who undergo surgery do not achieve curative (R0) resection [6].

Patients with SBA have a poor prognosis even after curative resection, with a 5-year survival of 40–65%, and most patients who undergo curative resection experience recurrence [7]. Regarding the role of adjuvant chemotherapy and/or radiotherapy, a phase 3 trial is ongoing, and some retrospective studies have shown controversial results. Therefore, there is no consensus on an optimal perioperative therapy. A meta-analysis that included 15 studies of 5986 patients showed no survival benefit of adjuvant chemotherapy and/or radiation therapy for patients with SBA [8]. However, the National Comprehensive Cancer Network (NCCN) recommends 6 months of adjuvant systemic therapy for stage III SBA [1]. For stage II SBA with microsatellite-stable or proficient mismatch repair, NCCN recommends the option of 6 months of adjuvant systemic therapy or close observation [1]. In cases of locally unresectable or medically inoperable SBA, neoadjuvant systemic therapy may be considered to convert the resectable state [9]; however, if the conversion to the resectable state could not be achieved, palliative chemotherapy should be considered.

Stage IV. Adenocarcinoma

The most common sites for distant metastases of SBA include the peritoneal cavity and liver. Although resectable metastases are rare for SBA, limited metastases to visceral organs can be considered for metastasectomy with a multidisciplinary team approach such as colorectal cancer. In a cohort study, long-term survivors are observed after metastatic SBA resection [10]. The treatment option for unresectable peritoneal or distant metastases is palliative systemic therapy. No randomized controlled trials have been conducted evaluating systemic therapy, with the exception of several retrospective studies or small phase 2 trials. Based on these limited results, several systemic therapy regimens are recommended for the treatment of metastatic SBA, regimens that include (1) cytotoxic chemotherapy such as gemcitabine, 5-FU, capecitabine, doxorubicin, mitomycin C, and irinotecan; (2) targeted therapy with a vascular endothelial growth factor-A (VEGF-A) inhibitor (bevacizumab) and epidermal growth factor receptor (EGFR) inhibitor (cetuximab); and (3) immune checkpoint inhibitors such as anti-PD-1 inhibitor (pembrolizumab, nivolumab) and anti-CTLA4 inhibitor (ipilimumab). The overview of treatment options according to the stage of SBA is summarized in Table 1.

Table 1 Overview of treatment of small bowel adenocarcinoma

Stage	Features	Recommendation
Tis		Endoscopic resection if feasible or surgical resection
Stage I	• T1aN0	Endoscopic resection if feasible or surgical resection
	• T1bN0 or T2N0	Surgical resection alone
Stage II	• MSI-H or dMMR	Surgical resection alone
	• MSS or pMMR and/or high-risk features including T4 stage, positive surgical margins, few lymph node exploration, tumor perforation	Surgical resection with or without 6 months of adjuvant systemic therapy
Stage III	• Locally resectable status	Surgical resection with 6 months of adjuvant systemic therapy
	• Locally unresectable state or medically inoperable condition	Neoadjuvant systemic therapy with surgical resection if feasible or definite systemic therapy
Stage IV	• Resectable distant metastases	Metastasectomy with adjuvant systemic therapy if feasible
	• Unresectable distant metastases	Definite systemic therapy

MSI-H microsatellite-instability high; *dMMR* deficient mismatch repair; *MSS* microsatellite-stable; *pMMR* proficient mismatch repair

Gastrointestinal Stromal Tumor and Sarcomas

Gastrointestinal stromal tumor (GIST) has activating mutations in the c-*KIT* (CD117) oncogene. *c-KIT* mutations are observed in about 60–85% of all GISTs, and a subset of GISTs lacking *c-KIT* mutations (about 5–10% of all GISTs) has activating mutations in a related receptor tyrosine kinase, the platelet-derived growth factor receptor alpha (*PDGFRA*) [2]. Imatinib mesylate, a first-line tyrosine kinase inhibitor, blocks the KIT/PDGFRA signal pathway and was approved by the US Food and Drug Administration in Feb 2002 for this indication.

Complete segmental resection with negative margins is the standard treatment for primary resectable GIST and sarcomas [11]. Because these rarely metastasize to the regional lymph node, lymphadenectomy is usually not recommended [11]. In addition, aggressive resection of adjacent organs that have been invaded with tumor or liver metastases may be beneficial in survival. Preoperative imatinib is generally not recommended for resectable GIST because it interferes with an accurate assessment of the risk of recurrence. However, it could be considered when a reduction in surgical morbidity is expected by downstaging the tumor [12]. However, despite complete resection with negative margins, 45–80% of patients will experience local or peritoneal recurrence generally within 2 years [6]. The NCCN recommends adjuvant treatment with imatinib for patients with intermediate- or high-risk of recurrence, for patients who have received neoadjuvant therapy with imatinib, or for patients not undergoing curative resection [12]. Risk stratification was based on tumor behavior such as tumor size and mitotic count (Table 2) [13].

Patients who have advanced unresectable GIST should be treated with imatinib. Response rates in patients with a c-*KIT* exon 11 mutation or a c-*KIT* exon 9 mutation are 70% and 50%, respectively, and the latter can be improved by dose escalation [6]. Whether neoadjuvant therapy with imatinib has improved clinical outcomes for patients with resectable metastatic GIST is not known. However, surgical resection could be considered if complete resection can be obtained

Table 2 Risk stratification based on behavior and treatment overview of small bowel gastrointestinal stromal tumor

Risk	Behavior	Recommendation
Very low	• Size: <2 cm and mitotic index: <5/50 HPF	Endoscopic, if feasible, or surgical resection alone
Low	• Size: 2–5 cm and mitotic index: <5/50 HPF	Surgical resection alone
Intermediate	• Size: 5–10 cm and mitotic index: <5/50 HPF • Size: <5 cm and mitotic index: 6–10/50 HPF	Complete resection with postoperative imatinib
High	• Size: >5 cm and mitotic index: >5/50 HPF • Size: 10 cm and any mitotic index • Any size and mitotic index: >10/50 HPF • Tumor rupture • Resectable distant metastases	Complete resection with prolonged postoperative imatinib treatment
Unresectable	• Medically unfit for complete resection • Unresectable distant metastases	Definite medical therapy including imatinib or sunitinib

HPF high-power field

even if in the presence of primary metastatic GIST [12]. For most patients with metastatic GIST who are ineligible for surgery, continuous administration of imatinib is required. Patients who develop progression following imatinib treatment or who develop significant adverse effects to imatinib can be switched to another second-line multi-targeted tyrosine kinase inhibitor, sunitinib, which has been shown to achieve overall response rates in about half of these patients [14]. Regorafenib, a multi-kinase inhibitor, is recommended for patients who have failed treatment with imatinib and sunitinib. Several other multi-kinase inhibitors also include sorafenib, pazopanib, ponatinib, dasatinib, and nilotinib. Chemotherapy and/or radiotherapy for advanced GIST are ineffective for the treatment of patients with unresectable metastases and for patients with tumor recurrence.

Neuroendocrine Tumor

The small bowel neuroendocrine tumor (NET) has metastatic potential, although it usually shows an indolent nature in disease progression. Therefore, resection of the primary tumor with the removal of the adjacent mesentery and lymph node is generally recommended in surgery [11]. The presence of lymph node metastases correlates with the size of the small bowel NET. Curative resection is the standard treatment for small bowel NET. For small-sized localized duodenal NET less than 1 cm confined to the submucosal layer, endoscopic resection could be considered. One retrospective study reported an endoscopic en bloc resection rate of 95% with a pathological complete resection of 41% achieved in 41 small duodenal NETs [15]. For localized duodenal NET more than 1 cm, located in a difficult position or beyond the submucosal layer, primary excision, segmental resection, or pancreatoduodenectomy with or without lymphadenectomy could be considered for curative resection [16]. For jejunal and ileal NET, surgical segmentectomy with or without regional lymphadenectomy is recommended [16]. The surgical procedure is necessary for a thorough evaluation for a synchronous tumor because the incidence of synchronous lesions is reported up to one-third [6]. If surgical resection is planned in patients with carcinoid syndrome or with large, bulky serotonin-producing functional tumors, perioperative management using somatostatin analogs (SSAs) should be considered to prevent carcinoid crisis.

Surgical resection could be considered if complete concomitant resection of the primary and metastatic tumor is feasible even in metastatic disease status with supporting data that may improve long-term survival. For patients with unresectable disease status and/or symptoms (carcinoid syndrome), curative surgery is generally not considered and is reserved for only debulking or palliative surgery in patients with disease-related complication [11]. The spectrum of the small bowel NET is diverse from a non-functioning solid tumor to a functioning tumor arising from neuroendocrine secretory cells that produce peptide hormone. A large number of metastatic small bowel NETs secrete serotonin, which could cause carcinoid syndrome. SSAs, such as octreotide and lanreotide, are considered a first-line treatment for patients with unresectable metastatic small bowel NET for both control of carcinoid syndrome and tumor progression. SSAs showed efficacy and comparable safety in symptomatic carcinoid syndrome with flushing and diarrhea in approximately three-quarters of patients [2]. In patients with a failed response to first-line SSAs, interferon-α2a could be considered as a second-line medical therapy [6]. The efficacy of systemic cytotoxic chemotherapy for small bowel NET is poor.

Conclusion

Small bowel cancers require a different therapeutic approach depending on the histological types. Although there are limited data on treatment options due to the low incidence of small bowel cancers, future clinical trials and larger studies will be helpful in understanding the therapeutic prognosis of these cancers. Furthermore, the development of various drug pipelines is expected to improve the survival rate of small bowel cancers.

References

1. https://www.nccn.org/professionals/physician_gls/pdf/small_bowel.pdf.
2. Puccini A, Battaglin F, Lenz HJ. Management of advanced small bowel cancer. Curr Treat Options in Oncol. 2018;19:69.
3. Nonaka S, Oda I, Tada K, Mori G, Sato Y, Abe S, et al. Clinical outcome of endoscopic resection for nonampullary duodenal tumors. Endoscopy. 2015;47:129–35.
4. Overman MJ, Kopetz S, Lin E, Abbruzzese JL, Wolff RA. Is there a role for adjuvant therapy in resected adenocarcinoma of the small intestine. Acta Oncol. 2010;49:474–9.
5. Cloyd JM, Norton JA, Visser BC, Poultsides GA. Does the extent of resection impact survival for duodenal adenocarcinoma? Analysis of 1,611 cases. Ann Surg Oncol. 2015;22:573–80.
6. Feldman MFL, Brandt LJ. Sleisenger and fordtran's gastrointestinal and liver disease: pathophysiology, diagnosis, management, 11/e. Elsevier; 2020.
7. Kitahara H, Honma Y, Ueno M, Kanemitsu Y, Ohkawa S, Mizusawa J, et al. Randomized phase III trial of post-operative chemotherapy for patients with stage I/II/III small bowel adenocarcinoma (JCOG1502C, J-BALLAD). Jpn J Clin Oncol. 2019;49:287–90.
8. Ye X, Zhang G, Chen H, Yong L. Meta-analysis of postoperative adjuvant therapy for small bowel adenocarcinoma. PLoS One. 2018;13:e0200204.
9. Yeung RS, Weese JL, Hoffman JP, Solin LJ, Paul AR, Engstrom PF, et al. Neoadjuvant chemoradiation in pancreatic and duodenal carcinoma. A Phase II Study. Cancer. 1993;72:2124–33.
10. Rompteaux P, Gagnière J, Gornet JM, Coriat R, Baumgaertner I, Lecomte T, et al. Resection of small bowel adenocarcinoma metastases: results of the ARCAD-NADEGE cohort study. Eur J Surg Oncol. 2019;45:331–5.
11. Ocasio Quinones GA, Woolf A. Small bowel cancer. StatPearls. Treasure Island (FL): StatPearls Publishing LLC; 2022.
12. https://www.nccn.org/professionals/physician_gls/pdf/gist.pdf.
13. Fletcher CD, Berman JJ, Corless C, Gorstein F, Lasota J, Longley BJ, et al. Diagnosis of gastrointestinal stromal tumors: a consensus approach. Hum Pathol. 2002;33:459–65.
14. George S, Blay JY, Casali PG, Stephenson P, Deprimo SE, Harmon CS, et al. Clinical evaluation of continuous daily dosing of sunitinib malate in patients with advanced gastrointestinal stromal tumour after imatinib failure. Eur J Cancer. 2009;45:1959–68.
15. Kim GH, Kim JI, Jeon SW, Moon JS, Chung IK, Lee SR, et al. Endoscopic resection for duodenal carcinoid tumors: a multicenter, retrospective study. J Gastroenterol Hepatol. 2014;29:318–24.
16. https://www.nccn.org/professionals/physician_gls/pdf/neuroendocrine.pdf.

Staging and Treatment. II-3. Surgical Resection and Adjuvant Chemotherapy

Key Points

- The appropriate extent of bowel resection for localized small bowel cancer (stages I–III) depends on the anatomical location of the tumor.
- A multidisciplinary team approach is needed in locally unresectable or metastatic small bowel cancer because initially unresectable small bowel cancer could be converted to resectable disease after neoadjuvant chemotherapy or chemoradiation therapy demonstrating good results in selective cases.
- Adjuvant chemotherapy for small bowel cancer follows the colorectal cancer guideline until the results of the first randomized controlled trial (BALLAD) on the usefulness of adjuvant chemotherapy in stage I–III small bowel cancer are available.

Introduction

Since small bowel cancer is rarely encountered in clinical practice, surgical extent and adjuvant therapy have not been standardized until recently; some expert groups have suggested clinical guidelines for small bowel cancer. However, there are still some controversies about their clinical effectiveness because these guidelines were based on retrospective studies rather than randomized controlled studies (RCTs). Here, we will introduce several retrospective studies and ongoing RCTs investigating surgical and adjuvant therapy of small bowel cancer and review the treatment guidelines that have been published to date.

Small Bowel Adenocarcinoma

Surgical Treatment

All patients with stage I–III small bowel adenocarcinoma should be considered for complete surgical resection with en bloc lymphadenectomy down to the origin of feeding vessels with a margin of at least 5–10 cm on either side of the tumor [1, 2].

The appropriate extent of bowel resection to treat localized small bowel adenocarcinoma depends on the anatomical location of the tumor. Segmental resection of the small intestine is often the mainstay of treatment in jejunoileal adenocarcinoma, although duodenal adenocarcinoma may require pancreaticoduodenectomy or segmental duodenal resection. Pancreaticoduodenectomy (Whipple procedure or pylorus-preserving pancreaticoduodenectomy) is predominantly considered in cancers arising in the second portion of the duodenum

---

Woo Ram Kim is the lead author of this chapter.

H. J. Chun et al., *Gastrointestinal Cancer*, https://doi.org/10.1007/978-981-99-0815-8_23

or invading any portion of the ampulla or pancreas. The laparoscopic Whipple procedure could be used selectively in high-volume centers with experienced surgeons due to the technical complexity of this procedure, but the approach is not recommended in cases of T4 tumors or cases suspected of synchronous peritoneal carcinomatosis [1].

Limited resection may be considered in small bowel adenocarcinoma involving the first, third, and fourth part of the duodenum [3]. Although it is associated with low lymph node retrieval, limited resection is recommended in small bowel adenocarcinoma of less than 2 cm and mesenteric tumors due to comparable results regarding overall survival (OS) or disease-specific survival between radical and limited resections [4, 5]. However, surgeons should attempt to retrieve regional lymph nodes as much as possible for proper staging. Some studies demonstrate that a minimum of five and nine lymph nodes in duodenal and jejunoileal cancer should be harvested for adequate staging [6, 7]. French and American expert guidelines recommend that the goal for the number of retrieved lymph nodes should be at least 6 and 8 for proper staging in small bowel adenocarcinoma, respectively [1, 2].

Intraoperative exploration must include the mesentery, omentum, and peritoneum. Up to 30% of patients diagnosed with small bowel adenocarcinoma present at a later metastatic stage. Delicate surgical exploration is mandatory because cytoreductive surgery in some cases could improve oncologic outcomes in highly selective patients [8]. Although Elias et al. demonstrated similar and satisfactory results of hyperthermic intraperitoneal chemotherapy (HIPEC) in the treatment of peritoneal carcinomatosis in colon, rectum, and small bowel adenocarcinoma [9], the evidence of its application for the treatment of small bowel adenocarcinoma is still lacking and therefore would not be recommended as a standard procedure.

The prognosis of nonresectable metastatic small bowel adenocarcinoma is poor. The 5-year OS and median OS are known as 3–5% and 12.7 months, respectively [10]. Although stage IV small bowel adenocarcinoma is treated mainly with systemic chemotherapy, palliative surgical treatment should be considered in cases of symptomatic tumors (hemorrhage or obstruction).

Furthermore, initially nonresectable metastatic cases could be converted into resectable disease after neoadjuvant chemotherapy or chemoradiation therapy and show good results in selective cases [11, 12]. Therefore, a multidisciplinary team approach is needed in locally unresectable or metastatic small bowel adenocarcinoma.

The French guideline, which is the first intergroup consensus document reported in 2017 [1], and the American guideline, which is the second and published in 2019 [2], are two guidelines available for small bowel adenocarcinoma so far and are summarized in Table 1.

Adjuvant Therapy

Small bowel adenocarcinomas are very rare, so there is limited scientific research on whether adjuvant therapy is beneficial or not. To date, only retrospective case-control studies or meta-analysis has been conducted, and it is difficult to draw definitive conclusions due to the small number of patients in each study and the conflicting results [13–16]. Therefore, small bowel adenocarcinomas are often treated with the same treatments as colon cancer because they are similar to colon cancers.

Chemotherapy

Evidence supporting the benefits of adjuvant chemotherapy for stage I–III small bowel cancer is lacking. Some retrospective studies and meta-analyses showed a benefit [14], but others did not [13, 15, 16]. Therefore, the ongoing international phase III BALLAD trial (NCT02502370), which is the first prospective trial investigating the role

Table 1 Comparison of surgical guidelines for small bowel adenocarcinoma between French [1] and American expert group [2]

Principle of surgery	French	American (NCCN)
Resection margin	At least 5 cm on either side of tumor	At least 5–10 cm on either side of the tumor
Extent of surgery	En-bloc excision down to the origin of feeding vessels depending on the location of primary tumor	
Whipple or PPPD	Duodenum second portion or Invading tumors to the ampulla or pancreas	
Limited segmentectomy	Duodenum third/fourth portion of anti-mesenteric tumor or duodenum first portion located on the mesenteric side and for lesions <2cm in size jejunal or ileal tumor	
Ileocecal resection or right hemicolectomy	Tumors involving last ileal loop or ileocecal valve	
Recommended numbers of harvesting lymph nodes	At least 6	At least 8
CRS and HIPEC	Can be considered only for expert centers with macroscopically resectable peritoneal carcinomatosis (but not yet standardized procedure)	CRS can be considered in resectable peritoneal carcinomatosis but HIPEC is not recommended

PPPD pylorus-preserving pancreaticoduodenectomy; *CRS* cytoreductive surgery; *HIPEC* hyperthermic intraperitoneal chemotherapy

of adjuvant 5-FU/leucovorin (5-FU/LV) or 5-FU/LV plus oxaliplatin (FOLFOX) compared to observation alone for patients with stage I–III small bowel adenocarcinoma, is important. Unlike colon cancer, chemotherapeutic regimens are diverse, including 5-fluorouracil alone or in combination with doxorubicin, cisplatin, mitomycin C, cyclophosphamide, and oxaliplatin [17]. Until the results of the RCTs are available, adjuvant chemotherapy is recommended in patients with stage II/III according to the French and American guidelines and expert group suggestions based on the results so far. A more detailed treatment algorithm for stage I–III small bowel adenocarcinoma is presented in Figs. 1 and 2.

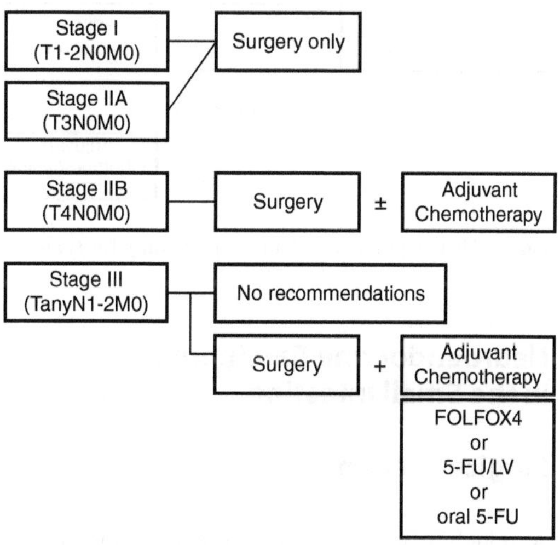

Fig. 1 French guideline of adjuvant therapy for stage I–III small bowel adenocarcinoma

Chemoradiation Therapy

The usefulness of chemoradiation for locally advanced duodenal adenocarcinoma has not yet been demonstrated. A multicenter study presented a survival benefit in patients treated with adjuvant chemoradiation therapy, compared to surgery alone [18]. However, a recent retrospective study of patients with nonmetastatic resected duodenal adenocarcinoma did not demonstrate a survival improvement between chemoradiation and chemotherapy alone [19]. Therefore, chemoradiation should only be considered in highly selected patients.

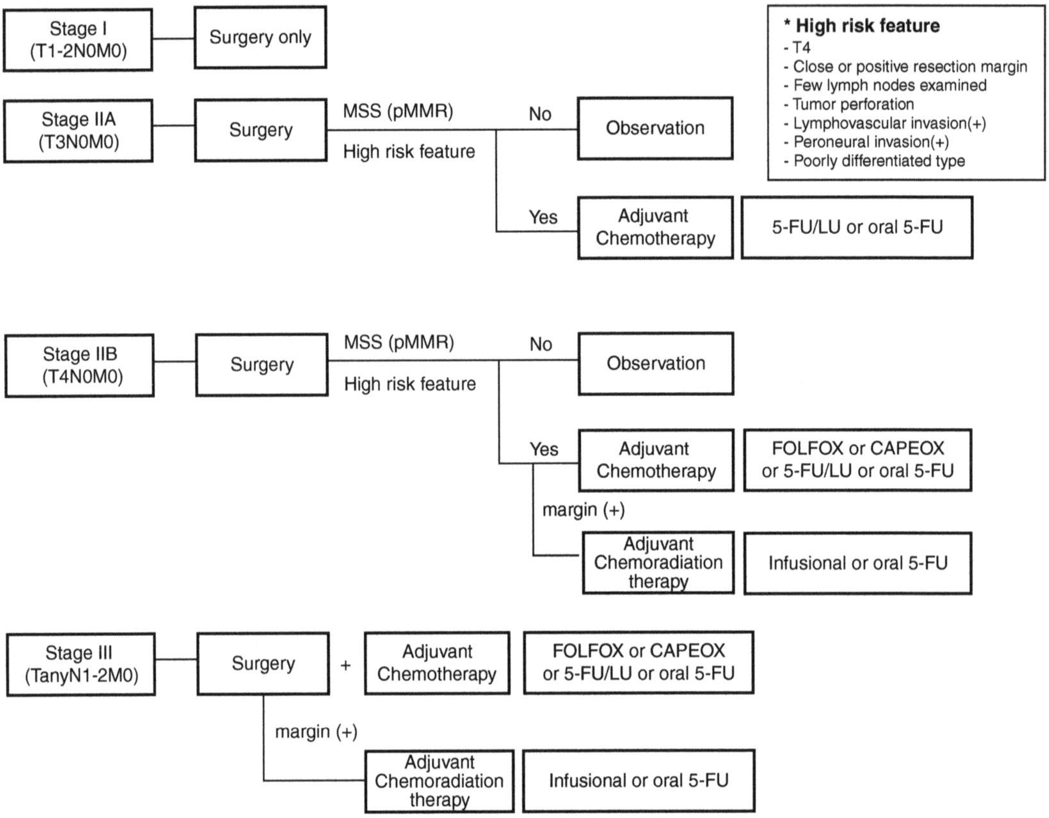

Fig. 2 NCCN guideline of adjuvant therapy for stage I–III small bowel adenocarcinoma

Neuroendocrine Carcinoma in the Small Intestine

Surgical Treatment

Although small intestine neuroendocrine tumors are small in size, regional and systemic metastases are quite common compared to other malignancies. Therefore, even for primary tumors less than 1 cm in size without regional lymph node metastasis, a segmental resection of the small intestine with adequate regional lymphadenectomy is required. However, if the tumor is larger than 1 cm in size or multicentric, or regional metastatic lymph nodes are suspected, wide excision of the bowel and mesentery along the vessel root is necessary [20]. In addition, simultaneous cholecystectomy is recommended because adjuvant antineoplastic therapy used in neuroendocrine tumors often causes gallstone-induced cholecystitis [21].

Recently, with the development of minimally invasive techniques, several retrospective studies have reported that laparoscopic or robotic surgery is safe and feasible in selective patients with small bowel neuroendocrine tumors [22–24]. The most appropriate indication for minimally invasive surgery is modest ileal and jejunal tumors of moderate size with limited nodal involvement. If the regional lymph nodes are too close to the main vessels to result in their incomplete removal, or if the lymph nodes are visible but the primary tumor is not clear or there is evidence of multicentric lesions, it is more suitable to choose open laparotomy rather than minimally invasive surgery [23].

Cytoreductive surgery (metastasectomy) for distant metastatic disease is routinely recommended in patients in whom more than 90% of the disease can be resected with or without ablation. This strategy is particularly appropriate for patients with stable and indolent disease but is not recommended for those with rapid progressive disease [20, 25]. Although recurrence occurs in 75% of patients, several studies presented an overall improved survival of up to 161 months when cytoreduction is performed [26]. In addition, metastasectomy can be considered in patients with hormonal syndromes for relief of symptoms.

Gastrointestinal Stroma Tumor in the Small Intestine

Surgical Treatment

Considering the rarity of intramural extension, limited surgery, including wedge or segmental resection, is often appropriate. Lymphadenectomy is usually not necessary due to the low incidence of nodal metastases. Because rupture of the gastrointestinal stromal tumor leads to devastating results, care must be taken not to injure the pseudocapsule of the tumor [27].

Laparoscopic surgery may be safe and feasible for selective patients with favorable anatomical locations and a modest size [28, 29]. If there is a possibility of rupturing the tumor during laparoscopic manipulation, minimally invasive surgery should never be performed.

In locally advanced and initially inoperable gastrointestinal stromal tumor, neoadjuvant imatinib could decrease tumor size, resulting in decreased morbidity and the potential for multivisceral resection [30]. When surgery is planned, imatinib can be suspended immediately before surgery, but other tyrosine-kinase inhibitors, such as sunitinib, regorafenib, ripretinib, or avapritinib, should be stopped at least 1 week prior to surgery [27].

Conclusion

Because of its rarity and the lack of available evidence, the standardization of surgical procedures and adjuvant therapy for SBA is difficult. Therefore, the two aforementioned guidelines are recommended for the treatment of SBA until various RCTs are performed. Neuroendocrine tumors and gastrointestinal tumors arising from small bowel are also rare, but surgical treatment is indisputable compared to SBA.

References

1. Locher C, Batumona B, Afchain P, Carrère N, Samalin E, Cellier C, et al. Small bowel adenocarcinoma: French intergroup clinical practice guidelines for diagnosis, treatments and follow-up (SNFGE, FFCD, GERCOR, UNICANCER, SFCD, SFED, SFRO). Dig Liver Dis. 2018;50:15–9.
2. Benson AB, Venook AP, Al-Hawary MM, Arain MA, Chen YJ, Ciombor KK, et al. Small Bowel Adenocarcinoma, Version 1.2020, NCCN Clinical Practice Guidelines in Oncology. J Natl Compr Cancer Netw. 2019;17:1109–33.
3. Kaklamanos IG, Bathe OF, Franceschi D, Camarda C, Levi J, Livingstone AS. Extent of resection in the management of duodenal adenocarcinoma. Am J Surg. 2000;179:37–41.
4. Platoff RM, Kellish AS, Hakim A, Gaughan JP, Atabek UM, Spitz FR, et al. Simple versus radical resection for duodenal adenocarcinoma: a propensity score matched analysis of national cancer database. Am Surg. 2021;87:266–75.
5. Cloyd JM, Norton JA, Visser BC, Poultsides GA. Does the extent of resection impact survival for duodenal adenocarcinoma? Analysis of 1,611 cases. Ann Surg Oncol. 2015;22:573–80.
6. Tran TB, Qadan M, Dua MM, Norton JA, Poultsides GA, Visser BC. Prognostic relevance of lymph node ratio and total lymph node count for small bowel adenocarcinoma. Surgery. 2015;158:486–93.
7. Wilhelm A, Müller SA, Steffen T, Schmied BM, Beutner U, Warschkow R. Patients with adenocarcinoma of the small intestine with 9 or more regional lymph nodes retrieved have a higher rate of positive lymph nodes and improved survival. J Gastrointest Surg. 2016;20:401–10.
8. Rompteaux P, Gagnière J, Gornet J-M, Coriat R, Baumgaertner I, Lecomte T, et al. Resection of small bowel adenocarcinoma metastases: results of the ARCAD-NADEGE cohort study. Eur J Surg Oncol. 2019;45:331–5.
9. Elias D, Glehen O, Pocard M, Quenet F, Goéré D, Arvieux C, et al. A comparative study of complete cytoreductive surgery plus intraperitoneal chemotherapy to treat peritoneal dissemination from colon, rectum, small bowel, and nonpseudomyxoma appendix. Ann Surg. 2010;251:896–901.
10. Aparicio T, Henriques J, Manfredi S, Tougeron D, Bouché O, Pezet D, et al. Small bowel adenocarcinoma: results from a nationwide prospective ARCAD-NADEGE cohort study of 347 patients. Int J Cancer. 2020;147:967–77.

11. Eigenbrod T, Kullmann F, Klebl F. Resection of small bowel adenocarcinoma liver metastasis combined with neoadjuvant and adjuvant chemotherapy results in extended disease-free period—a case report. Int J Gastrointest Cancer. 2006;37:94–7.
12. Rompteaux P, Gagnière J, Gornet JM, Coriat R, Baumgaertner I, Lecomte T, et al. Resection of small bowel adenocarcinoma metastases: results of the ARCAD-NADEGE cohort study. Eur J Surg Oncol. 2019;45:331–5.
13. Koo DH, Yun SC, Hong YS, Ryu MH, Lee JL, Chang HM, et al. Adjuvant chemotherapy for small bowel adenocarcinoma after curative surgery. Oncology. 2011;80:208–13.
14. Ecker BL, McMillan MT, Datta J, Mamtani R, Giantonio BJ, Dempsey DT, et al. Efficacy of adjuvant chemotherapy for small bowel adenocarcinoma: a propensity score-matched analysis. Cancer. 2016;122:693–701.
15. Aydin D, Sendur MA, Kefeli U, Unal OU, Tastekin D, Akyol M, et al. Evaluation of prognostic factors and adjuvant chemotherapy in patients with small bowel adenocarcinoma who underwent curative resection. Clin Colorectal Cancer. 2017;16:220–7.
16. Ye X, Zhang G, Chen H, Li Y. Meta-analysis of postoperative adjuvant therapy for small bowel adenocarcinoma. PLoS One. 2018;13:e0200204.
17. Singhal N, Singhal D. Adjuvant chemotherapy for small intestine adenocarcinoma. Cochrane Database Syst Rev. 2007;2007:Cd005202.
18. Narang AK, Miller RC, Hsu CC, Bhatia S, Pawlik TM, Laheru D, et al. Evaluation of adjuvant chemoradiation therapy for ampullary adenocarcinoma: the Johns Hopkins Hospital-Mayo Clinic collaborative study. Radiat Oncol. 2011;6:126.
19. Ecker BL, McMillan MT, Datta J, Lee MK, Karakousis GC, Vollmer CM Jr, et al. Adjuvant chemotherapy versus chemoradiotherapy in the management of patients with surgically resected duodenal adenocarcinoma: a propensity score-matched analysis of a nationwide clinical oncology database. Cancer. 2017;123:967–76.
20. Shah MH, Goldner WS, Benson AB, Bergsland E, Blaszkowsky LS, Brock P, et al. Neuroendocrine and Adrenal Tumors, Version 2.2021, NCCN Clinical Practice Guidelines in Oncology. J Natl Compr Cancer Netw. 2021;19:839–68.
21. Jayakrishnan TT, Groeschl RT, George B, Thomas JP, Clark Gamblin T, Turaga KK. Review of the impact of antineoplastic therapies on the risk for cholelithiasis and acute cholecystitis. Ann Surg Oncol. 2014;21:240–7.
22. Thomaschewski M, Neeff H, Keck T, Neumann HPH, Strate T, von Dobschuetz E. Is there any role for minimally invasive surgery in NET? Rev Endocr Metab Disord. 2017;18:443–57.
23. Baiu I, Visser BC. Minimally invasive small bowel cancer surgery. Surg Oncol Clin N Am. 2019;28:273–83.
24. Figueiredo MN, Maggiori L, Gaujoux S, Couvelard A, Guedj N, Ruszniewski P, et al. Surgery for small-bowel neuroendocrine tumors: is there any benefit of the laparoscopic approach? Surg Endosc. 2014;28:1720–6.
25. Bonds M, Rocha FG. Neuroendocrine tumors of the pancreatobiliary and gastrointestinal tracts. Surg Clin North Am. 2020;100:635–48.
26. Woltering EA, Voros BA, Beyer DT, Wang YZ, Thiagarajan R, Ryan P, et al. Aggressive surgical approach to the management of neuroendocrine tumors: a report of 1,000 surgical cytoreductions by a single institution. J Am Coll Surg. 2017;224:434–47.
27. Zhao WY, Zhao G, Wang M. [Updates and interpretations of the NCCN Clinical Practice Guidelines (2019 6th version) on gastrointestinal stromal tumor]. Zhonghua Wei Chang Wai Ke Za Zhi. 2020;23:866–71.
28. Chen K, Zhang B, Liang YL, Ji L, Xia SJ, Pan Y, et al. Laparoscopic versus open resection of small bowel gastrointestinal stromal tumors: systematic review and meta-analysis. Chin Med J. 2017;130:1595–603.
29. Gluzman MI, Kashchenko VA, Karachun AM, Orlova RV, Nakatis IA, Pelipas IV, et al. Technical success and short-term results of surgical treatment of gastrointestinal stromal tumors: an experience of three centers. Transl Gastroenterol Hepatol. 2017;2:56.
30. Rutkowski P, Gronchi A, Hohenberger P, Bonvalot S, Schöffski P, Bauer S, et al. Neoadjuvant imatinib in locally advanced gastrointestinal stromal tumors (GIST): the EORTC STBSG experience. Ann Surg Oncol. 2013;20:2937–43.

Staging and Treatment. II-4. Palliative Chemotherapy

Key Points

- FOLFOX, CAPEOX, or FOLFOXIRI regimens with or without bevacizumab are recommended as first-line therapy in advanced or metastatic small bowel cancers.
- Recent studies revealed a distinct genomic profile of small bowel cancers compared to colorectal and gastric cancers.
- Depending on MMR/MSI status, immunotherapies, FOLFIRI, or taxane-based chemotherapies could be options for second-line therapy.

Introduction

Approximately 32% of patients diagnosed with small bowel cancer have stage IV disease, of which 5-year survival is only 42% [1]. Few studies have specifically addressed the optimal management of small bowel cancers, and the general approach to the treatment of these tumors is based on the treatment principles established for metastatic colorectal cancer. However, more recently, new data are emerging on the molecular characterization of small bowel cancers and targeted treatment approaches in the advanced setting.

First-Line Therapy

In the absence of randomized studies performed to demonstrate the benefit of systemic therapy in patients with advanced or metastatic small bowel cancers, data supporting systemic therapy were limited mainly to retrospective studies with several small phase II trials [2]. Therapy is based on the goals of therapy, the type and timing of previous therapy, and the different toxicity profiles of the constituent drugs. Additionally, an evaluation of the efficacy and safety of these regimens should consider the performance status of the patient (Fig. 1) [3].

As first-line therapy in a patient suitable for intensive therapy without prior platinum resistance, the NCCN guidelines recommend a choice of three chemotherapy regimens, FOLFOX, CAPEOX, or FOLFOXIRI, all of which may be combined with bevacizumab [3].

The results of the retrospective studies showed an apparent advantage for systemic therapy, both in terms of median progression-free survival (PFS) and overall survival (OS) (6 vs. 1 month and 9–19 vs. 2–13 months, respectively) [4, 5].

Recent, despite relatively few, prospective phase II studies confirmed retrospective evidence. In a multicenter phase II study, a modified FOLFOX regimen (5-fluorouracil [5-FU] 2600 mg/m^2 continuous infusion for 46 h/on day 1, oxaliplatin 85 mg/m^2 on day 1, leucovorin

Hyun Jung Lee is the lead author of this chapter.

H. J. Chun et al., *Gastrointestinal Cancer*, https://doi.org/10.1007/978-981-99-0815-8_24

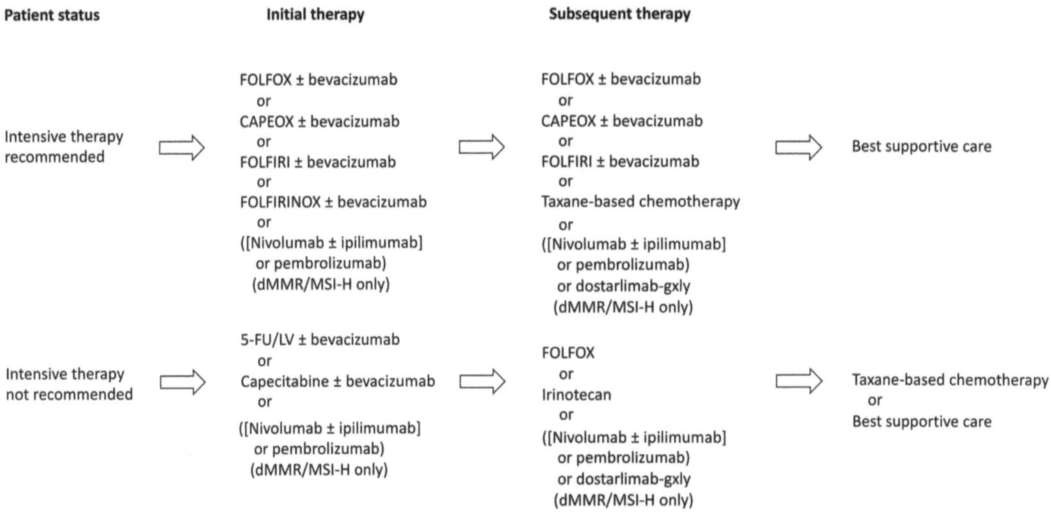

Fig. 1 Principles of systemic therapy for advanced or metastatic small bowel cancers. (Adapted from NCCN guidelines [14])

400 mg/m^2 on day 1, every 14 days) was administered to 33 patients with advanced or metastatic small bowel cancers that demonstrated an objective response rate of 48.5%, a median time to progression (TTP) of 7.8 months, and a median OS of 15.2 months [6]. In a single-institution study, the CAPEOX regimen (capecitabine 750 mg/m^2 twice daily on days 1 through 14 and oxaliplatin 130 mg/m^2 on day 1, every 21 days) also demonstrated a response rate of 52% and a median OS of 15.5 months [7]. In a recent study, among 33 patients with advanced small bowel cancers who received the CAPRINOX regimen dose adjusted according to the *UGT1A1* genotype, the objective response rate was 37.5%, and the median PFS and OS were 8.9 and 13.4 months, respectively [8].

Several retrospective analyses also have revealed favorable outcomes in patients treated with bevacizumab-containing regimens without adding significant toxicity [9, 10]. Based on these data, according to NCCN guidelines, a cytotoxic backbone regimen can be administered with or without bevacizumab [3].

For patients who are not appropriate for intensive therapy, treatment options would exclude the more toxic components of these regimens with 5-FU/LV or capecitabine with or without bevacizumab.

Second-Line Therapy

In second-line therapy, the FOLFIRI regimen has shown modest activity in patients after failure of initial platinum-based chemotherapy with an objective response rate of 20%, median PFS, and OS 3.2 months and 10.5 months, respectively [11]. Furthermore, a recent phase II trial including ten refractory small bowel cancers using nab-paclitaxel showed taxane sensitivity in patients with small bowel cancer [12].

To date, few data are available regarding the benefits of specific biological or targeted therapies in the treatment of advanced small bowel cancers. However, a recent large-scale genomic profiling study of a series of 317 small bowel cancers identified potentially targetable genomic alterations present in most small bowel cancer cases (91%) that showed a distinct difference from colorectal and gastric cancers [13]. *Point mutations in BRAF, ERBB2/HER2,* microsatellite instability (MSI), and high tumor mutational burden were all enriched in small bowel cancers.

Consequently, the NCCN guidelines recommend the choice of subsequent-line therapy depending on the mismatch repair (MMR) and MSI status of the tumor. For tumors with dMMR or MSI-H, checkpoint inhibitor therapy with anti-PD-1 inhibitors, alone or in combination with an anti-CTLA4 inhibitor, is recommended in the second-line setting. FOLFIRI (5-fluorouracil + leucovorin + irinotecan) or taxane-based chemotherapies are options in the second line for pMMR/MSS tumors or for patient's refractory to checkpoint inhibitor therapies [3].

Conclusion

Small bowel cancers are a rare but heterogeneous group of malignancies that require a personalized approach. Presently, the FOLFOX, CAPEOX, or FOLFOXIRI regimens are recommended as the first-line palliative chemotherapy. Further identification of multiple clinically relevant genomic alterations could reveal the greater importance of targeted or immunotherapies in a population with limited treatment options and poor prognosis.

References

1. Overman MJ, Hu CY, Kopetz S, Abbruzzese JL, Wolff RA, Chang GJ. A population-based comparison of adenocarcinoma of the large and small intestine: insights into a rare disease. Ann Surg Oncol. 2012;19:1439–45.
2. Puccini A, Battaglin F, Lenz HJ. Management of advanced small bowel cancer. Curr Treat Options in Oncol. 2018;19:69.
3. Cornes JS. Multiple lymphomatous polyposis of the gastrointestinal tract. Cancer. 1961;14:249–57.
4. Overman MJ, Kopetz S, Wen S, Hoff PM, Fogelman D, Morris J, et al. Chemotherapy with 5-fluorouracil and a platinum compound improves outcomes in metastatic small bowel adenocarcinoma. Cancer. 2008;113:2038–45.
5. Tsushima T, Taguri M, Honma Y, Takahashi H, Ueda S, Nishina T, et al. Multicenter retrospective study of 132 patients with unresectable small bowel adenocarcinoma treated with chemotherapy. Oncologist. 2012;17:1163–70.
6. Xiang XJ, Liu YW, Zhang L, Qiu F, Yu F, Zhan ZY, et al. A phase II study of modified FOLFOX as first-line chemotherapy in advanced small bowel adenocarcinoma. Anti-Cancer Drugs. 2012;23:561–6.
7. Overman MJ, Varadhachary GR, Kopetz S, Adinin R, Lin E, Morris JS, et al. Phase II study of capecitabine and oxaliplatin for advanced adenocarcinoma of the small bowel and ampulla of Vater. J Clin Oncol. 2009;27:2598–603.
8. McWilliams RR, Foster NR, Mahoney MR, Smyrk TC, Murray JA, Ames MM, et al. North Central Cancer Treatment Group N0543 (Alliance): a phase 2 trial of pharmacogenetic-based dosing of irinotecan, oxaliplatin, and capecitabine as first-line therapy for patients with advanced small bowel adenocarcinoma. Cancer. 2017;123:3494–501.
9. Takayoshi K, Kusaba H, Uenomachi M, Mitsugi K, Makiyama C, Makiyama A, et al. Suggestion of added value by bevacizumab to chemotherapy in patients with unresectable or recurrent small bowel cancer. Cancer Chemother Pharmacol. 2017;80:333–42.
10. Aydin D, Sendur MA, Kefeli U, Ustaalioglu BB, Aydin O, Yildirim E, et al. Evaluation of bevacizumab in advanced small bowel adenocarcinoma. Clin Colorectal Cancer. 2017;16:78–83.
11. Zaanan A, Gauthier M, Malka D, Locher C, Gornet JM, Thirot-Bidault A, et al. Second-line chemotherapy with fluorouracil, leucovorin, and irinotecan (FOLFIRI regimen) in patients with advanced small bowel adenocarcinoma after failure of first-line platinum-based chemotherapy: a multicenter AGEO study. Cancer. 2011;117:1422–8.
12. Overman MJ, Adam L, Raghav K, Wang J, Kee B, Fogelman D, et al. Phase II study of nab-paclitaxel in refractory small bowel adenocarcinoma and CpG island methylator phenotype (CIMP)-high colorectal cancer. Ann Oncol. 2018;29:139–44.
13. Schrock AB, Devoe CE, McWilliams R, Sun J, Aparicio T, Stephens PJ, et al. Genomic profiling of small-bowel adenocarcinoma. JAMA Oncol. 2017;3:1546–53.
14. National Comprehensive Cancer Network. NCCN Clinical Practice Guidelines in Oncology. small bowel cancers. ver 2.2021.

Part IV

Appendiceal Tumors

Epidemiology and Prevention

Key Points

- Approximately 1% of appendectomy specimens are diagnosed as appendiceal tumors.
- The most common types of appendiceal tumors are epithelial tumors and neuroendocrine tumors.
- The mean age of diagnosis for most appendix tumors is 50–60 years, except for neuroendocrine tumors (30 years).
- Older age and complicated appendicitis are suggested as risk factors for appendiceal tumor among patients with acute appendicitis.

Introduction

Primary appendiceal neoplasms are rare tumors that account for approximately 1% of all cancers [1]. They are mostly found incidentally in an appendectomy specimen [1, 2]. They can also be found during abdominal imaging or during colonoscopy, as only 30–50% of patients exhibit clinical manifestations such as acute appendicitis of these tumors [3, 4]. The epidemiology of appendiceal tumors has not been established due to these clinical characteristics. A recent analysis of the Surveillance, Epidemiology, and End Results (SEER) database reported that the age-adjusted annual inci-

Seung Yong Shin is the lead author of this chapter.

H. J. Chun et al., *Gastrointestinal Cancer*, https://doi.org/10.1007/978-981-99-0815-8_25

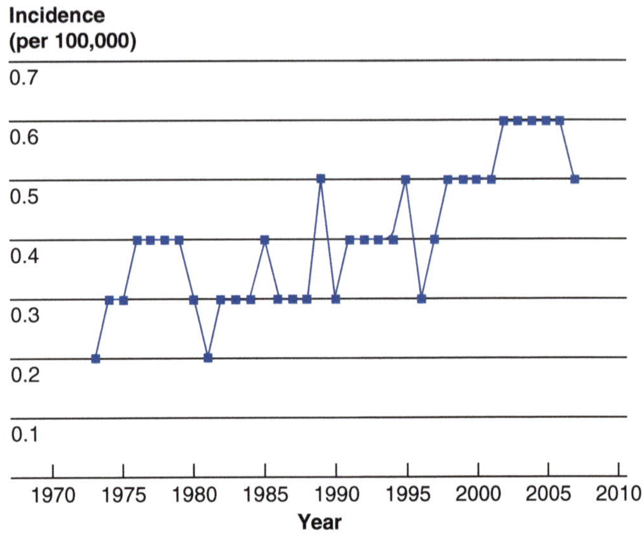

Fig. 1 Age-adjusted incidence rates for appendiceal tumors in the Surveillance, Epidemiology, and End Results (SEER) database from 1973 to 2007 (per 100,000 population) [3]

dence was 6 per 1,000,000 people in recent years [3], but the incidence has increased from 2 to 4 per 1,000,000 populations in the 1970s to 5–6 per 1,000,000 in 2006–2007 (Fig. 1). The reasons for these increases are unclear but may be associated with the development of imaging tools and colonoscopy [3, 5]. In this chapter, the epidemiology and risk factors will be introduced based on previous studies.

Mucinous Neoplasms

Epithelial tumors and neuroendocrine tumors (NETs) are known to be the most common appendiceal tumors. Approximately two-thirds of appendiceal tumors are epithelial tumors. Depending on whether mucin is produced or not, epithelial tumors are classified into mucus tumors and non-mucus tumors. Mucinous neoplasms have cytoplasmic mucin-containing epithelial cells that secrete mucin into the appendix lumen [6]. Epithelial neoplasms of the appendix have been detected in 0.2–2.0% of appendectomy specimens, and mucinous neoplasms comprised approximately 40% of all appendiceal tumors and 70% of the epithelial tumors of the appendix, respectively [2, 3]. Approximately 1000–2000 cases are reported annually in the United States [3, 7], and a recent study reported that the incidence of mucinous neoplasm has increased over time, from 0.6 cases per million persons in 1973 to 2.8 cases per million persons in 2011, with an annual percentage increase of 3.1% [7, 8].

The mean age of diagnosis is known to be about 60 years, but age at diagnosis has been reported to decrease with time [3, 8]. Females show a slightly higher incidence in both Western and Asian studies, but this difference is not significant [8–10].

Non-mucinous Neoplasms

Non-mucinous neoplasms also called colonic-type neoplasms are less common than mucinous neoplasms. Previous studies have reported that non-mucinous neoplasms comprise approximately 30% of appendiceal epithelial tumors [2]. They are commonly found in older patients in the sixth decade with male predominance [7].

Goblet Cell Carcinoma

Goblet cell carcinoma is extremely rare but occurs almost exclusively in the appendix. Approximately 5% of primary appendiceal neoplasms have been diagnosed as goblet cell tumors [3, 11]. They are often present in patients in the fifth to sixth decade and show a similar incidence between males and females [12, 13].

Neuroendocrine Tumor

Previous studies have reported that the appendix is the third or fourth most common site of NET occurrence [14, 15]. Neuroendocrine tumors were identified in 0.16–2.3% of appendectomy samples and comprised 43–57% of primary appendiceal tumors in previous studies [16, 17]. They are more common in young patients, and the mean age of the patients was about 30 years. Younger female patients were more frequent than in male patients in recent studies [18, 19]. These tumors are more often seen in female patients [20, 21].

Risk Factors

No definitive risk factors for appendiceal tumor have been established, but recent studies suggested age (>50 or ≥65) as independent risk factor for appendiceal tumor among patients with acute appendicitis [22, 23]. Complicated appendicitis and appendiceal inflammatory mass are also considered risk factors for appendiceal tumors, and interval appendectomies are strongly recommended in all adult patients, especially those 40 years or older and with indeterminate imaging, to determine the underlying cause of appendicitis [24–26]. Another study showed that diameter of the appendix in the sonography was ≥13 mm, and the absence of leukocytosis is a risk factor of appendiceal tumor [23].

Conclusion

Appendiceal tumor is rare disease, but the incidence has been increased overtime. Appendectomy should be considered in patients with risk factors for appendiceal tumor when acute appendicitis occurs.

References

1. Walid LS, Rita A, Ali S, Olatunji BA, Charles S, Bahar M, et al. Appendiceal mucinous neoplasms: diagnosis and management. Oncologist. 2017;22(9):1107–16.
2. Connor SJ, Hanna GB, Frizelle FA. Appendiceal tumors: retrospective clinicopathologic analysis of appendiceal tumors from 7,970 appendectomies. Dis Colon Rectum. 1998;41(1):75–80.
3. Turaga KK, Pappas SG, Gamblin T. Importance of histologic subtype in the staging of appendiceal tumors. Ann Surg Oncol. 2012;19(5):1379–85.
4. Deshmukh S, Verde F, Johnson PT, Fishman EK, Macura KJ. Anatomical variants and pathologies of the vermix. Emerg Radiol. 2014;21(5):543–52.
5. Schelomo M, Pamela RP, Todd MT, Beth AV. The rise in appendiceal cancer incidence: 2000-2009. J Gastrointest Surg. 2015;19(4):743–50.
6. Haroon AC, Reetesh KP. Management of mucinous appendiceal tumors. Ann Surg Oncol. 2018;25(8):2135–44.
7. Margaret EM, Timothy RC, Limin XC, Leslie HS. Primary malignant neoplasms of the appendix: a population-based study from the surveillance, epidemiology and end-results program, 1973-1998. Cancer. 2002;94(12):3307–12.
8. Walid LS, Michael G, Zhengjia C, Sungjin K, Edith B, Tanios BS, et al. Incidence and survival of appendiceal mucinous neoplasms: a SEER analysis. Am J Clin Oncol. 2017;40(6):569–73.
9. Han DK, Jae KJ. A prospective study of discrepancy between clinical and pathological diagnosis of appendiceal mucinous neoplasm. Ann Surg Treat Res. 2020;98(3):124–9.
10. Michael JO, Keith F, Chung-Yuan H, Cathy F, Melissa T, Richard R, et al. Improving the AJCC/TNM staging for adenocarcinomas of the appendix: the prognostic impact of histological grade. Ann Surg. 2013;257(6):1072–8.
11. Marcia LM, Melinda AM, Hakjung K, Jessica BO, Clifford YK. Malignancies of the appendix: beyond case series reports. Dis Colon Rectum. 2005;48(12):2264–71.
12. Payam SP, Rani K. Goblet cell carcinoid of the appendix. World J Surg Oncol. 2005;3:36.
13. Jorge AS, Donald EH, Kristen B. Pathologic classification and clinical behavior of the spectrum of goblet cell carcinoid tumors of the appendix. Am J Surg Pathol. 2009;33(8):1259–60.
14. Melinda AM, Jessica BO, Clifford YK. Updated population-based review of carcinoid tumors. Ann Surg. 2004;240(1):117–22.
15. Christine SL, Charles W, Charles RS, Kelly MM, Robert CG. Analysis of 900 appendiceal carcinoid tumors for a proposed predictive staging system. Arch Surg. 2008;143(7):664–70.
16. Dimitrios M, Diamantis IT, Stylianos V, Ioannis NS, Georgia-Sofia K, Alexandros P, et al. Neuroendocrine neoplasms of the appendix: a review of the literature. Anticancer Res. 2018;38(2):601–11.

17. Zulfu B, Yasin AY, Yesim A, Emre G, Fatih A, Baris M, et al. Appendix neuroendocrine tumor: retrospective analysis of 4026 appendectomy patients in a single center. Emerg Med Int. 2020;2020:4030527.
18. Krystallenia IA, Gregory AK, Simona GG, Eleftherios C, Ashley BG. Appendiceal neuroendocrine neoplasms: diagnosis and management. Endocr Relat Cancer. 2016;23(1):R27–41.
19. Hemminki K, Li X. Incidence trends and risk factors of carcinoid tumors: a nationwide epidemiologic study from Sweden. Cancer. 2001;92(8):2204–10.
20. Irvin MM, Kevin DL, Mark K. A 5-decade analysis of 13,715 carcinoid tumors. Cancer. 2003;97(4):934–59.
21. Nikhil P, Ashley KC, Helai O, Panagiotis D, Andrzej C, Rashpal F, et al. Surgical management of patients with neuroendocrine neoplasms of the appendix: appendectomy or more. Neuroendocrinology. 2018;106(3):242–51.
22. Stephen JS, Areg G, Joseph C, Steven M, Matthew B, Matthew D, et al. Risk factors for appendiceal cancer after appendectomy. Am Surg. 2021;87(6):994–8.
23. Maximilian B, Philipp L, Melanie L, Justus B, Christian K, Stephan K, et al. Risk factors for appendiceal neoplasm and malignancy among patients with acute appendicitis. Int J Color Dis. 2020;35(1):157–63.
24. Matthew JF, Mitchell C, Philip C, Laura AL. Increased risk of mucinous neoplasm of the appendix in adults undergoing interval appendectomy. JAMA Surg. 2013;148(8):703–6.
25. Sean CG, Wolfgang G, David S, Jennifer D, Karim A, Ian MP, et al. The American Society of Colon and Rectal Surgeons, Clinical Practice Guidelines for the management of appendiceal neoplasms. Dis Colon Rectum. 2019;62(12):1425–38.
26. Frederico JRT, Sérgio DCN, Eduardo HA, Edivaldo MU, Carlos AMM, Marcelo CR. Acute appendicitis, inflammatory appendiceal mass and the risk of a hidden malignant tumor: a systematic review of the literature. Acute appendicitis, inflammatory appendiceal mass and the risk of a hidden malignant tumor: a systematic review of the literature. World J Emerg Surg. 2017;12:12.

Pathological and Molecular Characteristics

Key Points

- Appendiceal mucinous neoplasm is classified into low-grade and high-grade appendiceal mucinous neoplasms. They are characterized by mucinous epithelial proliferation showing a distinct pushing border.
- Appendiceal adenocarcinoma and mucinous adenocarcinoma are malignant glandular neoplasms showing an infiltrative border.
- Appendiceal goblet cell adenocarcinoma is a malignant amphicrine tumor composed of goblet cell-like mucinous cells.
- Appendiceal neuroendocrine tumors (NET), which most commonly arise in the appendix tip, are graded based on the mitotic count and the Ki-67 proliferation index.

Introduction

Appendiceal tumors are rare gastrointestinal tumors that include a heterogeneous group of tumors. They are relatively difficult to diagnose, especially when neoplasms are limited to the appendix. Due to the recent development of imaging modalities and health screening, the incidence of appendiceal tumors has increased. There are four major histopathologic subtypes in appendiceal tumors: mucinous neoplasm (low-grade appendiceal mucinous neoplasm [LAMN], high-grade appendiceal mucinous neoplasm [HAMN]), adenocarcinoma (mucinous and non-mucinous), goblet cell adenocarcinoma, and neuroendocrine neoplasm.

Hee Young Na is the lead author of this chapter.

Appendiceal Mucinous Neoplasm

Definition

Appendiceal mucinous neoplasm is a neoplasm composed of mucinous epithelial proliferation which is associated with various degrees of extracellular mucin [1]. The margin of this neoplasm is typically of the pushing type. Appendiceal mucinous neoplasm is classified into LAMN and HAMN based on the grade of atypism of the neoplastic epithelium [1].

Histopathology

In LAMN, the villous, undulating, or flattened mucinous epithelium replaces the appendiceal mucosa. Cellular atypia is typically mild (Fig. 1). The wall of the appendix can show varying degrees of attenuated muscularis mucosa, fibrosis, and hyalinization. Although the epithelium can protrude into the appendiceal wall with a

H. J. Chun et al., *Gastrointestinal Cancer*, https://doi.org/10.1007/978-981-99-0815-8_26

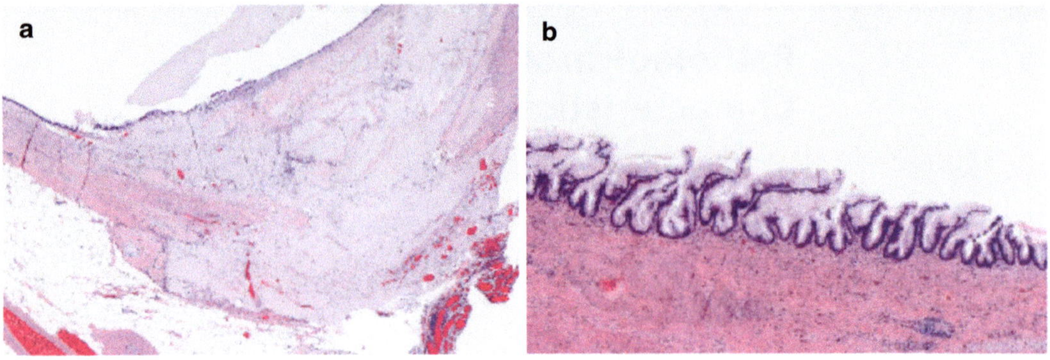

Fig. 1 Low-grade appendiceal mucinous neoplasm (**a**) Low-power view reveals LAMN with acellular mucin spillage in serosal surface. (**b**) The mucosa is replaced by mucinous epithelium showing villous pattern. *LAMN* low-grade appendiceal mucinous neoplasm

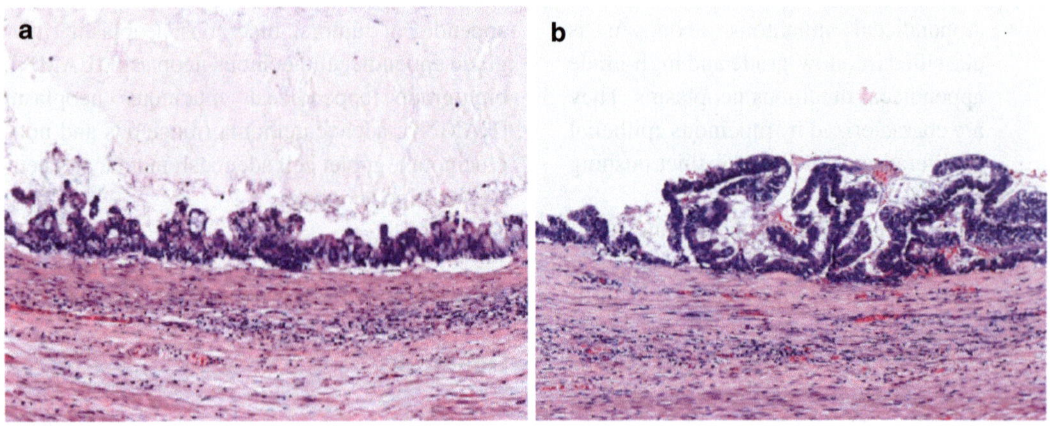

Fig. 2 High-grade appendiceal mucinous neoplasm. (**a**, **b**) The neoplastic epithelium in HAMN shows micropapillary or other complex growth pattern. Nuclear pleomorphism is observed. *HAMN* high-grade appendiceal mucinous neoplasm

pushing border (diverticulum-like growth), the infiltrative pattern of invasion is absent in appendiceal mucinous neoplasm. Extracellular mucin can dissect the appendiceal wall and extend to the peritoneal surface [2].

HAMN shares major histologic features with LAMN, such as subepithelial fibrosis, pushing border, and peritoneal dissemination. The difference of the HAMN from LAMN is that the epithelium in HAMN shows unequivocal high-grade dysplasia. In addition, more convoluted architectural patterns, such as micropapillary or cribriform patterns, can be observed (Fig. 2).

Molecular Characteristics

Mutations in *KRAS* and *GNAS* are common in appendiceal mucinous neoplasm [3–6]. Conversely, mutations in *APC, TP53,* and *SMAD4*, which are frequently observed in colorectal cancer, are not common [5–7]. A minority of cases show mutations in *FAT4, SMAD2, AKT1, MET, JAK3, PIK3CA, STK11,* and *RB1* genes [5–7]. Defective mismatch repair protein function or *BRAF* mutations are generally absent in appendiceal mucinous neoplasm [8, 9].

Appendiceal Adenocarcinoma

Definition

Appendiceal adenocarcinoma is a malignant glandular neoplasm, characterized by invasion [1]. Mucinous adenocarcinoma is diagnosed when >50% of the tumor is composed of extracellular mucin [1].

Histopathology

Non-mucinous adenocarcinoma shows irregular neoplastic glands that invade the wall of the appendix (Fig. 3). The morphology is generally similar to that of colorectal cancer, in which the epithelium shows columnar cells, containing hyperchromatic nuclei, and necrosis is common. Rarely are pancreatobiliary-type glands with columnar cells contain pale cytoplasm and irregular nuclei observed.

In mucinous adenocarcinoma, mucin pools often contain strips or clusters of neoplastic cells. When signet-ring cells constitute >50% of the tumor, the tumor is categorized as signet-ring cell adenocarcinoma.

Molecular Characteristics

Mucinous adenocarcinoma frequently harbors *KRAS* and *GNAS* mutations, while *BRAF* mutations or microsatellite instability is rare [4, 10]. Non-mucinous adenocarcinoma less often shows *KRAS* or *GNAS* mutations [10].

Appendiceal Goblet Cell Adenocarcinoma

Definition

Appendiceal goblet cell adenocarcinoma is a malignant amphicrine tumor composed of goblet cell-like mucinous cells, as well as variable numbers of endocrine cells and Paneth-like cells, typically arranged as tubules resembling intestinal crypts [1]. It was previously called a goblet cell carcinoid.

Histopathology

To be diagnosed as appendiceal goblet cell adenocarcinoma, a tumor must harbor a classic low-grade goblet cell adenocarcinoma component, which is composed of tubules of goblet-like cells [1]. Nuclear atypia is mild and mitosis is infrequent.

At least half of appendiceal goblet cell adenocarcinomas show high-grade features [11, 12], such as infiltrating single file structures, cribriform glands, diffusely infiltrating signet-ring cells, or sold sheets of cells [13]. Goblet cell adenocarcinoma is graded as grades 1 to 3, based

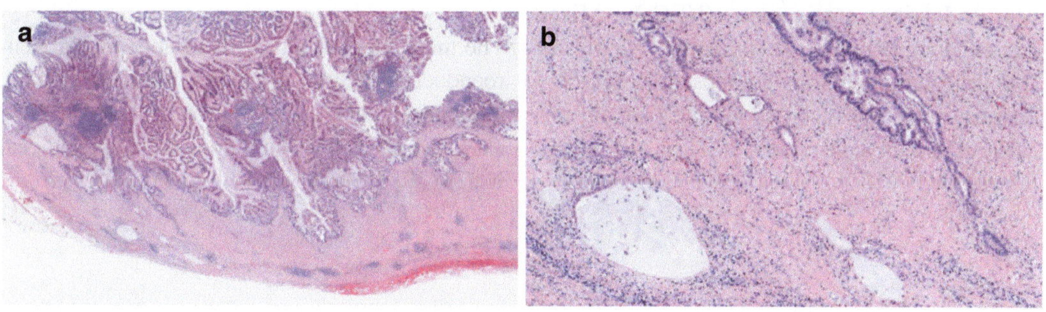

Fig. 3 Appendiceal adenocarcinoma shows infiltrative neoplastic glands in appendiceal wall. (**a**) Low-power and (**b**) high-power views

Table 1 The grading system of appendiceal goblet cell adenocarcinoma

Grade	Tubular or clustered growth (low-grade pattern)	Loss of tubular or clustered growth (any combination of high-grade patterns)
1	>75%	<25%
2	50–75%	25–50%
3	<50%	>50%

on the proportion of this high-grade pattern (loss of low-grade pattern) [12] (Table 1).

Molecular Characteristics

A recent study revealed mutations in Wnt-signaling-associated genes (*USP9X, NOTCH1, CTNNA1, CTNNB1, TRRAP*) in appendiceal goblet cell adenocarcinomas [14]. Mutations in chromatin remodeling genes (*ARID1A, ARID2, KDM6A, KMT2D*) are also observed [15, 16]. Mutations commonly associated with conventional colorectal adenocarcinomas (*TP53, KRAS, APC*) are rare to absent [14] in goblet cell adenocarcinoma, suggesting a distinct pathogenesis of this neoplasm.

Appendiceal Neuroendocrine Neoplasm

Definition

Appendiceal neuroendocrine neoplasms are epithelial neoplasms with neuroendocrine differentiation [1]. These include NETs and neuroendocrine carcinomas (NECs). Mixed neuroendocrine-non-neuroendocrine neoplasms (MiNEN) are neoplasms composed of neuroendocrine and non-neuroendocrine neoplasms, each of which constitutes 30% of the whole tumor [1].

Histopathology

Appendiceal NETs most commonly arise in appendiceal tip and can be classified as enterochromaffin-cell (EC-cell) (serotonin-producing) NETs, L-cell NETs, and tubular NETs (Fig. 4). EC-cell NETs are most common, and their histopathological features are similar to those of ileal EC-cell NETs [17], being composed of polyfocal cells in insular or solid growth pattern. S-100-positive sustentacular cells can also be found [18]. L-cell NETs show a trabecular or glandular pattern and produce GLP-1 and other proglucagon-derived peptides. Tubular NETs are arranged in small discrete tubules, occasionally with inspissated mucin, which should be distinguished from goblet cell adenocarcinoma and metastatic adenocarcinoma [19]. Appendiceal NETs are graded based on mitotic count and the Ki-67 proliferation index, similar to other NETs in the gastrointestinal tract.

Appendiceal NECs are morphologically identical to NECs in the colon and can be classified into small cell and large cell type.

Molecular Characteristics

The molecular pathogenesis of appendiceal neuroendocrine neoplasms is not fully understood, although recent studies have revealed *PTEN, EGFR, and c-KIT* point mutations in appendiceal NETs [20].

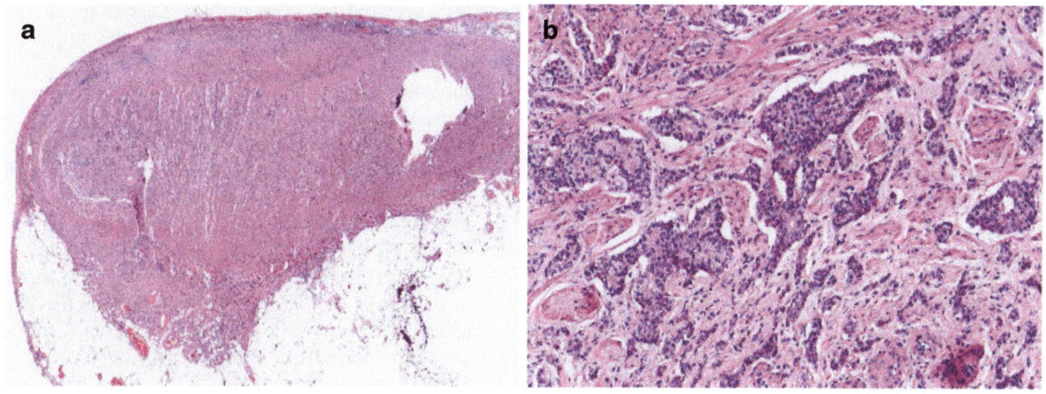

Fig. 4 Appendiceal neuroendocrine tumor. (**a**) NETs most commonly arise in the tip, and (**b**) solid and trabecular growth pattern is shown in this case. *NET* neuroendocrine tumor

Conclusion

Appendiceal tumors are rare tumors of the gastrointestinal tract. Appendiceal mucinous neoplasms show a typical pushing-type margin and are classified into LAMN and HAMN based on the atypism of the epithelium. Adenocarcinomas are malignant tumors with invasive growth and are divided into mucinous and non-mucinous adenocarcinomas according to the amount of mucin pool. Goblet cell adenocarcinomas are malignant amphicrine tumors that show both neuroendocrine and glandular differentiation in the same cell. Finally, appendiceal neuroendocrine neoplasms are categorized into NETs, NECs, and MiNENs.

References

1. Lokuhetty D, White V, Watanabe R, Cree I. WHO classification of digestive system tumors. Lyon: International Agency for Research on Cancer; 2018.
2. Bell PD, Huber AR, Drage MG, Barron SL, Findeis-Hosey JJ, Gonzalez RS. Clinicopathologic features of low-grade appendiceal mucinous neoplasm: a single-institution experience of 117 cases. Am J Surg Pathol. 2020;44(11):1549–55.
3. Hara K, Saito T, Hayashi T, Yimit A, Takahashi M, Mitani K, et al. A mutation spectrum that includes GNAS, KRAS and TP53 may be shared by mucinous neoplasms of the appendix. Pathol Res Pract. 2015;211(9):657–64.
4. Liao X, Vavinskaya V, Sun K, Hao Y, Li X, Valasek M, et al. Mutation profile of high-grade appendiceal mucinous neoplasm. Histopathology. 2020;76(3):461–9.
5. Liu X, Mody K, de Abreu FB, Pipas JM, Peterson JD, Gallagher TL, et al. Molecular profiling of appendiceal epithelial tumors using massively parallel sequencing to identify somatic mutations. Clin Chem. 2014;60(7):1004–11.
6. Amos CI, Wells WA, Tsongalis GJ. Molecular profiling of appendiceal epithelial tumors using massively parallel sequencing to identify somatic mutations. Clin Chem. 2014;60(7):1004–11.
7. Pengelly RJ, Rowaiye B, Pickard K, Moran B, Dayal S, Tapper W, et al. Analysis of mutation and loss of heterozygosity by whole-exome sequencing yields insights into pseudomyxoma peritonei. J Mol Diagn. 2018;20(5):635–42.
8. Misdraji J, Burgart LJ, Lauwers GY. Defective mismatch repair in the pathogenesis of low-grade appendiceal mucinous neoplasms and adenocarcinomas. Mod Pathol. 2004;17(12):1447–54.
9. Zauber P, Berman E, Marotta S, Sabbath-Solitare M, Bishop T. Ki ras gene mutations are invari

ably present in low-grade mucinous tumors of the vermiform appendix. Scand J Gastroenterol. 2011;46(7–8):869–74.
10. Davison JM, Choudry HA, Pingpank JF, Ahrendt SA, Holtzman MP, Zureikat AH, et al. Clinicopathologic and molecular analysis of disseminated appendiceal mucinous neoplasms: identification of factors predicting survival and proposed criteria for a three-tiered assessment of tumor grade. Mod Pathol. 2014;27(11):1521–39.
11. Tang LH, Shia J, Soslow RA, Dhall D, Wong WD, O'Reilly E, et al. Pathologic classification and clinical behavior of the spectrum of goblet cell carcinoid tumors of the appendix. Am J Surg Pathol. 2008;32(10):1429–43.
12. Taggart MW, Abraham SC, Overman MJ, Mansfield PF, Rashid A. Goblet cell carcinoid tumor, mixed goblet cell carcinoid-adenocarcinoma, and adenocarcinoma of the appendix: comparison of clinicopathologic features and prognosis. Arch Pathol Lab Med. 2015;139(6):782–90.
13. Burke AP, Sobin LH, Federspiel BH, Shekitka KM, Helwig EB. Goblet cell carcinoids and related tumors of the vermiform appendix. Am J Clin Pathol. 1990;94(1):27–35.
14. Jesinghaus M, Konukiewitz B, Foersch S, Stenzinger A, Steiger K, Muckenhuber A, et al. Appendiceal goblet cell carcinoids and adenocarcinomas ex-goblet cell carcinoid are genetically distinct from primary colorectal-type adenocarcinoma of the appendix. Mod Pathol. 2018;31(5):829–39.
15. Johncilla M, Stachler M, Misdraji J, Lisovsky M, Yozu M, Lindeman N, et al. Mutational landscape of goblet cell carcinoids and adenocarcinoma ex goblet cell carcinoids of the appendix is distinct from typical carcinoids and colorectal adenocarcinomas. Mod Pathol. 2018;31(6):989–96.
16. Wen KW, Grenert JP, Joseph NM, Shafizadeh N, Huang A, Hosseini M, et al. Genomic profile of appendiceal goblet cell carcinoid is distinct compared to appendiceal neuroendocrine tumor and conventional adenocarcinoma. Hum Pathol. 2018;77:166–74.
17. Klöppel G, Perren A, Heitz PU. The gastroenteropancreatic neuroendocrine cell system and its tumors: the WHO classification. Ann N Y Acad Sci. 2004;1014:13–27.
18. Carr NJ, Sobin LH. Neuroendocrine tumors of the appendix. Semin Diagn Pathol. 2004;21(2):108–19.
19. Kim JY, Hong SM. Recent updates on neuroendocrine tumors from the gastrointestinal and pancreatobiliary tracts. Arch Pathol Lab Med. 2016;140(5):437–48.
20. Park HY, Kwon MJ, Kang HS, Kim YJ, Kim NY, Kim MJ, et al. Targeted next-generation sequencing of well-differentiated rectal, gastric, and appendiceal neuroendocrine tumors to identify potential targets. Hum Pathol. 2019;87:83–94.

Staging and Treatment. II-1. Staging and Prognosis

Key Points

- The terminology and staging of appendiceal tumors remain controversial and often confusing.
- The prognosis of appendix tumors varies greatly depending on the type and stage of the tumor.
- Although appendiceal tumors are not usually diagnosed during colonoscopy, colonoscopy sometimes reveals lump-like bumps or mucinous or polyp lesions in the periappendix orifice.
- An imaging study using CT or magnetic resonance imaging should be performed to evaluate metastatic disease or the presence of pseudomyxoma peritonei.

Introduction

Accurate diagnosis and/or staging of appendiceal tumors is essential due to recent advances in treatment. However, the classification and terms of appendiceal tumors have been controversial for decades [1]. In general, appendiceal tumors can be classified as epithelial, such as adenomas or adenocarcinomas, or non-epithelial, such as neuroendocrine tumors. The epithelial tumor is subclassified as a mucinous neoplasm and a non-mucinous neoplasm. Appendiceal adenocarcinoma encompasses both mucinous and non-mucinous neoplasms. Non-epithelial appendiceal neoplasms include neuroendocrine neoplasms (NENs). Appendiceal NENs are usually asymptomatic and are found incidentally following appendectomy. Staging remains controversial and may be based on tumor size, depth of invasion, or degree of differentiation [2].

The fifth edition of the World Health Organization (WHO) classification published in 2019 broadly classified appendiceal tumors into serrated lesions and polyps, mucinous neoplasm, adenocarcinomas, and NENs [3]. Since most appendiceal neoplasms are asymptomatic, if symptoms such as fatigue or chronic abdominal pain appear, it is highly probable that the disease has already progressed.

Mucinous Neoplasm

Staging

The staging of appendiceal mucinous neoplasms is still challenging and often confusing. However, it has critical prognostic and therapeutic implications. Based on the Peritoneal Surface Oncology Group International (PSOGI) classification, nonneoplastic appendiceal mucinous lesions present simple mucoceles, while neoplastic appendiceal mucinous lesions present serrated polyps, mucinous neoplasms, and

Yoo Jin Lee is the lead author of this chapter.

H. J. Chun et al., *Gastrointestinal Cancer*, https://doi.org/10.1007/978-981-99-0815-8_27

Table 1 World Health Organization classification system of mucinous appendiceal neoplasm

WHO classification system of mucinous appendiceal neoplasms	
LAMN	G1
HAMN	G2
Mucinous adenocarcinoma	G2
Mucinous adenocarcinoma with signet-ring cells	G3

LAMN low-grade appendiceal mucinous neoplasm; *HAMN* high-grade appendiceal mucinous neoplasm. Adapted from Carr et al. [10]

mucinous adenocarcinomas [4, 5]. Appendiceal mucinous neoplasms can perforate and advance to peritoneal dissemination. This condition is characterized by a localized or generalized accumulation of thick, gelatinous material in the abdomen and/or pelvic peritoneal cavity, known as the pseudomyxoma peritonei [6].

In the eighth edition of the AJCC, appendiceal mucinous neoplasms are classified into serrated polyps with or without dysplasia, low-grade appendiceal mucinous neoplasm (LAMN), high-grade appendiceal mucinous neoplasm (HAMN), mucinous adenocarcinoma with or without signet-ring cells, and mucinous signet-ring cell carcinoma [7]. Table 1 summarizes the WHO grading system for mucinous appendiceal neoplasm. The AJCC eighth edition staging of mucinous neoplasm is presented in Table 2.

During staging, cross-sectional imaging with computed tomography (CT) or magnetic resonance (MRI is commonly used to evaluate the primary tumor and assess metastatic disease. The presence of pseudomyxoma peritonei can be found on CT scanning, but extraluminal mucin can be detected by MRI, which is more useful for detecting peritoneal disease than CT scanning [8]. The PET scan did not show an additional benefit for staging [9]. According to the Clinical Practice Guidelines of the American Society of Colon and Rectal Surgeons, obtaining serum tumor markers such as CEA, CA19-9, and CA125 is recommended for the diagnosis and monitoring of appendiceal neoplasms [2]. Since the implication of peritoneal cytology in its management and prognosis remains unclear, routine evaluation of peritoneal cytology is not recommended [2].

Table 2 American Joint Commission on Cancer eighth edition staging of mucinous neoplasm

T—primary tumor	
Tx	Primary tumor cannot be assessed
T0	No evidence of primary tumor
Tis	Carcinoma in situ (intramucosal carcinoma; invasion of the lamina propria or extension into but not through the muscularis mucosae)
Tis (LAMN)	Tumor confined by the muscularis propria; acellular mucin or mucinous epithelium may invade into the muscularis propria
T1	Tumor invades the submucosa (through the muscularis mucosa but not into the muscularis propria)
T2	Tumor invades the muscularis propria
T3	Tumor invades through the muscularis propria into the subserosa or the mesoappendix
T4b	Tumor directly invades or adheres to adjacent organs or structures
N—regional lymph nodes	
Nx	Regional lymph nodes cannot be assessed
N0	No regional lymph node metastasis
N1a	One regional lymph node is positive
N1b	Two or three regional lymph nodes are positive
N1c	No regional lymph nodes are positive, but there are tumor deposits in the subserosa or mesentery
N2	Four or more regional lymph nodes are positive
M—distant metastasis	
M0	No distant metastasis
M1a	Intraperitoneal acellular mucin, without identifiable tumor cells in the disseminated peritoneal mucinous deposits
M1b	Intraperitoneal metastasis only, including peritoneal mucinous deposits containing tumor cells
M1c	Metastasis to sites other than peritoneum

Note: T1 and T2 are not applicable to LAMN; acellular mucin or mucinous epithelium that extends into the subserosa or serosa should be classified as T3 or T4a, respectively

Adapted from Overman et al. [11]

Prognosis

The prognosis of appendiceal mucinous neoplasm varies according to its histology, classification, and staging [12, 13]. Appendiceal mucocele and serrated polyps are generally benign; therefore, the prognosis after surgical resection is excellent. Patients with LAMN without perforation or peritoneal involvement are typically cured by complete resection of the appendix and experience very low recurrence rates [14, 15]. However, patients with HAMNs should be careful to evaluate the presence of invasive adenocarcinoma through the meticulous histopathologic review of the entire surgical specimen [2]. The 10-year overall survival (OS) rate for pseudomyxoma peritonei is 63% after treatment [16]. The prognostic factors for appendiceal mucinous neoplasms are the presence of symptoms, perforation, increased tumor marker levels, and tumor involvement of surgical borders for appendiceal mucinous neoplasms [14, 17]. The prognosis of appendiceal mucinous adenocarcinoma is poor, with a 5-year overall survival rate of 53.6% [12].

Goblet Cell Tumor

Staging

There are several different classification/staging systems for goblet cell carcinoma or goblet cell carcinoid (GCC). First of all, the term of appendiceal GCC is no longer used in the fifth edition of the WHO classification of digestive system tumors. In this edition, GCCs are redefined as an adenocarcinoma subtype (goblet cell adenocarcinoma) rather than a NET and are staged accordingly [3, 18]. However, the term GCC is still used in several systems other than the WHO classification. The TNM staging for GCC proposed by the Union for International Cancer Control/American Joint Committee on Cancer (UICC/AJCC) is based on tumor size, nodal status, and metastatic disease [7, 19]. Tang et al. proposed a classification specific for appendiceal GCC based on the histological characteristics of the primary tumor [20]. In Tang's classification (Table 3), group A (typical GCC), group B (adenocarcinoma ex-GCC, signet-ring cell type), and group C (adenocarcinoma ex-GCC, poorly differentiated carcinoma) show progressively more aggressive phenotypes and a worse prognosis, demonstrating that this classification is useful for predicting clinical behavior and prognosis [20].

Prognosis

GCC is generally considered a low-grade malignancy, with a prognosis of GCCs lying somewhere between appendiceal neuroendocrine tumors. GCC has higher rates of peritoneal carcinomatosis and a lower OS compared to most appendiceal NET but has a better prognosis than appendiceal adenocarcinomas [21–23]. Although the majority of GCCs are identified incidentally after appendectomy, they often present with distant metastases involving the peritoneum, ovaries, omentum, liver, lymph nodes, and bones in approximately 10% of patients at diagnosis [24]. Since ovarian metastases are frequently observed, some groups recommend prophylactic oophorectomy in women diagnosed with GCC [20, 25, 26].

Table 3 Tang's classification

Group	Morphological criteria
A	Well-defined goblet cells arranged in clusters or cohesive linear pattern Minimal cytologic atypia Minimal to no desmoplasia Minimal architectural distortion of the appendiceal wall Degenerative change with extracellular mucin is acceptable
B	Goblet cells or signet-ring cells arranged in irregular large clusters but lack of confluent sheets of cells Discohesive single file or single cell infiltrating pattern Significant cytologic atypia Desmoplasia and associated destruction of the appendiceal wall
C	At least focal evidence of goblet cell morphology A component (>1 low-power field or 1 mm^2) not otherwise distinguishable from a poorly differentiated adenocarcinoma, which may appear as either (a) gland forming, (b) confluent sheets of signet-ring cells, or (c) undifferentiated carcinoma

Adapted from Tang et al. [20]

A 5-year survival rate (5-YSR) for all GCC ranges from 58 to 81% [20, 22, 27]. The prognosis is favorable for patients with early stage but worsens for patients with advanced disease. The survival of GCC is also slightly varied according to the classifications or staging systems used. Based on the AJCC staging system, the 5-YSR in stage 1 is 90–100%, but it significantly worsens to 14–22% in stage 4 [25, 28]. Based on the Tang classification, the 5-YSR in group A is 100% but drops to 36% for group B and 0% for group C with the Tang stages [20].

Neuroendocrine Neoplasm

Staging

Patients with appendiceal neuroendocrine tumor (NET) should be evaluated for the presence of symptoms that may be associated with carcinoid syndrome, such as hot flashes, diarrhea, and dyspnea. To evaluate possible liver metastasis, appendiceal NET requires staging by CT or MRI of the abdomen [29]. Colonoscopy is also necessary because NETs have been reported to accompany a synchronous neoplasm [2]. Because most appendiceal NETs express somatostatin receptors, somatostatin receptor scintigraphy (SRS) can be used to identify NET foci. However, SRS can be considered only in patients for whom a complete resection is not guaranteed and in patients with symptoms associated with carcinoid syndrome [30]. Some groups suggest that biochemical testing including chromogranin A and 5-hydroxyindoleacetic acid in a 24-h urine sample are recommended for patients with localized or metastatic appendiceal NETs for future surveillance and disease monitoring [2].

The AJCC guideline and ENETS classifications for primary appendiceal NET are shown in Table 4. These grading systems are limited by

Table 4 American Joint Commission on Cancer guideline and European Neuroendocrine Tumor Society classifications for primary appendiceal NET

AJCC guideline		ENETS classification	
Tumor			
		Tx	Primary tumor cannot be assessed
		T0	No evidence of primary tumor
T1a	Tumor ≤1 cm	T1	Tumor ≤1 cm with infiltration of the submucosa or muscularis propria
T1b	1–2 cm greatest diameter		
T2	Tumor >2 cm but ≤4 cm or with extension into the cecum	T2	Tumor ≤2 cm with infiltration of the submucosa, muscularis propria, and/or minimal (≤ 3 cm) of the subserosa and/or mesoappendix
T3	Tumor >4 cm or extension into the ileum	T3	Tumor >2 cm and/or > 3 mm infiltration of the serosa and/or mesoappendix
T4	Perforates peritoneum or invades other organs		Infiltration of the peritoneum and/or other neighboring organs
Nodes			
N0	No regional lymph node involvement	Nx	Nodes cannot be assessed
N1	Metastasis to regional nodes		
Metastasis			
M0	No distant metastasis	Mx	Distant metastasis not assessed
M1	Distant metastasis		
Stage			
–	–	0	Tis, N0, M0
I	T1, N0, M0	I	T1, N0, M0
II	T2.3, N0, M0	IIA	T2, N0, M0
III	T4, N0, M0	IIB	T3, N0, M0
	Any T, N1, M0	IIIA	T4, N0, M0
IV	Any T, ant N, M1	IIIB	Any T, N1, M0
		IV	Any T, any N, M1

Abbreviations: *AJCC* American Joint Commission on Cancer; *ENETS* European Neuroendocrine Tumor Society. Adapted from Pape et al. [30]

Table 5 Grading classification of NEN according to the World Health Organization 2019 classification (Adopted from "The 2019 WHO classification of tumors of the digestive system") [3]

Terminology	Differentiation	Grade	Mitotic rate (mitoses/2 mm^2)	Ki-67 index[a]
NET, G1	Well differentiated	Low	<2	<3%
NET, G2		Intermediate	2–20	3–20%
NET, G3		High	>20	>20%
NEC, small-cell type (SCNEC)	Poorly differentiated	High[b]	>20	>20%
NEC, large-cell type (LCNEC)			>20	>20%
MiNEN	Well or poorly differentiated	Variable[c]	Variable$	Variable$

LCNEC large-cell neuroendocrine carcinoma; *MiNEN* mixed neuroendocrine-non-neuroendocrine neoplasm; *NEC* neuroendocrine carcinoma; *NET* neuroendocrine tumor; *SCNEC* small-cell neuroendocrine carcinoma

[a] Mitotic rates are expressed as the number of mitoses/2 mm^2 as determined by counting in 50 fields of 0.2 mm^2 (i.e., in a total area of 10 mm^2); the Ki-67 proliferation index value is determined by counting at least 500 cells in the regions of highest labeling (hot spots), which are identified at scanning magnification; the final grade is based on whichever of the two proliferation indices places the neoplasm in the higher-grade category

[b] Poorly differentiated NECs are not formally graded but are considered high grade by definition

[c] In most MiNENs, both the neuroendocrine and non-neuroendocrine components are poorly differentiated, and the neuroendocrine component has proliferation indices in the same range as other NECs, but this conceptual category allows for the possibility that one or both components may be well differentiated; when feasible, each component should therefore be graded separately. Adapted from Nagtegaal et al. [3]

relying only on size and do not account for tumor grade and/or histopathological characteristics. Histopathological characteristics are crucial for the diagnosis and grading of appendiceal NENs. In the fifth edition of the WHO classification of NENs, grade 1 and 2 tumors are considered NETs, and neuroendocrine carcinomas (NECs) are all considered high-grade tumors (Table 5).

Table 6 Poor prognostic factors for appendiceal NEN

Factors [30]
Tumors >2 cm [34–36]
Localization in the base of the appendix [30, 37]
Ki-67 index >2% [37]
WHO grading: G2 [30]
Vascular or lymph vessel invasion [30]
Mesoappendiceal invasion >3 mm [30]
Positive resection margin (R1 resection) [30]

Prognosis

The majority of appendiceal NETs have an excellent prognosis, with a 5-year survival rate known to be nearly 100% [30, 31]. The prognosis of appendiceal NET is largely dependent on the size of the tumor. A tumor size <1 cm with clear surgical margins (R0 resection) is considered a good prognostic feature, and there is no further risk of recurrence after appendectomy [32]. A tumor >2 cm, located at the base of the appendix, a Ki-67 labeling index >2%, WHO grade G2, vascular or lymph vessel invasion, mesoappendiceal infiltration >3 mm, or positive resection margin has been reported to be associated with an aggressive disease course [32–34] (Table 6). An NEN with poor prognostic factors should be considered and discussed for further and more extensive surgery.

Conclusion

The accurate classification of the appendiceal tumor is important not only for determining treatment strategies but also for predicting prognosis. If lump-shaped protrusions or mucinous or polyp lesions are identified at the appendiceal orifice by colonoscopy, an appendiceal tumor should be carefully suspected. Imaging studies such as CT or MRI are essential to evaluate metastatic lesions and pseudomyxoma peritonei lesions. As the understanding of the molecular pathways of appendiceal tumors increases, their staging classification and prognosis are expected to be further developed in the future.

References

1. Valasek MA, Pai RK. An Update on the diagnosis, grading, and staging of appendiceal mucinous neoplasms. Adv Anat Pathol. 2018;25:38–60.
2. Glasgow SC, Gaertner W, Stewart D, Davids J, Alavi K, Paquette IM, et al. The American Society of Colon and Rectal Surgeons, clinical practice guidelines for the management of appendiceal neoplasms. Dis Colon Rectum. 2019;62:1425–38.
3. Nagtegaal ID, Odze RD, Klimstra D, Paradis V, Rugge M, Schirmacher P, et al. The 2019 WHO classification of tumours of the digestive system. Histopathology. 2020;76:182–8.
4. Carr NJ, Cecil TD, Mohamed F, Sobin LH, Sugarbaker PH, González-Moreno S, et al. A consensus for classification and pathologic reporting of pseudomyxoma peritonei and associated appendiceal neoplasia: the results of the Peritoneal Surface Oncology Group International (PSOGI) modified delphi process. Am J Surg Pathol. 2016;40:14–26.
5. Carr NJ, Bibeau F, Bradley RF, Dartigues P, Feakins RM, Geisinger KR, et al. The histopathological classification, diagnosis and differential diagnosis of mucinous appendiceal neoplasms, appendiceal adenocarcinomas and pseudomyxoma peritonei. Histopathology. 2017;71:847–58.
6. Van de Moortele M, De Hertogh G, Sagaert X, Van Cutsem E. Appendiceal cancer: a review of the literature. Acta Gastroenterol Belg. 2020;83:441–8.
7. Overman MAE, Compton C. Appendix carcinoma. In: Amin M, editor. AJCC cancer staging manual. 8th ed. Chicago: Springer; 2017.
8. Low RN, Barone RM, Lucero J. Comparison of MRI and CT for predicting the Peritoneal Cancer Index (PCI) preoperatively in patients being considered for cytoreductive surgical procedures. Ann Surg Oncol. 2015;22:1708–15.
9. Rohani P, Scotti SD, Shen P, Stewart JH, Russell GB, Cromer M, et al. Use of FDG-PET imaging for patients with disseminated cancer of the appendix. Am Surg. 2010;76:1338–44.
10. Carr NJ. Updates in appendix pathology: the precarious cutting edge. Surg Pathol Clin. 2020;13:469–84.
11. Overman MJAE, Compton CC. Appendix—carcinoma. In: American Joint Committee on Cancer. AJCC cancer staging manual. 8th ed. Springer; 2017.
12. Asare EA, Compton CC, Hanna NN, Kosinski LA, Washington MK, Kakar S, et al. The impact of stage, grade, and mucinous histology on the efficacy of systemic chemotherapy in adenocarcinomas of the appendix: analysis of the National Cancer Data Base. Cancer. 2016;122:213–21.
13. Misdraji J, Yantiss RK, Graeme-Cook FM, Balis UJ, Young RH. Appendiceal mucinous neoplasms: a clinicopathologic analysis of 107 cases. Am J Surg Pathol. 2003;27:1089–103.
14. Fournier K, Rafeeq S, Taggart M, Kanaby P, Ning J, Chen HC, et al. Low-grade appendiceal mucinous neoplasm of uncertain malignant potential (LAMN-UMP): prognostic factors and implications for treatment and follow-up. Ann Surg Oncol. 2017;24:187–93.
15. Morano WF, Gleeson EM, Sullivan SH, Padmanaban V, Mapow BL, Shewokis PA, et al. Clinicopathological features and management of appendiceal mucoceles: a systematic review. Am Surg. 2018;84:273–81.
16. Chua TC, Moran BJ, Sugarbaker PH, Levine EA, Glehen O, Gilly FN, et al. Early- and long-term outcome data of patients with pseudomyxoma peritonei from appendiceal origin treated by a strategy of cytoreductive surgery and hyperthermic intraperitoneal chemotherapy. J Clin Oncol. 2012;30:2449–56.
17. Shin R, Chai YJ, Park JW, Chang MS, Bae JM, Kim MJ, et al. Ultimate clinical outcomes of appendiceal mucinous neoplasm of uncertain malignant potential. Ann Surg Oncol. 2017;24:974–82.
18. Lioyd RV, Osamura RY, Kloppel G. WHO classification of tumours of endocrine organs. Lyon: International Agency for Research on Cancer; 2010.
19. Edge SB. AJCC cancer staging manual. 7th ed. New York: Springer; 2010.
20. Tang LH, Shia J, Soslow RA, Dhall D, Wong WD, O'Reilly E, et al. Pathologic classification and clinical behavior of the spectrum of goblet cell carcinoid tumors of the appendix. Am J Surg Pathol. 2008;32:1429–43.
21. Onyemkpa C, Davis A, McLeod M, Oyasiji T. Typical carcinoids, goblet cell carcinoids, mixed adenoneuroendocrine carcinomas, neuroendocrine carcinomas and adenocarcinomas of the appendix: a comparative analysis of survival profile and predictors. J Gastrointest Oncol. 2019;10:300–6.
22. Hsu C, Rashid A, Xing Y, Chiang YJ, Chagpar RB, Fournier KF, et al. Varying malignant potential of appendiceal neuroendocrine tumors: importance of histologic subtype. J Surg Oncol. 2013;107:136–43.
23. McCusker ME, Coté TR, Clegg LX, Sobin LH. Primary malignant neoplasms of the appendix: a population-based study from the surveillance, epidemiology and end-results program, 1973-1998. Cancer. 2002;94:3307–12.
24. Pape UF, Perren A, Niederle B, Gross D, Gress T, Costa F, et al. ENETS Consensus Guidelines for the management of patients with neuroendocrine neoplasms from the jejuno-ileum and the appendix including goblet cell carcinomas. Neuroendocrinology. 2012;95:135–56.
25. Pham TH, Wolff B, Abraham SC, Drelichman E. Surgical and chemotherapy treatment outcomes of goblet cell carcinoid: a tertiary cancer center experience. Ann Surg Oncol. 2006;13:370–6.

26. UKINETS. UKINETS bitesize guidance: Goblet Cell Carcinoma. http://www.ukinets.org/wp-content/uploads/UKINETSbitesize-guidance-GCC.pdf.
27. Turaga KK, Pappas SG, Gamblin T. Importance of histologic subtype in the staging of appendiceal tumors. Ann Surg Oncol. 2012;19:1379–85.
28. Fields AC, Lu P, Enzinger A, Goldberg J, Irani J, Bleday R, et al. Treatment patterns and outcomes in goblet cell carcinoid tumors of the appendix. J Surg Oncol. 2019;120:1096–101.
29. (NCCN) NCCN. NCCN clinical practice guidelines in oncology. https://www.nccn.org/professionals/physician_gls. Accessed 28 Nov 2021.
30. Pape UF, Niederle B, Costa F, Gross D, Kelestimur F, Kianmanesh R, et al. ENETS consensus guidelines for neuroendocrine neoplasms of the appendix (excluding goblet cell carcinomas). Neuroendocrinology. 2016;103:144–52.
31. Landry CS, Woodall C, Scoggins CR, McMasters KM, Martin RC 2nd. Analysis of 900 appendiceal carcinoid tumors for a proposed predictive staging system. Arch Surg. 2008;143:664–70; discussion 70.
32. Mullen JT, Savarese DM. Carcinoid tumors of the appendix: a population-based study. J Surg Oncol. 2011;104:41–4.
33. Shapiro R, Eldar S, Sadot E, Papa MZ, Zippel DB. Appendiceal carcinoid at a large tertiary center: pathologic findings and long-term follow-up evaluation. Am J Surg. 2011;201:805–8.
34. Fornaro R, Frascio M, Sticchi C, De Salvo L, Stabilini C, Mandolfino F, et al. Appendectomy or right hemicolectomy in the treatment of appendiceal carcinoid tumors? Tumori. 2007;93:587–90.
35. In't Hof KH, van der Wal HC, Kazemier G, Lange JF. Carcinoid tumour of the appendix: an analysis of 1,485 consecutive emergency appendectomies. J Gastrointest Surg. 2008;12:1436–8.
36. Moertel CG, Weiland LH, Nagorney DM, Dockerty MB. Carcinoid tumor of the appendix: treatment and prognosis. N Engl J Med. 1987;317:1699–701.
37. Moris D, Tsilimigras DI, Vagios S, Ntanasis-Stathopoulos I, Karachaliou GS, Papalampros A, et al. Neuroendocrine neoplasms of the appendix: a review of the literature. Anticancer Res. 2018;38:601–11.

Staging and Treatment. II-2. Overview of Treatment According to Stage

Key Points

- Prognosis and treatment of appendiceal cancer differs according to its histologic type.
- There is controversy on the treatment strategy due to the rarity of the disease and the lack of randomized controlled trials.
- Treatment of colonic-type adenocarcinoma of the appendix mirrors that of colon adenocarcinoma.
- For appendiceal goblet cell carcinoma, right hemicolectomy is recommended due to frequent peritoneal spread without nodal involvement.
- For low-grade localized appendiceal mucinous neoplasm (AMN), appendectomy or right hemicolectomy should be considered according to the individual risk, and for disseminated peritoneal AMN, cytoreduction surgery and hyperthermic intraperitoneal chemotherapy improve overall survival.
- For appendiceal neuroendocrine tumor (NET) <1 cm, appendectomy alone is recommended, and NET >2 cm or G3 should be treated with right hemicolectomy. Somatostatin analogs and everolimus are effective in metastatic unresectable appendiceal NET.

Introduction

The prognosis and treatment of appendiceal cancer differ according to histological type. There is controversy regarding the treatment strategy owing to the rarity of the disease and the lack of randomized controlled trials. Treatment guidelines have been established based on retrospective case series and expert opinions.

Appendiceal Colonic-Type Adenocarcinoma

Colonic-type adenocarcinoma is the most common cancer that arises in the appendix, comprising 60% of appendiceal cancers; however, it comprises only 0.5% of all gastrointestinal malignancies [1]. There are no standard staging or treatment guidelines because of the rarity of the disease; experts comply with colonic adenocarcinoma treatment indicated by the American Joint Commission on Cancer (AJCC), including the staging system and the National Comprehensive Cancer Network (NCCN) or European Society for Medical Oncology (ESMO) guidelines for colon cancer [2] (Tables 1 and 2).

For Tis or favorable T1 disease (negative section margin, grade 1 or 2, and no lymphovascular invasion), appendectomy alone might be sufficient [2]. Patients with unfavorable T1 (grade 3,

Yu Jin Kim is the lead author of this chapter.

H. J. Chun et al., *Gastrointestinal Cancer*, https://doi.org/10.1007/978-981-99-0815-8_28

Table 1 TNM staging system for goblet cell carcinomas of the appendix as per the UICC/AJCC guidelines—these are identical to those for appendiceal neuroendocrine neoplasms

Component	Criterion		
Primary tumor			
T0	No tumor evident		
T1a	Tumor ≤1 cm in greatest dimension		
T1b	Tumor >1 cm but ≤2 cm in greatest dimension		
T2	Tumor >2 cm but ≤4 cm, or with extension into the cecum		
T3	Tumor >4 cm, or with extension into the ileum		
T4	Tumor perforates peritoneum or invades other adjacent structures		
Regional lymph node metastases			
N0	None present		
N1	Present		
Distant metastases			
M0	None present		
M1	Present		
UICC/AJCC stage			
I	T1	N0	M0
II	T2–3	N0	M0
III	T4	N0	M0
	Any T	N1	M0
IV	Any T	Any N	M1

UICC Union for International Cancer Control; *AJCC* American Joint Committee on Cancer
Adapted from Pape et al. [6]

Table 2 TNM staging of mucinous adenocarcinoma of the appendix

Category	Definition
Primary tumor	
Tx	Primary tumor cannot be assessed
T0	No evidence of primary tumor
Tis	Carcinoma in situ: intraepithelial or invasion of lamina propria
T1	Tumor invades submucosa
T2	Tumor invades muscularis propria
T3	Tumor invades through muscularis propria into subserosa or mesoappendix
T4	Tumor penetrates visceral peritoneum, including peritoneal mucinous tumor within the right lower quadrant, and/or directly invades other organs or structures
T4a	Tumor penetrates visceral peritoneum, including peritoneal mucinous tumor within the right lower quadrant
T4b	Tumor directly invades other organs or structures
Regional lymph node metastases	
Nx	Regional lymph node cannot be assessed
N0	No regional lymph node metastasis
N1	Metastasis in one to three regional lymph nodes
N2	Metastasis in four or more regional lymph nodes
Distant metastases	
M0	No distant metastasis
M1	Distant metastasis
M1a	Intraperitoneal metastasis beyond the right lower quadrant, including PMP
M1b	Extraperitoneal metastasis
Histological grading	
Gx	Cannot be determined
G1	Well differentiated
G2	Moderately differentiated
G3	Poorly differentiated
G4	Undifferentiated

Adapted from Edge et al. [20]

lymphovascular invasion, and/or positive section margins) should be considered for right hemicolectomy [2]. For grade T2 or higher disease, lymph node dissection of ≥12 is recommended [2]. The rate of lymph node involvement in colonic-type adenocarcinoma or the appendix is 30% [1].

Adjuvant systemic chemotherapy is recommended for patients with positive regional lymph nodes, similar to that for colorectal adenocarcinoma. Adjuvant chemotherapy should be considered for stage II patients with high-risk features [3]. The incidence of distant metastasis at diagnosis is reported to be as high as 37% [1, 4].

Complete cytoreduction and hyperthermic intraperitoneal chemotherapy (HIPEC) should be considered for patients with peritoneal dissemination, including the ovaries, except for other organs. Metastasectomy for limited liver or lung lesions is acceptable as for colorectal adenocarcinoma [2, 3].

Appendiceal Goblet Cell Carcinoma

Due to the rarity of the disease and the lack of randomized controlled studies, controversy exists regarding treatment of appendiceal goblet cell carcinoma (GCC). Approximately 50–60% of GCC presents with acute appendicitis [5, 6], only 1% of GCCs undergo complete preoperative imaging studies before surgery, and most staging workups are performed after appendectomy [6, 7].

The North American and European Neuroendocrine Tumor Societies (NANETS and ENETS) recommend right hemicolectomy within 3 months after appendectomy [8, 9]. Evidence supporting right hemicolectomy in colorectal adenocarcinoma indicates that the rate of lymph node involvement in localized GCC of the appendix ranges from 20 to 40% [10], and peritoneal spread frequently occurs without nodal involvement due to submucosal growth patterns [11, 12].

In several studies, appendectomy alone is recommended in the early stage of GCC, that is, tumor size ≤1 cm, without serosal, mesoappendiceal, or cecal invasion, and with negative surgical section margins with typical group A histology [7, 13–15]. Based on Tang's classification, the 5-year overall survival (OS) was 100% in group A, 36% in group B, and 0% in group C [7]. The Surveillance, Epidemiology, and End Results (SEER) database has reported that approximately 40% of patients received right hemicolectomy [10]. However, the very early stages of GCC are rare, and the treatment strategy remains controversial.

Due to the high incidence of ovarian metastasis, some experts suggest prophylactic bilateral salpingo-oophorectomy [12], although its advantage remains unclear. Adjuvant chemotherapy must be considered for patients with stage III GCC [2]. For patients with metastatic peritoneal disease, cytoreductive surgery (CRS) and hyperthermic intraperitoneal chemotherapy (HIPEC) may be considered treatment options. In one prospective study, CRS with HIPEC was a significant factor in improving OS [12].

Most patients with metastatic disease are treated with chemotherapy regimens similar to those used in colonic adenocarcinoma, that is, regimens based on 5-fluorouracil (5-FU) [16]. Although evidence is limited, the ENETS recommends 5-FU-based chemotherapy, that is, FOLFOX, as used in colon adenocarcinoma for metastatic GCC [6]. Palliative chemotherapy, including various cytotoxic antiproliferative agents, has been reported to have efficacy in up to 50% of patients for 8–12 months [12, 17–19].

The 5-year OS rates based on the AJCC staging system were 100% for stage I, 76% for stage II, 22% for stage III, and 14% for stage IV cancer [20].

Mucinous Neoplasm of the Appendix

The prognosis and treatment of mucinous adenocarcinoma of the appendix (AMN) depend on the histological type, grading, and staging of the disease. In addition, ruptured or unruptured AMN should follow a different treatment strategy (Fig. 1).

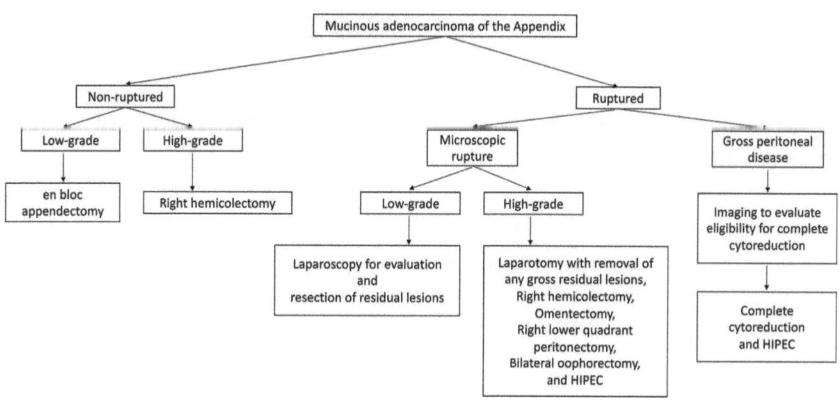

Fig. 1 Treatment of mucinous adenocarcinoma of the appendix. HIPEC, hyperthermic intraperitoneal chemotherapy. (Adapted from Kelly et al. [3])

Localized Mucinous Neoplasm of the Appendix

Non-ruptured localized low-grade AMN is cured by appendectomy with en bloc resection of the cyst regardless of the size of the lesion due to the low incidence of nodal involvement (2%) [21].

Right hemicolectomy should be considered in cases of nodal involvement after appendectomy, tumors involving the periappendiceal area, tumor size ≥2 cm, high-grade histology, or tumors that invade through the muscularis propria [22]. Another expert also recommended performing right hemicolectomy in the following situations [12]: degree of cellular undifferentiation, increased mitotic activity, involvement of the base of the appendix, lymph node metastasis, or tumor size >2 cm. In addition, patients with ruptured disease should be considered for hemicolectomy [23].

Since acellular and cellular mucin spillages have significantly different prognoses [12, 24, 25], cytoreduction surgery for diseases with localized cellular mucin spillage is recommended because of the high probability of progression to extensive intra-abdominal disease [12, 26, 27].

Adjuvant chemotherapy with a 5-FU-based regimen is recommended for patients with poorly differentiated tumors with lymph node involvement or perforation; however, this has been validated in prospective randomized trials.

Evidence for the effectiveness of adjuvant chemotherapy after localized AMN resection is still insufficient for poorly differentiated tumors (signet-ring histology), lymph node involvement or perforation, or low-grade tumors with lymphovascular invasion [23].

Appendiceal Mucinous Neoplasm with Peritoneal Metastasis

Based on a retrospective case series, complete cytoreduction with intraperitoneal chemotherapy is the optimal treatment for peritoneal dissemination. Therefore, a bilateral oophorectomy is recommended.

The completeness of cytoreduction is significantly correlated with prognosis, and the scores are defined as follows: complete resection (CCR) 0, no evidence of visible lesions; CCR 1, lesions <2.5 mm that could not be resected; CCR 2, lesions of 2.5–5 mm; and CCR 3, ≥5 mm of visible lesions left after surgery [23]. The peritoneal cancer index is an intraoperative score that assesses tumor burden in 13 areas and ranges from 1 to 39 [28].

Hyperthermic intraperitoneal chemotherapy (HIPEC) delivers a high dose of heated (to approximately 107 °F or 40–42 °C) chemotherapeutic agents into the peritoneum. The most commonly used agents are mitomycin C [29, 30], oxaliplatin, cisplatin, and 5-FU [30].

For AMN, the most commonly used agents are mitomycin C at 10–12.5 mg/m^2, oxaliplatin at 460 mg/m^2, cisplatin, and 5-FU, as single agents or a combination of two or more agents.

CRS and HIPEC are common treatment modalities for patients with disseminated low-grade neoplasms (G1, well differentiated) [30–32]. Although several retrospective case series have shown benefits for survival, no randomized trials have been performed to investigate CRS and HIPEC. In patients with complete CRS and HIPEC, the 5-year survival rate was 86% for disseminated peritoneal adenomucinosis (DPAM) and 50% for the more aggressive PMCA (indeterminate mucinous carcinomatosis) [33], compared to 20% in patients with incomplete cytoreduction. Two retrospective studies demonstrated the completeness of cytoreduction [34, 35]. Histopathology and HIPEC improved OS in peritoneal mucinous carcinomatosis (PMCA), and 15 had PMCA with indeterminate or discordant features [34].

Preoperative systemic chemotherapy is considered for high-grade appendiceal adenocarcinomas, in contrast to low-grade appendiceal mucinous neoplasms [23].

Palliative Systemic Chemotherapy

No randomized clinical trials have been conducted on palliative systemic chemotherapy. Systemic chemotherapy achieves a lower response rate in patients with stage IV low-grade mucinous neoplasms [36]; however, it improves the overall survival of patients with stage IV G2 or G3 mucinous adenocarcinoma. If tumor volume decreases after systemic chemotherapy, these patients receive subsequent CRC and HPEC treatment [30, 37, 38]. A single-center retrospective study showed that patients with unresectable high-grade adenocarcinoma (G2 or G3) responded to systemic chemotherapy, including the targeted agents irinotecan, platinum, capecitabine, gefitinib, bevacizumab, and cetuximab [39]. A single-center retrospective study reported that 44% of 78 patients with metastatic disease who underwent chemotherapy showed response [40].

Neuroendocrine Tumor of the Appendix

Surgical resection is the treatment of choice, and a simple appendicectomy or oncological right hemicolectomy is performed according to the staging and risk factors (Table 3 and Fig. 2) [9]. Appendectomy alone (in the case of R0 resection) is curative for appendiceal neuroendocrine tumor (NET) <1 cm. However, for NET <1 cm, which is located at the base of the appendix, or with invasion >3 mm, subsequent right hemicolectomy should be considered [6, 9, 41–47].

Lymph node or distant metastasis is unlikely but possible for tumors >1 cm and < 2 cm. The ENETS recommends right hemicolectomy if patients have one or more of the following risk factors: G2, vascular or lymph vessel invasion, and mesoappendiceal infiltration >3 mm [9]. For appendiceal NET >2 cm, right hemicolectomy with lymph node dissection is recom-

Table 3 TNM staging for appendiceal NET according to either the ENETS guidelines or the UICC/AJCC classification

	ENETS guidelines	UICC/AJCC classification
T—primary tumor		
x	Primary tumor not assessed/assessable	
0	No evidence of any primary tumor	
1	Tumor ≤1 cm with infiltration of the submucosa and muscularis propria	
1a		Tumor ≤1 cm
1b		Tumor >1 cm but ≤2 cm
2	Tumor ≤2 cm with infiltration of the submucosa, muscularis propria, and/or minimal (≤3 mm) infiltration of the subserosa and/or mesoappendix	Tumor >2 cm but ≤4 cm or with extension into the cecum
3	Tumor >2 cm and/or extensive (>3 mm) infiltration of the subserosa and/or mesoappendix	Tumor >4 cm or with extension into the ileum
4	Tumor with infiltration of the peritoneum and/or other neighboring organs	Tumor with perforation of the peritoneum or invasion of other adjacent structures
N		
Nx	Regional lymph nodes not assessed/assessable	
N0	No regional lymph node metastasis	
N1	Locoregional lymph node metastasis/–es	
M distant metastasis		
Mx	Distant metastasis not assessed/assessable	
M0	No distant metastasis	
M1	Distant metastasis/–es	

ENETS European Neuroendocrine Tumor Society; *UICC* Union for International Cancer Control; *AJCC* American Joint Committee on Cancer
Adapted from Pape et al. [9]

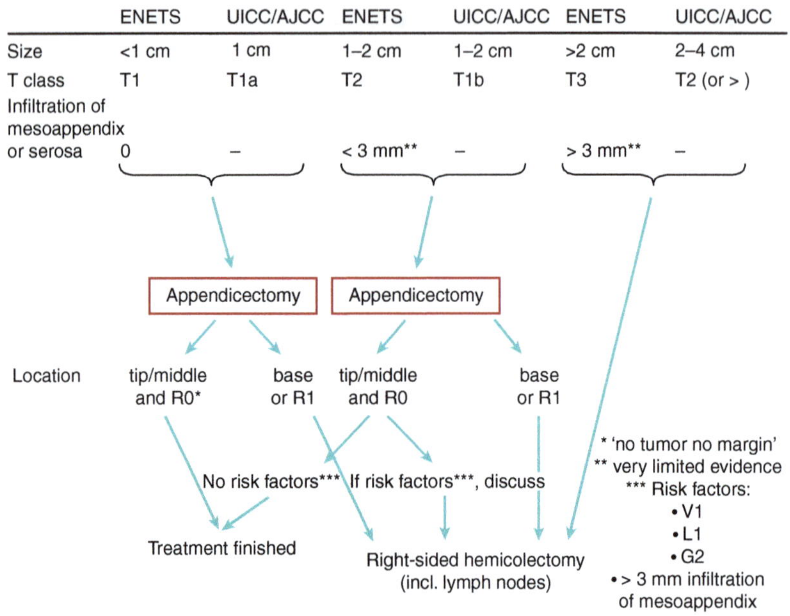

Fig. 2 Treatment for small appendiceal neuroendocrine tumor. V1 = vascular invasion; L1 = lymphatic invasion; G2 = grade 2 tumor (Ki-67: 3–20%) [9]

mended because of the high risk of lymph node metastasis, long-term recurrence, and/or distant metastasis [48]. Appendiceal G3 NET of any size should be treated using oncological right hemicolectomy and managed as adenocarcinomas [9].

In pediatric patients with appendiceal NET, the prognosis after resection is good, even in those ≥2 cm [9, 41, 49].

For unresectable appendiceal NET with distant metastases, somatostatin analogs play a role in improving progression-free survival [50]. Everolimus and peptide receptor radionuclide therapy, if available, may be treatment options for functional and nonfunctioning NETs [6, 8].

Conclusion

Appendiceal cancer accounts for <1% of all gastrointestinal cancers. The four common types of appendiceal cancer are colonic-type adenocarcinoma, goblet cell carcinoma, neoplasm of the appendix, and neuroendocrine tumors. The prognosis and treatment of appendiceal cancer differ according to the histological subtype. Treatment strategies have been established mostly based on expert opinion or retrospective studies owing to the rarity of the disease and few randomized clinical trials.

References

1. McCusker M, Coté T, Clegg L, Sobin L. Primary malignant neoplasms of the appendix: a population-based study from the surveillance, epidemiology and end-results program, 1973-1998. Cancer. 2002;94:3307–12.
2. Van de Moortele M, De Hertogh G, Sagaert X, Van Cutsem E. Appendiceal cancer: a review of the literature. Acta Gastroenterol Belg. 2020;83:441–8.
3. Kelly K. Management of appendix cancer. Clin Colon Rectal Surg. 2015;28:247–55.
4. Benedix F, Reimer A, Gastinger I, Mroczkowski P, Lippert H, Kube R. Primary appendiceal carcinoma—epidemiology, surgery and survival: results of a German multi-center study. Eur J Surg Oncol. 2010;36:763–71.
5. Olsen I, Holt N, Langer S, Hasselby J, Grønbæk H, Hillingsø J, et al. Goblet cell carcinoids: characteristics of a Danish cohort of 83 patients. PLoS One. 2015;10:e0117627.
6. Pape UF, Perren A, Niederle B, Gross D, Gress T, Costa F, et al. ENETS Consensus Guidelines for the management of patients with neuroendocrine neoplasms from the jejuno-ileum and the appendix including goblet cell carcinomas. Neuroendocrinology. 2012;95:135–56.

7. Tang LH, Shia J, Soslow RA, Dhall D, Wong WD, O'Reilly E, et al. Pathologic classification and clinical behavior of the spectrum of goblet cell carcinoid tumors of the appendix. Am J Surg Pathol. 2008;32:1429–43.
8. Boudreaux JP, Klimstra D, Hassan M, Woltering E, Jensen R, Goldsmith S, et al. The NANETS consensus guideline for the diagnosis and management of neuroendocrine tumors: well-differentiated neuroendocrine tumors of the Jejunum, Ileum, Appendix, and Cecum. Pancreas. 2010;39:753–66.
9. Pape UF, Niederle B, Costa F, Gross D, Kelestimur F, Kianmanesh R, et al. ENETS consensus guidelines for neuroendocrine neoplasms of the appendix (excluding goblet cell carcinomas). Neuroendocrinology. 2016;103:144–52.
10. Turaga K, Pappas S, Gamblin TC. Importance of histologic subtype in the staging of appendiceal tumors. Ann Surg Oncol. 2012;19:1379–85.
11. Lamarca A, Nonaka D, Lopez Escola C, Hubner R, O'Dwyer S, Chakrabarty B, et al. Appendiceal goblet cell carcinoids: management considerations from a reference peritoneal tumour service centre and ENETS centre of excellence. Neuroendocrinology. 2016;103:500–17.
12. Pahlavan P, Kanthan R. Goblet cell carcinoid of the appendix. World J Surg Oncol. 2005;3:36.
13. Bucher P, Gervaz P, Ris F, Oulhaci W, Egger J-F, Morel P. Surgical treatment of appendiceal adenocarcinoid (goblet cell carcinoid). World J Surg. 2005;29:1436–9.
14. Byrn J, Wang J-L, Divino C, Nguyen S, Warner RRP. Management of goblet cell carcinoid. J Surg Oncol. 2006;94:396–402.
15. Varisco B, McAlvin B, Dias J, Franga D. Adenocarcinoid of the appendix: is right hemicolectomy necessary? A meta-analysis of retrospective chart reviews. Am Surg. 2004;70:593–9.
16. Clift A, Frilling A. Neuroendocrine, goblet cell and mixed adeno-neuroendocrine tumours of the appendix: updates, clinical applications and the future. Expert Rev Gastroenterol Hepatol. 2017;11:237–47.
17. Toumpanakis C, Standish R, Baishnab E, Winslet M, Caplin M. Goblet cell carcinoid tumors (adenocarcinoid) of the appendix. Dis Colon Rectum. 2007;50:315–22.
18. Pham T, Wolff B, Abraham S, Drelichman E. Surgical and chemotherapy treatment outcomes of goblet cell carcinoid: a tertiary cancer center experience. Ann Surg Oncol. 2006;13:370–6.
19. Garin L, Corbinais S, Boucher E, Blanchot J, Le Guilcher P, Raoul J-L. Adenocarcinoid of the appendix vermiformis: complete and persistent remission after chemotherapy (folfox) of a metastatic case. Dig Dis Sci. 2002;47:2760–2.
20. Edge SB, Byrd DR, Carducci MA, Compton CC, Fritz A, Greene F. AJCC cancer staging manual. New York: Springer; 2010.
21. Yantiss R, Shia J, Klimstra D, Hahn H, Odze R, Misdraji J. Prognostic significance of localized extra-appendiceal mucin deposition in appendiceal mucinous neoplasms. Am J Surg Pathol. 2009;33:248–55.
22. González-Moreno S, Sugarbaker PH. Right hemicolectomy does not confer a survival advantage in patients with mucinous carcinoma of the appendix and peritoneal seeding. Br J Surg. 2004;91:304–11.
23. Shaib W, Assi R, Shamseddine A, Alese O, Staley C, Memis B, et al. Appendiceal mucinous neoplasms: diagnosis and management. Oncologist. 2017;22:1107–16.
24. Misdraji J, Yantiss R, Graeme Cook F, Balis U, Young R. Appendiceal mucinous neoplasms: a clinicopathologic analysis of 107 cases. Am J Surg Pathol. 2003;27:1089–103.
25. Carr NJ, McCarthy WF, Sobin LH. Epithelial noncarcinoid tumors and tumor-like lesions of the appendix. A clinicopathologic study of 184 patients with a multivariate analysis of prognostic factors. Cancer. 1995;75:757–68.
26. Pai R, Beck A, Norton J, Longacre T. Appendiceal mucinous neoplasms: clinicopathologic study of 116 cases with analysis of factors predicting recurrence. Am J Surg Pathol. 2009;33:1425–39.
27. Young R. Pseudomyxoma peritonei and selected other aspects of the spread of appendiceal neoplasms. Semin Diagn Pathol. 2004;21:134–50.
28. Jacquet P, Sugarbaker PH. Clinical research methodologies in diagnosis and staging of patients with peritoneal carcinomatosis. Cancer Treat Res. 1996;82:359–74.
29. Oleson JR, Calderwood SK, Coughlin CT, Dewhirst MW, Gerweck LE, Gibbs FA, et al. Biological and clinical aspects of hyperthermia in cancer therapy. Am J Clin Oncol. 1988;11:368–80.
30. Chua T, Moran B, Sugarbaker P, Levine E, Glehen O, Gilly F, et al. Early- and long-term outcome data of patients with pseudomyxoma peritonei from appendiceal origin treated by a strategy of cytoreductive surgery and hyperthermic intraperitoneal chemotherapy. J Clin Oncol. 2012;30:2449–56.
31. Davison J, Choudry H, Pingpank J, Ahrendt S, Holtzman M, Zureikat A, et al. Clinicopathologic and molecular analysis of disseminated appendiceal mucinous neoplasms: identification of factors predicting survival and proposed criteria for a three-tiered assessment of tumor grade. Mod Pathol. 2014;27:1521–39.
32. Barrios P, Losa F, Gonzalez Moreno S, Rojo A, Gómez Portilla A, Bretcha Boix P, et al. Recommendations in the management of epithelial appendiceal neoplasms and peritoneal dissemination from mucinous tumours (pseudomyxoma peritonei). Clin Transl Oncol. 2016;18:437–48.
33. Sugarbaker PH, Chang D. Results of treatment of 385 patients with peritoneal surface spread of appendiceal malignancy. Ann Surg Oncol. 1999;6:727–31.

34. Shaib W, Martin L, Choi M, Chen Z, Krishna K, Kim S, et al. Hyperthermic intraperitoneal chemotherapy following cytoreductive surgery improves outcome in patients with primary appendiceal mucinous adenocarcinoma: a pooled analysis from three tertiary care centers. Oncologist. 2015;20:907–14.
35. Dayal S, Taflampas P, Riss S, Chandrakumaran K, Cecil T, Mohamed F, et al. Complete cytoreduction for pseudomyxoma peritonei is optimal but maximal tumor debulking may be beneficial in patients in whom complete tumor removal cannot be achieved. Dis Colon Rectum. 2013;56:1366–72.
36. Asare E, Compton C, Hanna N, Kosinski L, Washington M, Kakar S, et al. The impact of stage, grade, and mucinous histology on the efficacy of systemic chemotherapy in adenocarcinomas of the appendix: analysis of the National Cancer Data Base. Cancer. 2016;122:213–21.
37. Teixeira MR, Qvist H, Giercksky KE, Bøhler PJ, Heim S. Cytogenetic analysis of several pseudomyxoma peritonei lesions originating from a mucinous cystadenoma of the appendix. Cancer Genet Cytogenet. 1997;93:157–9.
38. Sugarbaker PH, Bijelic L, Chang D, Yoo D. Neoadjuvant FOLFOX chemotherapy in 34 consecutive patients with mucinous peritoneal carcinomatosis of appendiceal origin. J Surg Oncol. 2010;102:576–81.
39. Shapiro JF, Chase JL, Wolff RA, Lambert LA, Mansfield PF, Overman MJ, et al. Modern systemic chemotherapy in surgically unresectable neoplasms of appendiceal origin: a single-institution experience. Cancer. 2010;116:316–22.
40. Lieu CH, Lambert LA, Wolff RA, Eng C, Zhang N, Wen S, et al. Systemic chemotherapy and surgical cytoreduction for poorly differentiated and signet ring cell adenocarcinomas of the appendix. Ann Oncol. 2012;23:652–8.
41. Boxberger N, Redlich A, Böger C, Leuschner I, von Schweinitz D, Dralle H, et al. Neuroendocrine tumors of the appendix in children and adolescents. Pediatr Blood Cancer. 2013;60:65–70.
42. In't Hof KH, van der Wal HC, Kazemier G, Lange JF. Carcinoid tumour of the appendix: an analysis of 1,485 consecutive emergency appendectomies. J Gastrointest Surg. 2008;12:1436–8.
43. Hsu C, Rashid A, Xing Y, Chiang Y-J, Chagpar R, Fournier K, et al. Varying malignant potential of appendiceal neuroendocrine tumors: importance of histologic subtype. J Surg Oncol. 2013;107:136–43.
44. Mullen J, Savarese DMF. Carcinoid tumors of the appendix: a population-based study. J Surg Oncol. 2011;104:41–4.
45. Shapiro R, Eldar S, Sadot E, Papa M, Zippel D. Appendiceal carcinoid at a large tertiary center: pathologic findings and long-term follow-up evaluation. Am J Surg. 2011;201:805–8.
46. Volante M, Daniele L, Asioli S, Cassoni P, Comino A, Coverlizza S, et al. Tumor staging but not grading is associated with adverse clinical outcome in neuroendocrine tumors of the appendix: a retrospective clinical pathologic analysis of 138 cases. Am J Surg Pathol. 2013;37:606–12.
47. Alexandraki KI, Griniatsos J, Bramis KI, Ballian N, Dimitriou N, Giannakakis T, et al. Clinical value of right hemicolectomy for appendiceal carcinoids using pathologic criteria. J Endocrinol Investig. 2011;34:255–9.
48. Bamboat Z, Berger D. Is right hemicolectomy for 2.0-cm appendiceal carcinoids justified? Arch Surg. 2006;141:349–52; discussion 352.
49. Henderson L, Fehily C, Folaranmi S, Kelsey A, McPartland J, Jawaid W, et al. Management and outcome of neuroendocrine tumours of the appendix-a two centre UK experience. J Pediatr Surg. 2014;49:1513–7.
50. Arnold R, Rinke A, Klose K-J, Müller H-H, Wied M, Zamzow K, et al. Octreotide versus octreotide plus interferon-alpha in endocrine gastroenteropancreatic tumors: a randomized trial. Clin Gastroenterol Hepatol. 2005;3:761–71.

Staging and Treatment. II-3. Surgical Resection for Appendiceal Neoplasms

Key Points

- The extent of surgical resection of appendiceal tumors depends on histopathologic subtypes, tumor sizes, localized/disseminated status of the appendix, and regional involvement.
- Appendiceal neuroendocrine neoplasms >2 cm or appendiceal adenocarcinoma are considered to perform right hemicolectomy in accordance with right-sided colon cancer.
- Cytoreductive surgery with hyperthermic intraperitoneal chemotherapy is considered the effective treatment for appendiceal mucinous neoplasms with pseudomyxoma peritonei.

Introduction

Appendiceal tumors are rare and generally detected in appendectomy specimens with an incidence of 0.7–1.4% [1, 2]. They are difficult to diagnose without surgical interventions such as appendectomy because of its anatomical location. In addition, appendiceal neoplasms consist of heterogeneous groups, which have different histopathological subtypes according to epithelial and non-epithelial origins. Appendiceal neuroendocrine neoplasms (NENs) are non-epithelial tumors. Conversely, appendiceal mucinous neoplasms, colonic-type adenocarcinomas, goblet cell adenocarcinomas, and signet-ring cell adenocarcinomas are regarded as appendiceal tumors of epithelial origin. Although there have been no unified terminologies and classifications of these diverse histopathologic features, treatment strategies for surgical treatments of appendiceal neoplasms should be decided considering histopathological subtypes and localized or disseminated tumor status.

Eun Jung Park is the lead author of this chapter.

Surgical Treatments for Appendiceal Neoplasms

Appendiceal Neuroendocrine Neoplasms

Surgical resection of appendiceal NENs is performed with the same treatment principles as those for carcinoid tumors. Although the prognosis for appendiceal NENs is favorable, the incidence of lymph node metastasis is relatively high. It is known that the incidence of lymph node metastasis is 15% in tumors <1 cm, 47% in tumors of 1–2 cm, and 86% >2 cm [3, 4]. Therefore, the surgeon should decide the extent of surgical resection according to the size, location, and histopathological grade of the tumor. Appendectomy is considered sufficient for the surgical treatment of tumors <1 cm, 1–2 cm with

H. J. Chun et al., *Gastrointestinal Cancer*, https://doi.org/10.1007/978-981-99-0815-8_29

low-risk characteristics (no lymphovascular or mesoappendiceal involvement), and well-distinguished NENs <2 cm. However, right hemicolectomy is recommended for appendiceal NENs >2 cm, or with incomplete resection or positive nodes due to increased risks of metastasis [5]. When appendiceal, NENs with peritoneal dissemination can be treated by cytoreductive surgery [6].

Appendiceal Adenocarcinoma

The principles of surgical treatment for appendiceal colonic-type adenocarcinoma are right hemicolectomy with regional lymph node dissection. Although appendiceal adenocarcinoma is not genetically different, surgical treatment is performed according to right-sided colon cancer. Goblet cell adenocarcinoma is not a typical adenocarcinoma but has mixed histological characteristics between neuroendocrine tumors and mucin-secreting gland malignant formation [7]. Appendectomy has been reported to be a curative surgical treatment for goblet cell adenocarcinoma <1 cm, not extended beyond appendiceal adventitia, and <2 mitoses/10 HPF [8]. However, right hemicolectomy is recommended to treat goblet cell adenocarcinoma in most cases. Signet-ring cell adenocarcinomas have more aggressiveness and poorer overall survival (OS) than goblet cell carcinoids and typical neuroendocrine tumors [9]. In the Surveillance, Epidemiology, and End Results (SEER) database from 1973 to 2007, the 5-year disease-specific survival rates of signet-ring cell adenocarcinoma were 27%, which was <93% of malignant carcinoid and 55% for colonic-type adenocarcinoma [10].

Appendiceal Mucinous Neoplasms and Pseudomyxoma Peritonei

In the surgical treatment of appendiceal mucinous neoplasms, there are several factors that determine the surgical strategy: histopathological grades, localized/disseminated status of appendix, and involvement of adjacent organs. Because the classifications for appendiceal mucinous neoplasms have been variable and confusing, the Peritoneal Surface Oncology Group International (PSOGI) provided a consensus for the classification and pathological reporting of appendiceal mucinous neoplasms and pseudomyxoma peritonei (PMP) [11]. It is important to categorize the histopathological grades of appendiceal mucinous neoplasm and PMP using both the PSOGI and the AJCC eighth editions: acellular mucin/mucin without epithelial cells; PMP with low-grade histologic features, grade 1, well-differentiated PMP with high-grade histologic features; grade 2, moderately differentiated PMP with signet-ring cells; and grade 3, poorly differentiated.

In localized, non-perforated low-grade appendiceal mucinous neoplasms, appendectomy is recommended. When there is appendiceal orifice involvement, cecectomy is considered to obtain a clear resection margin (Fig. 1). However, when appendiceal mucinous neoplasms are diagnosed as grade 2 or 3 histological grade, right hemicolectomy should be performed for oncologic safety.

PMP is the status of intraperitoneal accumulation of mucinous ascites and tumor nodules, which is disseminated from perforated appendiceal mucinous neoplasm (Fig. 2). Because intraperitoneal growth and mucin accumulation are asymptomatic, severe abdominal distention or intestinal obstruction can be established in patients with PMP (Fig. 3). The best standard surgical treatment for PMP from appendiceal mucinous neoplasm is regarded as cytoreductive surgery followed by hyperthermic intraperitoneal chemotherapy (HIPEC). Because mucinous tumor nodules are disseminated in intraperitoneal spaces, cytoreductive surgery aims to surgically remove visible macroscopic tumors by performing peritonectomy and resection of the involved organs (Fig. 4). HIPEC is used for the infiltration of chemotherapeutic agents into microscopic residual tumors in the peritoneal at 41–43 °C. HIPEC is performed for 30–90 min depending on the type of chemotherapeutic agent. Mitomycin-C is the most widely used chemotherapeutic drug for appendiceal and

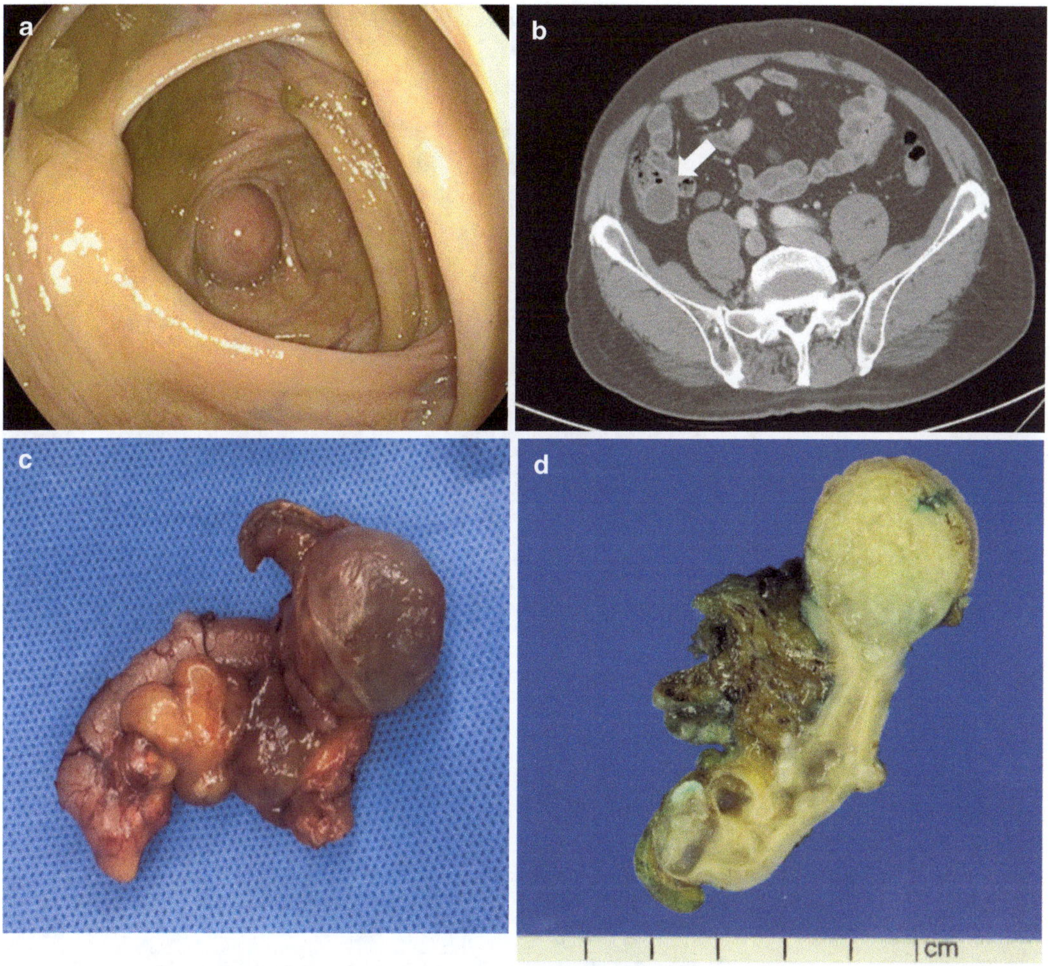

Fig. 1 Low-grade appendiceal mucinous neoplasms involving up to appendiceal orifice. (**a**) Colonoscopy findings. (**b**) Abdominopelvic computed tomography (CT). (**c**) Surgical specimen of appendix. (**d**) The cross section of appendix

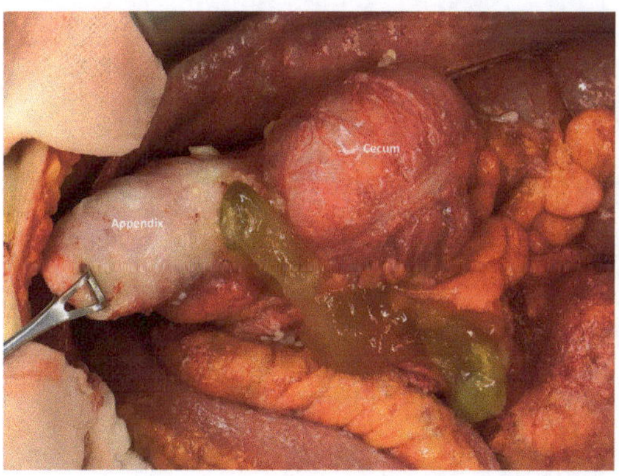

Fig. 2 Perforated appendiceal mucinous neoplasm with PMP

colorectal neoplasms for HIPEC. After unfavorable oncologic reports after PRODIGE-7 trials, the use of mitomycin-C has increased [12, 13]. The HIPEC technique consists of open (coliseum) or closed techniques (Fig. 5). In the recent study to evaluate results after cytoreductive surgery and HIPEC using mitomycin-C and cisplatin compared to cytoreductive surgery alone in patients with PMP, patients who received HIPEC had better OS than cytoreductive surgery alone [14]. Previous chemotherapy treatment, histopathological subtypes, major postoperative complications, high peritoneal cancer index, and completeness of cytoreduc-

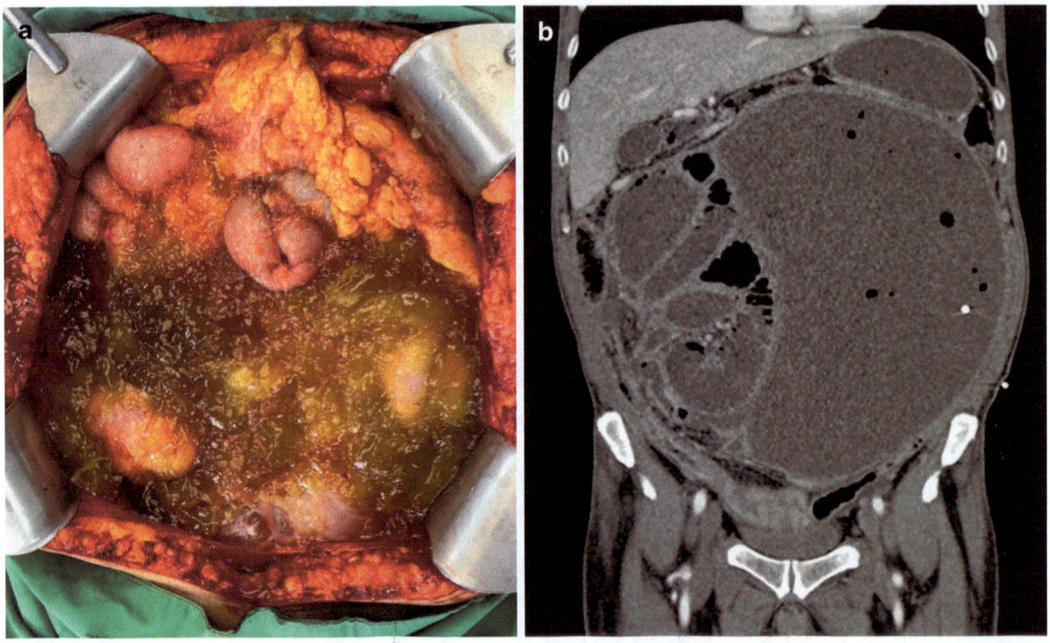

Fig. 3 (**a**) "Jelly-belly" features of PMP. (**b**) Computed tomography for distended and loculated low-grade appendiceal mucinous neoplasm

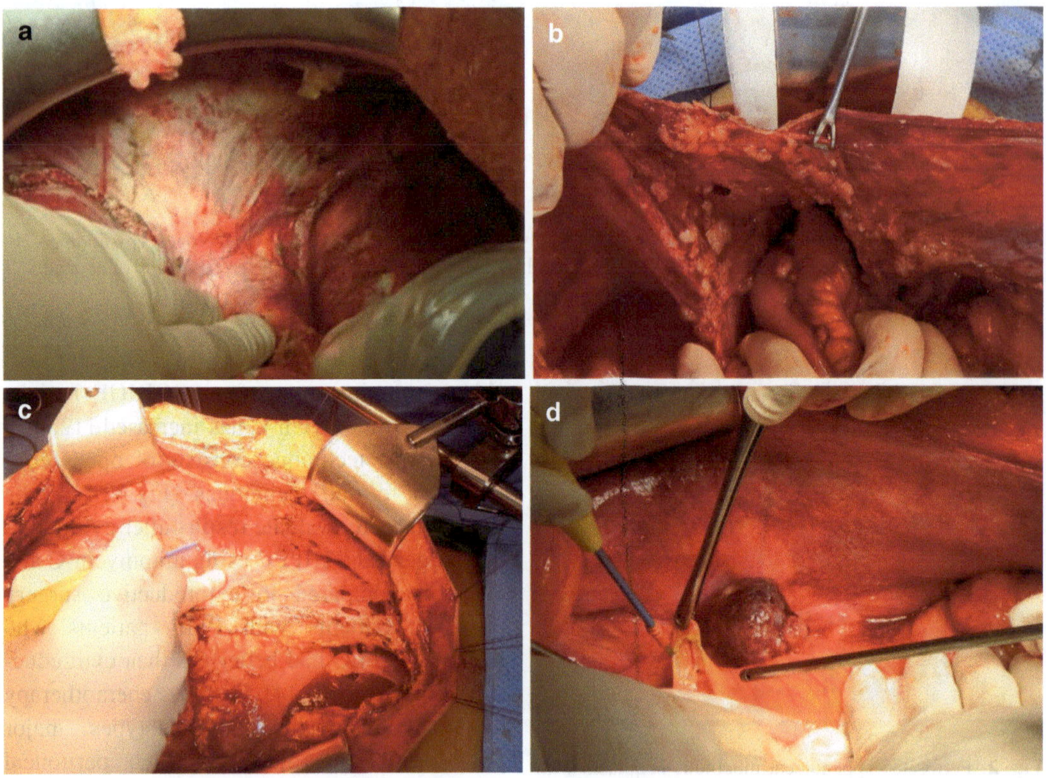

Fig. 4 Cytoreductive surgery for peritoneal metastasis. (**a**) Diaphragmatic peritonectomy. (**b**) Pelvic peritonectomy. (**c**) Parietal peritonectomy. (**d**) Excision of metastatic nodules

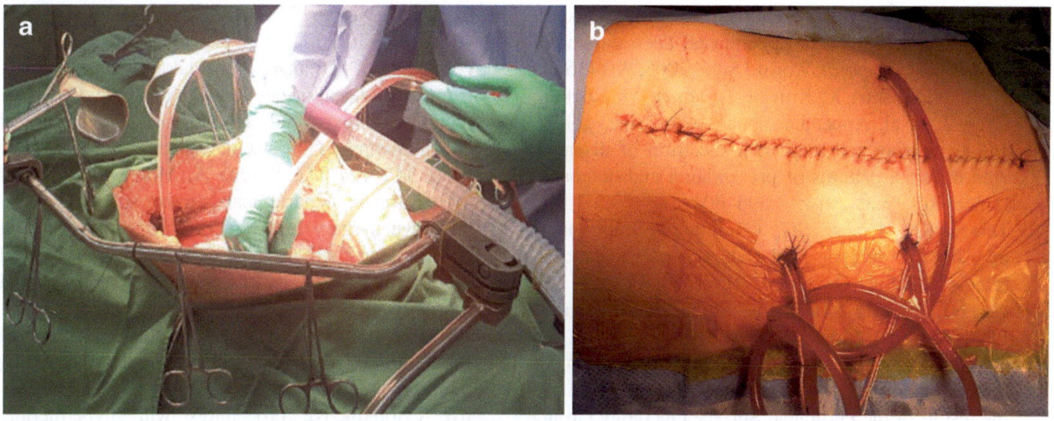

Fig. 5 HIPEC techniques. (**a**) Open (coliseum) technique. (**b**) Closed technique

tion are considered independent prognostic factors of OS after cytoreductive surgery followed by HIPEC in patients with PMP of appendiceal origins [15]. Cytoreductive surgery and HIPEC are associated with relatively high rates of morbidity and mortality, with 5–10% mortality and 30–40% major morbidity rates reported [16–19]. Therefore, proper patient selection and meticulous surgical procedures are required for successful oncologic outcomes.

Adjuvant Chemotherapy

Although there is no specific guideline, the same systemic chemotherapy regimens for appendiceal colonic-type adenocarcinoma as in colon cancer are recommended and include the use of the combination 5-fluorouracil, leucovorin, and oxaliplatin (FOLFOX). There is no role for adjuvant chemotherapy for low-grade appendiceal mucinous neoplasm. However, appendiceal mucinous neoplasm and PMP with grades 2–3 are required for adjuvant chemotherapy, as is the case for colon cancer [20].

Conclusion

Appendiceal tumors are rare and have various histopathologic and biologic features. Surgical treatments for appendiceal neoplasms should be considered based on the histopathologic subtypes, tumor size, lymph node involvement, and the extent of tumors. Cytoreductive surgery followed by HIPEC is effective for the treatment of PMP of appendiceal origin. Tailored surgical strategies are required as curative treatments and to improve survivals.

References

1. Overman MJ, Fournier K, Hu CY, Eng C, Taggart M, Royal R, et al. Improving the AJCC/TNM staging for adenocarcinomas of the appendix: the prognostic impact of histological grade. Ann Surg. 2013;257:1072–8.
2. Whitfield CG, Amin SN, Garner JP. Surgical management of primary appendiceal malignancy. Color Dis. 2012;14:1507–11.
3. Mullen JT, Savarese DM. Carcinoid tumors of the appendix: a population-based study. J Surg Oncol. 2011;104:41–4.
4. Stinner B, Kisker O, Zielke A, Rothmund M. Surgical management for carcinoid tumors of small bowel, appendix, colon, and rectum. World J Surg. 1996;20:183–8.
5. Boudreaux JP, Klimstra DS, Hassan MM, Woltering EA, Jensen RT, Goldsmith SJ, et al. The NANETS consensus guideline for the diagnosis and management of neuroendocrine tumors: well-differentiated neuroendocrine tumors of the Jejunum, Ileum, Appendix, and Cecum. Pancreas. 2010;39:753–66.
6. Elias D, David A, Sourrouille I, Honoré C, Goéré D, Dumont F, et al. Neuroendocrine carcinomas: optimal surgery of peritoneal metastases (and associated intra-abdominal metastases). Surgery. 2014;155:5–12.
7. Hoehn RS, Rieser CJ, Choudry MH, Melnitchouk N, Hechtman J, Bahary N. Current management of appendiceal neoplasms. Am Soc Clin Oncol Educ Book. 2021;41:1–15.

8. Bucher P, Gervaz P, Ris F, Oulhaci W, Egger JF, Morel P. Surgical treatment of appendiceal adenocarcinoid (goblet cell carcinoid). World J Surg. 2005;29:1436–9.
9. Shaib W, Krishna K, Kim S, Goodman M, Rock J, Chen Z, et al. Appendiceal neuroendocrine, goblet and signet-ring cell tumors: a spectrum of diseases with different patterns of presentation and outcome. Cancer Res Treat. 2016;48:596–604.
10. Turaga KK, Pappas SG, Gamblin T. Importance of histologic subtype in the staging of appendiceal tumors. Ann Surg Oncol. 2012;19:1379–85.
11. Carr NJ, Cecil TD, Mohamed F, Sobin LH, Sugarbaker PH, González-Moreno S, et al. A consensus for classification and pathologic reporting of pseudomyxoma peritonei and associated appendiceal neoplasia: the results of the Peritoneal Surface Oncology Group International (PSOGI) modified delphi process. Am J Surg Pathol. 2016;40:14–26.
12. Quénet F, Elias D, Roca L, Goéré D, Ghouti L, Pocard M, et al. Cytoreductive surgery plus hyperthermic intraperitoneal chemotherapy versus cytoreductive surgery alone for colorectal peritoneal metastases (PRODIGE 7): a multicentre, randomised, open-label, phase 3 trial. Lancet Oncol. 2021;22:256–66.
13. van de Vlasakker VCJ, Lurvink RJ, Cashin PH, Ceelen W, Deraco M, Goéré D, et al. The impact of PRODIGE 7 on the current worldwide practice of CRS-HIPEC for colorectal peritoneal metastases: a web-based survey and 2021 statement by Peritoneal Surface Oncology Group International (PSOGI). Eur J Surg Oncol. 2021.
14. Kusamura S, Barretta F, Yonemura Y, Sugarbaker PH, Moran BJ, Levine EA, et al. The role of hyperthermic intraperitoneal chemotherapy in pseudomyxoma peritonei after cytoreductive surgery. JAMA Surg. 2021;156:e206363.
15. Chua TC, Moran BJ, Sugarbaker PH, Levine EA, Glehen O, Gilly FN, et al. Early- and long-term outcome data of patients with pseudomyxoma peritonei from appendiceal origin treated by a strategy of cytoreductive surgery and hyperthermic intraperitoneal chemotherapy. J Clin Oncol. 2012;30:2449–56.
16. Chua TC, Yan TD, Saxena A, Morris DL. Should the treatment of peritoneal carcinomatosis by cytoreductive surgery and hyperthermic intraperitoneal chemotherapy still be regarded as a highly morbid procedure?: a systematic review of morbidity and mortality. Ann Surg. 2009;249:900–7.
17. Desantis M, Bernard JL, Casanova V, Cegarra-Escolano M, Benizri E, Rahili AM, et al. Morbidity, mortality, and oncological outcomes of 401 consecutive cytoreductive procedures with hyperthermic intraperitoneal chemotherapy (HIPEC). Langenbeck's Arch Surg. 2015;400:37–48.
18. Foster JM, Sleightholm R, Patel A, Shostrom V, Hall B, Neilsen B, et al. Morbidity and mortality rates following cytoreductive surgery combined with hyperthermic intraperitoneal chemotherapy compared with other high-risk surgical oncology procedures. JAMA Netw Open. 2019;2:e186847.
19. Votanopoulos KI, Newman NA, Russell G, Ihemelandu C, Shen P, Stewart JH, et al. Outcomes of Cytoreductive Surgery (CRS) with hyperthermic intraperitoneal chemotherapy (HIPEC) in patients older than 70 years; survival benefit at considerable morbidity and mortality. Ann Surg Oncol. 2013;20:3497–503.
20. Anonymous. The Chicago Consensus on peritoneal surface malignancies: management of appendiceal neoplasms. Cancer. 2020;126:2525–33.

Staging and Treatment. II-4. Palliative Chemotherapy: First-Line and Second-Line Chemotherapy Regimens

Key Points

- Unlike colorectal cancer, peritoneal metastases are more common than distant metastases in appendiceal cancer.
- The standard treatment for appendiceal cancer with peritoneal metastasis includes cytoreductive surgery and hyperthermic intraperitoneal chemotherapy, and systemic palliative chemotherapy is limited to patients who are ineligible for surgery due to disease recurrence or distant metastasis.
- To date, no optimal guidelines or recommendations for systemic chemotherapy for appendiceal cancer are available, due to the rarity of the disease itself and limited clinical studies.
- Systemic palliative chemotherapy for appendiceal cancer should be determined individually according to the histological type, severity of the disease, and general conditions of the patient.

Introduction

Appendiceal cancer is very rare and accounts for only 1% of all colorectal cancers [1, 2]. It is a heterogeneous disease with various clinical features ranging from early cancer confined to the appendix to advanced cancer with peritoneal or distant dissemination. Peritoneal dissemination is more likely than distant metastasis due to the anatomical location of the appendix and the biological characteristics of the tumor [3]. This is quite different from colorectal cancer, where peritoneal metastases account for 15% of all metastases, which is relatively rare. Distant metastases of appendiceal cancer are very rare, with only 2% of lymph node metastases and 2% of liver or lung metastases [4]. Standard treatment for appendiceal cancer with peritoneal dissemination is cytoreductive surgery and hyperthermic intraperitoneal chemotherapy (HIPEC) without preoperative systemic chemotherapy. When recurrence occurs, it occurs primarily within the peritoneal cavity and usually progresses slowly; repeated debulk or complete cytoreduction and HIPEC are reasonable.

Systemic palliative chemotherapy is reserved for patients ineligible for surgery due to recurrent disease or distant metastases. Although first- and second-line systemic chemotherapy for colorectal cancer is well established, there is no strong evidence or recommendations for systemic chemotherapy for appendiceal cancer due to low prevalence, few clinical studies, and poor therapeutic response. Therefore, systemic palliative chemotherapy for appendiceal cancer should be determined individually according to the histological type, the severity of the disease, and the general conditions of the patient. Appendiceal

Jun Lee is the lead author of this chapter.

H. J. Chun et al., *Gastrointestinal Cancer*, https://doi.org/10.1007/978-981-99-0815-8_30

cancer can be divided into four subtypes according to histological characteristics: mucinous adenocarcinoma, colonic adenocarcinoma, goblet cell carcinoma, or neuroendocrine carcinoma. Signet-ring cells may or may not be present in colonic adenocarcinoma or mucinous adenocarcinoma and therefore are not classified separately. In this chapter, we discuss palliative chemotherapy for appendiceal cancer, focusing on recently published literature.

Peritoneal Metastasis: Hyperthermic Intraperitoneal Chemotherapy

Standard treatment for appendiceal cancer with peritoneal metastases is cytoreductive surgery and hyperthermic intraperitoneal chemotherapy (HIPEC). In cytoreductive surgery, all lesions are completely removed, or, in principle, residual lesions (<2.5 mm) are as few as possible. Generally, cytoreductive surgery involves complete omentectomy, peritonectomy of the right lower quadrant, and bilateral oophorectomy, except in women of childbearing age. HIPEC is administered intraoperatively in a single dose of chemotherapeutic agents to eradicate residual microscopic cancer cells. The most used and recommended drug is mitomycin C (40 mg in 3 L), which is injected for 90 min while maintaining the inflow temperature of 40–42 °C (30 mg in the first 60 min and 10 mg in the last 30 min) [5]. Other chemotherapeutic agents, 5-fluorourcil (5-FU), oxaliplatin, and cisplatin, are also used in single or in combination (Table 1), although there are presently no studies that compare the superiority of chemotherapeutic agents. Complete cytoreductive surgery and HIPEC are the most important factors in determining a patient's prognosis and survival. Sugarbaker et al. [6] reported that the 5-year survival rate of patients with appendiceal malignancy who underwent complete cytoreduction and HIPEC is 86% (adenomucinosis by pathology) and 50% (adenomucinosis and carcinomatosis by pathology).

Another treatment option is early postoperative intraperitoneal chemotherapy, which involves inserting a subcutaneous port into the abdomen after surgery and administering an anticancer agent at normal temperature for 1–7 days. Although there have been few clinical studies, the therapeutic effect is known to be similar to that of HIPEC. Recurrence after cytoreductive surgery and HIPEC is almost confined to the peritoneal cavity and slow in growth, so repeated debulk or complete cytoreductive surgery and HIPEC are reasonable.

Table 1 First-line regimens of intraperitoneal chemotherapy for appendiceal cancer with peritoneal metastasis

Regimen	Dosing method
Mitomycin	30 mg at start, 60 min, followed by 10 mg for 30 min
	30 mg/m² for 90–120 min
Mitomycin + doxorubicin	Mitomycin at 15 mg/m² plus doxorubicin at 15 mg/m². For 90 min
Oxaliplatin	At 300 mg/m² for 30 min
Oxaliplatin +5-FU/LV	Oxaliplatin 360–460 mg/m² for 30 min 5-Fluorouracil 400 mg/m² and leucovorin 20 mg/m² + N/S 250 mL for 60 min

5-FU 5-fluorouracil; *LV* leucovorin; *iv* intravenously; *N/S* normal saline

Distant Metastasis: Palliative Systemic Chemotherapy

Evidence for the role of systemic chemotherapy in appendiceal cancer is limited, and there are no precise guidelines for chemotherapy regimens, including the first- and second-line treatments. Furthermore, appendiceal cancer is rare and heterogeneous, making it difficult to investigate the effectiveness of chemotherapy [7]. Palliative systemic chemotherapy is a treatment option for patients with appendiceal cancer who are no longer candidates for surgery due to recurrent disease or distant metastases. Although the classification varies according to the histological type of appendiceal cancer, we describe palliative chemotherapy for appendiceal cancer by subdividing tumors into epithelial cancer and neuroendocrine tumors to facilitate understanding and application.

Appendiceal Epithelial Cancer

Original epithelial cancer of the appendix consists of colonic-type adenocarcinoma and mucinous adenocarcinoma. As there is no prospective randomized trial for any epithelial-derived appendiceal cancer subtypes, no standard chemotherapy regimen has been established. Most appendiceal epithelial cancer chemotherapy regimens have been adopted and are used in chemotherapy regimens for metastatic colorectal cancer (Table 2).

5-FU-based chemotherapy is the most commonly used and reported. In 39 patients with appendiceal tumor with pseudomyxoma peritonei, combination therapy with capecitabine and mitomycin C showed a response in 15 patients (38%) and a decrease in tumor markers in more than 50% [8]. In another study, 54 patients who were not indicated for cytoreductive surgery and HIPEC received 5-FU-based chemotherapy. Thirty patients (55.6%) responded to treatment, with a complete response, partial response, or stable disease [9]. Furthermore, 20 patients were treated with FOLFOX (oxaliplatin, leucovorin, and 5-FU) chemotherapy, and a partial response occurred in 20%. With median progression-free survival (PFS) and overall survival (OS) reported at 8 and 26 months, respectively, FOLFOX chemotherapy is well tolerated and active in patients with peritoneal pseudomyxoma whose disease is considered unresectable or recurrent after cytoreductive surgery and HIPEC [10].

Table 2 First-line regimens of systemic palliative chemotherapy for appendiceal epithelial cancer

Regimen	Dosing method
FOLFOX (every 2 weeks)	Oxaliplatin 85 mg/m^2 iv over 2 h, day 1 Leucovorin 400 mg/m^2 iv over 2 h, day 1 5-FU 400 mg/m^2 bolus, iv day 1, followed by 1200 mg/m^2 days 1–2
CAPEOX (every 3 weeks)	Oxaliplatin 130 mg/m^2 iv day 1 Capecitabine 1000 mg/m^2 po twice daily for 14 days
FOLFIRI (every 2 weeks)	Irinotecan 180 mg/m^2 iv over 30–90 min, day 1 Leucovorin 400 mg/m^2 iv infusion to match duration of irinotecan, day 1 5-FU 400 mg/m^2 bolus, iv day 1, followed by 1200 mg/m^2 days 1–2
5-FU/LV (every 1 week)	Leucovorin 200 mg/m^2 iv over 2 h 5-FU 500 mg/m^2 bolus, iv 1 h after the start of leucovorin
Capecitabine (every 3 weeks)	Capecitabine 850–1250 mg/m^2 po twice daily for 14 days

5-FU 5-fluorouracil; *LV* leucovorin; *iv* intravenously

For colorectal cancer patients who can receive intensive treatment, the use of a targeted agent in systemic chemotherapy for advanced and metastatic disease is the first-line option. However, to date, there is no precise evidence or guidelines for the use of targeted agents in appendiceal cancer. Logan-Collins et al. [11] reported that mean vascular endothelial growth factor count was correlated with survival and this correlation was stronger in patients with relapse. Prospective studies on targeted agents such as epidermal growth factor inhibitor (EGF) and anti-vascular endothelial growth factor (VEGF) for inoperable, advanced, or metastatic appendiceal cancer are needed.

Existing evidence regarding the effects of chemotherapy is very limited; however, a recent Surveillance, Epidemiology, and End Results (SEER)-based study reported that the outcome of chemotherapy has improved in recent years [12]. In particular, better survival rates have been reported in patients with mucinous adenocarcinoma, colonic adenocarcinoma, and signet-ring cell carcinoma.

Appendiceal Neuroendocrine Tumor

Because appendiceal neuroendocrine tumor (APN) is usually asymptomatic and is discovered incidentally, appendectomy is the main treatment for removal. Patients with tumors >2 cm or with incomplete resection or positive nodes are risk factors for local or distant metastasis and require right hemicolectomy. Because advanced, distant metastatic APN is very rare, treatment is generally the same as that of neuroendocrine tumor of

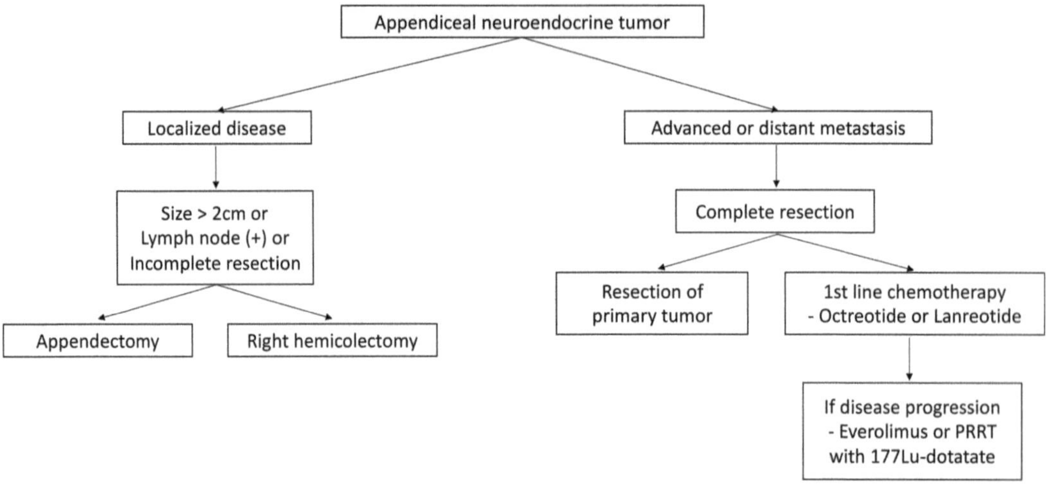

Fig. 1 Summary of the treatment algorithm for appendiceal neuroendocrine tumor. *PPRT* peptide receptor radionuclide therapy

other GI tracts. In patients with liver metastases or other limited metastases, regional therapy or cytoreductive surgery may be considered as therapeutic options [13]. However, most patients with resected metastatic disease are very likely to experience relapse eventually [14, 15].

For unresectable, metastatic appendiceal neuroendocrine carcinoma with significant tumor burden or progressive disease, octreotide LAR or lanreotide is the first-line treatment. The prospective randomized study, PROMID, compared octreotide LAR with placebo in 85 patients with metastatic neuroendocrine tumors [16]. After 6 months of treatment, stable disease was observed in 66.7% of patients in the octreotide LAR group and in 37.2% of patients in the placebo group. In addition, octreotide LAR was excellent in the median time to tumor progression (14.6 vs. 6 months). In the randomized, controlled study CLARINET, which compared lanreotide with placebo in 204 patients with enteropancreatic neuroendocrine tumor [17], lanreotide achieved a prolonged PFS (not reached vs. 18.0 months) and an estimated PFS at 24 months (65.1 vs. 33.0). If disease progression occurs after administration of octreotide LAR or lanreotide, everolimus or peptide receptor radionuclide therapy with 177Lu-dotate can be used as the second-line therapeutic option. The treatment algorithm for appendiceal neuroendocrine tumors is shown in Fig. 1.

The goblet cell tumor is a mixed tumor of adenocarcinoma of epithelial origin and neuroendocrine origin. It is characterized by the presence of intestinal-type goblet cells, accounting for approximately 14% of all appendiceal cancers [18]. Goblet cell tumors have a more aggressive behavior and a worse prognosis, so the 5-year survival rate for metastatic disease is <20% [19, 20]. In general, goblet cell tumors are more similar to colorectal adenocarcinoma than neuroendocrine tumor in clinical features, tumor behavior, and response to treatment, so colorectal adenocarcinoma treatment is adopted [21]. Therefore, systemic palliative chemotherapy for goblet cell tumors is the same as appendiceal epithelial cancer. Only in cases with no response, although evidence is lacking, somatostatin analogues or radionuclide therapy may be considered.

Conclusion

For appendiceal cancer, peritoneal dissemination is the most common, and cytoreductive surgery with HIPEC is the standard treatment. Systemic chemotherapy may be considered for inoperable, advanced disease, or distant metastases. Presently, there are very few accurate guidelines or recommendations for systemic chemotherapy of appendiceal cancer. Appendiceal epithelial cancer is generally treated by applying systemic chemotherapy for colorectal cancer and appendiceal neuroendocrine tumors by applying treatments of other gastrointestinal neuroendocrine tumors. More prospective studies are needed to confirm the effectiveness and prognosis of systemic chemotherapy for appendiceal cancer and to establish an optimal chemotherapy regimen.

References

1. Marmor S, Portschy PR, Tuttle TM, Virnig BA. The rise in appendiceal cancer incidence: 2000-2009. J Gastrointest Surg. 2015;19:743–50.
2. Siegel RL, Miller KD, Fuchs HE, Jemal A. Cancer Statistics, 2021. CA Cancer J Clin. 2021;71:7–33.
3. Carr NJ, Bibeau F, Bradley RF, Dartigues P, Feakins RM, Geisinger KR, et al. The histopathological classification, diagnosis and differential diagnosis of mucinous appendiceal neoplasms, appendiceal adenocarcinomas and pseudomyxoma peritonei. Histopathology. 2017;71:847–58.
4. González-Moreno S, Sugarbaker PH. Right hemicolectomy does not confer a survival advantage in patients with mucinous carcinoma of the appendix and peritoneal seeding. Br J Surg. 2004;91:304–11.
5. Turaga K, Levine E, Barone R, Sticca R, Petrelli N, Lambert L, et al. Consensus guidelines from The American Society of Peritoneal Surface Malignancies on standardizing the delivery of hyperthermic intraperitoneal chemotherapy (HIPEC) in colorectal cancer patients in the United States. Ann Surg Oncol. 2014;21:1501–5.
6. Sugarbaker PH, Chang D. Results of treatment of 385 patients with peritoneal surface spread of appendiceal malignancy. Ann Surg Oncol. 1999;6:727–31.
7. Asare EA, Compton CC, Hanna NN, Kosinski LA, Washington MK, Kakar S, et al. The impact of stage, grade, and mucinous histology on the efficacy of systemic chemotherapy in adenocarcinomas of the appendix: analysis of the National Cancer Data Base. Cancer. 2016;122:213–21.
8. Farquharson AL, Pranesh N, Witham G, Swindell R, Taylor MB, Renehan AG, et al. A phase II study evaluating the use of concurrent mitomycin C and capecitabine in patients with advanced unresectable pseudomyxoma peritonei. Br J Cancer. 2008;99:591–6.
9. Shapiro JF, Chase JL, Wolff RA, Lambert LA, Mansfield PF, Overman MJ, et al. Modern systemic chemotherapy in surgically unresectable neoplasms of appendiceal origin: a single-institution experience. Cancer. 2010;116:316–22.
10. Pietrantonio F, Maggi C, Fanetti G, Iacovelli R, Di Bartolomeo M, Ricchini F, et al. FOLFOX-4 chemotherapy for patients with unresectable or relapsed peritoneal pseudomyxoma. Oncologist. 2014;19:845–50.
11. Logan-Collins JM, Lowy AM, Robinson-Smith TM, Kumar S, Sussman JJ, James LE, et al. VEGF expression predicts survival in patients with peritoneal surface metastases from mucinous adenocarcinoma of the appendix and colon. Ann Surg Oncol. 2008;15:738–44.
12. Wang G, Li Q, Chen W. Chemotherapy in the treatment of different histological types of appendiceal cancers: a SEER based study. BMC Cancer. 2021;21:778.
13. Lesurtel M, Nagorney DM, Mazzaferro V, Jensen RT, Poston GJ. When should a liver resection be performed in patients with liver metastases from neuroendocrine tumours? A systematic review with practice recommendations. HPB (Oxford). 2015;17:17–22.
14. Mayo SC, de Jong MC, Pulitano C, Clary BM, Reddy SK, Gamblin TC, et al. Surgical management of hepatic neuroendocrine tumor metastasis: results from an international multi-institutional analysis. Ann Surg Oncol. 2010;17:3129–36.
15. Saxena A, Chua TC, Perera M, Chu F, Morris DL. Surgical resection of hepatic metastases from neuroendocrine neoplasms: a systematic review. Surg Oncol. 2012;21:e131–41.
16. Rinke A, Müller HH, Schade-Brittinger C, Klose KJ, Barth P, Wied M, et al. Placebo-controlled, double-blind, prospective, randomized study on the effect of octreotide LAR in the control of tumor growth in patients with metastatic neuroendocrine midgut tumors: a report from the PROMID Study Group. J Clin Oncol. 2009;27:4656–63.
17. Caplin ME, Pavel M, Ćwikła JB, Phan AT, Raderer M, Sedláčková E, et al. Lanreotide in metastatic enteropancreatic neuroendocrine tumors. N Engl J Med. 2014;371:224–33.
18. McCusker ME, Coté TR, Clegg LX, Sobin LH. Primary malignant neoplasms of the appendix: a population-based study from the surveillance, epidemiology and end-results program, 1973-1998. Cancer. 2002;94:3307–12.
19. Landry CS, Woodall C, Scoggins CR, McMasters KM, Martin RC 2nd. Analysis of 900 appendiceal carcinoid tumors for a proposed predictive staging system. Arch Surg. 2008;143:664–70. discussion 70
20. Tang LH, Shia J, Soslow RA, Dhall D, Wong WD, O'Reilly E, et al. Pathologic classification and clinical behavior of the spectrum of goblet cell carcinoid tumors of the appendix. Am J Surg Pathol. 2008;32:1429–43.
21. Rossi RE, Luong TV, Caplin ME, Thirlwell C, Meyer T, Garcia-Hernandez J, et al. Goblet cell appendiceal tumors—management dilemmas and long-term outcomes. Surg Oncol. 2015;24:47–53.

Part V

Colorectal Cancer

Epidemiology and Prevention. I-1. Epidemiology and Risk Factors

Key Points

- Colorectal cancer (CRC) was the third most diagnosed cancer in men and the second in women worldwide in 2020.
- CRC incidence and mortality rates vary markedly around the world. In Korea, CRC is the third highest among male cancers and the third highest among female cancers in 2018.
- Non-modifiable risk factors of CRC are age, male sex, ethnicity, family history, inflammatory bowel disease, genetics, and diabetes mellitus.
- Modifiable risk factors for CRC are diet, obesity, physical inactivity, smoking, and alcohol consumption.

Introduction

Colorectal cancer (CRC) is a common and lethal disease. The risk of developing CRC is influenced by both environmental and genetic factors. The epidemiology of CRC and risk factors for its development will be discussed here.

Bun Kim is the lead author of this chapter.

Epidemiology

The incidence and mortality rates of CRC vary markedly around the world (Fig. 1) [1]. Globally, CRC is the third most diagnosed cancer in men and the second in women, according to the World Health Organization (WHO) GLOBOCAN database [2]. Rates of both incidence and mortality are substantially higher in males than in females (Fig. 2). Mortality rates from CRC have progressively declined since the mid-1980s in the United States and many other western countries [3, 4]. This improvement in outcome can be attributed, at least in part, to the detection and removal of colonic polyps, the detection of CRCs at an earlier stage, and more effective primary and adjuvant treatments.

In Korea, according to the data from the Central Cancer Registry published in 2020, there were 243,837 new cancers in 2018. Of these, colorectal cancer ranked fourth with 27,909 cases among both men and women, representing 11.4% of the total [5]. CRC was more common in men, with a male-to-female ratio of 1.5:1. The number of cases was 16,686 in men, the third highest among male cancers, and 11,223 in women, the third highest among female cancers (Fig. 3). By age group, men and women in their 70s accounted for the highest proportion with 26.0%, followed by those in their 60s (25.9%) and those in their 50s (20.4%) [3]. As a result of an international comparison of the net 5-year survival rate of cancer (2010–2014), the survival rate of colon cancer and rectal cancer in

H. J. Chun et al., *Gastrointestinal Cancer*, https://doi.org/10.1007/978-981-99-0815-8_31

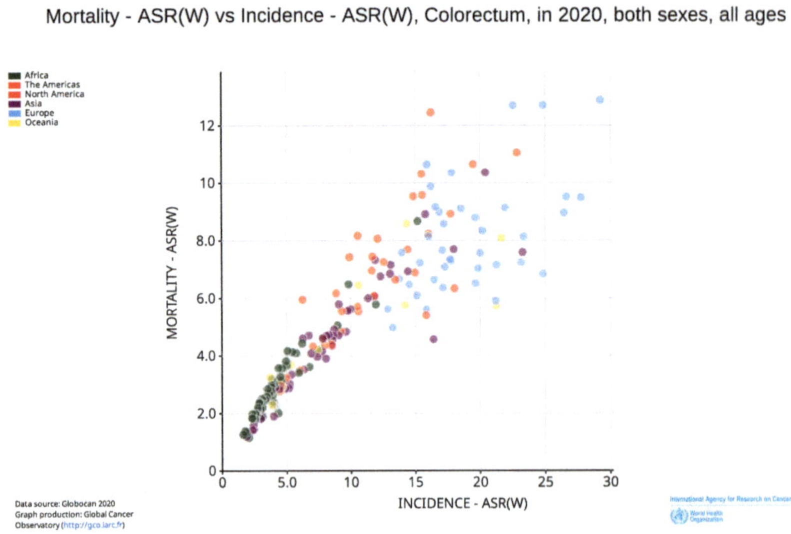

Fig. 1 Standardized incidence and mortality rates for CRC for both sexes in 2020, per 100,000 [2]

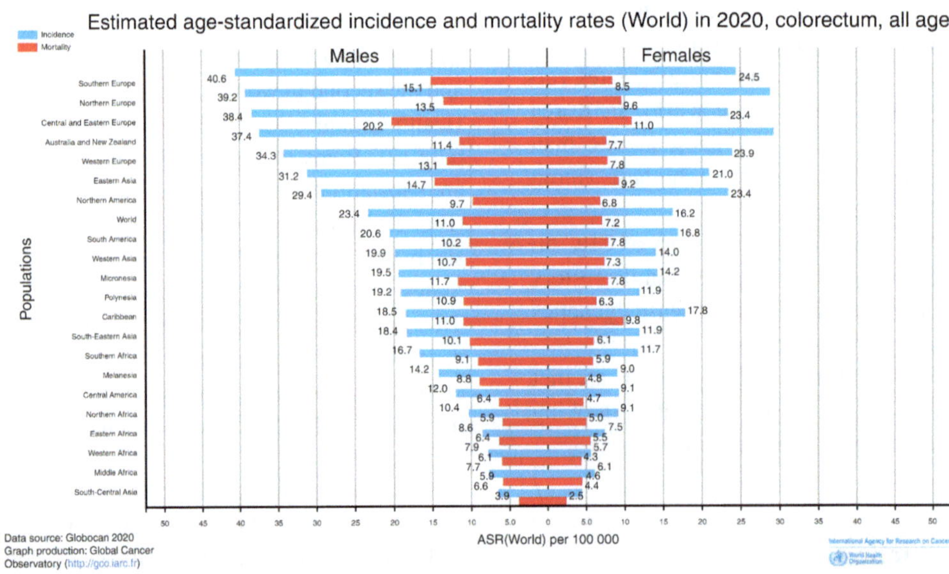

Fig. 2 Age-standardized (world) incidence and mortality rates for colorectal cancer, by sex [2]

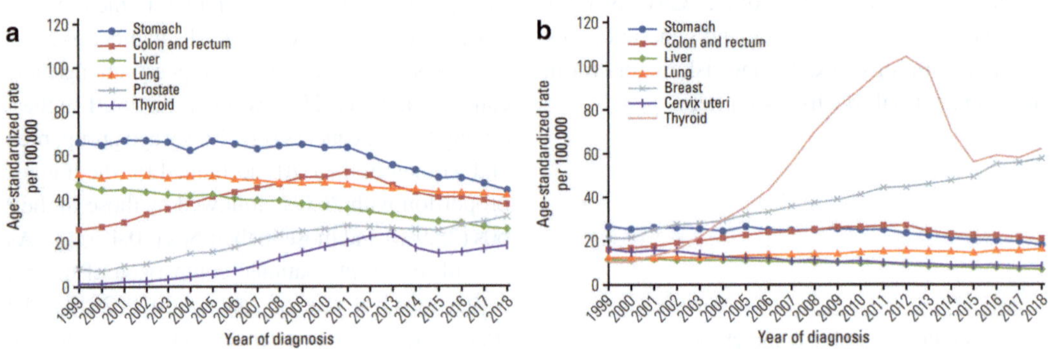

Fig. 3 Trends in age-standardized incidences of selected cancers by sex from 1999 to 2018 in Korea. (**a**) Men. (**b**) Women. Age standardization was based on Segi's world standard population [3]

Table 1 International comparison of 5-year survival rates for cancer ('2010–'2014)

Cancer type	Republic of Korea	USA	England	Japan
Colon	71.8	64.9	60.0	67.8
Rectum	71.1	64.1	62.5	64.8

Adapted from Allemani et al. [6]

Korea was higher than in the United States, United Kingdom, or Japan (Table 1) [6].

Risk Factors

Environmental and genetic factors can increase the likelihood of developing CRC. There are multiple non-modifiable factors (age, male sex, ethnicity, family history, inflammatory bowel disease, genetics, and diabetes mellitus) and modifiable factors (diet, obesity, physical inactivity, cigarette smoking, and alcohol consumption) of CRC (Table 2) [9].

Table 2 Risk factors for colorectal cancer

Non-modifiable risk factors	Modifiable risk factors
Age ≥ 50 years	Smoking
Male sex	Excessive alcohol consumption
Ethnicity	High consumption of red meats
Family history (colorectal cancer or colorectal polyp)	High consumption of processed foods
History of inflammatory bowel disease	Low intake of fruits and vegetables
Type 2 DM	Body fat and obesity
	Low physical activity

DM diabetes mellitus
Adapted from Emily et al. [7]

Age

Older age is one of the most significant factors influencing the risk of developing colorectal cancer [8, 9]. It is estimated that individuals after 65 years of age are approximately three times more likely to develop colorectal cancer compared to those aged 50–64 years and have approximately 30-fold higher risk than individuals aged 25–49 years [10].

Male Sex

According to the American Cancer Society, men have about 30% higher risk of developing colorectal cancer compared to women. Furthermore, men diagnosed with colorectal cancer have a worse prognosis and approximately 40% higher mortality compared to women [11]. The reasons for sex disparity are not fully understood; it is considered that they may be related to differences in exposure to risk factors (e.g., alcohol and tobacco), diet patterns, and sex hormone levels [11, 12].

Ethnicity

The incidence of colorectal cancer varied substantially by race. Non-Hispanic Black individuals experience one of the highest incidence rates of all racial groups. The incidence rate of colorectal cancer in non-Hispanic Black individuals is estimated to be approximately 50% higher than in Asian/Pacific Islanders and approximately 20% higher than in non-Hispanic Whites [11, 13].

Family History of Colorectal Cancer

A family history of colorectal cancer significantly increased the risk of developing colorectal cancer. This phenomenon shares both inherited genetic predisposition and lifestyle factors. The risk of CRC development is significantly higher if a relative is diagnosed before the age of 60. Moreover, a higher number of affected relatives (not only first-degree but also second- and third-degree relatives) also increase the risk of the disease [8, 9, 11].

Inflammatory Bowel Disease

Inflammatory bowel disease (IBD) is ranked as the third highest risk condition for the development of colorectal cancer, behind hereditary non-polyposis colorectal cancer (HNPCC) and familial adenomatous polyposis (FAP). Due to the fact that chronic inflammation promotes tumor growth and progression, individuals with IBD have about two to six times higher risk of developing CRC in comparison to healthy individuals. The risk of CRC increases with the duration of IBD and the anatomic extent and severity of the disease [8, 14, 15].

Genetics

It is estimated that 2–8% of colorectal cancer cases arise as a result of inherited syndromes. HNPCC is an autosomal dominant disease caused by mutations in genes known as mismatch repair errors. Patients with HNPCC have about 20% risk of developing CRC by age 50 and about 80% risk of developing CRC by age 85 [10, 16].

FAP is caused by defects in the adenomatous polyposis coli (*APC*) gene. *APC* is classified as a tumor suppressor gene. Individuals with FAP start to develop hundreds or even thousands of colon polyps in their mid-teens, and, with high probability, most of these colon polyps will evolve into cancer. It is assumed that almost all patients with the earlier unrecognized and untreated FAP syndrome will be diagnosed with colorectal cancer before the age of 35–40.

The increased risk of CRC development is also associated with the appearance of Peutz-Jeghers syndrome, juvenile polyposis syndrome, *PTEN* hamartoma tumor syndrome, and *MUTYH*-associated polyposis.

Diabetes Mellitus

Epidemiological data indicate that diabetes is an independent risk factor for various gastrointestinal cancers, including CRC [17, 18]. Individuals with type 2 diabetes have approximately two to three times greater risk of developing CRC compared to the nondiabetic population [19, 20]. The development of CRC is believed to be related to an increase in insulin concentration and inflammation associated with the disease [17, 21].

Diet High in Red and Processed Meat

Studies have shown that regular consumption of processed and red meat is an important risk factor for the development of CRC [10, 22]. The risk of CRC is estimated to increase by approximately 17% for each 100 g of red meat and by approximately 18% for each 50 g of processed meat eaten daily [23–25]. The exact mechanism by which consumption of red and processed meat may contribute to the development of CRC is still under investigation. Several factors that are believed to influence the occurrence of cancer are heterocyclic amines (HACs), polycyclic aromatic hydrocarbons (PAHs), and N-nitroso compounds (NOCs), which are harmful substances that can be produced during high-temperature or open-fire cooking of meat (e.g., panfrying, grilling, and roasting) [26, 27]. The other factor that is believed to contribute to the malignant transformation of colon cells is heme, an iron-containing porphyrin present in large amounts in red meat [22, 25, 28]. It should also be emphasized that consumption of high-fat, processed, and red meat contributes to obesity, insulin resistance, and increased bile acid secretion, which acts as an aggressive surfactant for the mucosa and increases the risk of developing CRC.

Diet Low in Fruits and Vegetables

Fruits and vegetables are great sources of fiber, which is known as a protective factor against CRC. In addition to fiber intake, the consumption of fruits and vegetables provides a large number of bioactive compounds, such as vitamins, minerals, folate, plant sterols, and protease inhibitors. Many of these compounds exhibit potent antioxidant and anti-inflammatory properties, which could inhibit DNA and cellular damage. The results of several studies demonstrated that a high intake of fruits and vegetables may be associated with a lower development of CRC risk [11, 22].

Obesity

A condition of abnormal or excessive fat accumulation is a convincing risk factor for the development of CRC. Overweight/obese men and women have a 50% and 20% higher risk of developing colorectal cancer compared to people of normal weight, respectively. It is estimated that the overall risk of CRC increases by 3% for every 5 kg of weight gain [29, 30]. The mechanisms underlying the induction of carcinogenesis in overweight/obese people are not fully understood. One possible mechanism was that abnormal or excessive fat accumulation causes alternations in adipose tissue hormone and cytokine secretions. Adipose tissue from overweight/obese people releases more factors (e.g., leptin, resistin, TNF-alpha, IL-1, IL-6, IL-7, and IL-8), which are known to exhibit mitogenic effects on epithelial cells, inhibit cell apoptosis, promote oxidative stress, suppress immune response, and reduce IGF-1 axis activity and have been associated with cancer development and progression [22, 28].

Physical Inactivity

Physically inactive people are estimated to have up to 50% higher risk of developing colorectal cancer compared to those who are most physically active [30]. Regular physical exercises have been shown to improve immune system function, reduce inflammation, reduce stress, optimize the metabolic rate, help regulate hormone levels, and prevent obesity and, as a result, may help protect against cancer development.

Cigarette Smoking

Individuals who smoke cigarettes have to two- to threefold higher risk of developing CRC than nonsmokers, and the risk increases with dose and duration of exposure [31]. Furthermore, cigarette smoking is considered to be attributed to up to 12% of colorectal cancer deaths [32]. Tobacco smoke contains a mixture of a thousand chemicals, and of the 60 are well-established carcinogens (e.g., N-nitrosamines, polycyclic aromatic hydrocarbons, aromatic amines, aldehydes, and metals) that are known to damage DNA.

Alcohol Consumption

Consumption of two to three drinks per day is estimated to increase the risk of CRC by approximately 20%, while the consumption of more than three alcoholic beverages increases this risk by approximately 40% [10, 11]. The various mechanisms involved include the production of reactive oxygen species and nitrogen species (during the oxidative metabolism of ethanol), production of mutagenic acetaldehyde (the first metabolite of ethanol), depletion of S-adenosylmethionine (epigenetic alternations), inactivation of tumor suppressor genes, hormonal imbalance, reduction in folate concentration, and impairment of retinoic acid metabolism [12, 33].

Conclusion

As mentioned above, there are several known epidemiological risk factors of CRC. More clinical studies are needed to understand the mechanisms of carcinogenesis; the impact of lifestyle; behavioral, environmental, and genetic factors; or the synergistic action of the different aspects to increase the efficacy of preventive/treatment and survival for patients with CRC.

References

1. Sawicki T, Ruszkowska M, Danielewicz A, Niedźwiedzka E, Arłukowicz T, Przybyłowicz KE. A review of colorectal cancer in terms of epidemiology, risk factors, development, symptoms and diagnosis. Cancers (Basel). 2021;13(9):2025.

2. Globocan. 2020. https://gco.iarc.fr/today/data/factsheets/cancers/10_8_9-Colorectum-fact-sheet.pdf.
3. Islami F, Ward EM, Sung H, Cronin KA, Tangka FKL, Sherman RL, et al. Annual report to the nation on the status of cancer, part 1: national cancer statistics. J Natl Cancer Inst. 2021;113(12):1648–69.
4. Siegel RL, Miller KD, Fuchs HE, Jemal A. Cancer statistics, 2021. CA Cancer J Clin. 2021;71:7–33.
5. Hong S, Won YJ, Lee JJ, Jung KW, Kong HJ, Im JS, et al. Cancer statistics in Korea: incidence, mortality, survival, and prevalence in 2018. Cancer Res Treat. 2021;53(2):301–15.
6. Allemani C, Matsuda T, Di Carlo V, Harewood R, Matz M, Nikšić M, et al. Global surveillance of trends in cancer survival 2000-14 (CONCORD-3): analysis of individual records for 37,513,025 patients diagnosed with one of 18 cancers from 322 population-based registries in 71 countries. Lancet. 2018;391(10125):1023–75.
7. Emily M, Ambizas. The pharmacist's role in colorectal cancer screening. US Pharm. 2020;45(4):5–8.
8. Amersi F, Agustin M, Ko CY. Colorectal cancer: epidemiology; risk factors, and health services. Clin Colon Rectal Surg. 2005;18:133–40.
9. Thelin C, Sikka S. Epidemiology of colorectal cancer—incidence, lifetime risk factors statistics and temporal trends. London, UK: Intech; 2015.
10. Rawla P, Sunkara T, Barsouk A. Epidemiology of colorectal cancer: incidence, mortality; survival, and risk factors. Gastroenterol Rev. 2019;14(2):89–103.
11. American Cancer Society. Colorectal cancer facts & figures 2017–2019. Atlanta, GA: American Cancer Society; 2017.
12. Keum N, Giovannucci E. Global burden of colorectal cancer: emerging trends, risk factors and prevention strategies. Nat Rev Gastroenterol Hepatol. 2019;16(12):713–32.
13. Ellis L, Abrahão R, McKinley M, Yang J, Somsouk M, Marchand LL, et al. Colorectal cancer incidence trends by age, stage, and racial/ethnic group in California, 1990-2014. Cancer Epidemiol Biomark Prev. 2018;27:1011–8.
14. Gandomani H, Yousefi S, Aghajani M, Mohammadian-Hafshejani A, Tarazoj A, Pouyesh V, et al. Colorectal cancer in the world: incidence, mortality and risk factors. Biomed Res Ther. 2017;4(10):1656–75.
15. Keller DS, Windsor A, Cohen R, Chand M. Colorectal cancer in inflammatory bowel disease: review of the evidence. Tech Coloproctol. 2019;23(1):3–13.
16. Win AK, Macinnis RJ, Hopper JL, Jenkins MA. Risk prediction model for colorectal cancer: a review. Cancer Epidemiol Biomark Prev. 2012;21(3):398–410.
17. Ma Y, Yang W, Song M, Smith-Warner SA, Yang J, Li Y, et al. Type 2 diabetes and risk of colorectal cancer in two large U.S. prospective cohorts. Br J Cancer. 2018;119(11):1436–42.
18. Pang Y, Kartsonaki C, Guo Y, Chen Y, Yang L, Bian Z, et al. Diabetes, plasma glucose and incidence of colorectal cancer in Chinese adults: a prospective study of 0.5 million people. J Epidemiol Community Health. 2018;72(10):919–25.
19. Yao C, Nash GF, Hickish T. Management of colorectal cancer and diabetes. J R Soc Med. 2014;107(3):103–9.
20. Peeters PJ, Bazelier MT, Leufkens HG, de Vries F, De Bruin ML. The risk of colorectal cancer in patients with type 2 diabetes: associations with treatment stage and obesity. Diabetes Care. 2015;38(3):495–502.
21. Brzacki V, Nagorni A, Kallistratos M, Manolis A, Lovic D. Diabetes mellitus: a clinical condition associated with metabolic syndrome and colorectal cancer risk. Curr Pharmacol Rep. 2019;5:205–9.
22. World Cancer Research Fund/American Institute for Cancer Research. Continuous Update Project Expert Report 2018. Diet, Nutrition, Physical Activity and Colorectal Cancer. https://www.wcrf.org/dietandcancer.
23. Chan DS, Lau R, Aune D, Vieira R, Greenwood DC, Kampman E, et al. Red and processed meat and colorectal cancer incidence: meta-analysis of prospective studies. PLoS One. 2011;6(6):e20456.
24. Aykan NF. Red meat and colorectal cancer. Oncol Rev. 2015;9(1):288.
25. Aran V, Victorino AP, Thuler LC, Ferreira CG. Colorectal cancer: epidemiology, disease mechanisms and interventions to reduce onset and mortality. Clin Colorectal Cancer. 2016;15(3):195–203.
26. Cascella M, Bimonte S, Barbieri A, Del Vecchio V, Caliendo D, Schiavone V, et al. Dissecting the mechanisms and molecules underlying the potential carcinogenicity of red and processed meat in colorectal cancer (CRC): an overview on the current state of knowledge. Infect Agents Cancer. 2018;13:3.
27. Hur SJ, Yohan Y, Jo C, Jeong JL, Lee KT. Effect of dietary red meat on colorectal cancer risk-a review. Compr Rev Food Sci Food Saf. 2019;18(6):1812–24.
28. Murphy N, Moreno V, Hughes DJ, Vodicka L, Vodicka P, Aglago EK, et al. Lifestyle and dietary environmental factors in colorectal cancer susceptibility. Mol Asp Med. 2019;69:2–9.
29. Ferlay J, Ervik M, Lam F, Colombet M, Mery L, Piñeros M, et al. Global cancer observatory: cancer today. Lyon, France: International Agency for Research on Cancer. https://gco.iarc.fr/today.
30. Fidler MM, Soerjomataram I, Bray F. A global view on cancer incidence and national levels of the Human Development Index. Int J Cancer. 2016;139(1):2436–46.

31. Giovannucci E. An updated review of the epidemiological evidence that cigarette smoking increases risk of colorectal cancer. Cancer Epidemiol Biomark Prev. 2001;10(7):725–31.
32. Wong MCS, Huang J, Lok V, Wang J, Fung F, Ding H, et al. Differences in incidence and mortality trends of colorectal cancer worldwide based on sex, age, and anatomic location. Clin Gastroenterol Hepatol. 2021;19(5):955–66.
33. Rossi M, Jahanzaib Anwar M, Usman A, Keshavarzian A, Bishehsari F. Colorectal cancer and alcohol consumption-populations to molecules. Cancers. 2018;10(2):38.

Epidemiology and Prevention. I-2. Prevention: Risk Reduction (Primary Prevention) and Screening (Secondary Prevention)

Key Points

- To reduce colorectal cancer risk, healthy dietary habits (characterized by high intake of fruits, vegetables, whole grains, nuts and legumes, fish or other seafood, and low-fat milk and other dairy products), maintenance of healthy body weight, physical activity, reducing alcohol consumption, and smoking cessation are recommended.
- The long-term use of aspirin can be considered in select individuals (based on age, cardiovascular risk, bleeding risk, and Lynch syndrome) for the prevention of colorectal cancer.
- Stool-based tests (FIT, gFOBT) and colonoscopy are primarily recommended for the screening of colorectal cancer in adults with average risk.
- A more intensive screening program is suggested for high-risk adults (i.e., a personal history or family history of colorectal cancer, hereditary colorectal cancer syndrome).

Introduction

Colorectal cancer (CRC) is the third most common cancer worldwide. The incidence of CRC tends to increase with societal and economic development and to stabilize or decrease in highly developed countries with higher rates compared to other countries [1]. This phenomenon is probably attributable to the changing risk factors (e.g., dietary patterns, physical inactivity, visceral fat, alcohol intake, and smoking) and increased CRC screening programs [2]. Furthermore, the progression of carcinogenesis is divided into the stage of initiation, promotion, and progression [3]. In most cases of colorectal carcinogenesis, genetic and epigenetic alterations are involved in each step originating from a benign precursor lesion, defined as a polyp [4]. A classic pathway, the sequence of adenoma-carcinoma (85–90% of sporadic CRC) [5, 6], the serrated pathway (10–15% of sporadic CRC) [7, 8], and the inflammatory pathway (<2% of all CRC) [9, 10] are three distinct pathways of colorectal carcinogenesis. Therefore, primary prevention of CRC should focus on modification

Ji Soo Park is the lead author of this chapter.

H. J. Chun et al., *Gastrointestinal Cancer*, https://doi.org/10.1007/978-981-99-0815-8_32

of the modifiable lifestyle and nutritional risk factors (approximately 47% of CRC in the United States of America and 45% in the United Kingdom are likely attributable to modifiable risk factors [11]) and chemoprevention of known mechanisms of colorectal carcinogenesis. Furthermore, the optimal timing and method of CRC screening could contribute to the secondary prevention of CRC.

Risk Reduction (Primary Prevention)

Healthy Dietary Patterns

In previous studies on dietary patterns and CRC risk, a "healthy" pattern (characterized by high intake of fruits, vegetables, whole grains, nuts and legumes, fish or other seafood, and low-fat milk and other dairy products) and an "unhealthy" pattern (characterized by high intake of red and processed meat, sugar-sweetened beverages, refined grains, desserts, and potatoes) have been consistently observed [12]. The overall CRC risk increases by 12% for each 100 g/day of red and processed meat intake (95% confidence interval (CI), 4–21%) and 7% for each 10 g/day of ethanol intake in alcoholic drink (95% CI, 5–9%) and decreases by 17% for each 90 g/day of dairy product intake (95% CI, 11–21%) and by 13% for each 400 g/day of dairy products intake (95% CI, 10–17%) [13]. Especially, in 2015, the International Agency for Research on Cancer (IARC) expert panel stipulated processed meat as a group 1 carcinogen and red meat as a group 2A carcinogen based on evidence of increased risk of CRC [14, 15]. The World Cancer Research Fund (WCRF)/American Institute for Cancer Research (AICR) report concluded that processed meat intake increased the risk of CRC with convincing evidence [11]. The Dietary Guidelines published by the United States Department of Health and Human Services (HHS) and the United States Department of Agriculture (USDA) recommended low red and processed meat and salted food patterns [16], and the American Cancer Society (ACS) also recommended a healthy eating pattern that included foods high in a variety of vegetables, fruits, and whole grains and to limit red and processed meats, sugar-sweetened beverages, or highly processed foods and refined grain products [17].

Control Obesity and Physical Inactivity

Excess adiposity, which is commonly measured by body mass index (BMI) and waist circumference (WC), is established as a distinctive risk factor for CRC [11]. Among the abdominal fat compartments, visceral adipose tissue (VAT) secretes more pro-inflammatory adipokines and less adiponectin [18] and is infiltrated with more immune cells [19], compared to subcutaneous adipose tissue (SAT). VAT-related inflammatory conditions, insulin resistance, and subsequent hyperinsulinemia are suspected to promote colorectal carcinogenesis [20]. Although the cancer preventive effect of intentional weight loss by caloric or dietary restriction is still limited in humans, the effect of the absence of excess body fat is sufficiently supported by previous research [21]. Furthermore, physical activity is associated with a lower risk of colon cancer [22], possibly due to its beneficial effect on gut motility, inflammation, metabolic hormones, and the immune system [23]. The ACS recommended that adults perform 150–300 min of moderate-intensity physical activity (3–5.9 metabolic equivalents of task [MET]), or 75–150 min of vigorous-intensity physical activity (≥6 MET), or an equivalent combination (achieving or exceeding the upper limit of 300 min is optimal) per week [17]. Therefore, achieving and maintaining a healthy body weight and physical activeness are recommended for CRC prevention [2, 11, 17].

Reducing Alcohol Consumption and Smoking Cessation

Ethanol in alcoholic beverages is a well-established risk factor for many kinds of cancer. In 1988, the IARC expert working group first classified alcohol consumption as carcinogenic to humans, based on the causality of carcinogenesis in oral cavity and pharynx, esophagus, liver, and larynx [24]. Subsequently, different studies confirmed the group 1 carcinogenicity of alcohol consumption and specified "ethanol in alcoholic beverages" as carcinogenic, with sufficient evidence of causality also for CRC risk [25–27]. The WCRF/AICR defined consumption of alcohol drinks as a convincing cause of CRC, based on the evidence of intake above 30 g of ethanol per day (two drinks per day) [11]. The ACS recommended that "it is best not to drink alcohol" and to limit alcohol consumption to no more than 1 drink per day for women and two drinks per day for men [17]. One type of alcoholic beverage is not less risky for the development of cancer than others [17].

Cigarette smoking is another well-established carcinogen for humans [27]. In previous studies, CRC risk increased with pack-years (relative risk [RR] for 30 pack-years: 1.26, 95% CI 1.17–1.36) [28] and was especially associated with elevated risk of proximal colon cancer (RR 1.19, 95% CI 1.05–1.34), rectal cancer (RR 1.27, 95% CI 1.14–1.42) [29], and MSI-high, CIMP-high, and *BRAF*-mutant subtypes [30]. Considering its carcinogenicity and harmful effects on the cardiovascular, respiratory, and immune systems, smoking cessation should be strongly recommended [31].

Chemoprevention

Aspirin, a nonsteroidal anti-inflammatory drug, is the most extensively studied drug for the prevention of CRC. Previous large, randomized trials and cohort studies have shown that daily use of aspirin was associated with a reduced risk of general cancers, especially CRC [32, 33]. In the Women's Health Study, long-term use of alternative day low-dose aspirin (100 mg) was associated with a reduction in CRC risk after 10 years, with a posttrial reduction of 42% (HR 0.58, 95% CI 0.42–0.80) of CRC [34, 35], probably because aspirin could prevent the early stage of colorectal carcinogenesis [2]. However, the optimal dose and duration of aspirin treatment for the prevention of CRC remains inconclusive. Furthermore, recent large randomized clinical trials evaluating aspirin failed to show its intrinsic efficacy in primary prevention of cardiovascular disease and improvement in survival improvement and even identified an increased risk of major bleeding [36–39], which made the preventive use of aspirin more difficult. Present guidelines recommend low-dose aspirin in people aged 50–69 years with a cardiovascular disease risk of $\geq$10% over the next 10 years, who do not have an increased risk of bleeding, and who are willing to take aspirin for at least 10 years to reduce the risk of CRC [40]. In contrast, the chemopreventive role of aspirin receives more attention in patients with hereditary nonpolyposis colorectal cancer syndrome (Lynch syndrome). In the CaPP2 study, daily intake of 600 mg of aspirin was associated with a reduced risk of CRC among participants with Lynch syndrome (HR 0.65, 95% CI 0.43–0.97), especially in those who achieved a minimum of 2 years of treatment (HR 0.58, 95% CI 0.39–0.87) [41]. Dose optimization is also expected in the ongoing CaPP3 study.

Screening (Secondary Prevention)

The objectives of CRC screening are to remove adenomas and sessile serrated lesions before they become carcinoma and to detect early-stage CRC to improve treatment outcome [40]. In general, CRC screening guidelines are provided for the following "average-risk" adults: individuals without a personal history or family history of CRC or colorectal adenoma, a personal history of inflammatory bowel disease, a confirmed or suspected hereditary CRC syndrome, or a personal history of receiving radiation therapy to the abdomen or pelvic area [42].

The ACS, the American College of Gastroenterology (ACG), and the United States Preventive Services Task Force (USPSTF) recommend screening for CRC in all adults aged 45–49 years (recommendation B) as well as the adults aged 50–75 years (recommendation A) [40, 43, 44]. They suggest screening for CRC in adults aged 76–85 years should be selectively offered by the clinicians' decision based on patient preference, life expectancy, health status, and prior screening history [40, 43, 44].

Stool-Based Tests

The fecal immunochemical test (FIT) or high-sensitivity, guaiac-based fecal occult blood test (gFOBT) can be recommended annually, and positive results on stool-based screening tests require following colonoscopy [31, 40, 43, 44]. FITs use antibodies that selectively detect the globin component of human hemoglobin [43]. Furthermore, the multitarget stool DNA test (mt-sDNA test) combines an immunochemical assay for hemoglobin; aberrantly methylated *BMP3, NDRG,* and *NDRG4*; mutated *K-Ras*; and *β-Actin*, which can be tested every 3 years.

Direct Visualization Tests

Colonoscopy is one of the most commonly used CRC screening modalities. Although there is a risk of overdetection and removal of small polyps with a low probability of progressing to cancer and its complications, including perforation and bleeding, previous studies have confirmed the efficacy of colonoscopy screening in lowering the risk of CRC incidence and mortality [45, 46]. If adenomatous polyps, serrated sessile polyps, traditional serrated adenoma, or large hyperplastic polyps (≥1 cm) are found at colonoscopy, proper management and short-term follow-up tests are recommended [31]. Otherwise, colonoscopy screening can be repeated every 10 years [31, 40, 43, 44]. Computed tomography (CT) colonography and flexible sigmoidoscopy can be selected for individuals in some setting, which will be repeated every 5 years. In addition, if alarm symptoms such as iron deficiency anemia, rectal bleeding, or a change in bowel habit are detected even in individuals <45 years of age, prompt evaluation using colonoscopy or flexible sigmoidoscopy should be conducted [31].

The Korean Guideline for CRC Screening

In 2015, a multi-society expert committee for the revision of the national Korean cancer screening guidelines published a revised CRC screening guideline. They recommended (1) an annual or biannual FIT in asymptomatic patients, beginning at 45 years of age and continuing until 80 years (recommendation B); (2) the lack of evidence for the risks or benefits of FIT in adults older than 80 years (recommendation I); (3) selective use of colonoscopy for colorectal cancer screening, taking into account individual preferences and the risk of colorectal cancer (recommendation C); (4) the lack of evidence for the risks or benefits of double-contrast barium enema for colorectal cancer screening in asymptomatic adults (recommendation I); and (5) the lack of evidence for the risks or benefits of computed tomographic colonography for colorectal cancer screening in asymptomatic adults (recommendation I) [47]. Nonetheless, the National Cancer Screening Program of Korea still provides annual FIT for adults 50 years of age or older and offers subsequent colonoscopy only for those with a positive FIT result.

Special Consideration for Individuals with an Increased Risk of CRC

The ACG suggests initiating CRC screening with a colonoscopy at age 40 or 10 years before the youngest affected relative (whichever earlier), for individuals with CRC or advanced polyp in 1 first-degree relative (FDR) at age <60 years, or CRC or advanced polyp in ≥2 FDR at any age with 5-year interval [31, 40]. For an individual with a personal history of inflammatory bowel disease, colonoscopy screening is recommended initiating 8 years after the onset of symptoms [31]. If an individual has a known genetic mutation related to hereditary CRC syndrome (i.e., Lynch syndrome, familial adenomatous polyposis [FAP], MUTYH-associated polyposis, Peutz-Jeghers syndrome, juvenile polyposis syndrome, serrated polyposis syndrome, Cowden syndrome,

PTEN hamartoma tumor syndrome, or Li-Fraumeni syndrome), early-initiated and short-interval colonoscopy screening should be recommended [48].

Conclusion

Some pathological mechanisms of CRC carcinogenesis can be prevented by lifestyle modification, while screening and appropriate management of colon adenoma and early-stage CRC confer a second preventive effect of CRC. A more personalized approach and clinical implementation of CRC prevention are needed.

References

1. Arnold M, Sierra MS, Laversanne M, Soerjomataram I, Jemal A, Bray F. Global patterns and trends in colorectal cancer incidence and mortality. Gut. 2017;66:683–91.
2. Keum N, Giovannucci E. Global burden of colorectal cancer: emerging trends, risk factors and prevention strategies. Nat Rev Gastroenterol Hepatol. 2019;16:713–32.
3. Pitot HC. The molecular biology of carcinogenesis. Cancer. 1993;72:962–70.
4. Conteduca V, Sansonno D, Russi S, Dammacco F. Precancerous colorectal lesions (review). Int J Oncol. 2013;43:973–84.
5. Fearon ER, Vogelstein B. A genetic model for colorectal tumorigenesis. Cell. 1990;61:759–67.
6. Vogelstein B, Fearon ER, Hamilton SR, Kern SE, Preisinger AC, Leppert M, et al. Genetic alterations during colorectal-tumor development. N Engl J Med. 1988;319:525–32.
7. Leggett B, Whitehall V. Role of the serrated pathway in colorectal cancer pathogenesis. Gastroenterology. 2010;138:2088–100.
8. Kedrin D, Gala MK. Genetics of the serrated pathway to colorectal cancer. Clin Transl Gastroenterol. 2015;6:e84.
9. Itzkowitz SH, Yio X. Inflammation and cancer IV. Colorectal cancer in inflammatory bowel disease: the role of inflammation. Am J Physiol Gastrointest Liver Physiol. 2004;287:G7–G17.
10. Jess T, Rungoe C, Peyrin-Biroulet L. Risk of colorectal cancer in patients with ulcerative colitis: a meta-analysis of population-based cohort studies. Clin Gastroenterol Hepatol. 2012;10:639–45.
11. WCRF/AICR. Continuous update project expert report 2018. Diet, nutrition, physical activity and colorectal cancer. World Cancer Research Fund International; 2018.
12. Tabung FK, Brown LS, Fung TT. Dietary patterns and colorectal cancer risk: a review of 17 years of evidence (2000-2016). Curr Colorectal Cancer Rep. 2017;13:440–54.
13. Vieira AR, Abar L, Chan DSM, Vingeliene S, Polemiti E, Stevens C, et al. Foods and beverages and colorectal cancer risk: a systematic review and meta-analysis of cohort studies, an update of the evidence of the WCRF-AICR continuous update project. Ann Oncol. 2017;28:1788–802.
14. Bouvard V, Loomis D, Guyton KZ, Grosse Y, Ghissassi FE, Benbrahim-Tallaa L, et al. Carcinogenicity of consumption of red and processed meat. Lancet Oncol. 2015;16:1599–600.
15. IARC. Red meat and processed meat. IARC monographs on the evaluation of carcinogenic risks to humans. 2018;114:1–511.
16. DGA Committee. Scientific report of the 2020 Dietary Guidelines Advisory Committee: advisory report to the Secretary of Agriculture and the Secretary of Health and Human Services. https://www.dietaryguidelines.gov/2020-advisory-committee-report. Accessed 7 Nov 2021.
17. Rock CL, Thomson C, Gansler T, Gapstur SM, McCullough ML, Patel AV, et al. American Cancer Society guideline for diet and physical activity for cancer prevention. CA Cancer J Clin. 2020;70:245–71.
18. Samaras K, Botelho NK, Chisholm DJ, Lord RV. Subcutaneous and visceral adipose tissue gene expression of serum adipokines that predict type 2 diabetes. Obesity (Silver Spring). 2010;18:884–9.
19. Bruun JM, Lihn AS, Pedersen SB, Richelsen B. Monocyte chemoattractant protein-1 release is higher in visceral than subcutaneous human adipose tissue (AT): implication of macrophages resident in the AT. J Clin Endocrinol Metab. 2005;90:2282–9.
20. Calle EE, Kaaks R. Overweight, obesity and cancer: epidemiological evidence and proposed mechanisms. Nat Rev Cancer. 2004;4:579–91.
21. Lauby-Secretan B, Scoccianti C, Loomis D, Grosse Y, Bianchini F, Straif K, et al. Body fatness and cancer—viewpoint of the IARC Working Group. N Engl J Med. 2016;375:794–8.
22. Rezende LFM, Sa TH, Markozannes G, Rey-Lopez JP, Lee IM, Tsilidis KK, et al. Physical activity and cancer: an umbrella review of the literature including 22 major anatomical sites and 770 000 cancer cases. Br J Sports Med. 2018;52:826–33.
23. Ruiz-Casado A, Martin-Ruiz A, Perez LM, Provencio M, Fiuza-Luces C, Lucia A. Exercise and the hallmarks of cancer. Trends Cancer. 2017;3:423–41.
24. IARC. Alcoholic beverages. 1988.
25. IARC. Alcohol consumption and ethyl carbamate. 2010.
26. IARC. Personal habits and indoor combustions. 2012.
27. Secretan B, Straif K, Baan R, Grosse Y, El Ghissassi F, Bouvard V, et al. A review of human carcinogens—

Part E: tobacco, areca nut, alcohol, coal smoke, and salted fish. Lancet Oncol. 2009;10:1033–4.
28. Johnson CM, Wei C, Ensor JE, Smolenski DJ, Amos CI, Levin B, et al. Meta-analyses of colorectal cancer risk factors. Cancer Causes Control. 2013;24:1207–22.
29. Murphy N, Ward HA, Jenab M, Rothwell JA, Boutron-Ruault MC, Carbonnel F, et al. Heterogeneity of colorectal cancer risk factors by anatomical subsite in 10 European countries: a multinational cohort study. Clin Gastroenterol Hepatol. 2019;17:1323–31.e6.
30. Limsui D, Vierkant RA, Tillmans LS, Wang AH, Weisenberger DJ, Laird PW, et al. Cigarette smoking and colorectal cancer risk by molecularly defined subtypes. J Natl Cancer Inst. 2010;102:1012–22.
31. National Comprehensive Cancer Network. Colorectal cancer screening (version 2.2021). 2021.
32. Cao Y, Nishihara R, Wu K, Wang M, Ogino S, Willett WC, et al. Population-wide impact of long-term use of aspirin and the risk for cancer. JAMA Oncol. 2016;2:762–9.
33. Rothwell PM, Wilson M, Elwin C-E, Norrving B, Algra A, Warlow CP, et al. Long-term effect of aspirin on colorectal cancer incidence and mortality: 20-year follow-up of five randomised trials. Lancet. 2010;376:1741–50.
34. Cook NR, Lee IM, Gaziano JM, Gordon D, Ridker PM, Manson JE, et al. Low-dose aspirin in the primary prevention of cancer: the Women's health study: a randomized controlled trial. JAMA. 2005;294:47–55.
35. Cook NR, Lee IM, Zhang SM, Moorthy MV, Buring JE. Alternate-day, low-dose aspirin and cancer risk: long-term observational follow-up of a randomized trial. Ann Intern Med. 2013;159:77–85.
36. Raber I, McCarthy CP, Vaduganathan M, Bhatt DL, Wood DA, Cleland JGF, et al. The rise and fall of aspirin in the primary prevention of cardiovascular disease. Lancet. 2019;393:2155–67.
37. ASCEND Study Collaborative Group Group, Bowman L, Mafham M, Wallendszus K, Stevens W, Buck G, et al. Effects of aspirin for primary prevention in persons with diabetes mellitus. N Engl J Med. 2018;379:1529–39.
38. Gaziano JM, Brotons C, Coppolecchia R, Cricelli C, Darius H, Gorelick PB, et al. Use of aspirin to reduce risk of initial vascular events in patients at moderate risk of cardiovascular disease (ARRIVE): a randomised, double-blind, placebo-controlled trial. Lancet. 2018;392:1036–46.
39. McNeil JJ, Nelson MR, Woods RL, Lockery JE, Wolfe R, Reid CM, et al. Effect of aspirin on all-cause mortality in the healthy elderly. N Engl J Med. 2018;379:1519–28.
40. Shaukat A, Kahi CJ, Burke CA, Rabeneck L, Sauer BG, Rex DK. ACG clinical guidelines: colorectal cancer screening 2021. Am J Gastroenterol. 2021;116:458–79.
41. Burn J, Sheth H, Elliott F, Reed L, Macrae F, Mecklin J-P, et al. Cancer prevention with aspirin in hereditary colorectal cancer (Lynch syndrome), 10-year follow-up and registry-based 20-year data in the CAPP2 study: a double-blind, randomised, placebo-controlled trial. Lancet. 2020;395:1855–63.
42. Winawer SJ, Schottenfeld D, Flehinger BJ. Colorectal cancer screening. J Natl Cancer Inst. 1991;83:243–53.
43. Wolf AMD, Fontham ETH, Church TR, Flowers CR, Guerra CE, LaMonte SJ, et al. Colorectal cancer screening for average-risk adults: 2018 guideline update from the American Cancer Society. CA Cancer J Clin. 2018;68:250–81.
44. US Preventive Services Task Force, Davidson KW, Barry MJ, Mangione CM, Cabana M, Caughey AB, et al. Screening for colorectal cancer: US preventive services task force recommendation statement. JAMA. 2021;325:1965–77.
45. Nishihara R, Wu K, Lochhead P, Morikawa T, Liao X, Qian ZR, et al. Long-term colorectal-cancer incidence and mortality after lower endoscopy. N Engl J Med. 2013;369:1095–105.
46. Knudsen AB, Zauber AG, Rutter CM, Naber SK, Doria-Rose VP, Pabiniak C, et al. Estimation of benefits, burden, and harms of colorectal cancer screening strategies: modeling study for the US preventive services task force. JAMA. 2016;315:2595–609.
47. Sohn DK, Kim MJ, Park Y, Suh M, Shin A, Lee HY, et al. The Korean guideline for colorectal cancer screening. J Korean Med Assoc. 2015;58:420–32.
48. National Comprehensive Cancer Network. Genetic/familial high-risk assessment: colorectal (version 1.2021). https://www.nccn.org/professionals/physician_gls/pdf/genetics_colon.pdf. Accessed 7 Nov 2021.

Epidemiology and Prevention. I-3. Pathologic and Molecular Characteristics of Colorectal Cancer

Key Points

- Colorectal cancers present as exophytic or ulcerative lesions.
- More than 90% of CRCs are adenocarcinomas.
- Important general prognostic pathologic features are the depth of invasion and the status of lymph node metastasis.
- Recently, the development of tailored medicine is underway based on the identification of molecular profiles of patients with CRC.

Introduction

Colorectal cancer (CRC) has shown the tendency to increase year by year. CRC was the second most common tumor in males and the third most common among females in Korea in 2018, according to the National Cancer Registration Statistics.

Molecular Characteristics

CRCs evolve sequentially through a multistep cumulative carcinogenic process in which genetic and epigenetic alterations occur. The most (~84%) sporadic CRCs develop from the traditional carcinogenesis pathway through the classic adenoma-carcinoma sequence that is activated by the *APC*/β-catenin pathway, and the remainder develop through the hypermutant serrated pathway (about 13%) or the ultramutant pathway (about 3%). Various types of molecular classification of CRCs have been described [1, 2].

Genomic Classification

CRC is classified into two main groups according to mutation rate: hypermutated and non-hypermutated cancers. Hypermutated cases (~15% of CRCs) have a high frequency of mutations, and most show microsatellite instability (MSI) due to defective DNA mismatch repair, including Lynch syndrome with 2–3% of ultramutated cancers related to DNA polymerase epsilon (POLE). Non-hypermutated cases (~85% of CRCs) have a low frequency of mutations and are microsatellite-stable (MSS), but they have a high frequency of DNA somatic copy number alterations (SCNAs) including *APC* (80%), *TP53* (60%), *KRAS* (45%), *SMAD4*, and *PIK3CA*.

Transcriptomic Profiling

The Colorectal Cancer Subtyping Consortium (CRCSC) suggested four main consensus molecular subtype (CMS) groups in 2015 [2], based on

So-Young Jin is the lead author of this chapter.

H. J. Chun et al., *Gastrointestinal Cancer*, https://doi.org/10.1007/978-981-99-0815-8_33

biological processes by gene expression patterns: CMS1 (MSI immune, 14%), CMS2 (canonical, 37%), CMS3 (metabolic, 13%), CMS4 (mesenchymal, 23%), and mixed (13%) subtypes. This classification might potentially be applied to subtype-based targeted interventions, although further studies are required to validate this.

Pathological Characteristics

Traditionally, colorectal carcinomas are divided by location; right-sided or proximal colon cancer (from cecum to transverse colon), left-sided colon cancer (from splenic flexure to the sigmoid colon), and rectal cancer. Tumors in the right colon often grow as polypoid masses (Fig. 1a). Because lesions occur in the large-caliber colon, they rarely cause obstruction. On the contrary, carcinomas in the left colon are presented as ulcers with rolled edges (Fig. 1b). Because these are characterized as near-total circumferential "napkin ring"-type constrictions, they frequently result in obstruction.

CRC is defined as an invasion of tumor cells through the muscularis mucosae into the submucosa. The majority (90%) of CRCs are adenocarcinoma. The general microscopic characteristics of right- and left-sided colonic adenocarcinomas are similar. Tumor glands consist of mucin-containing columnar epithelium containing pencil-like nuclei in picket fence appearance (Fig. 2).

CRC has also been traditionally graded as moderate or poor according to the percentage of gland formation. Presently, two-tiered grading is recommended: low-grade (formerly well to moderately differentiated) and high-grade (formerly poorly differentiated) tumors. The least differentiated component should be considered.

Although morphology cannot reliably define the underlying molecular events, certain correlations have been associated with MSI status. CRCs with MSI often have prominent mucinous differentiation and peritumoral lymphocytic infiltrates. These tumors, as well as those with a CpG island hypermethylation phenotype, are frequently located in the right colon. CRCs with MSI can be recognized by loss of immunohistochemical staining for mismatch repair (MMR) proteins in the nuclei of tumor cells or by genetic analysis of MMR genes.

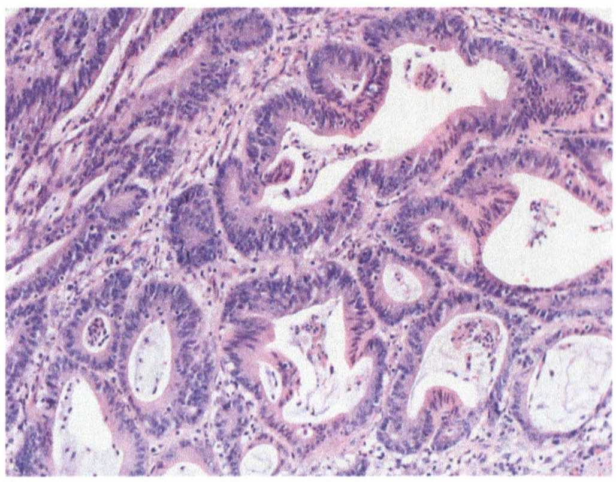

Fig. 2 Usual microscopic finding of moderately differentiated colonic adenocarcinoma is characterized as columnar cell-lined neoplastic gland (H-E, ×200)

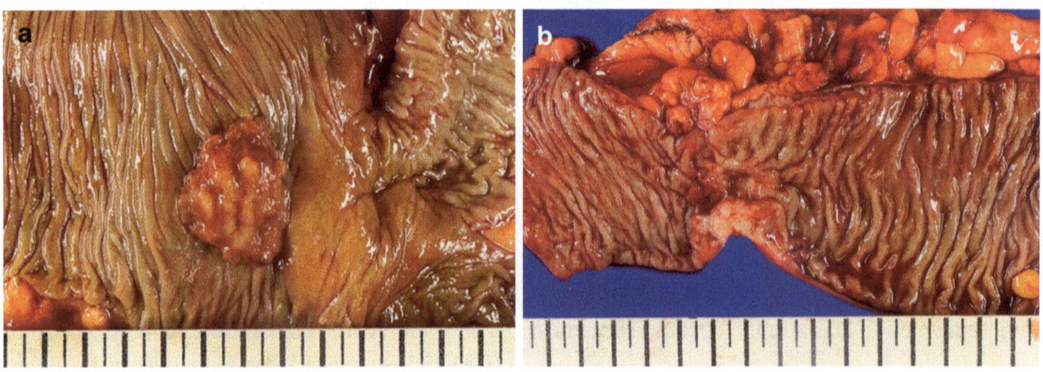

Fig. 1 Macroscopic findings of CRCs. A polypoid exophytic mass is seen in the right colon (**a**), and an annular napkin ring-type constrictive ulcerative lesion is seen in the left colon (**b**)

Table 1 World Health Organization classification of colorectal adenocarcinoma 2019

WHO classification of colorectal adenocarcinoma, 2019
Adenocarcinoma, NOS
Serrated adenocarcinoma
Adenoma-like adenocarcinoma
Micropapillary adenocarcinoma
Mucinous adenocarcinoma
Poorly cohesive carcinoma
Signet-ring cell carcinoma
Medullary adenocarcinoma
Adenosquamous carcinoma
Carcinoma, undifferentiated, NOS
Carcinoma with a sarcomatoid component

NOS not otherwise specified
Adapted from the World Health Organization (WHO) Classification of Tumors: Digestive System Tumors. 5th ed.

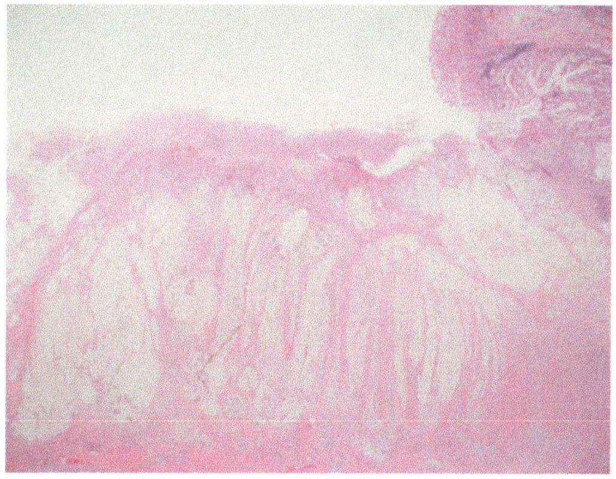

Fig. 3 Mucinous carcinoma consists of abundant extracellular mucin in most tumor mass (H-E, ×12.5)

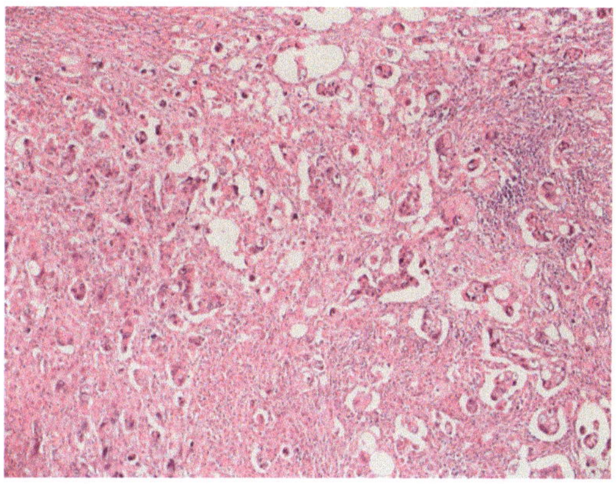

Fig. 4 Micropapillary carcinoma is characterized by arborizing glands within empty lymphatic-like spaces (H-E staining, ×40)

The World Health Organization (WHO) classification of colorectal adenocarcinoma was revised in 2019 [3] (Table 1). Characteristic histological findings of common types are as follows: mucinous adenocarcinoma and signet-ring cell carcinoma can be diagnosed when extracellular mucins are over 50% of tumor areas (Fig. 3) and signet-ring cells are over 50% of the tumor component, respectively. Medullary carcinoma is a rare histological type characterized by solid or sheet-like structures and profound lymphocytic infiltration. Micropapillary adenocarcinoma can be diagnosed when small tumor cell clusters are surrounded by empty spaces, simulating lymphatic or small vessel invasion (Fig. 4). This type of cancer has an increased risk of lymphovascular invasion and nodal metastasis and is often associated with poor prognostic factors such as lymphatic and vascular invasion. Serrated adenocarcinoma is a special subtype of CRC that is morphologically similar to serrated polyps and is characterized by neoplastic glands with prominent epithelial serrations, low nucleus-cytoplasm ratio, abundant eosinophilic cytoplasm, and vesicular nuclei. Adenosquamous carcinoma is diagnosed when an area of definite squamous differentiation is present in the tumor. Undifferentiated carcinoma is diagnosed when the epithelial tumor lacks morphological, immunohistochemical, and molecular evidence of specific differentiation. Adenoma-like adenocarcinoma, also called villous adenocarcinoma, is composed of villous adenoma-like well-differentiated tumors in the invasive portion, with pushing border and minimal desmoplasia. Some tumors may display features of neuroendocrine differentiation.

Important essential histological findings include lymphatic invasion (Fig. 5), intramural and extramural vascular invasion, and perineural invasion. Tumor budding is defined as single cells or clusters of up to four tumor cells at the invasive margin of the tumor (Fig. 6), which is determined by hematoxylin-eosin (H-E) staining in a hotspot on the invasive front using a three-

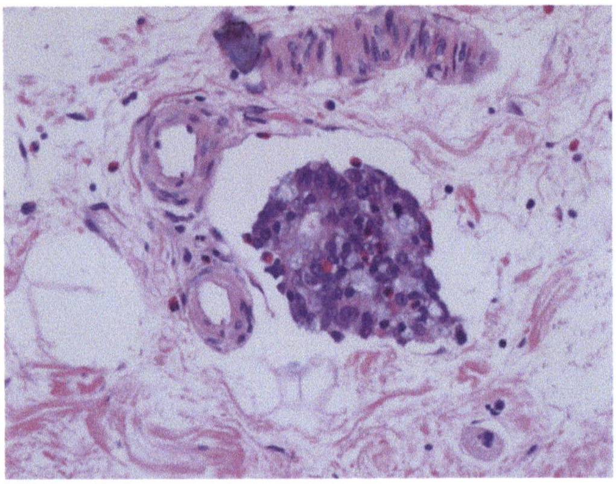

Fig. 5 A tumor embolus is visible in the lymphatic space (H-E, ×400)

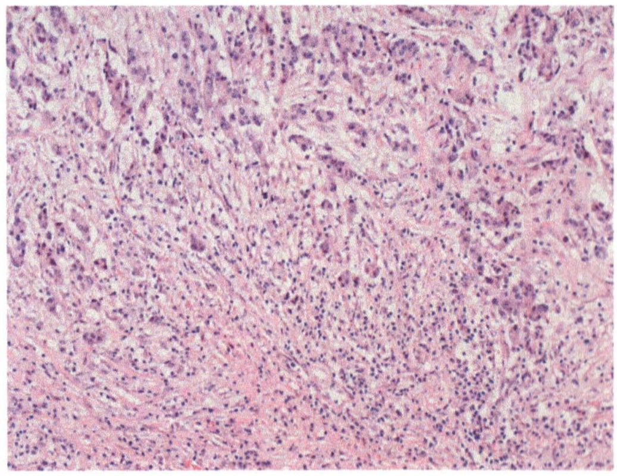

Fig. 6 Many tumor budding foci are visible in the invasive front of colon cancer (H-E, ×100)

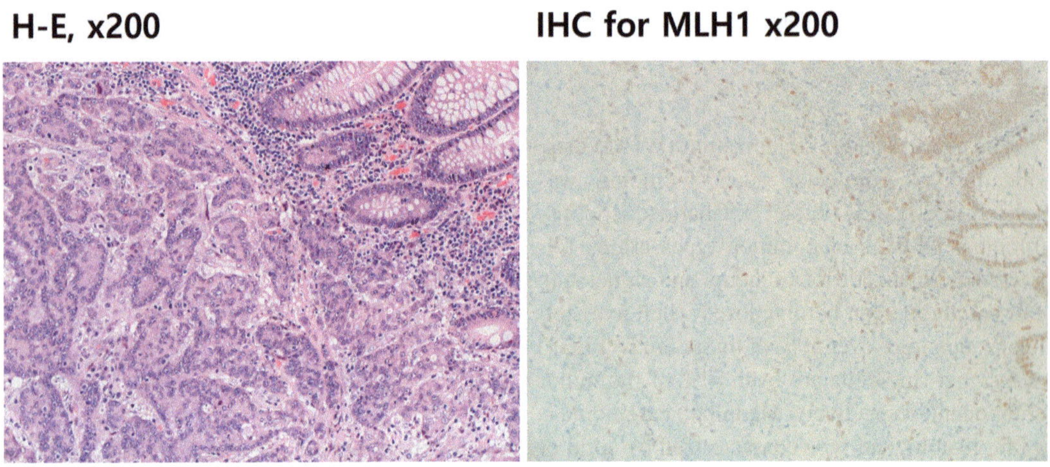

Fig. 7 Tumor cell nuclei are negative for MLH1 MMR protein on immunohistochemistry

tier scoring system according to an international consensus [4]. Higher budding scale is associated with a worse prognosis. Intratumoral lymphocytes and a Crohn-like reaction are associated with a better outcome. PD1/PDL1 status can be used as an index for cancer immunotherapy.

Complete resection of the neoplastic mass is essential. The circumferential radial resection margin (considered positive if the distance between tumor and edge of resection is ≤1 mm) is important, particularly in rectal cancer, and is closely related to local recurrence and overall survival.

MSI results from defective MMR mechanisms leading to predisposition to mutations. MSI is a reference test for the diagnosis of Lynch syndrome. The National Cancer Institute (NCI) recommends a set of five genetic markers: *BAT25, BAT26, D2S123, D5S346,* and *D17S250* [5]. Comparison of DNA from both the tumor and the normal counterpart is needed for MSI analysis. MMR status can also be identified using immunohistochemistry for a panel of four MMR proteins, including MLH1, MSH2, PMS2, and MSH6 (Fig. 7).

Liquid biopsy refers to the analysis of the components found on the patient peripheral blood (circulating tumor cells, exosomes, or cell-free DNA) and is a promising diagnostic tool for the identification of the metastatic CRC and to detect predictive markers of therapeutic response. The detection of *RAS* and *BRAF* mutations is likely to become widely acceptable in the near future.

Conclusion

The role of pathologists is transitioning toward the identification of the specific molecular profile of individual patients with CRC in addition to a more traditional morphological diagnosis. The pathology report guidelines of the CRC Gastrointestinal Study Group of the Korean Society of Pathologists have suggested to include standard data elements and conditional data elements of resected colorectal cancers according to a checklist developed in 2021 [6].

References

1. Guinney J, Dienstmann R, Wang X, de Reynies A, Schlicker A, Soneson C, et al. The consensus molecular subtypes of colorectal cancer. Nat Med. 2015;21:1350–6.
2. Muller MF, Ibrahim AEK, Arends MJ. Molecular pathological classification of colorectal cancer. Virchows Arch. 2016;469:125–34.
3. WHO Classification of Tumours Editorial Board. WHO classification of tumours: digestive system tumours. 5th ed. Geneva: World Health Organization; 2019.
4. Lugli A, Kirsch R, Ajioka Y, Bosman F, Cathomas G, Dawson H, et al. Recommendations for reporting tumor budding in colorectal cancer based on the international tumor budding consensus conference (ITBCC) 2016. Mod Pathol. 2017;30:1299–311.
5. Boland CR, Thibodeau SN, Hamilton SR, Sidransky D, Eshleman JR, Burt RW, et al. A National Cancer Institute workshop on microsatellite instability for cancer detection and familial predisposition: development of international criteria for the determination of microsatellite instability in colorectal cancer. Cancer Res. 1998;58:5248–57.
6. Kim B-H, Kim JM, Kang GH, Chang HJ, Kang DW, Kim JH, et al. Standardized pathology report for colorectal cancer, 2nd edition. J Pathol Transl Med. 2020;54:1–19.

Staging and Treatment. II-1. Staging and Prognosis

Key Points

- The goal of diagnosis and treatment is to decide the appropriate treatment methods and to increase survival in patients with colorectal cancer.
- The best treatment can be performed only by closely observing the patient's signs and symptoms, choosing appropriate diagnostic methods, and determining the exact stage.

Introduction

Early colon cancer is generally asymptomatic. Colorectal cancer (CRC) screening plays a key role in the diagnosis of curable cancerous lesions. If a diagnosis is made through screening or a patient comes to the hospital because of specific symptoms, it is important to properly assess the signs and symptoms and implement an appropriate diagnostic strategy to differentiate diagnosis and the correct stage in order to determine the correct treatment method. In this chapter, the physical examination, diagnostic methods, and staging for the diagnosis of patients with CRC will be reviewed, and the prognosis according to each stage will be reviewed.

Diagnosis for Colon Cancer

The diagnosis of CRC is closely related to symptoms. There are no exact symptoms suggestive of CRC. Each symptom of CRC may appear depending on the location of the CRC. Symptoms of right CRC were diarrhea and anemia due to bleeding, and symptoms such as abdominal pain due to obstruction may appear, but the symptom of right colon cancer appears later than in left CRC. This is because right colon cancer has a large luminal diameter and loose intestinal contents, so changes in bowel habits do not occur until the colon lumen is almost completely occluded by the tumor. Conversely, in the case of the left colon, since the stool is hard, abdominal pain and nausea due to intestinal obstruction more frequently occur than on right-side colon [1]. Additionally, changes in stool habits, such as constipation or diarrhea, bloody stool, or mucus stool, may appear. In the case of rectal lesions, this pattern is more pronounced [2]. Abdominal pain or tenesmus may appear during and after defecation. In addition, nonspecific symptoms such as palpable abdominal mass, general weakness, and weight loss may appear. Additionally, pathological fracture due to bone metastasis, liver failure, jaundice due to liver metastasis, and Sister Mary Joseph's nodule due to peritoneal metastasis can appear.

Yoonjae Kim is the lead author of this chapter.

H. J. Chun et al., *Gastrointestinal Cancer*, https://doi.org/10.1007/978-981-99-0815-8_34

Physical examination is an important diagnostic method for CRC. Abdominal distension and palpable mass caused by CRC can be observed. In most cases, cancerous masses are usually hard to touch. However, with colon cancer of the transverse colon or the sigmoid colon, the palpable mass can move. Furthermore, metastatic lymph nodes could be palpable.

In the case of rectal cancer, a digital rectal examination can be a crucial test for diagnosis. In the case of lower rectal cancer, the cancer can be diagnosed only by a digital rectal examination. The size, shape, and location of the rectal cancer can be reported. In the case of metastatic CRC, the rectal shelf can be palpable [3].

The fecal occult blood test (FOBT) or fecal immunochemical test (FIT) can be used as screening tests for CRC, but these are not frequently used for diagnosis or staging of CRC. In a meta-analysis of CRC, the sensitivity for detecting CRC was 92.3% with DNA testing and 73.8% with FIT [4].

Barium enema is a radiological examination of the colonic mucosa. CRC appears when there is a lesion in the colon mucosa and usually appears in the form of a polyp or a mass that narrows the lumen of the colon. When colonic stenosis progresses, it can present in the shape of an "apple core appearance" which is a typical shape of advanced CRC. For barium enema, the sensitivity is 81%, and the specificity is 96% for adenomas larger than 1 cm [5].

Colonoscopy has the advantage of obtaining tissue, and thus it has an important position in the diagnosis of CRC. For diagnostic purposes of CRC, other than screening tests, rectal endoscopy or sigmoidoscopy is not frequently used. Through colonoscopy, the shape, size, and distance from the anal axis can be determined. During colonoscopy, polyps can be removed, and other synchronous colon cancer can be detected before surgery. On perioperative clearing colonoscopy, synchronous high-risk adenomas (number $\geq$3, size $\geq$10 mm, high-grade dysplasia, villous histology, and serrated adenoma $\geq$10 mm) were detected in 95 patients (32.4%) in one study. A full colonoscopy is recommended before treatment for CRC. If the entire colon cannot be seen due to obstruction, a colonoscopy is recommended within 6 months after surgery. If the lesion is small, tattooing or clipping can be performed to accurately identify the location of the lesion during the preoperative examination [6, 7].

Computed tomography (CT) is the most important test for determining preoperative staging. In one meta-analysis, the specificity and sensitivity for the T staging were 86% and 78%, and the specificity and sensitivity for lymph node detection were 70% and 78%, respectively, while the sensitivity for the N staging was much lower, less than 50% [8, 9]. If CRC is diagnosed, CT should include not only the abdomen but also the pelvis and chest in the imaging range to detect distant metastases. CT colonoscopy can be used when the colonoscopy cannot pass close to the CRC or when the colonoscopy is difficult; this examination also requires colon preparation. Therefore, CT colonoscopy is useful as a preoperative examination when a stent is inserted. However, it is impossible to obtain tissue by biopsy or to remove polyps by CT colonoscopy [10].

Magnetic resonance imaging (MRI) is sometimes used as a substitute for CT when a patient is allergic to CT contrast agents, but usually two types of MRI are used for staging. First, liver MRI can be used to provide with additional confirmation if liver metastasis of CRC is suspected, but it is not an essential staging workup method as defined by the existing guidelines. Pelvic (rectal) MRI is one of the most important tests for staging rectal cancer [11]. If the stage 1 cancer is confirmed, there is no need to conduct pelvic MRI, and if the patient is unable to undergo surgery for several reasons, it is not an indication for MRI examination. It is possible to accurately predict the T stage before surgery, and the presence of the lymph node metastasis can also be accurately detected by MRI.

Endorectal ultrasound can identify the T stage and N stage of the rectal cancer very accurately. However, the results will vary depending on the skill of the operator, and due to the high accuracy of pelvic MRI, an endorectal ultrasound is mainly recommended when MRI cannot be used due to the presence of a pacemaker or for other reasons.

Positron emission tomography/computed tomography (PET/CT) is not routinely indicated.

Its usefulness has been proven when it shows equivocal findings on CT or MRI or when it is contraindicated with a contrast medium for CT or MRI [12]. Furthermore, since metastasectomy is possible in CRC, it can be used if it is an indication for potentially surgically curable M1 disease or image-guided liver-directed therapy for liver metastasis, such as ablation or embolization. When such image-guided liver-directed therapy is used, it can be useful for response assessment and recurrence monitoring.

In addition, the complete blood test, the biochemistry profile, and CEA test findings are required, while the determination of the gene mutation status for *RAS* and *BRAF* and HER2 amplifications, universal mismatch repair (MMR), and microsatellite instability (MSI) testing through biopsy of the tumor should be performed.

Staging and Prognosis

Since the tumor stage is closely related to prognosis, it is important to determine the stage of CRC and establish a treatment strategy accordingly for the treatment of CRC. Treatment of CRC and rectal cancer is carried out according to the stages T, N, and M, as with most other cancers. T, N, and M staging defines the extent (size) of the tumor (T), the spread to nearby lymph nodes (N), and the spread (metastasis) to distant sites (M).

The staging of CRC is generally established according to the guidelines of the American Joint Committee on Cancer (AJCC) (Tables 1 and 2). The most recent AJCC version is the eighth edition [13–16], released in 2017. First, the T stage is classified according to the depth of the lesion.

Table 1 American Joint Committee on Cancer (AJCC) TNM staging system eighth ed., 2017

Primary tumor (T)	
Tx	Primary tumor cannot be assessed
T0	No evidence of primary tumor
Tis	Carcinoma in situ, intramucosal carcinoma (involvement of lamina propria with no extension through muscularis mucosa)
T1	Tumor invades the submucosa (through the muscularis mucosa but not into the muscularis propria)
T2	Tumor invades the muscularis propria
T3	Tumor invades through the muscularis propria into pericolorectal tissues
T4	Tumor invades the visceral peritoneum or invades or adheres to adjacent organ or structure
T4a	Tumor invades through the visceral peritoneum (including gross perforation of the bowel through tumor and continuous invasion of tumor through areas of inflammation to the surface of the visceral peritoneum)
T4b	Tumor directly invades or adheres to adjacent organs or structures
Regional lymph nodes (N)	
Nx	Regional lymph nodes cannot be assessed
N0	No regional lymph node metastasis
N1	One to three regional lymph nodes are positive (tumor in lymph nodes measuring ≥0.2 mm), or any number of tumor deposits are present and all identifiable lymph nodes are negative
N1a	One regional lymph node is positive
N1b	Two or three regional lymph nodes are positive
N1c	No regional lymph nodes are positive, but there are tumor deposits in the subserosa, mesentery, or nonperitonealized pericolic or perirectal/mesorectal tissues
N2	Four or more regional lymph nodes are positive
N2a	Four to six regional lymph nodes are positive
N2b	Seven or more regional lymph nodes are positive
Distant metastasis (M)	
M0	No distant metastasis by imaging
M1	Metastasis to one or more distant sites or organs or peritoneal metastasis is identified
M1a	Metastasis to one site or organ is identified without peritoneal metastasis
M1b	Metastasis to two or more sites or organs is identified without peritoneal metastasis
M1c	Metastasis to the peritoneal surface is identified alone or with other site or organ metastasis

The difference from other gastrointestinal adenocarcinomas is that CRC distributed to the muscular mucosa is not included in stage 1 but is classified as Tis and classified as stage 0. Stage T4 is divided into T4a and T4b. Stage N refers to regional lymph nodes, and stage N is classified according to the number of lymph nodes. According to the number, N1 staging is classified as N1a, N1b, and N1c, and N2 staging is classified as N2a and N2b. The M stage is classified into M1a, M1b, and M1c. Since metastasectomy is possible for CRC, the stage M is also subdivided and organized, and each stage is subdivided according to the number of metastatic lesions and peritoneal invasions.

Table 2 American Joint Committee on Cancer (AJCC) TNM staging system eighth ed., 2017

Stage grouping	
0	Tis N0 M0
I	T1–T2 N0 M0
IIA	T3 N0 M0
IIB	T4a N0 M0
IIC	T4b N0 M0
IIIA	T1–T2 N1/N1c M0 T1 N2a M0
IIIB	T3–T4a N1/N1c M0 T2–T3 N2a M0 T1–T2 N2b M0
IIIC	T4a N2a M0 T3–T4a N2b M0 T4b N1–N2 M0
IVA	AnyT AnyN M1a
IVB	AnyT AnyN M1b
IVC	AnyT AnyN M1c

Cancer prognosis is classified by the American National Cancer Institute Surveillance Epidemiology and End Results (SEER) program. Prognosis is classified into localized (disease is in the organ of origin), regional (invasion to surrounding tissues or metastasis to regional lymph nodes), and distant (metastasis to distant organ) to establish nationwide statistics.

Figure 1 shows the annual change in prognostic statistics in Korea [17]. Table 3 shows the prognostic statistics for CRC for a similar period in the United States [18].

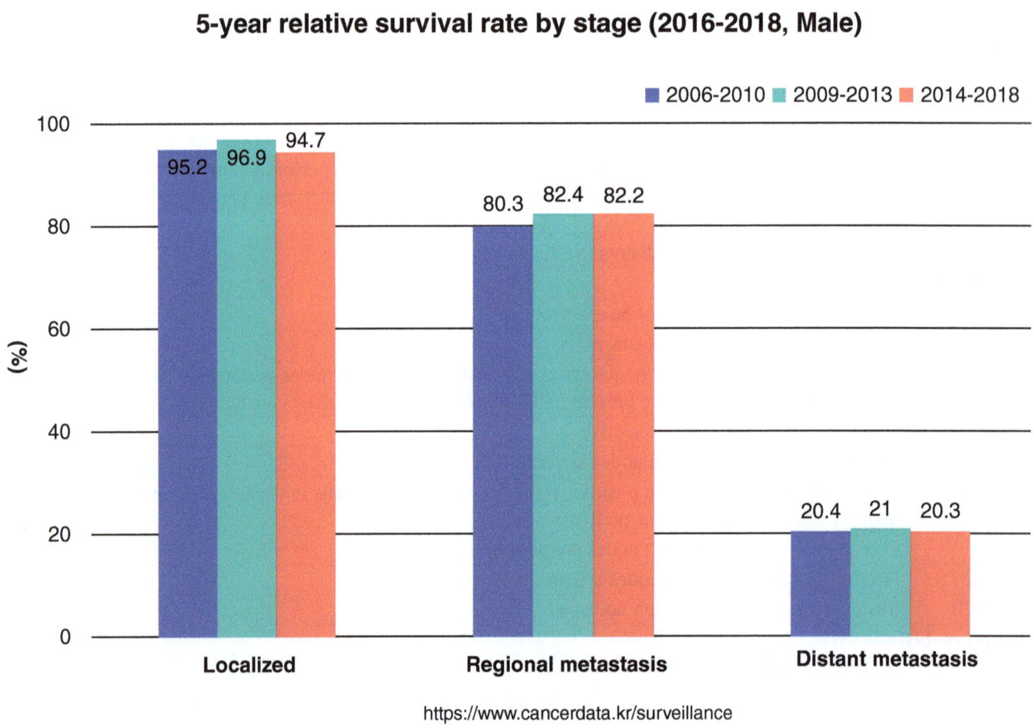

Fig. 1 Survival rates for colorectal cancer of Korea

Table 3 Survival rates for colorectal cancer of the United States

SEER stage	Colon cancer 5-year relative survival rate (%)	Rectal cancer 5-year relative survival rate (%)
Localized	91	89
Regional	72	72
Distant	14	16

Conclusion

In conclusion, stage of diagnosis is a very important prognostic factor for survival in colon cancer. Since symptoms and signs of CRC are varied, through physical exam and clinical suspicion, gastroenterologists should select the appropriate test and determine the stage for best treatment.

References

1. Baran B, Mert Ozupek N, Yerli Tetik N, Acar E, Bekcioglu O, Baskin Y. Difference between left-sided and right-sided colorectal cancer: a focused review of literature. Gastroenterology Res. 2018;11:264–73.
2. Tamas K, Walenkamp AM, de Vries EG, van Vugt MA, Beets-Tan RG, van Etten B, et al. Rectal and colon cancer: not just a different anatomic site. Cancer Treat Rev. 2015;41:671–9.
3. Recio-Boiles A, Kashyap S, Tsoris A, Babiker HM. Rectal cancer. StatPearls. Treasure Island: StatPearls Publishing, StatPearls Publishing LLC; 2021.
4. Imperiale TF, Ransohoff DF, Itzkowitz SH, Levin TR, Lavin P, Lidgard GP, et al. Multitarget stool DNA testing for colorectal-cancer screening. N Engl J Med. 2014;370:1287–97.
5. Glick S. Double-contrast barium enema for colorectal cancer screening: a review of the issues and a comparison with other screening alternatives. AJR Am J Roentgenol. 2000;174:1529–37.
6. Nam K, Shin JE. Risk factors of advanced metachronous neoplasms in surveillance after colon cancer resection. Korean J Intern Med. 2021;36:305–12.
7. Dua A, Liem B, Gupta N. Lesion retrieval, specimen handling, and endoscopic marking in colonoscopy. Gastrointest Endosc Clin N Am. 2019;29:687–703.
8. Korsbakke K, Dahlbäck C, Karlsson N, Zackrisson S, Buchwald P. Tumor and nodal staging of colon cancer: accuracy of preoperative computed tomography at a Swedish high-volume center. Acta Radiol Open. 2019;8:2058460119888713.
9. Dighe S, Purkayastha S, Swift I, Tekkis PP, Darzi A, A'Hern R, et al. Diagnostic precision of CT in local staging of colon cancers: a meta-analysis. Clin Radiol. 2010;65:708–19.
10. Pickhardt PJ, Hassan C, Halligan S, Marmo R. Colorectal cancer: CT colonography and colonoscopy for detection—systematic review and meta-analysis. Radiology. 2011;259:393–405.
11. Horvat N, Carlos Tavares Rocha C, Clemente Oliveira B, Petkovska I, Gollub MJ. MRI of rectal cancer: tumor staging, imaging techniques, and management. Radiographics. 2019;39:367–87.
12. Kijima S, Sasaki T, Nagata K, Utano K, Lefor AT, Sugimoto H. Preoperative evaluation of colorectal cancer using CT colonography, MRI, and PET/CT. World J Gastroenterol. 2014;20:16964–75.
13. Weiser MR. AJCC 8th edition: colorectal cancer. Ann Surg Oncol. 2018;25:1454–5.
14. Amin MB, Edge SB, Greene F, Byrd DR, Brookland RK, Washington MK, Gershenwald JE, Compton CC, Hess KR, Sullivan DC. AJCC cancer staging manual. New York: Springer; 2017.
15. NCC Network. NCCN clinical practice guidelines in oncology (NCCN guidelines®): colon cancer, 2021. https://www.nccn.org/professionals/physician_gls/default.aspx.
16. NCC Network. NCCN clinical practice guidelines in oncology (NCCN guidelines®): rectal cancer, 2021. https://www.nccn.org/professionals/physician_gls/default.aspx.
17. Hong S, Won Y-J, Lee JJ, Jung K-W, Kong H-J, Im J-S, et al. Cancer statistics in Korea: incidence, mortality, survival, and prevalence in 2018. Cancer Res Treat. 2021;53:301–15.
18. American Cancer Society. Cancer facts & figures 2020. Atlanta: American Cancer Society; 2020.

Staging and Treatment. II-2. Overview of Treatment of CRC

Key Points

- If there is no evidence of unfavorable risk factors, endoscopic resection of polyp containing adenocarcinoma is available.
- Surgical resection is the only curative treatment for colorectal cancer.
- Adjuvant chemotherapy is needed in patients with stage III (node-positive) disease and stage II with MSS/pMMR and high-risk features.
- Treatment for rectal cancer is similar to that for colon cancer, except for the option of radiotherapy.
- Genetic testing including *KRAS, NRAS, BRAF, MSI-MMR, and Her2* is essential before chemotherapy to determine the chemotherapy approach.

Introduction

Colorectal cancer (CRC) is the third most diagnosed cancer and is the fourth leading cause of death worldwide [1]. Surgical resection is the curative treatment of colorectal cancer. However, endoscopic resection is a reasonable modality for early colon cancer. In addition, therapeutic options for metastatic disease have been rapidly evolving, and physicians now have access to several drugs with activity in the first-, second-, and even third-line settings. It is important to understand these drugs and their roles in the treatment of metastatic disease. In this chapter, we will provide an overview of the treatment of colon cancer including rectal cancer.

Seun Ja Park is the lead author of this chapter.

Management of Malignant Polyps

Most colon cancers arise from polyps (adenomas). Nonmalignant adenoma or carcinoma (no evidence of invasive cancer, defined as invasion into the submucosa) can be effectively managed by endoscopic resection.

On occasion, an endoscopically removed polyp may reveal an invasive adenocarcinoma within the adenoma. Treatment recommendations in this situation should be individualized based on tumor characteristics, including negative margins, no evidence of invasion beyond the submucosa, well- or moderately differentiated adenocarcinoma, and no evidence of lymphatic or vascular invasion. In this setting, the risk of lymph node metastases is low (5%), and follow-up with periodic colonoscopic examinations is reasonable [2]. The presence of any of the unfavorable risk factors (poorly differentiated adenocarcinoma, lymphovascular invasion, submucosal invasion) should prompt the consideration of colectomy with en bloc removal of the regional lymph nodes [3, 4].

H. J. Chun et al., *Gastrointestinal Cancer*, https://doi.org/10.1007/978-981-99-0815-8_35

Malignant polyps that have occurred in the lower rectum may cause difficulties when deciding on additional surgery. This is due to problems such as the anus sphincter preservation procedure and frequent local recurrence.

Definitive surgical resection should be considered for a resected rectal polyp without clear margins or with adverse pathologic features. If a rectal polyp is resected with equivocal margins and there is no evidence of muscle invasion, transanal excision may be considered feasible [5, 6].

Occasionally, chemoradiation can be considered an option if surgery is refused or if there are medical comorbidities that prevent surgery [7].

Surgical Resection for Localized Colon Cancer

Resection for localized colon cancer removes the affected segment of the bowel, the adjacent mesentery, and the draining lymph nodes [8].

Surgery may consist of segmental resection or subtotal colectomy, depending on the underlying colonic pathology (multifocal cancer, familial adenomatous polyposis, and hereditary nonpolyposis colorectal cancer). Therefore, all patients with colorectal cancer should be informed of their family history prior to therapy, as an inherited predisposition to colorectal cancer [9].

Laparoscopic colectomy was not inferior to open colectomy in several prospective randomized studies, with the laparoscopic surgery group having shorter perioperative recovery, hospital stay, and duration of parenteral narcotic use and oral analgesics, as well as comparable intraoperative complications and postoperative mortality [10, 11]. Patients who have potentially resectable and non-obstructing disease should undergo colectomy with removal of regional lymph nodes. Potentially resectable obstructing disease may be considered for one-stage colectomy with removal of the regional lymph nodes or for two-stage colectomy with removal of the regional lymph nodes after diversion or stent [12].

Neoadjuvant Chemotherapy or Chemoradiotherapy of Colon Cancer

Patients with bulky nodal disease or clinically T4b may be considered for neoadjuvant FOLFOX or CAPEOX [13]. Chemotherapy (5-fluorouracil/leucovorin or capecitabine) with radiotherapy is an option for locally unresectable or medically inoperable disease. Subsequently, patients should be re-evaluated for conversion to resectable disease [14].

Adjuvant Chemotherapy of Colon Cancer

After curative surgical resection, adjuvant chemotherapy eradicates micrometastases and reduces the possibility of recurrence. Survival benefits have been demonstrated in patients with stage III (node-positive) disease and stage II with MSS/pMMR and high-risk features, including pT4, poorly differentiated/undifferentiated histology, lymphovascular invasion, perineural invasion, bowel obstruction, localized perforation, insufficient number of lymph nodes examined, close/indeterminate/positive margins, or tumor budding. FOLFOX (6 months), CAPEOX (3 months), capecitabine (6 months), or 5-FU/leucovorin (6 months) is recommended [15–18].

Treatment for Metastatic Disease of Colon Cancer

Patients with metastatic disease are not surgical candidates, and palliative chemotherapy is mostly recommended. Patients who present with unresectable metastatic disease with an imminent risk of obstruction, significant bleeding, or perforation may be considered for colon resection [19].

Limited Metastatic Disease, Predominantly in the Liver and Lung

Surgery may be considered a potentially curative option for patients with limited metastatic disease, predominantly in the liver and lung. Patients with potentially resectable, synchronous liver and/or lung metastases can be considered for synchronous or staged colectomy with liver or lung resection and/or local therapy (radiofrequency ablation or SBRT) [20]. Neoadjuvant chemotherapy followed by synchronous or staged colectomy and resection of metastatic disease is another option. Furthermore, it is another option that colectomy followed by chemotherapy and staged resection of metastatic disease can be considered.

Palliative Chemotherapy

Patients with unresectable metastatic disease are not surgical candidates, and palliative chemotherapy is recommended primarily. Genetic testing including *KRAS, NRAS, BRAF, MSI-MMR,* and *Her2* is essential before chemotherapy to determine which strategy to use [21].

Treatment of Rectal Cancer

The treatment of rectal cancer is usually similar to that of colon cancer, but there are some differences. Because the rectum has a narrow space and is close to the anus, on occasion recurrence occurs after surgery. Furthermore, it is also difficult to preserve the anus. Therefore, it is necessary to determine the treatment method through pelvic MRI and/or rectal EUS, and a multidisciplinary team evaluation before surgery is warranted [22].

Patients with clinical stage T1, N0 based on the assessment of the pelvic MRI or endorectal ultrasound may be considered for transanal local excision or transabdominal resection. Neoadjuvant therapy (long-course chemotherapy, radiotherapy, or short-course radiotherapy) is an option for patients with clinical stage T3, N any with clear circumferential resection margin (CRM) by MRI, or T1–2/N1–2. After completion of radiation therapy, it is necessary to re-evaluate at the eighth week when the response is the best and decide whether to have surgery or not [23–25]. Restaging is needed following long-course chemotherapy/radiotherapy or chemotherapy alone, in the locally unresectable or medically inoperable rectal cancer.

Patients who present with potentially resectable, synchronous liver-only and/or with lung-only metastases may be considered for neoadjuvant chemotherapy and/or radiotherapy. Restaging followed by synchronous or staged colectomy and resection of metastatic disease is another option. For patients with unresectable synchronous metastases, the treatment is the same as for colon cancer. The treatment approach for rectal cancer with unresectable metastases is similar to that of colon cancer, with the exception of radiation therapy which may be considered as an option.

Conclusion

Choosing the appropriate treatment for CRC patients has an important effect on the patient's prognosis. Surgical resection is only a curative treatment for colorectal cancer. The survival rate of colorectal cancer is increasing remarkably through surgery, appropriate chemotherapy, and radiation therapy. It is necessary to determine the appropriate treatment method well and use the newly developed anticancer drug, including target agents and immunotherapy, appropriately.

References

1. Goodarzi E, Beiranvand R, Naemi H, Momenabadi V, Khazaei Z. Worldwide incidence and mortality of colorectal cancer and human development index (HDI): an ecological study. WCRJ. 2019;6:e1433–40.
2. Skibber J, Minsky B, Hoff P. Cancer of the colon and rectum. In: DeVita VT Jr, Hellmann S, Rosenberg SA, editors. Cancer: principles and practice of oncology. 6th ed. Philadelphia: Lippincott Willams & Wilkins; 2001:1216–1271.
3. Pai RK, Cheng YW, Jakubowski MA, Shadrach BL, Plesec TP, Par RK. Colorectal carcinomas with submucosal invasion (pT1): analysis of histopathological and molecular factors predicting lymph node metastasis. Mod Pathol. 2017;30:113–22.
4. Shaukat A, Kaltenbach T, Dominitz JA, Robertson DJ, Anderson JC, Cruise M, et al. Endoscopic recognition and management strategies for malignant colorectal polyps: recommendations of the US Multi-Society Task Force on Colorectal Cancer. Gastroenterology. 2020;159:1916–34.
5. Mellgren A, Sirivongs P, Rothenberger DA, Madoff RD, Garcia-Aguilar J. Is local excision adequate therapy for early rectal cancer? Dis Colon Rectum. 2000;43:1064–71.
6. Sengupta S, Tjandra JJ. Local excision of rectal cancer: what is the evidence? Dis Colon Rectum. 2001;44:1345–61.
7. Rombouts AJM, Al-Najami I, Abbott NL, Appeit A, Baatrup G, Bach S, et al. Can we save the rectum by watchful waiting or transanal microsurgery following (chemo) radiotherapy versus total mesorectal excision for early REctal cancer (STAR-TREC study)?: protocol for a multicentre, randomised feasibility study. BMJ Open. 2017;28(7):e019474.
8. Vogel JD, Eskicioglu C, Weiser MR, Feingold DL, Steele SR. The American Society of Colon and Rectal Surgeons clinical practice guidelines for the treatment of colon cancer. Dis Colon Rectum. 2017;60:999–1017.
9. Stoffel EM, Mangu PB, Gruber SB, Hamilton SR, Kalady MF, Lau MWY, et al. Hereditary colorectal cancer syndromes: American Society of Clinical Oncology clinical practice guideline endorsement of the familial risk-colorectal cancer: European Society for Medical Oncology clinical practice guidelines. J Clin Oncol. 2015;33:209–17.
10. Clinical Outcomes of Surgical Therapy Study Group, Nelson H, Sargent DJ, Wieand HS, Fleshman J, Anvari M, Stryker SJ, et al. A comparison of laparoscopically assisted and open colectomy for colon cancer. N Engl J Med. 2004;350:2050–9.
11. Fleshman J, Sargent DJ, Green E, Anvari M, Stryker SJ, Beart RW Jr, et al. Laparoscopic colectomy for cancer is not inferior to open surgery based on 5-year data from the COST Study Group trial. Ann Surg. 2007;246:655–64.
12. Malakorn S, Stein SL, Lee JH, You YN. Urgent management of obstructing colorectal cancer: divert, stent, or resect? J Gastrointest Surg. 2019;23:425–32.
13. Body A, Prenen H, Latham S, Lam M, Tipping-Smith S, Raghunath A, et al. The role of neoadjuvant chemotherapy in locally advanced colon cancer. Cancer Manag Res. 2021;13:2567–79.
14. Hakins AT, Ford MM, Geiger TM, Hopkins MB, Kachnic LA, Muldoon RL, et al. Neoadjuvant radiation for clinical T4 colon cancer: a potential improvement to overall survival. Surgery. 2019;165:469–75.
15. Andre T, Boni C, Mounediji-Boudiaf L, Navarro M, Tabernero J, Hichish T, et al. Oxaliplatin, fluorouracil, and leucovorin as adjuvant treatment for colon cancer. N Engl J Med. 2004;350:2342–51.
16. Quasar Collaborative Group, Gray R, Barnwell J, McConkey C, Hills RK, Williams NS, Kerr DJ. Adjuvant chemotherapy versus observation in patients with colorectal cancer: a randomised study. Lancet. 2007;370:2020–9.
17. Tournigand C, Andre T, Bonnetain F, Chibaudel B, Lledo G, Hickish T, et al. Adjuvant therapy with fluorouracil and oxaliplatin in stage II and elderly patients (between ages 70 and 75 years) with leucovorin in the adjuvant treatment of colon cancer trial. J Clin Oncol. 2012;30:3353–60.
18. Quah HM, Chou JF, Gonen M, Shia J, Schrag D, Landmann RG, et al. Identification of patients with high-risk stage II colon cancer for adjuvant therapy. Dis Colon Rectum. 2008;51:503–7.
19. Pisano M, Zorcolo L, Merli C, Cimbanassi S, Poiasina E, Ceresoli M, et al. 2017 WSES guidelines on colon and rectal cancer emergencies: obstruction and perforation. World J Emerg Surg. 2018;13:36.
20. Molla M, Fernandez-Plana J, Albiol S, Fondevila C, Vollmer I, Cases C, et al. Limited liver or lung colorectal cancer metastases. Systemic treatment, surgery, ablation or SBRT. J Clin Med. 2021;10:2131–46.
21. Afrăsânie VA, Marinca MV, Alexa-Stratulat T, Gafton B, Păduraru M, Adavidoaiei AM, et al. KRAS, NRAS, BRAF, HER2 and microsatellite instability in metastatic colorectal cancer—practical implications for the clinician. Radiol Oncol. 2019;53:265–74.
22. Ruppert R, Kube R, Strassburg J, Lewin A, Baral J, Maurer CA, et al. Avoidance of overtreatment of rectal cancer by selective chemoradiotherapy: results of the optimized surgery and MRI-based multimodal therapy trial. J Am Coll Surg. 2020;231:413–25.
23. Sauer R, Becker H, Hohenberger W, Rodel C, Wittekind C, Fietkau R, et al. Preoperative versus postoperative chemoradiotherapy for rectal cancer. N Engl J Med. 2004;351:1731–40.
24. O'Connell MJ, Colangelo LH, Beart RW, Petrelli NJ, Allegra CJ, Sharif S, et al. Capecitabine and oxaliplatin in the preoperative multimodality treatment of rectal cancer: surgical end points from National Surgical Adjuvant Breast and Bowel Project trial R-04. J Clin Oncol. 2014;32:1927–34.
25. Gerard J, Azria D, Gourgou-Bourgade S, Martel-Laffay I, Hennequin C, Etienne PL, et al. Randomized multicenter phase III trial comparing two neoadjuvant chemoradiotherapy (CT-RT) regimens (RT45-Cap versus RT50-Capox) in patients (pts) with locally advanced rectal cancer (LARC): results of the ACCORD 12/0405-Prodige 2. J Clin Oncol. 2010;28:1638–44.

Staging and Treatment. II-3. Endoscopic Treatment: Indication, Outcome

Key Points

- Non-pedunculated malignant polyps are considered high risk for residual or recurrent cancer if they have any of the following characteristics: poor histological types (poorly differentiated adenocarcinoma, signet ring cell carcinoma, and mucinous carcinoma), submucosal invasion depth >1 mm, lymphovascular invasion, intermediate- to high-grade tumor budding, and tumor involvement of the cautery margin.
- Pedunculated malignant polyps are considered at high risk of residual or recurrent cancer if they have any of the following features: poor tumor differentiation, lymphovascular invasion, and tumor within 1 mm of the resection margin.
- ESD can be considered for colorectal lesions, particularly if the lesions are >20 mm or cannot be removed otherwise by en bloc resection using snare EMR.

Introduction

Early colorectal cancer (CRC) is defined as cancer that is confined to the mucosa or submucosal layer regardless of lymph node metastasis that does not invade the muscularis mucosa. The possibility of lymph node metastasis in intramucosal cancer is extremely rare and negligible and can be curatively resected by endoscopic procedure [1]. However, if cancer invades the submucosal layer, the possibility of lymph node metastasis is reported to be 6–13% [2]. The depth of invasion of the submucosal layer is associated with the possibility of lymph node metastasis, and it should be determined whether endoscopic procedures are to be performed. In this chapter, we will discuss indications and procedures for early CRC that can be treated with endoscopy.

The Risks of Lymph Node Metastasis

Presently, there are at least two classification systems to predict lymph node metastasis. The Kikuchi classification system is used for non-polypoid lesions and divides submucosal tissue into three layers: sm1, sm2, and sm3 (Fig. 1). The frequency of lymph node metastasis in sm1 and sm2 has been reported to be 2% and 8%, and the risk of lymph node metastasis in sm3 has been described as 12–25%. For non-pedunculated polyps, the depth of invasion >1 mm is widely accepted as a cutoff point for deep submucosal involvement and increased risk of LNM. A meta-analysis of studies investigating risk factors for LNM found that deep submucosal infiltration (>1 mm) was an independent risk

Yunho Jung is the lead author of this chapter.

H. J. Chun et al., *Gastrointestinal Cancer*, https://doi.org/10.1007/978-981-99-0815-8_36

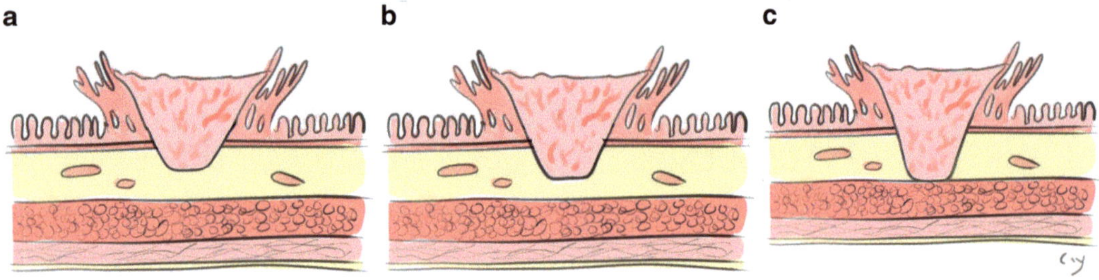

Fig. 1 The Kikuchi classification system is used for non-polypoid lesions and divides submucosal tissue into three layers. (**a**) sm1, upper third of submucosal tissue; (**b**) sm2, central third of submucosal tissue; and (**c**) sm3, lower third of submucosal tissue (adapted from Shaukat et al. [3])

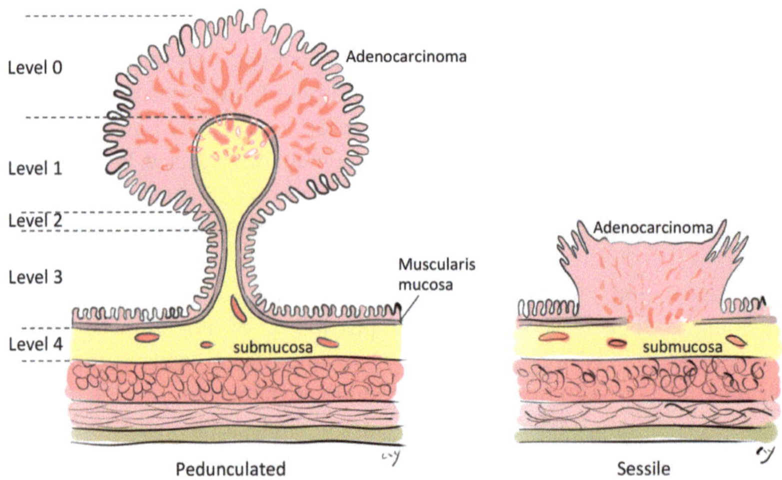

Fig. 2 Haggitt's classification is applicable in pedunculated polypoid lesions and defines the depth of invasion according to the following criteria: level 1, carcinoma invading through the muscularis mucosae but limited to the head of the polyp; level 2, carcinoma invading to the level of the neck (the junction of the head and stalk); level 3, carcinoma invading any part of the stalk; and level 4, carcinoma invading into the submucosa of the bowel wall below the level of the stalk but above the muscularis propria (adapted from Shaukat et al. [3])

factor for LNM (OR, 3.00; 95% CI, 1.36–6.62) [4]. The Korean Society of Gastrointestinal Endoscopy (KSGE) Task Force on Clinical Practice Guidelines and the US Multi-Society Task Force on Colorectal Cancer (MSTF) recommended that non-pedunculated malignant polyps be considered high risk for residual or recurrent cancer if they have any of the following features: poor histologic types (poorly differentiated adenocarcinoma, signet ring cell carcinoma, and mucinous carcinoma), submucosal invasion depth >1 mm, lymphovascular invasion, intermediate- to high-grade tumor growth, and tumor involvement of the cautery margin [3, 5]. Haggitt's classification is applicable in pedunculated polypoid lesions and defines the depth of invasion according to the following criteria: level 1 = carcinoma invading limited to the head of the polyp, level 2 = the neck, level 3 = stalk, and level 4 = the submucosa of the bowel wall below the level of the stalk but above the muscularis propria (Fig. 2). Invasion of Haggitt's levels 1 and 2 is known to have a low risk of lymph node metastasis, but level 3 is controversial according to the study results. The risk of lymph node metastasis at level 4 of Haggitt's classification is known to be about 27%. The US MSTF recommended that pedunculated malignant polyps should be considered at high risk of residual or recurrent cancer if they have any of the following features: poor tumor differentiation, lymphovascular invasion, and tumor within 1 mm of the resection margin [3].

Tumor Size and Morphology

Larger tumors have an increased risk of submucosal invasion. If the size of the lesion is <1.0 cm, the risk of submucosal invasion is <1%. However, in the case of polypoid lesions (type 0-Ip or 0-Is) with a diameter >2.0 cm, the risk of submucosal invasion is reported to be approximately 30% [6]. Laterally spreading tumors (LSTs) are classified as granular (LST-G) and nongranular (LST-NG) types, depending on the presence or absence of a granular surface pattern. Kudo et al. [7] proposed a subclassification of LSTs, in which LST-Gs are classified as homogeneous (LST-G-H) and nodular mixed subtypes (LST-G-N) and LST-NGs are classified as flat elevated (LST-NG-F) and pseudo-depressed subtypes (LST-NG-PD) (Fig. 3). According to the results of a recent study analyzing 2822 LSTs, the rates of submucosal invasive carcinoma were 0.8% in the LST-G-H, 15.2% in the LST-G-M, 8.0% in the LST-NG-F, and 42.5% in LST-NG-PD [9]. LST-Gs with a low submucosal invasion rate (7%) are generally observed under the largest nodules or depression and can be used to predict submucosal invasion before endoscopic treatment [10].

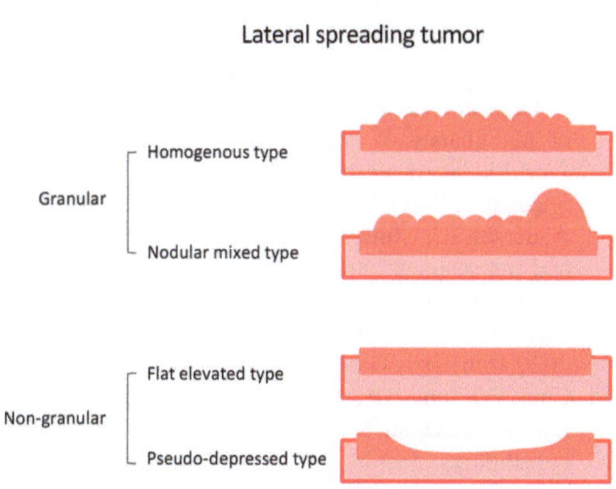

Fig. 3 Laterally spreading tumor (LST) and its subclassification in relation to macroscopic-type classification (adapted from Tanaka et al. [8])

Preoperative Evaluation of Lesions

Endoscopic findings with white light imaging suggestive of submucosal cancer were reported as loss of lobulation, excavation, swelling of the stalk, depressed delimitation area, fullness, fold convergence, and sign of non-lift [11]. As observed in the pit pattern classified by Kudo et al. [7], type Vi contains irregularly arranged pits that can be invasive mucosal or superficial submucosal invasive cancer and should be determined as appropriate between endoscopic and surgical treatments. The type Vn pit pattern contains unstructured pits. It presents with a large submucosal invasive cancer and requires surgical resection with lymph node dissection [12]. Narrowband imaging is an optical imaging technique that can enhance real-time visualization of mucosal surface structures, and vascular patterns can determine whether a lesion is neoplastic or non-neoplastic and its infiltration depth. The NBI International Colorectal Endoscopic (NICE) classification system has been well validated as a reliable and accurate measure for neoplasia classification and depth assessment [13]. In the case of NICE classification type 3, the risk of deep submucosal invasion is 93.5%, so surgical treatment is appropriate [12].

Endoscopic Resection Techniques

En bloc resection is the optimal treatment for colorectal tumors, especially adenocarcinomas, facilitating histopathological diagnosis and allowing proper assessment of vascular invasion and depth of vascular invasion. In addition, en bloc resection shows a lower recurrence rate than piecemeal resection [14].

Endoscopic Mucosal Resection

Endoscopic mucosal resection (EMR) is performed using a snare, usually after lifting the submucosal tissue of the lesion by fluid injection. Different sizes of snares and braids are available, depending on the size and morphology of the lesion. EMR is usually indicated for benign adenomas and small lesions (<20 mm) [15]. In these lesions, an en bloc resection rate of up to 80% can be achieved. The main advantages of EMR are the relatively short procedure times and an acceptable complication rate, with delayed bleeding in 0.9% and a perforation rate between 0.4 and 1.3% [16]. A recent meta-analysis reported that the mean risk of recurrence after EMR of non-pedunculated colorectal lesions is 15%, occurring in 3% of en bloc resections and 20% of piecemeal resections [14]. Therefore, the indication for EMR in CRC is for potential en bloc resection of lesions <20 mm.

Endoscopic Submucosal Dissection

Endoscopic submucosal dissection (ESD) involves the circumferential mucosal incision around the lesion or tumor followed by the stepwise dissection of the submucosa underneath the tumor and just above the proper muscle layer. Special knives are used depending on the preference of the endoscopist. This technique has advantages that enable en bloc resection regardless of tumor size. Pathologists can accurately assess the resection margins of the tissue removed en bloc in all directions. However, colorectal ESD is technically difficult due to the anatomical features of the colon, such as thin walls, folds and flexures, and colonic peristalsis. This technical difficulty is likely to be associated with complications, especially perforation. ESD has significantly better clinical outcomes than EMR with low recurrence rates of approximately 1.2% [17]. According to a recent meta-analysis evaluating the outcome of ESD in colorectal neoplasia, the en bloc resection rate was 91%, the R0 resection rate was 82.9%, the delayed bleeding rate was 2.7%, and the perforation rate was 5.2% [18]. ESD can be considered for colorectal lesions, particularly if the lesions are larger than 20 mm or cannot be removed otherwise by en bloc resection using snare EMR [19].

Table 1 Indications for endoscopic submucosal dissection of colorectal tumors

Lesions for which endoscopic en bloc resection is required
1. Lesions for which en bloc resection with snare EMR is difficult to apply
(a) LST-NG, particularly LST-NG (PD)
(b) Lesions showing a VI-type pit pattern
(c) Carcinoma with shallow T1 (SM) invasion
(d) Large depressed-type tumors
e) Large protruded-type lesions suspected to be carcinoma[a]
2. Mucosal tumors with submucosal fibrosis[b]
3. Sporadic tumors in conditions of chronic inflammation such as ulcerative colitis
4. Local residual or recurrent early carcinomas after endoscopic resection

EMR endoscopic mucosal resection, *LST-G* laterally spreading tumor granular type, *LST-NG* laterally spreading tumor nongranular type, *PD* pseudo-depressed, *SM* submucosal

Adapted from Tanaka et al. [19]

[a] Including LST-G, nodular mixed type

[b] As a result of a previous biopsy or prolapse caused by peristalsis of the intestine

Conclusion

To perform an appropriate endoscopic treatment for CRC, it is necessary to assess whether endoscopic treatment is possible considering lymph node metastasis through endoscopic findings, pit pattern, NBI findings, and imaging modalities. The appropriate endoscopic procedure should be selected according to the size and shape of the lesion (Table 1).

References

1. Morson BC, Whiteway JE, Jones EA, Macrae FA, Williams CB. Histopathology and prognosis of malignant colorectal polyps treated by endoscopic polypectomy. Gut. 1984;25:437–44.
2. Matsuda T, Saito Y, Fujii T, Uraoka T, Nakajima T, Kobayashi N, et al. Size does not determine the grade of malignancy of early invasive colorectal cancer. World J Gastroenterol. 2009;15:2708–13.
3. Shaukat A, Kaltenbach T, Dominitz JA, Robertson DJ, Anderson JC, Cruise M, et al. Endoscopic recognition and management strategies for malignant colorectal polyps: recommendations of the US Multi-Society Task Force on Colorectal Cancer. Gastroenterology. 2020;159:1916–34.e2.
4. Choi JY, Jung SA, Shim KN, Cho WY, Keum B, Byeon JS, et al. Meta-analysis of predictive clinicopathologic factors for lymph node metastasis in patients with early colorectal carcinoma. J Korean Med Sci. 2015;30:398–406.
5. Park CH, Yang DH, Kim JW, Kim JH, Kim JH, Min YW, et al. Clinical practice guideline for endoscopic

resection of early gastrointestinal cancer. Clin Endosc. 2020;53:142–66.
6. Anonymous. The Paris endoscopic classification of superficial neoplastic lesions: esophagus, stomach, and colon: November 30 to December 1, 2002. Gastrointest Endosc. 2003;58:S3–S43.
7. Kudo S, Lambert R, Allen JI, Fujii H, Fujii T, Kashida H, et al. Nonpolypoid neoplastic lesions of the colorectal mucosa. Gastrointest Endosc. 2008;68:S3–S47.
8. Tanaka S, Terasaki M, Hayashi N, Oka S, Chayama K. Warning for unprincipled colorectal endoscopic submucosal dissection: accurate diagnosis and reasonable treatment strategy. Dig Endosc. 2013;25:107–16.
9. Ishigaki T, Kudo SE, Miyachi H, Hayashi T, Minegishi Y, Toyoshima N, et al. Treatment policy for colonic laterally spreading tumors based on each clinicopathologic feature of 4 subtypes: actual status of pseudo-depressed type. Gastrointest Endosc. 2020;92:1083–94.e6.
10. Uraoka T, Saito Y, Matsuda T, Ikehara H, Gotoda T, Saito D, et al. Endoscopic indications for endoscopic mucosal resection of laterally spreading tumours in the colorectum. Gut. 2006;55:1592–7.
11. Ikehara H, Saito Y, Matsuda T, Uraoka T, Murakami Y. Diagnosis of depth of invasion for early colorectal cancer using magnifying colonoscopy. J Gastroenterol Hepatol. 2010;25:905–12.
12. Tanaka S, Hayashi N, Oka S, Chayama K. Endoscopic assessment of colorectal cancer with superficial or deep submucosal invasion using magnifying colonoscopy. Clin Endosc. 2013;46:138–46.
13. Hewett DG, Kaltenbach T, Sano Y, Tanaka S, Saunders BP, Ponchon T, et al. Validation of a simple classification system for endoscopic diagnosis of small colorectal polyps using narrow-band imaging. Gastroenterology. 2012;143:599–607.e1.
14. Belderbos TD, Leenders M, Moons LM, Siersema PD. Local recurrence after endoscopic mucosal resection of nonpedunculated colorectal lesions: systematic review and meta-analysis. Endoscopy. 2014;46:388–402.
15. Nakajima T, Saito Y, Tanaka S, Iishi H, Kudo SE, Ikematsu H, et al. Current status of endoscopic resection strategy for large, early colorectal neoplasia in Japan. Surg Endosc. 2013;27:3262–70.
16. Holmes I, Friedland S. Endoscopic mucosal resection versus endoscopic submucosal dissection for large polyps: a Western colonoscopist's view. Clin Endosc. 2016;49:454–6.
17. De Ceglie A, Hassan C, Mangiavillano B, Matsuda T, Saito Y, Ridola L, et al. Endoscopic mucosal resection and endoscopic submucosal dissection for colorectal lesions: a systematic review. Crit Rev Oncol Hematol. 2016;104:138–55.
18. Fuccio L, Hassan C, Ponchon T, Mandolesi D, Farioli A, Cucchetti A, et al. Clinical outcomes after endoscopic submucosal dissection for colorectal neoplasia: a systematic review and meta-analysis. Gastrointest Endosc. 2017;86:74–86.e17.
19. Tanaka S, Kashida H, Saito Y, Yahagi N, Yamano H, Saito S, et al. Japan Gastroenterological Endoscopy Society guidelines for colorectal endoscopic submucosal dissection/endoscopic mucosal resection. Dig Endosc. 2020;32:219–39.

Staging and Treatment. II-4. Surgical Treatment

Key Points

- The principles of oncologic resection include harvesting of adequate lymph nodes, ligating the supplying vessels at their origin, and obtaining adequate margins.
- Local excision of benign polyps and highly selected early rectal cancers is technically feasible and is associated with markedly reduced morbidity and mortality compared to radical surgery.
- With the introduction of total mesorectal excision and complete mesocolic excision, the outcome of colorectal cancer surgery has improved significantly.
- Several randomized controlled trials support the efficacy of minimally invasive colorectal cancer surgery with improved short-term results and noninferior oncologic outcomes compared to open surgery.

Introduction

Surgery is the mainstay curative treatment for patients with nonmetastatic colorectal cancer. Standardized surgical techniques have been developed to facilitate training and improve oncological outcomes. The introduction of total mesorectal excision (TME) resulted in a better postoperative outcome, a reduced local recurrence rate, and better overall survival (OS) for rectal cancer [1, 2].

The most significant contribution to improving the outcome of rectal cancer surgery may be the standardization and widespread implementation of TME. However, complete mesocolic excision (CME) for colon cancer surgery has not yet been universally adopted by surgeons, and data on long-term oncological outcomes are awaited. One of the most substantial recent developments in colorectal cancer (CRC) surgery is the implementation of a minimally invasive approach [3]. Randomized controlled trials have demonstrated the comparability of laparoscopic versus open surgery for CRC. With the recent evidence, noninferiority of the laparoscopic approach for TME could not be proven. In an attempt to improve the quality of TME, new surgical techniques, such as transanal total mesorectal excision and robotic surgery, are now widely performed [4, 5]. However, long-term oncological data is lacking.

In this chapter, the surgical management of nonmetastatic CRC will be reviewed.

Preoperative Planning: Tumor Localization

Tumor localization before planned surgery is necessary, especially with a minimally invasive approach when a tactile assessment is not an option for palpating a mass [6]. A tumor that does

Seung Yoon Yang is the lead author of this chapter.

H. J. Chun et al., *Gastrointestinal Cancer*, https://doi.org/10.1007/978-981-99-0815-8_37

not involve serosa is invisible intraoperatively, and manual palpation of the tumor during laparoscopy is impossible. Therefore, the accurate localization of the neoplastic infiltrate remains one of the most important tasks prior to elective laparoscopic surgery. India ink tattooing aids in intraoperative localization with a low risk of associated morbidity [7]. Although different techniques are used for tattooing, it is essential to be consistent in the marking method used and to record it in the colonoscopy report. Submucosal infiltration is critical for identification because tattooing in the mesentery or transmurally in the peritoneal cavity can obscure accurate marking. Intraoperative colonoscopy with laparoscopic assistance can be used when preoperative localization measures fail.

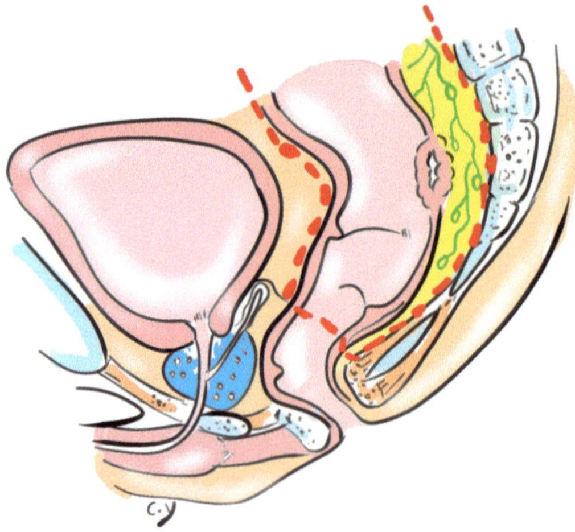

Fig. 1 Sagittal views of the rectum and mesorectum showing the correct plane for total mesorectal excision (adapted from Nelson et al. [9])

Oncologic Principles of Colorectal Cancer Surgery

Whatever the approach, minimally invasive or open, the basic principles for the oncologic resection of CRC include en bloc lymphadenectomy, ligation at the origin of the feeding vessels, and adequate proximal and distal resection margins [1, 2]. The purpose of central ligation of the primary feeding vessel is to maximize lymph node harvesting and excise all potential mesenteric nodal disease due to lateral migration of tumor cells within lymphatic drainage [8].

The introduction of total mesorectal excision by Sir Richard Heald revolutionized the surgical treatment for rectal cancer [2]. The fundamental principles of TME involve a sharp dissection under direct vision of the rectum with the mesorectum under the cover of the fascia propria, and a clear circumferential margin could be achieved. Sharp dissection was performed down to the levator muscles with the rectum and mesorectum excised at this level. By sharp dissection, excessive blood loss was avoided, which commonly occurs with blunt dissection and tearing of the presacral venous plexus. Regarding autonomic nerve preservation, sharp dissection enabled identification and preservation of the hypogastric nerves, as well as sacral nerves, in the bloodless operating field (Fig. 1). Thus, bladder and sexual functions have been significantly improved using this technique [10].

Heald hypothesized that local recurrence often resulted from microscopic tumor deposits within the mesorectum distal to the primary tumor. They proposed that excision of the entire mesorectum, total mesorectal excision (TME), would reduce the rate of local recurrence [2, 11]. Quirke et al. demonstrated that traditional pathological evaluation of rectal cancer specimens ignored the importance of the circumferential radial margin (CRM) [12]. They developed and promoted pathologic emphasis on evaluating the completeness of the mesorectal excision and the status of the radial margins.

CME technique is a newer concept that advocates sharp dissection of the visceral fascia from the parietal fascia of the retroperitoneum and central ligation of the primary vasculature [1]. This technique was first described by Hohenberger, who demonstrated a decrease in 5-year local recurrence and an improvement in 5-year survival from 6.5% to 3.6% and 82.1% to 89.1%, respectively. The adoption of CME is based on the learning from rectal cancer and the concept that cancers grow circumferentially and extend radially rather than longitudinally toward the embryologic planes of the specimen; therefore, the preservation of these planes of resection can decrease the risk of shedding tumor during dissection. CME with high ligation reports higher rates of lymph node harvest and increased resection of extranodal tumor deposits and upstaging, which improve locoregional control and survival [8, 13]. This technique has no confirmed benefit in prospective randomized trials and is not consistently adopted primarily because it is more technically demanding and requires extensive dissection, especially for right colectomy, in which the head of the pancreas and the anterior surface of the superior mesenteric vein and the superior mesenteric artery are exposed to perform a true central ligation of the ileocolic and middle colic vasculature [14, 15].

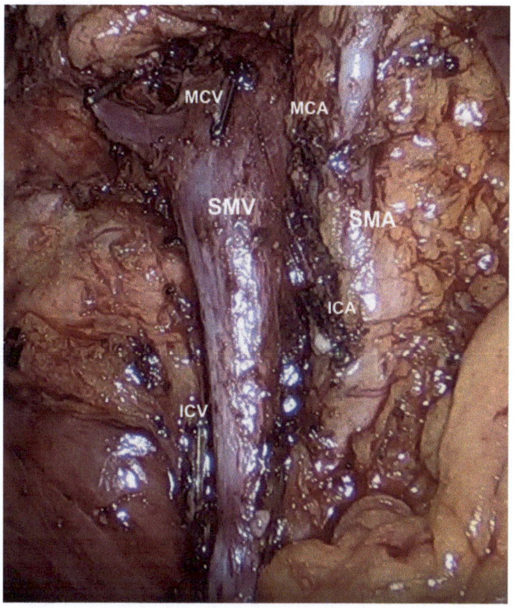

Fig. 2 Overview of the complete mesocolic excision procedure with the site of vascular ligation. Ascending colon cancer: only the right branch of the middle colic artery is ligated. Lymphadenectomy around the origin of the colic artery with complete exposure of the superior mesenteric vein (SMV)

Surgical Approach to Colon Cancers

Right Colon Cancers

Right colectomy is the procedure recommended for tumors proximal to the proximal transverse colon. The surgeon should explore the abdominal cavity to determine whether there is any distant metastasis, including liver, peritoneal, mesenteric, or pelvic metastases. CME is performed in either a lateral-to-medial or medial-to-lateral fashion, according to the surgeon's preference. The separation of the visceral fascia from the parietal fascia can be achieved through sharp dissection and ligation of the supplying vessels at their origin (Fig. 2). If the tumor infiltrates or adheres to the duodenum or perinephric fat tissue, to clear a possible tumor spread, complete Kocherization may be necessary. If the tumor is locally advanced, the entire prerenal soft tissue behind Gerota's fascia may need to be cleared, especially for tumors that grow posteriorly. After identifying the root of the middle colic artery, the site of vascular ligation depends on the location of the tumors. When the tumor is located in the cecum and ascending colon, only the right branch of the middle colic artery is ligated. If the tumor is present at these latter sites, the root of the middle colic artery is ligated. If the tumor is located in the ascending proximal colon or cecum, a suitable amount of branches of the distal ileum to the superior mesenteric artery (SMA) are needed in the specimen to obtain a longer distal ileum. As a result, the length of the distal ileum is determined by the extent of mesenteric dissection.

Transverse Colon Cancers

Transverse colon cancers are anatomically variable by the relationship of the tumor to two collateralizing vascular supplies with attendant variable lymphatic basins. Mobilization of the transverse colon is technically challenging due to the often foreshortened mesocolon that surrounds the pancreas and fragile middle colic vessels that are at risk of avulsion [16].

Until now, transverse colon cancer has been poorly studied, and transverse colon cancer cases are often excluded from large prospective randomized trials due to their complexity and the potentially high rate of complications [17]. For transverse colon cancer, a transverse colectomy or an extended hemicolectomy can be performed. For a colonic resection for transverse colon cancer to be complete, technically complicated passages are required to achieve lymph node dissection around the middle colic artery and to perform the difficult reconstruction of the bowel continuity. Presently, the best surgical approach for transverse colon cancer has not yet been established. Due to the lack of consistent data to compare the two approaches, the choice of which to perform must be based on the preference and experience of the surgeon.

Left Colon Cancers

The basic steps of left colectomy for colon cancer include abdominal examination to determine distant disease, ligation of the left colic artery and the inferior mesenteric vein at the inferior border of the pancreas with visualization and protection of the left ureter during these maneuvers, and complete mobilization of the left colon and splenic flexure to allow tension-free anastomosis. Various approaches can be used for proximal and distal transection. This procedure can be performed in an open approach through the handport. Alternatively, resection and anastomosis can be performed intracorporeally.

Surgical Approach to Rectal Cancers

Local Excision

Early rectal cancer management includes Tis, T1, and some selected T2 tumor lesions that undergo appropriate clinical preoperative evaluation [18]. Local excision can be defined as an organ preservation strategy that involves minimal dissection of early rectal cancer with good resection margins. Rectal dissection can be performed submucosally for benign lesions and in full thickness for neoplastic or malignant lesions. Local excision of these lesions with an acceptable rate of recurrence can be achieved by various transanal endoscopic techniques such as transanal endoscopic microsurgery (TEM) and minimally invasive transanal surgery (TAMIS) that are superior to simple transanal excision (TAE) [19, 20].

Local excision of early rectal cancers does not adequately remove or sample regional mesorectal lymph nodes. Preoperative prediction of lymph node positivity is crucial. Increased risk factors for lymph node metastasis and local recurrence include depth of invasion, lymphatic or vascular invasion, poor differentiation, tumor budding, and abnormal lymph nodes identified on imaging [21]. Due to imprecise staging and possibly a higher chance of positive resection margins, local excision results in a higher incidence of local recurrence compared to radical surgery. Patients who are unfit or unwilling to undergo radical surgery may choose an oncologically less sound local excision option to avoid the increased surgical complications related to radical surgery.

Low Anterior Resection

Dissection begins with medial to lateral mobilization of the left colon, including full mobilization of the splenic flexure and ligation of the inferior mesenteric vessels. TME requires a circumferential sharp dissection of the contents of the mesorectal fascia, beginning at the sacral promontory and proceeding to the pelvic floor. The pelvic splanchnic nerves and ureters are positioned laterally and must be protected from injury. The anterolateral ligaments that contain the middle hemorrhoidal vessels and splanchnic nerve branches are identified with medial traction of the rectum and should be divided away from the lateral pelvic sidewall to prevent damage to the nerve trunks. Sharp or cautery devices allow for precise dissection. For posterior tumors, anterior dissection begins immediately behind the Denonvilliers fascia, preserving nerves of sexual function that travel to the bladder, prostate, and sexual organs. For anterior tumors, dissection includes the Denonvilliers fascia, exposing the seminal vesicles or posterior vaginal wall to ensure a clear anterior margin at the expense of potential damage to urogenital function nerves (Fig. 3). The subsequent dissection is guided by

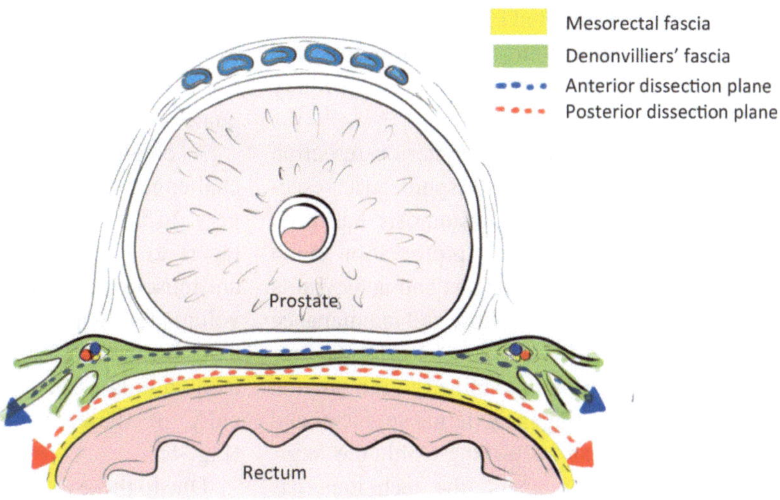

Fig. 3 Schematic representation of the relationships of the correct surgical plane during an anterior total mesorectal excision to the Denonvilliers fascia in the male (adapted from Yang et al. [22])

the extent of the cancer as seen on preoperative imaging. Dissection may continue over the surface of the levators into the upper anal canal if ultralow resection is needed or through the levators if an extralevator abdominoperineal resection is indicated. The completed TME is a circumferentially encased fascial envelope with a bilobed configuration of the posterior mesorectum.

Transanal TME

Oncological outcomes, particularly local disease control, in rectal cancer depend heavily on the acquisition of a quality TME specimen with an intact mesorectum and adequate radial and distal margins [12]. In particular, visualization can be difficult in an obese patient with a bulky tumor and a narrow pelvis, leaving limited space for pelvic dissection. Having an anteriorly located distal tumor can also complicate the situation for these patients by predisposing them to a higher risk of CRM involvement [23]. Furthermore, difficult introduction of instruments and poor ergonomics of the stapler in the pelvis are obstacles in ensuring a secure distal margin, which require multiple stapler firings that can result in asymmetrical staple lines and increased risk of anastomotic leakage [24].

In response to these challenges, transanal TME (taTME), referred to as "bottom-to-up" TME, was developed to provide a more direct approach to the most complicated phases of dissection in the distal rectum, to ensure an adequate distal resection margin, and to facilitate preservation of the sphincter [4, 5, 25]. Over the years, the taTME technique has undergone gradual refinements to allow for careful excision of low rectal tumors.

Penna et al. summarized the procedure in five essential steps: (1) placement of a distal circumferential purse string, (2) full-thickness rectotomy, (3) TME, (4) specimen extraction, and (5) anastomosis [26].

A recent meta-analysis recently showed that taTME was a feasible and safe method compared to lapTME for patients with mid- and low-rectal cancer, as patients undergoing taTME had a longer and lower positive CRM, a higher quality of resected TME, and shorter postoperative hospital stays [27]. Nonetheless, multicenter randomized controlled trials are needed to further assess the safety and efficiency of taTME.

Intersphincteric Resection and Coloanal Anastomosis

A better understanding of the anatomy of the sphincter, improved surgical techniques, and advances in CRT have led to the evolution of rectal cancer treatment from abdominoperineal resection (APR) to sphincter-preserving surgery (SPS) [28].

In recent years, ultralow anterior resection (uLAR) with or without intersphincteric resection (ISR) and coloanal anastomosis has been performed, allowing anal preservation with secure distal and radial margins and achieving a balance between oncologic cure and maintenance of anal function [29]. ISR is indicated for patients with distal rectal tumors confined to the internal sphincter, not affecting the external sphincter and located below the anorectal ring within the surgical canal. In recent years, the technique has undergone significant refinements and modifications. Partial removal of the external sphincter is also performed if there is invasion of the intersphincteric space and/or external sphincter muscles [30, 31] (Fig. 4a, b). The introduction of the ISR technique has challenged the conventional belief that adequate fecal continence requires the preservation of an intact internal sphincter. Moreover, it has offered a feasible alternative for patients who would otherwise need an APR. Despite the introduction of anal preservation with ISR, anal dysfunction remains a major concern. Low anterior resection syndrome (LARS), consisting of symptoms of stool frequency, fecal incontinence, or urgency, occurs frequently after sphincter-preserving operations [31]. Therefore, an assessment of anal function should be performed before planning this type of surgery and should take into account the patient's age and level of activity.

Abdominoperineal Resection

Traditionally, abdominoperineal resection (APR) has been deemed the standard surgical treatment for low-lying rectal cancers [33]. Advances in preoperative CRT and refinements in surgical skills led to a reduction in the number of patients undergoing the procedure; however, it is still indicated in patients with tumor invasion of the external anal sphincter and levator muscles and in those with poor anorectal function and inadequate response to CRT [28, 34].

A combination of anatomical and surgical challenges complicates conventional APR surgery. In the distal rectum, the mesorectal tissue tapers to approximately 2 cm above the levator ani muscles; thus, there is less protective tissue volume for the tumor to traverse before involving the CRM [35]. Moreover, the conventional APR technique is associated with the technical difficulty of dissecting deep in the pelvis [36] (Fig. 4c).

Due to these inherent challenges, APR is associated with oncologic outcomes that are inferior to those of low anterior resection, as well as with higher risks of intraoperative perforations and CRM involvement [35, 36].

The ELAPE surgical technique closely resembles Miles' original operation, which involves careful mobilization of the mesorectum to the level of the levator muscles; however, in this approach, the abdominal and perineal dissections meet just above the levator muscles, leaving the levators attached to the mesorectum and creating a cylindrical specimen with more tissue covering the tumor in the distal rectum [36] (Fig. 4d). The perineal phase of the procedure is executed with the patient in the prone position. The extended perineal dissection follows the inferior surface of the levator muscles up to the level of the abdominal dissection termination. To enhance visualization, the coccyx is usually removed along with the main specimen. In cases where primary closure is not feasible, a reconstruction of the gluteus maximus flap of the pelvic floor is performed to cover the perineal defect [37]. The results of a randomized trial of a single institution and a recent meta-analysis of several case series indicate that ELAPE is associated with lower rates of intraoperative perforation, lower rates of positive CRM and local recurrence, and similar complication rates compared to conventional APR [38, 39].

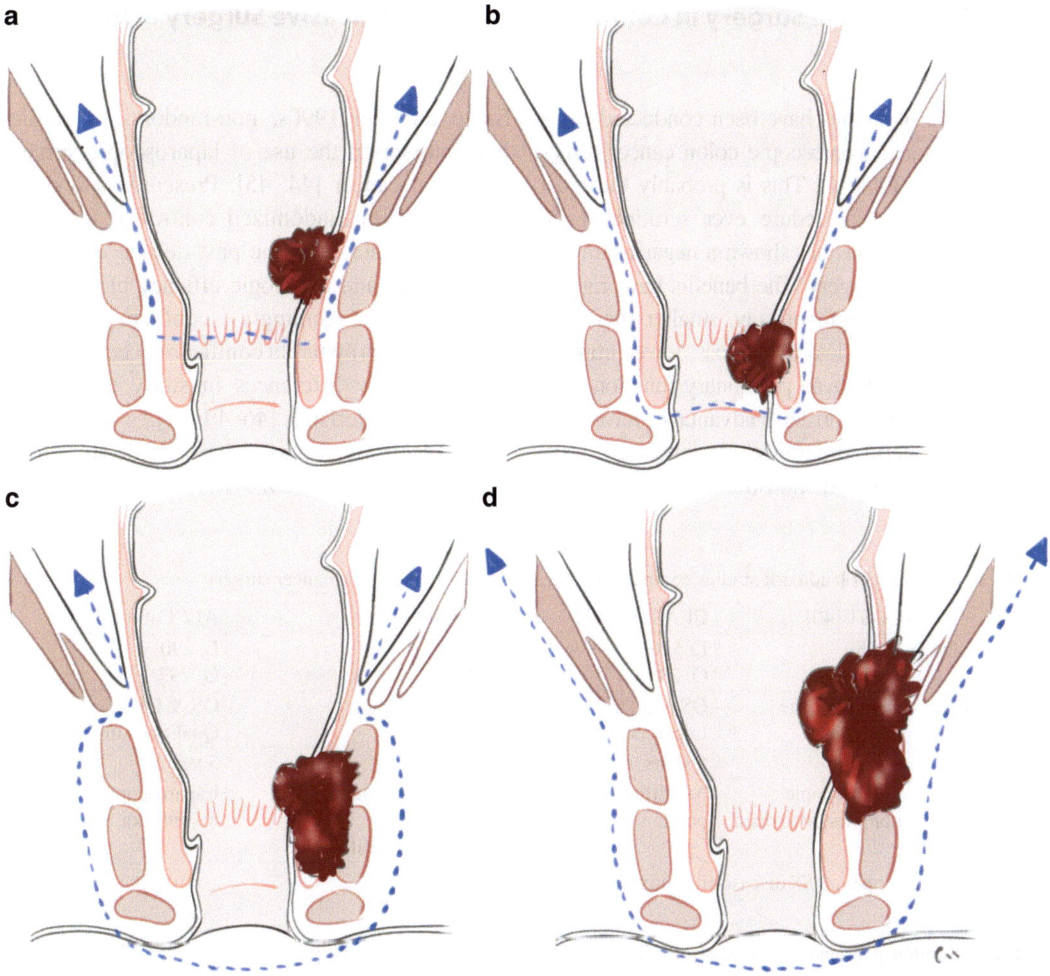

Fig. 4 Schematic of surgical options for low-lying rectal cancer. (**a**) Partial ISR, (**b**) total ISR for a tumor invading the internal sphincter, and (**c**) abdominal perineal resection for a tumor invading beyond the internal sphincter. (**d**) Extralevator abdominoperineal resection for a tumor invading both the levator ani muscle and the external sphincter muscle (adapted from Noh et al. [32]). *ISR* intersphincteric resection

Minimally Invasive Colorectal Cancer Surgery

In traditional open abdominal surgeries, surgeons typically make an incision 6–12 inches in length, large enough to offer adequate visibility, provide access to the abdominal organs, and allow the use of handheld surgical instruments. Minimally invasive surgical approaches have been developed to perform operations through smaller incisions, reducing the discomfort and healing complications associated with long incisions. Minimally invasive surgery can be used to effectively treat a variety of common benign and malignant colon and rectal conditions. All minimally invasive techniques require advanced surgical skills and specialized equipment.

Minimally Invasive Surgery in Colon Cancer

A multitude of studies have been conducted comparing open and laparoscopic colon cancer resection [40–43] (Table 1). This is probably the most intensely studied procedure ever scrutinized. In none of these studies has shown a negative impact on laparoscopic surgery. The benefits have ranged from decreased length of stay, smaller incisions, less narcotic usage, less blood loss, lower transfusion rates, and improved pulmonary function after surgery. Although short-term advantages have been shown, long-term differences in oncologic outcomes have not been demonstrated.

Minimally Invasive Surgery in Rectal Cancer

Since the late 1990s, non-randomized studies have supported the use of laparoscopic surgery for rectal cancer [44, 45]. Presently, a body of research from randomized controlled trials has been accumulated in the past decade evaluating the surgical and oncologic efficacy of this technique with seemingly conflicting results (Table 2). This apparent conflict may be explained by significant differences in study design and patient characteristics [46–49, 51].

The Robotic versus Laparoscopic Resection for Rectal Cancer (ROLARR) trial investigated

Table 1 Summary of landmark studies comparing open and laparoscopic colon cancer surgery

Trial	COST [40]	CLASSIC [41]	COLOR [42]	ALCCaS [43]
Sample size	L: 289 O: 287	L: 526 O: 268	L: 627 O: 621	L: 290 O: 297
End points	Quality of life DFS	OS and DFS Local recurrence	DFS	OS & DFS Quality of life
Follow-up	3 years	5 years	5 years	5 years
Conclusions	Laparoscopic noninferior to open	No difference in end points	Unable to conclude noninferior Small clinical difference	Laparoscopic noninferior to open

L laparoscopic, *O* open, *DFS* disease-free survival, *OS* overall survival

Table 2 Summary of landmark studies of minimally invasive rectal cancer surgery

Trial	COLOR II [46]	COREAN [47]	ALaCaRt [48]	ACOSOG Z6051 [49]	ROLARR [50]
Sample size	L: 739 O: 364	L: 170 O: 170	L: 238 O: 237	L: 240 O: 222	R: 237 L: 234
End points	Short-term outcomes Genitourinary function Oncologic outcomes	Involvement of CRM Completeness of TME Recovery of bowel function Quality of life	Oncologic outcomes	CRM, DRM Completeness of TME Oncologic outcomes	Conversion to open Short-term outcomes Pathological outcomes Quality of life Genitourinary function
Follow-up	3 years	3 years	N.A	47.9 months (median)	30 days, 6 months
Conclusions	• Similar safety, resection margins • Improved recovery after laparoscopy • No change in genitourinary function • Similar DFS	• Equivalent quality of resection • Improved short-term outcomes (laparoscopic) • Similar DFS	• Laparoscopic noninferior to open	• Use of laparoscopy compared to open surgery failed to meet the criteria for noninferiority • Similar oncologic outcomes	• Robotic surgery did not significantly reduce the risk of conversion to open surgery

L laparoscopic, *O* open, *R* robotic, *CRM* circumferential resection margin, *TME* total mesorectal excision, *DRM* distal resection margin, *DFS* disease-free survival

the safety, efficacy, and outcomes of robotic versus laparoscopic rectal cancer surgery [50]. This international, multicenter, prospective, randomized controlled trial compared the two minimally invasive approaches for the risk of conversion to open procedure, with secondary end points that included intraoperative and postoperative complications, as well as pathological, functional, and short-term oncologic outcomes. The initial results of the study found that the robotic approach did not significantly reduce the risk of conversion to open procedure compared to laparoscopic resection, suggesting that robotic-assisted surgery, performed by surgeons with varying degrees of experience, did not offer an advantage over laparoscopy.

Conclusion

The surgical management of CRC has evolved substantially in the past 100 years and continues to progress as surgeons seek the best treatment. With the introduction of total mesorectal excision and CME, the outcome of CRC surgery has improved significantly. Furthermore, the increasing surgical treatment options for CRC and quality of life have become a major issue; therefore, tailored treatment that takes into account both oncological and anticipated functional outcomes is essential.

References

1. Hohenberger W, Weber K, Matzel K, Papadopoulos T, Merkel S. Standardized surgery for colonic cancer: complete mesocolic excision and central ligation—technical notes and outcome. Color Dis. 2009;11:354–64; discussion 64–5.
2. Heald RJ, Husband EM, Ryall RD. The mesorectum in rectal cancer surgery—the clue to pelvic recurrence? Br J Surg. 1982;69:613–6.
3. Addison P, Agnew JL, Martz J. Robotic colorectal surgery. Surg Clin North Am. 2020;100:337–60.
4. Simillis C, Hompes R, Penna M, Rasheed S, Tekkis PP. A systematic review of transanal total mesorectal excision: is this the future of rectal cancer surgery? Color Dis. 2016;18:19–36.
5. Sylla P, Rattner DW, Delgado S, Lacy AM. NOTES transanal rectal cancer resection using transanal endoscopic microsurgery and laparoscopic assistance. Surg Endosc. 2010;24:1205–10.
6. Cho YB, Lee WY, Yun HR, Lee WS, Yun SH, Chun HK. Tumor localization for laparoscopic colorectal surgery. World J Surg. 2007;31:1491–5.
7. Botoman VA, Pietro M, Thirlby RC. Localization of colonic lesions with endoscopic tattoo. Dis Colon Rectum. 1994;37:775–6.
8. West NP, Morris EJ, Rotimi O, Cairns A, Finan PJ, Quirke P. Pathology grading of colon cancer surgical resection and its association with survival: a retrospective observational study. Lancet Oncol. 2008;9:857–65.
9. Nelson H, Sargent DJ. Refining multimodal therapy for rectal cancer. N Engl J Med. 2001;345:690–2.
10. Junginger T, Kneist W, Heintz A. Influence of identification and preservation of pelvic autonomic nerves in rectal cancer surgery on bladder dysfunction after total mesorectal excision. Dis Colon Rectum. 2003;46:621–8.
11. Heald RJ, Ryall RD. Recurrence and survival after total mesorectal excision for rectal cancer. Lancet. 1986;1:1479–82.
12. Quirke P, Durdey P, Dixon MF, Williams NS. Local recurrence of rectal adenocarcinoma due to inadequate surgical resection. Histopathological study of lateral tumour spread and surgical excision. Lancet. 1986;2:996–9.
13. West NP, Hohenberger W, Weber K, Perrakis A, Finan PJ, Quirke P. Complete mesocolic excision with central vascular ligation produces an oncologically superior specimen compared with standard surgery for carcinoma of the colon. J Clin Oncol. 2010;28:272–8.
14. Sun KK, Zhao H. Vascular anatomical variation in laparoscopic right hemicolectomy. Asian J Surg. 2020;43:9–12.
15. Rosenberg J, Fischer A, Haglind E. Current controversies in colorectal surgery: the way to resolve uncertainty and move forward. Color Dis. 2012;14:266–9.
16. Milone M, Manigrasso M, Elmore U, Maione F, Gennarelli N, Rondelli F, et al. Short- and long-term outcomes after transverse versus extended colectomy for transverse colon cancer. A systematic review and meta-analysis. Int J Color Dis. 2019;34:201–7.
17. Sjo OH, Lunde OC, Nygaard K, Sandvik L, Nesbakken A. Tumour location is a prognostic factor for survival in colonic cancer patients. Color Dis. 2008;10:33–40.
18. Morino M, Risio M, Bach S, Beets-Tan R, Bujko K, Panis Y, et al. Early rectal cancer: the European Association for Endoscopic Surgery (EAES) clinical consensus conference. Surg Endosc. 2015;29:755–73.
19. Rai V, Mishra N. Transanal approach to rectal polyps and cancer. Clin Colon Rectal Surg. 2016;29:65–70.
20. Lee L, Edwards K, Hunter IA, Hartley JE, Atallah SB, Albert MR, et al. Quality of local excision for rectal neoplasms using transanal endoscopic microsurgery versus transanal minimally invasive surgery: a multi-

institutional matched analysis. Dis Colon Rectum. 2017;60:928–35.
21. São Julião GP, Celentano JP, Alexandre FA, Vailati BB. Local excision and endoscopic resections for early rectal cancer. Clin Colon Rectal Surg. 2017;30:313–23.
22. Yang SY, Kim HS, Cho MS, Kim NK. Three-dimensional anatomy of the Denonvilliers' fascia after micro-CT reconstruction. Sci Rep. 2021;11:21759.
23. Perez RO, Habr-Gama A, São Julião GP, Proscurshim I, Fernandez LM, de Azevedo RU, et al. Transanal endoscopic microsurgery (TEM) following neoadjuvant chemoradiation for rectal cancer: outcomes of salvage resection for local recurrence. Ann Surg Oncol. 2016;23:1143–8.
24. Suwanabol PA, Maykel JA. Transanal total mesorectal excision: a novel approach to rectal surgery. Clin Colon Rectal Surg. 2017;30:120–9.
25. Marks JH, Myers EA, Zeger EL, Denittis AS, Gummadi M, Marks GJ. Long-term outcomes by a transanal approach to total mesorectal excision for rectal cancer. Surg Endosc. 2017;31:5248–57.
26. Penna M, Cunningham C, Hompes R. Transanal total mesorectal excision: why, when, and how. Clin Colon Rectal Surg. 2017;30:339–45.
27. Xu W, Xu Z, Cheng H, Ying J, Cheng F, Xu W, et al. Comparison of short-term clinical outcomes between transanal and laparoscopic total mesorectal excision for the treatment of mid and low rectal cancer: a meta-analysis. Eur J Surg Oncol. 2016;42:1841–50.
28. Smith JJ, Garcia-Aguilar J. Advances and challenges in treatment of locally advanced rectal cancer. J Clin Oncol. 2015;33:1797–808.
29. Schiessel R, Karner-Hanusch J, Herbst F, Teleky B, Wunderlich M. Intersphincteric resection for low rectal tumours. Br J Surg. 1994;81:1376–8.
30. Akagi Y, Kinugasa T, Oka Y, Mizobe T, Yoshida T, Yuge K, et al. External sphincter resection for lower rectal and anal canal adenocarcinoma: achieving anal preservation with oncological and functional satisfaction. Surg Today. 2014;44:1385–8.
31. Akagi Y, Kinugasa T, Shirouzu K. Intersphincteric resection for very low rectal cancer: a systematic review. Surg Today. 2013;43:838–47.
32. Noh GT, Han K, Cheong C, Han YD, Kim NK. Novel anal sphincter saving procedure with partial excision of levator-ani muscle in rectal cancer invading ipsilateral pelvic floor. Ann Surg Treat Res. 2017;93:195–202.
33. Miles WE. A method of performing abdomino-perineal excision for carcinoma of the rectum and of the terminal portion of the pelvic colon (1908). CA Cancer J Clin. 1971;21:361–4.
34. Hawkins AT, Albutt K, Wise PE, Alavi K, Sudan R, Kaiser AM, et al. Abdominoperineal resection for rectal cancer in the twenty-first century: indications, techniques, and outcomes. J Gastrointest Surg. 2018;22:1477–87.
35. Nagtegaal ID, van de Velde CJ, Marijnen CA, van Krieken JH, Quirke P. Low rectal cancer: a call for a change of approach in abdominoperineal resection. J Clin Oncol. 2005;23:9257–64.
36. West NP, Finan PJ, Anderin C, Lindholm J, Holm T, Quirke P. Evidence of the oncologic superiority of cylindrical abdominoperineal excision for low rectal cancer. J Clin Oncol. 2008;26:3517–22.
37. Holm T, Ljung A, Häggmark T, Jurell G, Lagergren J. Extended abdominoperineal resection with gluteus maximus flap reconstruction of the pelvic floor for rectal cancer. Br J Surg. 2007;94:232–8.
38. Han JG, Wang ZJ, Wei GH, Gao ZG, Yang Y, Zhao BC. Randomized clinical trial of conventional versus cylindrical abdominoperineal resection for locally advanced lower rectal cancer. Am J Surg. 2012;204:274–82.
39. Yu HC, Peng H, He XS, Zhao RS. Comparison of short- and long-term outcomes after extralevator abdominoperineal excision and standard abdominoperineal excision for rectal cancer: a systematic review and meta-analysis. Int J Color Dis. 2014;29:183–91.
40. Weeks JC, Nelson H, Gelber S, Sargent D, Schroeder G. Short-term quality-of-life outcomes following laparoscopic-assisted colectomy vs open colectomy for colon cancer: a randomized trial. JAMA. 2002;287:321–8.
41. Jayne DG, Thorpe HC, Copeland J, Quirke P, Brown JM, Guillou PJ. Five-year follow-up of the Medical Research Council CLASICC trial of laparoscopically assisted versus open surgery for colorectal cancer. Br J Surg. 2010;97:1638–45.
42. Buunen M, Veldkamp R, Hop WC, Kuhry E, Jeekel J, Haglind E, et al. Survival after laparoscopic surgery versus open surgery for colon cancer: long-term outcome of a randomised clinical trial. Lancet Oncol. 2009;10:44–52.
43. Bagshaw PF, Allardyce RA, Frampton CM, Frizelle FA, Hewett PJ, McMurrick PJ, et al. Long-term outcomes of the australasian randomized clinical trial comparing laparoscopic and conventional open surgical treatments for colon cancer: the Australasian Laparoscopic Colon Cancer Study trial. Ann Surg. 2012;256:915–9.
44. Baik SH, Kwon HY, Kim JS, Hur H, Sohn SK, Cho CH, et al. Robotic versus laparoscopic low anterior resection of rectal cancer: short-term outcome of a prospective comparative study. Ann Surg Oncol. 2009;16:1480–7.
45. Patriti A, Ceccarelli G, Bartoli A, Spaziani A, Biancafarina A, Casciola L. Short- and medium-term outcome of robot-assisted and traditional laparoscopic rectal resection. JSLS. 2009;13:176–83.
46. van der Pas MH, Haglind E, Cuesta MA, Furst A, Lacy AM, Hop WC, et al. Laparoscopic versus open surgery for rectal cancer (COLOR II): short-term outcomes of a randomised, phase 3 trial. Lancet Oncol. 2013;14:210–8.

47. Kang SB, Park JW, Jeong SY, Nam BH, Choi HS, Kim DW, et al. Open versus laparoscopic surgery for mid or low rectal cancer after neoadjuvant chemoradiotherapy (COREAN trial): short-term outcomes of an open-label randomised controlled trial. Lancet Oncol. 2010;11:637–45.
48. Stevenson AR, Solomon MJ, Lumley JW, Hewett P, Clouston AD, Gebski VJ, et al. Effect of laparoscopic-assisted resection vs open resection on pathological outcomes in rectal cancer: the ALaCaRT randomized clinical trial. JAMA. 2015;314:1356–63.
49. Fleshman J, Branda M, Sargent DJ, Boller AM, George V, Abbas M, et al. Effect of laparoscopic-assisted resection vs open resection of stage II or III rectal cancer on pathologic outcomes: the ACOSOG Z6051 randomized clinical trial. JAMA. 2015;314:1346–55.
50. Jayne D, Pigazzi A, Marshall H, Croft J, Corrigan N, Copeland J, et al. Effect of robotic-assisted vs conventional laparoscopic surgery on risk of conversion to open laparotomy among patients undergoing resection for rectal cancer: the ROLARR randomized clinical trial. JAMA. 2017;318:1569–80.
51. Bonjer HJ, Deijen CL, Abis GA, Cuesta MA, van der Pas MH, de Lange-de Klerk ES, et al. A randomized trial of laparoscopic versus open surgery for rectal cancer. N Engl J Med. 2015;372:1324–32.

Staging and Treatment. II-5. Adjuvant Chemotherapy

Key Points

- The goal of postoperative (adjuvant) therapy is to eradicate these micrometastases, thus increasing the cure rate of colorectal cancer.
- The benefits of adjuvant chemotherapy have been demonstrated most clearly in stage III colorectal cancer.
- We recommend a course of adjuvant chemotherapy in addition to chemoradiotherapy after resection of stage II or III rectal cancer (grade 1A).
- For patients who can tolerate it, in keeping with the NCCN guidelines, an oxaliplatin-containing regimen (oxaliplatin plus short-term 5-FU infusion and leucovorin [FOLFOX] or capecitabine plus oxaliplatin [CAPOX]) is recommended for patients with node-positive or T4 disease (grade 2B).

Introduction

Carcinoma of the colon or rectum (colorectal cancer [CRC]) is a common and lethal disease in Korea and the United States. Global- and country-specific data on incidence and mortality are available from the World Health Organization (WHO) GLOBOCAN database.

Surgical resection is the primary treatment modality for early-stage CRC (stages I through III), and the most powerful tool to assess prognosis after potentially curative surgery is pathologic analysis of the resected specimen. In addition, the pathology of CRC and the major determinants of prognosis after surgical resection are important to decide next-step treatment (Table 1).

The clinical and postoperative pathological findings are considered the clinicopathologic factors that define "high-risk" stage II colon cancer by the ASCO [1], NCCN [2], or the ESMO guidelines [3] (Table 2).

The prognostic value of a wide variety of promising and potentially clinically applicable molecular markers has been studied in CRC [4] (Table 3), including:

- DNA content (aneuploidy)
- Tumor suppressor genes (LOH 1p, LOH 8p, LOH 5q, *SMAD4*, *TP53* gene)
- Oncogenes other than *RAS* and *BRAF* (e.g., *c-MYC*)
- Apoptosis/cell suicide-related genes (*Bcl-2*; *BAX*; apoptosis protease-activating factor-1 [*APAF1*])
- DNA synthesis-related genes (thymidylate synthetase; thymidine phosphorylase)
- Growth factors and growth factor receptor genes (transforming growth factors a and b, human epidermal growth factor receptor-2 [*HER2*])

Eun Sun Kim is the lead author of this chapter.

H. J. Chun et al., *Gastrointestinal Cancer*, https://doi.org/10.1007/978-981-99-0815-8_38

Table 1 World Health Organization (WHO) classification of tumors of the colon and rectum

Benign epithelial tumors and precursors	Malignant epithelial tumors
Serrated dysplasia, low grade	Adenocarcinoma NOS
Serrated dysplasia, high grade	Serrated adenocarcinoma
Hyperplastic polyp, microvesicular type	Adenoma-like adenocarcinoma
Hyperplastic polyp, goblet cell	Micropapillary adenocarcinoma
Adenomatous polyp, low-grade dysplasia	Mucinous adenocarcinoma
Adenomatous polyp, high-grade dysplasia	Poorly cohesive carcinoma
Tubular adenoma, low grade	Signet-ring cell carcinoma
Tubular adenoma, high grade	Medullary adenocarcinoma
Villous adenoma, low grade	Adenosquamous carcinoma
Villous adenoma, high grade	Carcinoma, undifferentiated, NOS
Tubulovillous adenoma, low grade	Carcinoma with sarcomatoid component
Tubulovillous adenoma, high grade	Neuroendocrine tumor NOS
Advanced adenoma	Neuroendocrine tumor, grade 1
Glandular intraepithelial neoplasia, low grade	Neuroendocrine tumor, grade 2
Glandular intraepithelial neoplasia, high grade	Neuroendocrine tumor, grade 1
	L cell tumor
	Glucagon-like peptide-producing tumor
	PP/PYY-producing tumor
	Enterochromaffin cell carcinoid
	Serotonin-producing tumor
	Neuroendocrine carcinoma NOS
	Large-cell neuroendocrine carcinoma
	Small-cell neuroendocrine carcinoma
	Mixed neuroendocrine-non-neuroendocrine neoplasm (MiNEN)

NOS not otherwise specified, *PP* pancreatic polypeptide, *PYY* peptide YY
Adapted from WHO classification of Tumours, Digestive System Tumours, 5th ed.

Table 2 Definitions of "high-risk" stage II colon cancer from expert groups

	ASCO [1]	NCCN [2]	ESMO [3]
T4 primary tumor	+	+	+ (major)
Inadequately sampled nodes	+ (<13)	+ (<12)	+ (major) (<12)
Poorly differentiated tumor	+	+	+ (minor)
Perforation	+	+ (localized)	+ (major)
Obstruction		+	+ (minor)
Lymphovascular invasion	+	+	+ (minor)
Perineural invasion	+	+	+ (minor)
Close/indeterminate or positive margins		+	
High preoperative levels of serum CEA			+ (minor)

ASCO American Society of Clinical Oncology, *NCCN* National Comprehensive Cancer Network, *ESMO* European Society for Medical Oncology, *CEA* carcinoembryonic antigen

- Cyclins and cyclin-dependent kinase inhibitor genes (p27; p21)
- Angiogenesis-related genes (vascular endothelial growth factor [VEGF])
- Adhesion molecule and glycoprotein genes (CD44; E-cadherin [*CDH1*]; sialo-Tn antigen)
- Matrix metalloproteinases and their inhibitors (MMPs; urokinase-type plasminogen activator)
- Metastasis suppressor genes (e.g., *NM23H1B*)
- Overexpression of and high circulating levels of microRNA
- Epigenetic aberrations such as methylation levels
- Peroxisome proliferator-activated receptor-gamma (*PPARG*)
- Circulating tumor DNA
- Soluble type IV collagen
- Deletions in 18q

Table 3 Molecular classification of colorectal carcinoma

	Chromosomal instability pathway	Mismatch repair pathway	Serrated//CIMP pathway		Hybrid pathway
Heredity	Hereditary and sporadic	Hereditary	Hereditary and sporadic		Sporadic
CIMP status	Negative	Negative	High	High	Low
MSI status	MSS	MSI-H	MSI-H	MSI-L	MSI-L or MSS
Chromosomal instability	Present	Absent	Absent	Absent	Present
KRAS mutation	Present	Present or absent	Absent	Absent	Present
BRAF mutation	Absent	Absent	Present	Present	Absent
MLH1 status	Normal	Mutation	Methylated	Partial methylation	Normal

CIMP CpG island methylator phenotype, *MSS* microsatellite stability, *MSI* microsatellite instability, *MSI-H* high-level microsatellite instability, *MSI-L* low-level microsatellite instability
Adapted from Noffsinger et al. [4]

Most tumors of the colon and rectum are carcinomas. Other histological types (neuroendocrine neoplasms, hamartomas, mesenchymal tumors, and lymphomas) are relatively unusual. Of the carcinomas, more than 90% are adenocarcinomas. Cytokeratin (CK) 20 and caudal-type homeobox 2 (CDX2) are two of the most sensitive and specific markers of intestinal differentiation and are extremely useful immunohistochemical (IHC) markers to correctly identify colorectal origin adenocarcinomas [5–7]. IHC for CK20 and CK7 can be particularly helpful in the differential diagnosis of a primary appendiceal malignancy versus mucinous ovarian cancer.

The most important pathological characteristics are the presence of distant metastases, local tumor extent, nodal positivity (particularly the number of lymph nodes), residual disease, extramural tumor deposits, lymphovascular and perineural invasion, histologic differentiation grade, and, for patients treated with neoadjuvant therapy prior to rectal cancer resection, tumor regression grade.

Among patients receiving neoadjuvant (presurgical) treatment for rectal cancer, the posttreatment stage is a more accurate predictor of outcome than the pretreatment clinical stage. Five-year survival according to pathological stage after chemoradiotherapy for rectal cancer is outlined in Table 4 [8].

Surgical resection is the only curative treatment for locoregional colon cancer. The outcome is more closely related to the extent of the disease at the time of presentation.

Table 4 The 5- and 10-year disease-free survival (DFS) according to posttreatment pathological stage (yp) and tumor regression grade (TRG) at resection after neoadjuvant chemoradiotherapy in the German Rectal Cancer Study Group (CAO/ARO/AIO-94) trial

yp category	5-year DFS (%)	10-year DFS (%)
ypT		
T0	86	90
T1	95	95
T2	81	78
T3	65	66
T4	42	40
ypN		
N0	85	84
N1	65	59
N2	18	28
TRG		
4	86	90
2–3	75	74
0–1	63	63

Adapted from Fokas et al. [8]

Adjuvant Therapy for Stage III (Node-Positive) Resected Colon Cancer

The goal of postoperative (adjuvant) therapy is to eradicate these micrometastases, thus increasing the cure rate. The benefits of adjuvant chemotherapy have been demonstrated most clearly in stage

III, in which fluoropyrimidine-based adjuvant chemotherapy provides an approximately 30% reduction in the risk of disease recurrence and a 22–32% reduction in mortality [9]. The European Society of Medical Oncology suggests that adjuvant therapy should be initiated as soon as possible after surgery and ideally no later than 8 weeks [2]. We recommend an oxaliplatin-based regimen, rather than a fluoropyrimidine-based regimen alone, for fit patients with resected stage III disease who are younger than 70 years of age and likely to tolerate oxaliplatin and for those whose tumors are mismatch repair enzyme deficient (dMMR) or microsatellite unstable. In the context of dMMR colon cancer, fluoropyrimidines alone are ineffective for adjuvant therapy. FOLFOX (oxaliplatin plus leucovorin [LV] and short-term infusion of 5-fluorouracil [FU]) is a widely accepted standard regimen for stage III resected colon cancer and represents our preferred regimen when 6 months of adjuvant therapy is chosen. Oxaliplatin plus oral capecitabine (CAPOX, also known as XELOX) may be more toxic, but it may be selected over FOLFOX if a shorter course of adjuvant therapy (e.g., 3 months) is chosen or if an ambulatory infusion pump is not feasible.

The optimal duration of adjuvant oxaliplatin chemotherapy for patients with stage III colon cancer is evolving, and the following issues inform the decision:

- Based on the MOSAIC and NSABP C-07 trials and an analysis of the International Duration Evaluation of Adjuvant Chemotherapy (IDEA) collaboration (six separate randomized trials of 6 versus 3 months of adjuvant oxaliplatin-based therapy), we continue to suggest 6 months of therapy for individuals with high-risk cancers (T4N2). The International Duration Evaluation of Adjuvant Chemotherapy (IDEA) analysis suggests limiting adjuvant therapy to 3 months in patients with low-risk disease (T1-3N1) and suggests that CAPOX/XELOX may be a better choice than FOLFOX for adjuvant therapy of 3 months [9]. The cumulative and dose-limiting peripheral neuropathy associated with oxaliplatin (13% grade 3 neuropathy with 6 months of FOLFOX in the MOSAIC trial [10]) indicated that a shorter duration of therapy might be advantageous if equally effective. For patients with preexisting neuropathy or who are considered unlikely to tolerate oxaliplatin or who do not have deficient mismatch repair (dMMR) status, a fluoropyrimidine alone is an acceptable option compared to 6 months of short-term infusional FU/LV.

Adjuvant Chemotherapy for Resected Stage II Colon Cancer

When assessing the risk of recurrence and the potential benefit of chemotherapy, factors that should be considered include: the number of lymph nodes analyzed; the presence of high-risk clinicopathologic features (such as fewer than 12 nodes in the surgical specimen, T4 or perforated/obstructed lesion, poorly differentiated histology [including signet-ring and mucinous, as long as they are not microsatellite instability (MSI)-unstable], lymphovascular or perineural invasion); MMR status; the presence of a V600E BRAF mutation (for patients with proficient MMR [pMMR]/microsatellite stable tumors); and evaluation of other comorbidities and anticipated life expectancy.

Based on the available data, adjuvant chemotherapy cannot be considered a standard of care for all patients with resected stage II disease according to the guidelines of the National Comprehensive Cancer Network (NCCN) [2, 11] (Table 5).

Table 5 Predicted 5-year DFS estimates for patients with node-negative colon cancer

	Low grade		High grade	
Disease stage	Surgery, alone (%)	Surgery and chemotherapy (%)	Surgery, alone (%)	Surgery and chemotherapy (%)
T3N0	73 (69–76)	77 (74–80)	65 (60–70)	70 (65–74)
T4N0	60 (54–68)	66 (59–73)	51 (43–60)	57 (49–66)

Adapted from Gill et al. [11]

Patients without high-risk characteristics who have high MSI (MSI-H)/dMMR tumors have a favorable prognosis and are unlikely to derive significant benefit from adjuvant fluoropyrimidine-based therapy. We suggest observation alone for these patients.

We suggest adjuvant chemotherapy for most patients with pMMR tumors and clinicopathological high-risk features, particularly those with T4 cancers or multiple high-risk features.

For patients with T3 pMMR tumors and without high-risk clinicopathological characteristics, the use of the 12-gene recurrence score assay is an option for those who consider that a difference in a predicted 5-year recurrence risk of 21% versus 11% (for recurrence score, respectively, corresponding to an estimated 6% versus 3% absolute reduction in mortality) would change their decision to take or not take adjuvant therapy. In stage II and III disease, 3 months of CAPOX is not inferior to 6 months of oxaliplatin-based therapy, while 3 months of FOLFOX is not inferior to 6 months of FOLFOX.

Conclusion

We recommend a course of adjuvant chemotherapy in addition to chemoradiotherapy after resection of stage II or III rectal cancer (grade 1A). For patients who can tolerate treatment, according to NCCN guidelines, we suggest an oxaliplatin-containing regimen (oxaliplatin plus short-term FU infusion and leucovorin [FOLFOX] or capecitabine plus oxaliplatin [CAPOX]) for those with node-positive or T4 disease (grade 2B).

References

1. Benson AB 3rd, Schrag D, Somerfield MR, Cohen AM, Figueredo AT, Flynn PJ, et al. American Society of Clinical Oncology recommendations on adjuvant chemotherapy for stage II colon cancer. J Clin Oncol. 2004;22(16):3408–19.
2. National Comprehensive Cancer Network (NCCN). NCCN clinical practice guidelines in oncology. https://www.nccn.org/professionals/physician_gls. Accessed 9 Nov 2021.
3. Argiles G, Tabernero J, Labianca R, Hochhauser D, Salazar R, Iveson T, et al. Localised colon cancer: ESMO clinical practice guidelines for diagnosis, treatment and follow-up. Ann Oncol. 2020;31(10):1291–305.
4. Noffsinger AE. Serrated polyps and colorectal cancer: new pathway to malignancy. Annu Rev Pathol. 2009;4:343–64.
5. Werling RW, Yaziji H, Bacchi CE, Gown AM. CDX2, a highly sensitive and specific marker of adenocarcinomas of intestinal origin: an immunohistochemical survey of 476 primary and metastatic carcinomas. Am J Surg Pathol. 2003;27(3):303–10.
6. Moll R, Zimbelmann R, Goldschmidt MD, Keith M, Laufer J, Kasper M, et al. The human gene encoding cytokeratin 20 and its expression during fetal development and in gastrointestinal carcinomas. Differentiation. 1993;53(2):75–93.
7. Landau MS, Kuan SF, Chiosea S, Pai RK. BRAF-mutated microsatellite stable colorectal carcinoma: an aggressive adenocarcinoma with reduced CDX2 and increased cytokeratin 7 immunohistochemical expression. Hum Pathol. 2014;45(8):1704–12.
8. Fokas E, Liersch T, Fietkau R, Hohenberger W, Beissbarth T, Hess C, et al. Tumor regression grading after preoperative chemoradiotherapy for locally advanced rectal carcinoma revisited: updated results of the CAO/ARO/AIO-94 trial. J Clin Oncol. 2014;32(15):1554–62.
9. Sargent D, Sobrero A, Grothey A, O'Connell MJ, Buyse M, Andre Y, et al. Evidence for cure by adjuvant therapy in colon cancer: observations based on individual patient data from 20,898 patients on 18 randomized trials. J Clin Oncol. 2009;27(6):872–7.
10. Andre T, Boni C, Navarro M, Tabernero J, Hickish T, Topham C, et al. Improved overall survival with oxaliplatin, fluorouracil, and leucovorin as adjuvant treatment in stage II or III colon cancer in the MOSAIC trial. J Clin Oncol. 2009;27(19):3109–16.
11. Gill S, Loprinzi CL, Sargent DJ, Thome SD, Alberts SR, Haller DG, et al. Pooled analysis of fluorouracil-based adjuvant therapy for stage II and III colon cancer: who benefits and by how much? J Clin Oncol. 2004;22(10):1797–806.

Staging and Treatment. II-6. Palliative Chemotherapy

Key Points

- The goal of palliative therapy is to increase the possibility of resection in patients with metastatic CRC and, therefore, increase the survival rate.
- The selection of biological agents for patients with metastatic CRC is based on tumor location and molecular testing, including *KRAS, NRAS,* and *BRAF* mutations and MSI. The second-line chemotherapeutic regimen could be selected based on the first-line regimen.
- Although the optimal chemotherapeutic regimen for third line or beyond in patients with metastatic CRC is not yet known, various attempts are made to develop novel therapy for these patients to improve prognosis.

Introduction

Colorectal cancer (CRC) is the third most frequently diagnosed in Korea, and the age-standardized incidence rate per 100,000 CRC was 25.6 in 2020 [1]. Almost 50% of all diagnosed CRC patients can be cured by surgery; however, 40–50% of newly diagnosed patients will eventually develop metastatic disease [2]. Despite recent developments in the treatment of CRC, median overall survival (OS) in patients with metastatic CRC is less than 30 months. Approximately 20–30% of patients with metastatic CRC have been reported to be potentially resectable, and 60–70% of patients with metastatic CRC cannot be resected [3]. The goal of palliative therapy is to increase the possibility of resection in patients with metastatic CRC and therefore increase the survival rate. The National Comprehensive Cancer Network (NCCN) guidelines recommend evaluating the possibility of resection every 2 months while conducting chemotherapy [4]. In this chapter, we will provide an overview of palliative chemotherapy in patients with metastatic CRC.

Jae Hyun Kim is the lead author of this chapter.

Selection of Palliative Chemotherapeutic Regimens as First-Line Treatment

For the treatment of patients with metastatic CRC, FOLFIRI (5-fluorouracil + leucovorin + irinotecan) or FOLFOX (5-fluorouracil + leucovorin + oxaliplatin) is a regimen based on palliative chemotherapy as first line. Because there was no difference in progression-free survival (PFS), OS, and overall response rate between FOLFIRI and FOLFOX, both regimens are considered an option in first-line treatment [5]. FOLFIRI could cause gastrointestinal disturbance and alopecia, while FOLFOX could result in peripheral neuropathy and thrombocytopenia. To select the biological

H. J. Chun et al., *Gastrointestinal Cancer*, https://doi.org/10.1007/978-981-99-0815-8_39

agent for palliative chemotherapy, two factors are important: tumor location and molecular testing. According to the NCCN guidelines, anti-epidermal growth factor receptor (EGFR) antibody (cetuximab or panitumumab) is recommended only for patients with wild-type *KRAS* (Kirsten rat sarcoma viral oncogene homolog), wild-type *NRAS* (neuroblastoma RAS viral oncogene homolog), wild-type *BRAF* (v-Raf murine sarcoma viral oncogene homolog B1), and left-sided tumors, while anti-vascular endothelial growth factor receptor (VEGFR) antibody (bevacizumab) is recommended for other cases [4].

The criteria for dividing the location of tumors are generally based on the splenic flexure; a tumor located from the cecum to the distal transverse colon is classified as a right-sided tumor, while a tumor located from the splenic flexure to the rectum is classified as a left-sided tumor. Because CRC has molecular heterogeneity by sidedness, the biological agent should be selected considering the location of primary tumor. A pooled analysis of metastatic CRC patients with a wild-type RAS gene included six randomized trials (CRYSTAL, FIRE-3, CALGB 80405, PRIME, PEAK, and 20050181) and reported a significant benefit for chemotherapy plus anti-EGFR antibody among patients with left-sided tumors in terms of OS and PFS but not in patients with right-sided tumors [6]. Based on these results, the NCCN guideline recommends anti-EGFR antibody in patients with left-sided tumors.

Molecular testing including *KRAS, NRAS, BRAF*, and microsatellite instability (MSI) is also essential to select the biological agent for patients with metastatic CRC. Recently, commonly available next-generation sequencing (NGS) provides multigene panels including these molecular tests. In the PRIME, OPUS, and CRYSTAL trials, chemotherapy plus cetuximab or panitumumab showed an improvement in OS and PFS in patients with wild-type *RAS* compared to patients with mutated *RAS* [7–12], and subsequently the NCCN guidelines recommended treatment with an anti-EGFR antibody in patients with wild-type *RAS*. Among patients with wild-type *KRAS*, none of the BRAF-mutated patients responded to cetuximab or panitumumab and had significantly shorter OS and PFS than wild-type BRAF patients [13]. Therefore, wild-type BRAF could be a criterion to select anti-EGFR antibody treatment in patients with metastatic CRC [14, 15]. According to these results, cetuximab or panitumumab is recommended only for wild-type KRAS, wild-type NRAS, wild-type BRAF, and left-sided tumors, while bevacizumab is recommended for other cases. Recently, programmed death-1 (PD-1) blockade has emerged as highly effective therapy for patients with MSI-high/deficient mismatch repair gene (dMMR) metastatic CRC that is refractory to standard chemotherapy combinations. In the KEYNOTE-177 and KEYNOTE-164 trials, pembrolizumab led to significantly longer PFS than standard chemotherapy with a manageable safety profile in patients with MSI-high/dMMR metastatic CRC [16, 17]. The CheckMate-142 trial showed that nivolumab + ipilimumab had high response rates, PFS, and OS with a manageable safety [18]. Based on these results, the NCCN guidelines recommend nivolumab ± ipilimumab or pembrolizumab in patients with MSI-high/dMMR metastatic CRC. However, the potential for immunotherapy is not common in CRC patients, because the incidence of MSI-high is low (4–5%) among patients with metastatic CRC [19, 20]. A flowchart for choosing the first-line treatments in patients with metastatic CRC is summarized in Fig. 1.

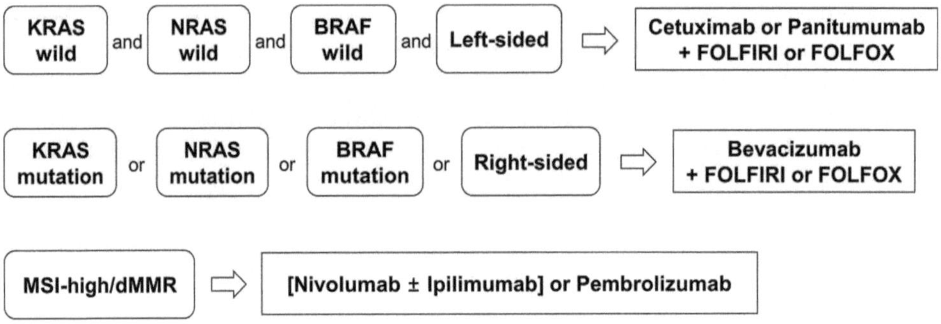

Fig. 1 Selection of first-line regimens for patients with metastatic CRC

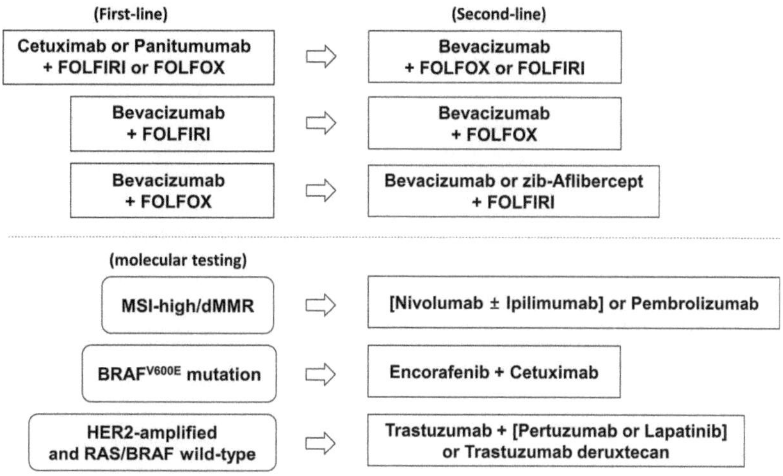

Fig. 2 Selection of second-line regimens for patients with metastatic CRC

Second-Line Treatment

The second-line chemotherapeutic regimen should be selected based on the first-line regimen. If cetuximab or panitumumab plus FOLFORI or FOLFOX was selected as first-line regimen, bevacizumab plus FOLFOX or FOLFIRI could be a second-line regimen. If bevacizumab plus FOLFIRI were selected as the first-line regimen, bevacizumab plus FOLFOX could be the second-line regimen, while if bevacizumab plus FOLFOX was selected as the first-line regimen, bevacizumab or zib-aflibercept plus FOLFIRI could be selected as the second-line regimen [21]. When a patient with CRC has *BRAF*^{V600E} mutations, encorafenib (a recently approved BRAF inhibitor) plus cetuximab could represent the standard care regimen. In the BEACON trial, the combination of encorafenib and cetuximab improved the overall response rate and OS with a manageable safety profile in patients with *BRAF*^{V600E}-mutated metastatic CRC [22, 23]. As with the first-line treatment, if a patient with metastatic CRC has MSI high/dMMR, either nivolumab + ipilimumab or pembrolizumab could be selected as the second-line regimen. Recently, HER2-targeted combination therapy has been introduced as a therapy for patients with metastatic CRC. Although HER2 amplification and/or overexpression is detected in only 2–6% of patients with stage III/IV CRC [24, 25], the efficacy increases notably with combination HER2-targeted regimens, including trastuzumab + pertuzumab or lapatinib or trastuzumab deruxtecan in metastatic CRC patients with HER2-amplified and wild-type *RAS* and wild-type *BRAF* [26, 27].

The flow of choosing second-line treatments in patients with metastatic CRC is summarized in Fig. 2.

Third-Line or Beyond Treatment

Survival of patients with metastatic CRC has gradually increased in recent years, reaching a median of 25–30 months. Subsequently, the number of patients with metastatic CRC to receive a third-line or beyond treatment is growing; however, the optimal chemotherapeutic regimen is still unknown. For these patients, there are presently several options [28, 29]: (1) two oral agents, including regorafenib, which targets VEGFR, and trifluridine/tipiracil, which causes DNA dysfunction; (2) irinotecan + cetuximab or panitumumab for patients with wild-type *RAS*; (3) traditionally preferred agents including capecitabine and 5-FU; and (4) trastuzumab + pertuzumab or lapatinib or trastuzumab deruxtecan for patients with HER2-amplified and wild-type *RAS* and wild-type *BRAF* or pembrolizumab or nivolumab ± ipilimumab for patients with MSI-high/dMMR. Unfortunately, the median PFS of metastatic CRC patients who received third-line or beyond treatment is still under 4 months, despite these new treatment introductions. Common toxicities associated with third-line or beyond treatments are hand-foot skin reaction, fatigue, diarrhea, thrombocytopenia, and leucopenia; therefore, patients who receive third-line or beyond treatments should be monitored for adverse events. Continuous efforts through clinical trials of new treatment combinations or new regimens could improve long-term outcomes for patients with metastatic CRC. It is important to share opinions with experts on best practice for treatment selection and management that could improve long-term outcomes for patients with metastatic CRC.

Conclusion

Choosing an appropriate treatment for patients with metastatic CRC has an important effect on the patient's prognosis. Therefore, it is important to select the appropriate patient for treatment and to choose treatment regimens according to the guidelines for palliative therapy. With the development of NGS techniques, numerous trials are evaluating the molecular biological characteristics of CRC and the effective application of targeted therapy and immunotherapy. As a result, individualized precision medical care for CRC patients is expected in the near future. Establishing an appropriate treatment plan for patients with metastatic CRC by gathering newer and more diverse information will play a crucial role in reducing the recurrence rate and increasing the survival rate of patients with metastatic CRC.

References

1. Jung KW, Won YJ, Hong S, Kong HJ, Im JS, Seo HG. Prediction of cancer incidence and mortality in Korea, 2021. Cancer Res Treat. 2021;53:316–22.
2. Xie YH, Chen YX, Fang JY. Comprehensive review of targeted therapy for colorectal cancer. Signal Transduct Target Ther. 2020;5:22.
3. Saif MW. Secondary hepatic resection as a therapeutic goal in advanced colorectal cancer. World J Gastroenterol. 2009;15:3855–64.
4. Anonymous. National Comprehensive Cancer Network. NCCN clinical practice guidelines in oncology. Colon cancer ver 3.2021.
5. Colucci G, Gebbia V, Paoletti G, Giuliani F, Caruso M, Gebbia N, et al. Phase III randomized trial of FOLFIRI versus FOLFOX4 in the treatment of advanced colorectal cancer: a multicenter study of the Gruppo Oncologico Dell'Italia Meridionale. J Clin Oncol. 2005;23:4866–75.
6. Arnold D, Lueza B, Douillard JY, Peeters M, Lenz HJ, Venook A, et al. Prognostic and predictive value of primary tumour side in patients with RAS wild-type metastatic colorectal cancer treated with chemotherapy and EGFR directed antibodies in six randomized trials. Ann Oncol. 2017;28:1713–29.
7. Douillard JY, Oliner KS, Siena S, Tabernero J, Burkes R, Barugel M, et al. Panitumumab-FOLFOX4 treatment and RAS mutations in colorectal cancer. N Engl J Med. 2013;369:1023–34.
8. Douillard JY, Siena S, Cassidy J, Tabernero J, Burkes R, Barugel M, et al. Final results from PRIME: randomized phase III study of panitumumab with FOLFOX4 for first-line treatment of metastatic colorectal cancer. Ann Oncol. 2014;25:1346–55.
9. Bokemeyer C, Bondarenko I, Hartmann JT, de Braud F, Schuch G, Zubel A, et al. Efficacy according to biomarker status of cetuximab plus FOLFOX-4 as first-line treatment for metastatic colorectal cancer: the OPUS study. Ann Oncol. 2011;22:1535–46.
10. Bokemeyer C, Köhne CH, Ciardiello F, Lenz HJ, Heinemann V, Klinkhardt U, et al. FOLFOX4 plus cetuximab treatment and RAS mutations in colorectal cancer. Eur J Cancer. 2015;51:1243–52.
11. Van Cutsem E, Köhne CH, Láng I, Folprecht G, Nowacki MP, Cascinu S, et al. Cetuximab plus irinotecan, fluorouracil, and leucovorin as first-line treatment for metastatic colorectal cancer: updated analysis of overall survival according to tumor KRAS and BRAF mutation status. J Clin Oncol. 2011;29:2011–9.
12. Van Cutsem E, Lenz HJ, Köhne CH, Heinemann V, Tejpar S, Melezínek I, et al. Fluorouracil, leucovorin, and irinotecan plus cetuximab treatment and RAS mutations in colorectal cancer. J Clin Oncol. 2015;33:692–700.
13. Di Nicolantonio F, Martini M, Molinari F, Sartore-Bianchi A, Arena S, Saletti P, et al. Wild-type BRAF is required for response to panitumumab or cetuximab in metastatic colorectal cancer. J Clin Oncol. 2008;26:5705–12.
14. Pietrantonio F, Petrelli F, Coinu A, Di Bartolomeo M, Borgonovo K, Maggi C, et al. Predictive role of BRAF mutations in patients with advanced colorectal cancer receiving cetuximab and panitumumab: a meta-analysis. Eur J Cancer. 2015;51:587–94.
15. Bokemeyer C, Van Cutsem E, Rougier P, Ciardiello F, Heeger S, Schlichting M, et al. Addition of cetuximab to chemotherapy as first-line treatment for KRAS wild-type metastatic colorectal cancer: pooled analysis of the CRYSTAL and OPUS randomised clinical trials. Eur J Cancer. 2012;48:1466–75.
16. André T, Shiu K-K, Kim TW, Jensen BV, Jensen LH, Punt C, et al. Pembrolizumab in microsatellite-instability–high advanced colorectal cancer. N Engl J Med. 2020;383:2207–18.
17. Le DT, Kim TW, Van Cutsem E, Geva R, Jäger D, Hara H, et al. Phase II open-label study of Pembrolizumab

in treatment-refractory, microsatellite instability-high/mismatch repair-deficient metastatic colorectal cancer: KEYNOTE-164. J Clin Oncol. 2020;38:11–9.
18. Overman MJ, Lonardi S, Wong KYM, Lenz HJ, Gelsomino F, Aglietta M, et al. Durable clinical benefit with Nivolumab plus Ipilimumab in DNA mismatch repair-deficient/microsatellite instability-high metastatic colorectal cancer. J Clin Oncol. 2018;36:773–9.
19. Battaglin F, Naseem M, Lenz HJ, Salem ME. Microsatellite instability in colorectal cancer: overview of its clinical significance and novel perspectives. Clin Adv Hematol Oncol. 2018;16:735–45.
20. Goldstein J, Tran B, Ensor J, Gibbs P, Wong HL, Wong SF, et al. Multicenter retrospective analysis of metastatic colorectal cancer (CRC) with high-level microsatellite instability (MSI-H). Ann Oncol. 2014;25:1032–8.
21. Yamada Y, Matsuhashi N, Fujii H, Makiyama A, Iihara H, Takahashi T, et al. Impact of anti-angiogenic agents on chemotherapy efficacy in patients with metastatic colorectal cancer: second-line FOLFIRI plus bevacizumab or Aflibercept. Anticancer Res. 2021;41:533–41.
22. Tabernero J, Grothey A, Van Cutsem E, Yaeger R, Wasan H, Yoshino T, et al. Encorafenib plus Cetuximab as a new standard of care for previously treated BRAF V600E-mutant metastatic colorectal cancer: updated survival results and subgroup analyses from the BEACON study. J Clin Oncol. 2021;39:273–84.
23. Kopetz S, Grothey A, Yaeger R, Van Cutsem E, Desai J, Yoshino T, et al. Encorafenib, binimetinib, and cetuximab in BRAF V600E–mutated colorectal cancer. N Engl J Med. 2019;381:1632–43.
24. Ingold Heppner B, Behrens HM, Balschun K, Haag J, Krüger S, Becker T, et al. HER2/neu testing in primary colorectal carcinoma. Br J Cancer. 2014;111:1977–84.
25. Ross JS, Fakih M, Ali SM, Elvin JA, Schrock AB, Suh J, et al. Targeting HER2 in colorectal cancer: the landscape of amplification and short variant mutations in ERBB2 and ERBB3. Cancer. 2018;124:1358–73.
26. Siena S, Di Bartolomeo M, Raghav K, Masuishi T, Loupakis F, Kawakami H, et al. Trastuzumab deruxtecan (DS-8201) in patients with HER2-expressing metastatic colorectal cancer (DESTINY-CRC01): a multicentre, open-label, phase 2 trial. Lancet Oncol. 2021;22:779–89.
27. Meric-Bernstam F, Hurwitz H, Raghav KPS, McWilliams RR, Fakih M, VanderWalde A, et al. Pertuzumab plus trastuzumab for HER2-amplified metastatic colorectal cancer (MyPathway): an updated report from a multicentre, open-label, phase 2a, multiple basket study. Lancet Oncol. 2019;20:518–30.
28. Fernández-Montes A, Grávalos C, Pericay C, Safont MJ, Benavides M, Élez E, et al. Current options for third-line and beyond treatment of metastatic colorectal cancer. Spanish TTD group expert opinion. Clin Colorectal Cancer. 2020;19:165–77.
29. Bekaii-Saab T, Kim R, Kim TW, O'Connor JM, Strickler JH, Malka D, et al. Third- or later-line therapy for metastatic colorectal cancer: reviewing best practice. Clin Colorectal Cancer. 2019;18:e117–29.

Staging and Treatment. II-7. Overview of Treatment of Rectal Cancer

Key Points

- Preoperative chemoradiation therapy is a standard of care for locally advanced rectal cancer patient.
- Both conventional long-course chemoradiotherapy and short-course radiotherapy can be used for preoperative treatment.

Introduction

Radiotherapy is a local treatment and is commonly used as an adjuvant treatment before or after surgery for rectal cancer with a high probability of recurrence, that is, stage II or III. In the case of distant metastasis that can be resected even in stage IV, adjuvant radiation therapy can be performed and can be used to prevent recurrence after local excision of stage I cancer or as a first-line treatment when surgery is impossible or difficult. In addition, if surgery to preserve anal function is difficult due to the location or size of the tumor, radiation therapy before surgery can reduce the extent of the tumor and preserve the anus.

Postoperative Radiation Therapy and Chemoradiation Therapy

Although the primary treatment for rectal cancer is surgery, it is a disease with a high tendency of local recurrence even after curative resection. For this reason, many studies have been conducted to evaluate the benefits of adjuvant therapy. Early studies, such as NSABP R-01, have attempted to improve treatment outcome by adding radiation therapy after surgery [1]. Results from many randomized trials show that surgery with radiotherapy significantly reduced local recurrence (LR) compared to surgery alone but had only marginally better overall survival (OS) [2, 3].

There were two studies that showed improvement of OS following combined chemotherapy with radiotherapy after surgery. The Mayo-North Central Cancer Treatment Group study was conducted to compare postoperative radiation therapy with or without chemotherapy. A total of 204 patients with pT3–4 or N+ rectal cancer were randomly allocated to postoperative radiotherapy-alone group (45–50.4 Gy) or to radiotherapy plus chemotherapy with fluorouracil group. After a median follow-up of more than 7 years, postoperative chemoradiotherapy (CRT) reduced LR,

Sun Young Ma is the lead author of this chapter.

H. J. Chun et al., *Gastrointestinal Cancer*, https://doi.org/10.1007/978-981-99-0815-8_40

distant metastasis, cancer-related deaths, and overall death rate [4]. According to the Gastrointestinal Tumor Study Group study (GITSG 7175), although the trial was prematurely terminated due to high acute toxicity of the CRT group, OS was improved in the postoperative CRT group compared to the surgery-alone group (45% vs. 27%, 10 years) [5]. On the other hand, studies such as NSABP R-02 have conducted comparisons between a group that received chemotherapy alone after surgery and a group that added radiation therapy to chemotherapy after surgery. Results from the NSABP R-02 study showed that the addition of radiotherapy with 50.4 Gy to postoperative chemotherapy in Dukes' B and C rectal cancers reduced locoregional recurrence compared to postoperative chemotherapy alone (8% vs. 13% at 5 years) but no benefit for DFS or OS [6].

Preoperative Radiation Therapy and Chemoradiation Therapy

Radiation therapy before surgery is intended to increase the resectability of surgical resection by lowering the stage of the tumor, and it also increases the possibility of sphincter preservation on distal rectal cancer surgery. In the Swedish rectal cancer study, 1168 patients with resectable Dukes' A to C rectal cancer were randomly assigned to a group that underwent surgery 1 week after receiving 5 Gy radiotherapy and to a group that underwent surgery only. After 5 years of follow-up, preoperative radiotherapy reduced the LR rate (11% vs. 27%) and improved OS (58% vs. 8%) compared to the surgery-alone group without increased postoperative mortality [7]. The long-term follow-up result of this study also showed benefits of preoperative radiotherapy [8]. The LR rate of the surgery-alone group was too high, but the surgical method was not total mesorectal excision (TME). A Dutch trial multicenter phase 3 study involved 1861 patients who were randomly allocated into a group that received 5 Gy radiotherapy before TME or a group with TME alone. The 2-year OS and sphincter preservation rate were same in both groups. The 2-year LR rate was 2.4% in the preoperative radiotherapy plus TME group and 8.2% in the TME-alone group; it showed that preoperative radiotherapy was effective for reducing LR rate even with standardized total mesorectal excision [9]. There was significant difference in 10-year cumulative LR rate (5% vs. 11%, $p < 0.0001$) and 10-year survival (50% vs. 40%, $p = 0.032$) but no OS difference [10].

The French study (FFCD 9203) and EORTC 22921 study compared preoperative radiation therapy with preoperative CRT (45 Gy of radiation alone versus radiation with concurrent bolus 5-FU plus leucovorin followed by surgery) in resectable T3–4 rectal cancer. The preoperative CRT group showed increased tumor downstaging, lower LR, and higher acute toxicity but no difference in OS compared to the preoperative radiotherapy group [11, 12]. The results from meta-analysis studies that compared preoperative radiation therapy with preoperative CRT in patients with resectable stage II or III rectal cancer are also similar [13, 14]. Based on these findings, due to improved local control rate despite the lack of OS benefit and increased acute toxicity, preoperative CRT was performed as a suitable treatment for locally advanced rectal cancer.

Preoperative Vs. Postoperative Treatment

Several phase III prospective trials have been conducted comparing preoperative CRT and postoperative CRT. The NSABPR-03 study was terminated early, but 5-year DFS was significantly improved in the preoperative CRT group, and 5-year OS also showed a trend of improvement.

The German Rectal Cancer Group trial (CAO/ARO/AIO-94) evaluated 823 patients with T3–4 or N+ rectal cancer, randomized into two groups. In both groups, 50.4 Gy of radiotherapy was delivered in 28 fractions, and a boost of 5.4 Gy was delivered in the postoperative group. 5-FU(1 g/m^2/day) was given in a 120-h continuous intravenous infusion during the first and fifth weeks of radiotherapy; surgery was performed 6 weeks after the completion of CRT 1 month after surgery, and four 5-day cycles of fluorouracil (500 mg/m^2/day for 5 days every 4 weeks) were given in both groups. As a result, preoperative CRT had a lower LR (6% vs. 13%, 5 years), higher sphincter preservation (39% vs. 19%), lower grade 3 or 4 acute toxic effects (27% vs. 40%), and lower late toxic effects (14% vs. 24%) than postoperative CRT group but did not improve OS [15].

A Korean trial was conducted in 240 patients with locally advanced (T3–4 or N+) rectal cancer, compared two groups of preoperative and postoperative CRT. CRT consisted of 50 Gy in 25 fractions and concurrent capecitabine (825 mg/m^2 twice per day, without weekend breaks). In the postoperative group, chemotherapy consisted of four cycles of capecitabine (2500 mg/m^2/day for 14 days, followed by a 1-week break) or four cycles of bolus 5-FU/leucovorin (375 mg 5-FU/m^2/day and 20 mg leucovorin/m^2/day for 5 days every 4 weeks), and total mesorectal excision was performed. Results of this study show no significant difference in DFS and OS between the two groups, but the preoperative CRT group had a higher rate of sphincter preservation (68% vs. 42%) for the patients with low-lying tumors [16].

The MRC CR07 trial compared short-course preoperative radiotherapy versus initial surgery with selective postoperative CRT. A total of 1350 patients of resectable rectal cancer were randomly allocated to short-course preoperative radiotherapy (25 Gy in five fractions) or to initial surgery with selective postoperative CRT (45 Gy in 25 fractions with concurrent 5-FU) restricted to patients with involvement of the circumferential resection margin. LR at 3 years was significantly lower (4.4% vs. 10.6%), and 3-year DFS was improved in the preoperative therapy group (77.5% vs. 71.5%) but no difference in OS. These results showed short-course preoperative radiotherapy was superior to postoperative CRT in patients with close or involved circumferential resection margin [17].

Song et al. performed a meta-analysis with three randomized phase III trials, which compared preoperative CRT to postoperative CRT for stage II–III resectable rectal cancer. The meta-analysis results showed significantly lower 5-year locoregional recurrence rate in the preoperative CRT group than in the postoperative CRT group, but no significant difference of distant metastasis or survival between two groups, and similar chronic toxicity and sphincter preservation rate [18]. The results from these studies support the evidence that preoperative treatment is more effective than postoperative treatment for locally advanced rectal cancer.

Radiation Dose and Fractionation

Long-Course Chemoradiotherapy Vs. Short-Course Radiotherapy

After the German trial, conventionally fractionated CRT, irradiating 50–50.4 Gy in 1.8–2.0 Gy per fraction, has become the standard of care for reducing the risk of recurrence and increasing the rate of sphincter-sparing surgery in locally advanced rectal cancer [13, 15, 16, 19]. Typically, a dose of 45 Gy in 25 fractions of radiation is applied to the pelvis, including the primary tumor and regional lymph node areas, followed by a boost of 5.4 Gy of radiation therapy in three fractions to the tumor bed with a 2 cm margin for preoperative radiation therapy or 5.4-9 Gy in three to five fractions to the surgical bed in postoperative cases. When performing boost irradiation after 45 Gy, the small intestine should be excluded to minimize toxicity. For unresectable tumors, radiation doses higher than 54 Gy may be required if technically feasible [20]. Conversely, hypofractionated radiotherapy was adopted in some parts of Europe, for example, in the Swedish and the Dutch trial, patients of the preoperative radiotherapy group irradiated 25 Gy in five fractions for a week, followed by surgery 1 week after radiation therapy. The results of both studies showed a significant improvement in local control in the preoperative short-course radiotherapy group compared to the surgery-alone group [7–10]. These trials provide a rationale for preoperative short-course radiation therapy without concurrent chemotherapy as alternative preoperative radiation therapy. In a Polish trial and TROG trial comparing preoperative short-course radiation therapy to long-course CRT, there was no difference of local recurrence rate between two groups [21, 22].

Interval Between Surgeries After Neoadjuvant Therapy

The standard interval between surgeries after preoperative radiation therapy has not been established. In the Stockholm III trial, patients with resectable rectal cancer were randomly allocated into three groups for evaluating optimal fractionation and time to surgery after radiation, each treated with 5 Gy × 5 radiotherapy followed by surgery within 1 week, 5 Gy × 5 followed by surgery after 4–8 weeks, and 2 Gy × 25 followed by surgery after 4–8 weeks. This study shows similar results of oncologic outcome in all three groups, but in the short-course radiotherapy with delayed surgery group, postoperative complications were significantly fewer than in the immediate surgery group. Based on this result, the authors concluded that delay to surgery after short-course radiotherapy is more optimal than immediate surgery [23].

The GRECCAR6 study evaluated the effect of increasing the interval between preoperative CRT and surgery on pathologic complete response (pCR) rate. Patients with cT3–4 or N+ rectal cancer who had received CRT (45–50 Gy with fluorouracil or capecitabine) were randomly assigned to the 7-week or the 11-week after completion of CRT groups. As a result, the pCR rate after resection did not increase but also increased morbidity and had a worse quality of mesorectal resection in the 11-week group [24].

Nonoperative Management (NOM)

With increasing interest in patients' quality of life, watch-and-wait approaches without radical resection for organ preservation in patients with clinical complete response (cCR) after preoperative CRT are being attempted [25–28]. In selected patients with cCR after preoperative treatment who refuse surgery due to permanent colostomy or inadequate bowel continence after TME, NOM can be considered, but with conditions. These patients should receive close follow-up by a multidisciplinary team [29]. For NOM or local excision after definitive or preoperative CRT, 50–54 Gy in 25–30 fractions is recommended [30–33].

Radiation Therapy Technique

Radiation Treatment Volume

External beam radiation therapy for rectal cancer treats the primary tumor and potentially at-risk regional lymph nodes and is determined in detail by the conditions of each stage of the disease, such as the tumor('s) invasion status, location, and lymph node involvement.

Generally, for clinical T3N1–2 rectal cancer patients, it is recommended to include the tumor bed with a 2–5 cm margin, the mesorectum, the presacral lymph nodes, internal iliac lymph nodes, and obturator lymph nodes in the treatment volume [20]. If the primary tumor has invaded the anus or the anterior organs such as the bladder, prostate, or vagina, it should be included in the treatment field for inguinal lymph nodes or external iliac lymph nodes according to lymphatic drainage of the involved organ [34, 35]. In cases with abdominoperineal resection, perineal wounds should be included.

Positioning of Patient

In most cases, rectal cancer patients are treated in a prone position to reduce the volume of the small intestine included in the treatment field during radiation therapy. In addition, a device such as a belly board designed to drop the intestines of the abdomen forward may be used [36, 37]. Patients whose treatment volume includes inguinal lymph nodes or who have a stoma may need to be treated in a supine position; whether the patient is treated in a supine or prone position, treatment with a full-filled bladder can further reduce the dose to the small intestine [29].

Various Techniques of Radiotherapy

Three-Dimensional Conformal Radiation Therapy (3D-CRT)

In 3D-CRT, a four-field box technique or a three-field technique with both lateral fields and a posterior field is typically used. The lateral fields are useful for sparing volumes of the bladder and small bowel.

Intensity-Modulated Radiation Therapy (IMRT) and Volumetric Modulated Arc Therapy (VMAT)

Modulated radiation therapy is a state-of-the-art technology that can properly distribute maximum radiation to the target volume and minimize radiation to surrounding normal tissues by adjusting the radiation intensity differently for each area even in the same radiation field. There is a possibility of reducing treatment-related side effects in normal organs such as the bladder, colon, and small intestine [38–43].

Image-Guided Radiation Therapy (IGRT)

IGRT is a treatment technique that allows for more accurate radiation therapy by taking images such as cone-beam CT or MRI before each treatment to confirm the location of the patient's organs or tumors.

Stereotactic Body Radiation Therapy (SBRT)

Also known as stereotactic ablative body radiation (SABR), it is a treatment method that precisely irradiates a tumor with high doses of radiation using numerous radiation beams from different directions. It can be considered in patients with small-sized oligometastatic tumors in the liver or lungs.

Intraoperative Radiation Therapy (IORT)

IORT is a method of delivering a high dose of radiation once to the tumor bed during surgery. It has the advantage of exposing normal organs to less radiation than external beam radiation therapy. It can be used on very close or positive margins after resection and as boost irradiation in locally advanced or recurrent rectal cancer patients [44–46].

Complications of Radiation Therapy

As radiation therapy techniques become more varied and advanced, it is difficult to interpret complications of radiation therapy. Surgery itself can cause side effects such as urinary dysfunction, and chemotherapy also has side effects; careful evaluation of the side effects of radiation therapy is necessary [47–49].

Symptoms due to early adverse effect of radiation include pelvic pain, changes in bowel habits, urinary dysfunction, anal pain, and perianal skin reactions. Onset occurs during treatment, and effects are usually temporary and disappear within 2–4 weeks after completion of treatment.

Late bowel and anorectal dysfunction such as chronic diarrhea, fecal incontinence, and rectal emptying problems may occur [50]. In this case, antidiarrheal medication may be helpful; avoiding raw vegetables and low-fat diets or probiotic supplementation is also helpful [51]. The incidence of long-term urinary incontinence varies with surgical methods and does not appear to be increased with radiation therapy. The Dutch trial reported that there were no differences in rates of difficulty with bladder emptying in the group receiving radiotherapy before surgery compared with the group not receiving radiotherapy [47]. Few studies have evaluated the risk of radiation-induced secondary malignancies in rectal cancer patients and show different results, some suggesting it increases the risk of second malignancies and some are not [52]. Other late complications such as sexual dysfunction and pelvic bone fractures may occur [53].

Conclusion

For locally advanced rectal cancer patients, preoperative CRT is recommended rather than initial surgery followed by adjuvant therapy. In addition, short-course preoperative radiation therapy can also be considered [20, 29]. The timing of surgery after preoperative radiotherapy or CRT is preferably 4–8 weeks to achieve the benefit of downstaging [23, 24, 29].

References

1. Fisher B, Wolmark N, Rockette H, Redmond C, Deutsch M, Wickerham DL, et al. Postoperative adjuvant chemotherapy or radiation therapy for rectal cancer: results from NSABP protocol R-01. J Natl Cancer Inst. 1988;80(1):21–9.
2. Colorectal Cancer Collaborative Group. Adjuvant radiotherapy for rectal cancer: a systematic overview of 8,507 patients from 22 randomised trials. Lancet. 2001;358(9290):1291–304.
3. Glimelius B, Grönberg H, Järhult J, Wallgren A, Cavallin-Ståhl E. A systematic overview of radiation therapy effects in rectal cancer. Acta Oncol. 2003;42:476–92.
4. Krook JE, Moertel CG, Gunderson LL, Wieand HS, Collins RT, BeartKubista RW, et al. Effective surgical adjuvant therapy for high-risk rectal carcinoma. N Engl J Med. 1991;324(11):709–15.
5. Thomas PR, Lindblad AS. Adjuvant postoperative radiotherapy and chemotherapy in rectal carcinoma: a review of the Gastrointestinal Tumor Study Group experience. Radiother Oncol. 1988;13(4):245–52.
6. Wolmark N, Wieand HS, Hyams DM, Colangelo L, Dimitrov NV, Romond EH, et al. Randomized trial of postoperative adjuvant chemotherapy with or without radiotherapy for carcinoma of the rectum: National Surgical Adjuvant Breast and Bowel Project Protocol R-02. J Natl Cancer Inst. 2000;92(5):388–96.
7. Cedermark B, Dahlberg M, Glimelius B, Påhlman L, Rutqvist LE, Wilking N. Swedish rectal cancer trial: improved survival with preoperative radiotherapy in resectable rectal cancer. N Engl J Med. 1997;336(14):980–7.
8. Folkesson J, Birgisson H, Pahlman L, Cedermark B, Glimelius B, Gunnarsson U. Swedish rectal cancer trial: long lasting benefits from radiotherapy on survival and local recurrence rate. J Clin Oncol. 2005;23(24):5644–50.
9. Kapiteijn E, Marijnen CA, Nagtegaal ID, Putter H, Steup WH, Wiggers T, et al.; Dutch Colorectal Cancer Group. Preoperative radiotherapy combined with total mesorectal excision for resectable rectal cancer. N Engl J Med. 2001;345:638–646.
10. van Gijn W, Marijnen CAM, Nagtegaal ID, Kranenbarg EMK, Putter H, Wiggers T, et al. Preoperative radiotherapy combined with total mesorectal excision for resectable rectal cancer: 12-year follow-up of the multicentre, randomised controlled TME trial. Lancet Oncol. 2011;12(6):575–82.
11. Gerard JP, Conroy T, Bonnetain F, Bouche O, Chapet O, Closon-Dejardin MT, et al. Preoperative radiotherapy with or without concurrent fluorouracil and leucovorin in T3–4 rectal cancers: results of FFCD 9203. J Clin Oncol. 2006;24(28):4620–5.
12. Jean-François B, Laurence C, Gilles C, Laurent M, Philippe M, Ljiljana RJ, et al. Chemotherapy with preoperative radiotherapy in rectal cancer. N Engl J Med. 2006;355(11):1114–23.
13. Ceelen WP, Van Nieuwenhove Y, Fierens K, Pattyn P. Preoperative chemoradiation versus radiation alone for stage II and III resectable rectal cancer. Cochrane Database Syst Rev. 2009;(1):CD006041.
14. Fiorica F, Cartei F, Licata A, Enea M, Ursino S, Colosimo C, et al. Can chemotherapy concomitantly delivered with radiotherapy improve survival of patients with resectable rectal cancer? A meta-analysis of literature data. Cancer Treat Rev. 2010;36:539–49.
15. Sauer R, Becker H, Hohenberger W, Rödel C, Wittekind C, Fietkau R, et al.; Rectal Cancer Study Group. Preoperative versus postoperative chemoradiotherapy for rectal cancer. N Engl J Med. 2004;351:1731–1740.
16. Park J, Yoon SM, Yu CS, Kim JH, Kim TW, Kim JC. Randomized phase 3 trial comparing preoperative and postoperative chemoradiotherapy with capecitabine for locally advanced rectal cancer. Cancer. 2011;117(16):3703–12.
17. Sebag-Montefiore D, Stephens RJ, Steele R, Monson J, Grieve R, Khanna S, et al. Preoperative radiotherapy versus selective postoperative chemoradiotherapy in patients with rectal cancer (MRC CR07 and NCIC-CTG C016): a multicentre, randomised trial. Lancet. 2009;373(9666):811–20.
18. Song JH, Jeong JU, Lee JH, Kim SH, Cho HM, Um JW, et al.; Korean Clinical Practice Guideline for Colon and Rectal Cancer Committee. Preoperative chemoradiotherapy versus postoperative chemoradiotherapy for stage II-III resectable rectal cancer: a meta-analysis of randomized controlled trials. Radiat Oncol. 2017;35(3):198–207.
19. Sauer R, Liersch T, Merkel S, Fietkau R, Hohenberger W, Hess C, et al. Preoperative versus postoperative chemoradiotherapy for locally advanced rectal cancer: results of the German CAO/ARO/AIO-94 randomized phase III trial after a median follow-up of 11 years. J Clin Oncol. 2012;30:1926–33.
20. NCCN clinical practice guidelines in oncology (NCCN guidelines), rectal cancer. Version 2. 2021.
21. Bujko K, Nowacki MP, Nasierowska-Guttmejer A, Michalski W, Bebenek M, Kryj M. Long-term results of a randomized trial comparing preoperative short-course radiotherapy with preoperative conventionally fractionated chemoradiation for rectal cancer. Br J Surg. 2006;93:1215–23.
22. Ngan SY, Burmeister B, Fisher RJ, Solomon M, Goldstein D, Joseph D, et al. Randomized trial of short-course radiotherapy versus long-course chemoradiation comparing rates of local recurrence in patients with T3 rectal cancer: trans-Tasman radiation oncology group trial 01.04. J Clin Oncol. 2012;30:3827–33.

23. Erlandsson J, Holm T, Pettersson D, Berglund Å, Cedermark B, Radu C, et al. Optimal fractionation of preoperative radiotherapy and timing to surgery for rectal cancer (Stockholm III): a multicentre, randomised, non-blinded, phase 3, non-inferiority trial. Lancet Oncol. 2017;18(3):336–46.
24. Lefevre JH, Mineur L, Kotti S, et al. Effect of interval (7 or 11 weeks) between neoadjuvant radiochemotherapy and surgery on complete pathologic response in rectal cancer: a multicenter, randomized, controlled trial (GRECCAR-6). J Clin Oncol. 2016;34:3773–80.
25. Dossa F, Chesney TR, Acuna SA, Baxter NN. A watch-and-wait approach for locally advanced rectal cancer after a clinical complete response following neoadjuvant chemoradiation: a systematic review and meta-analysis. Lancet Gastroenterol Hepatol. 2017;2(7):501–13.
26. van der Valk MJM, Hilling DE, Bastiaannet E, Meershoek-Klein Kranenbarg E, Beets GL, Figueiredo NL, et al.; WWD Consortium. Long-term outcomes of clinical complete responders after neoadjuvant treatment for rectal cancer in the International Watch & Wait Database (IWWD): an international multicentre registry study. Lancet. 2018;391(10139):2537.
27. Smith JJ, Strombom P, Chow OS, Roxburgh CS, Lynn P, Eaton A, et al. Assessment of a watch-and-wait strategy for rectal cancer in patients with a complete response after neoadjuvant therapy. JAMA Oncol. 2019;5(4):e185896.
28. Sanford NN, Dee EC, Ahn C, Kazmi SA, Beg MS, Folkert MR, rt al. Recent trends and overall survival of young versus older adults with stage II to III rectal cancer treated with and without surgery in the United States, 2010-2015. Am J Clin Oncol. 2020;43(10):694–700.
29. Wo JY, Anker CJ, Ashman JB, Bhadkamkar NA, Bradfield L, Chang DT, et al. Radiation therapy for rectal cancer: executive summary of an ASTRO clinical practice guideline. Pract Radiat Oncol. 2021;11:13–25.
30. Rullier E, Rouanet P, Tuech JJ, Valverde A, Lelong B, Rivoire M, et al. Organ preservation for rectal cancer (GRECCAR 2): a prospective, randomised, open-label, multicentre, phase 3 trial. Lancet. 2017;390(10093):469–79.
31. Stijns RCH, de Graaf EJR, Punt CJA, Nagtegaal ID, Nuyttens JJME, van Meerten E, et al. Long-term oncological and functional outcomes of chemoradiotherapy followed by organ-sparing transanal endoscopic microsurgery for distal rectal cancer: the CARTS study. JAMA Surg. 2019;154:47–54.
32. Creavin B, Ryan E, Martin ST, Hanly A, O'Connell PR, Sheahan K, et al. Organ preservation with local excision or active surveillance following chemoradiotherapy for rectal cancer. Br J Cancer. 2017;116:169–74.
33. Habr-Gama A, Lynn PB, Jorge JM, São Julião GP, Proscurshim I, Gama-Rodrigues J, et al. Impact of organ-preserving strategies on anorectal function in patients with distal rectal cancer following neoadjuvant chemoradiation. Dis Colon Rectum. 2016;59:264–9.
34. Roels S, Duthoy W, Haustermans K, Penninckx F, Vandecaveye V, Boterberg T, et al. Definition and delineation of the clinical target volume for rectal cancer. Int J Radiat Oncol Biol Phys. 2006;65:1129–42.
35. Valentini V, Gambacorta MA, Barbaro B, Chiloiro G, Coco C, Das P, et al. International consensus guidelines on Clinical Target Volume delineation in rectal cancer. Radiother Oncol. 2016;120:195–201.
36. Gallagher MJ, Brereton HD, Rostock RA, Zero JM, Zekoski DA, Poyss LF, et al. A prospective study of treatment techniques to minimize the volume of pelvic small bowel with reduction of acute and late effects associated with pelvic irradiation. Int J Radiat Oncol Biol Phys. 1986;12(9):1565–73.
37. Nuyttens JJ, Robertson JM, Yan D, Martinez A. The position and volume of the small bowel during adjuvant radiation therapy for rectal cancer. Int J Radiat Oncol Biol Phys. 2001;51(5):1271–80.
38. Dröge LH, Weber HE, Guhlich M, Leu M, Conradi LC, Gaedcke J, et al. Reduced toxicity in the treatment of locally advanced rectal cancer: a comparison of volumetric modulated arc therapy and 3-D conformal radiotherapy. BMC Cancer. 2015;15:750.
39. Regnier A, Ulbrich J, Münch S, Oechsner M, Wilhelm D, Combs SE, et al. Comparative analysis of efficacy, toxicity, and patient-reported outcomes in rectal cancer patients undergoing preoperative 3-D conformal radiotherapy or VMAT. Front Oncol. 2017;7:225.
40. Stuyck C, Wegge M, Bulens P, Joye I, Haustermans K, et al. Moderate dose escalation with volumetric modulated arc therapy improves outcome in rectal cancer. Acta Oncol. 2017;56:1501–6.
41. Ng SY, Colborn KL, Cambridge L, Hajj C, Yang TJ, Wu AJ, et al. Acute toxicity with intensity modulated radiotherapy versus 3-dimensional conformal radiotherapy during preoperative chemoradiation for locally advanced rectal cancer. Radiother Oncol. 2016;121:252–7.
42. Wee CW, Kang HC, Wu HG, Chie EK, Choi N, Park JM, et al. Intensity-modulated radiotherapy versus three-dimensional conformal radiotherapy in rectal cancer treated with neoadjuvant concurrent chemoradiation: a metaanalysis and pooled-analysis of acute toxicity. Jpn J Clin Oncol. 2018;48:458–66.
43. Yu M, Jang HS, Jeon DM, Cheon GS, Lee HC, Chung MJ, et al. Dosimetric evaluation of tomotherapy and four-box field conformal radiotherapy in locally advanced rectal cancer. Radiat Oncol J. 2013;31(4):252–9.
44. Haddock MG. Intraoperative radiation therapy for colon and rectal cancers: a clinical review. Radiat Oncol. 2017;12(1):11.
45. Nakfoor BM, Willett CG, Shellito PC, Kaufman DS, Daly WJ. The impact of 5-fluorouracil and intraoperative electron beam radiation therapy on the outcome of patients with locally advanced primary rectal and rectosigmoid cancer. Ann Surg. 1998;228(2):194–200.

46. Mathis KL, Nelson H, Pemberton JH, Haddock MG, Gunderson LL. Unresectable colorectal cancer can be cured with multimodality therapy. Ann Surg. 2008;248(4):592–8.
47. Lange MM, Maas CP, Marijnen CA, Wiggers T, Rutten HJ, Kranenbarg EK, et al. Urinary dysfunction after rectal cancer treatment is mainly caused by surgery. Br J Surg. 2008;95(8):1020–8.
48. Vironen JH, Kairaluoma M, Aalto AM, Kellokumpu IH. Impact of functional results on quality of life after rectal cancer surgery. Dis Colon Rectum. 2006;49:568–78.
49. Birgisson H, Påhlman L, Gunnarsson U, Glimelius B, Swedish Rectal Cancer Trial Group. Adverse effects of preoperative radiation therapy for rectal cancer: long-term follow-up of the Swedish rectal cancer trial. J Clin Oncol. 2005;23:8697–705.
50. Peeters KC, van de Velde CJ, Leer JW, Martijn H, Junggeburt JM, Kranenbarg EK, et al. Late side effects of short-course preoperative radiotherapy combined with total mesorectal excision for rectal cancer: increased bowel dysfunction in irradiated patients—a Dutch colorectal cancer group study. J Clin Oncol. 2005;23(25):6199–206.
51. McGough C, Baldwin C, Frost G, Andreyev HJ. Role of nutritional intervention in patients treated with radiotherapy for pelvic malignancy. Br J Cancer. 2004;90(12):2278–87.
52. Wiltink LM, Nout RA, Fiocco M, Meershoek-Klein Kranenbarg E, Jürgenliemk-Schulz IM, Jobsen JJ, et al. No increased risk of second cancer after radiotherapy in patients treated for rectal or endometrial cancer in the randomized TME, PORTEC-1, and PORTEC-2 trials. J Clin Oncol. 2015;33(15):1640–6.
53. Marijnen CA, van de Velde CJ, Putter H, van den Brink M, Maas CP, Martijn H, et al. Impact of short-term preoperative radiotherapy on health-related quality of life and sexual functioning in primary rectal cancer: report of a multicenter randomized trial. J Clin Oncol. 2005;23(9):1847–58.

Part VI

Anal Cancer

Epidemiology and Prevention. I-1. Epidemiology and Risk Factors

Key Points

- Anal cancer is a rare malignancy.
- Risk factors for anal cancer include sexual activity (more than ten sexual partners, anal receptive intercourse, sexually transmitted disease [STD]), human papillomavirus [HPV] infection, human immunodeficiency virus (HIV) infection, chronic immunosuppression, and smoking.
- The incidence of anal cancer is increasing and is related to an increase in the incidence of HPV infection and a longer survival in HIV-infected patients.
- An HPV vaccine is available and may reduce the risk of anal cancer in high-risk populations.

Introduction

Anal cancer is a rare cancer; most cases are HPV-related cancer types that arise from the squamous epithelium of the anus. About 85% of anal cancers are squamous cell carcinomas (SCCs), the remaining 10% are adenocarcinoma, and 5% are rare cancers such as small-cell carcinoma, melanoma, and metastatic cancer [1]. This chapter focuses on anal SCCs, which comprise most anal cancers.

Seong Jung Kim is the lead author of this chapter.

Epidemiology

In 2020, 331 cases of anal cancer occurred in Korea, accounting for 0.14% of all cancers, and it was ranked the 13th most common cancer. Ninety-five deaths from anal cancer occurred, with a cumulative risk of 1%. The cumulative prevalence of anal cancer in the past 5 years was 1080, with 67% diagnosed in patients over the age of 60, and 58% were females. The cumulative incidence rate is 2.1 per 100,000 person-years [2, 3].

According to recent reports of epidemiology of anal cancer, the incidence of anal cancer has increased over the past several decades. In the United States from 2001 to 2015, the incidence of anal cancer increased by a rate of 2.7%/year [4]. In Australia, the incidence of anal cancer increased to 3.4%/year in men and 1.9%/year in women from 1982 to 2005 [1]. In the period 1975 to 2002 in Scotland, the incidence of anal cancer doubled compared to the previous period [5].

This increase in the incidence of anal cancer in the general population may be related to changes in sexual practice, such as early sexual

H. J. Chun et al., *Gastrointestinal Cancer*, https://doi.org/10.1007/978-981-99-0815-8_41

intercourse and a large number of lifetime sexual partners [6].

Risk Factors

Sexual Activity

Case-control studies of the epidemiology of anal cancer have shown that homosexual men with more than ten lifetime sexual partners, a history of anal warts, as well as women with multiple sexual partners, anal receptive intercourse, and sexually transmitted disease (STD) such as herpes, chlamydia, gonorrhea, and syphilis are reported risk factors for anal cancer [7].

Human Papillomavirus

Anal human papillomavirus (HPV) infection is one of the leading causes of anal cancer, and this infection mainly results from anal sexual exposure to HPV [1]. Increasing evidence indicates that persistent infection with a high-risk form of HPV (subtypes 16 and 18) causes anal cancer as it is known to do in the cervix and head and neck [8]. A study of tumor samples of anal cancer in Denmark and Sweden found that HPV DNA was found in 88% of patients with anal cancer and none in rectal cancer [7]. In a systemic review published in 2007, the prevalence of HPV subtypes 16 and18 was shown to be 72% in patients with invasive anal cancer [9]. HPV-positive disease in head and neck cancer is a predictive factor for an improved prognosis, but the prognostic value of HPV infection in anal cancer is unknown [10].

Human Immunodeficiency Virus

HIV infection is a well-known risk factor for anal cancer, and this risk is not reduced even if the disease is well controlled with highly active antiretroviral therapy [11]. In general, some of the increase in the incidence of anal cancer may be due to improved survival in HIV-infected patients, as the risk of anal cancer increases with the length of HIV infection. A patient with a history of HIV for more than 15 years has a 12 times greater risk of anal cancer than patient with HIV for less than 5 years [12]. The incidence of anal canal cancer, which increased from 19.0 per 100,000 person-years from 1992 to 1995 to 78.2 per 100,000 person-years from 2000 to 2003, correlates with a natural history of coinfection with HIV and HPV that began during the HIV epidemic in the 1980s [13], and a recent study on the risk of anal cancer in HIV-infected patients reported an incidence of 131 per 100,000 person-years for HIV-infected males who have sex with males (MSM) and 3.9–30 per 100,000 person-years for females living with HIV [14, 15].

Chronic Immunosuppression

Anal cancer is well known to occur at an increased rate in patients with chronic immunosuppression due to hereditary or acquired immunodeficiency. The relative risk of anal cancer in kidney transplant patients is increased by a factor of 10- to 100-fold. Some of this risk is due to an increase in the rate of HPV infection in patients with new kidney transplants from 23 to 47% in patients with established kidney transplants [16]. Other immunosuppression, such as chronic use of steroids or immunomodulators, increases the likelihood of persistent HPV infection but is not clearly associated with anal cancer [17].

Smoking

Smoking has significantly increased the risk of developing anal cancer in many case-control studies. There appears to be a direct correlation between the amounts of cigarettes smoked and an increased relative risk. The relative risk for people with a 20-pack smoking history was 1.9, but the relative risk for people with a 50-pack smoking history was 5.2 [18]. Current smoking has the highest risk, with a relative risk of 9.4 for men and 7.7 for women [19].

Prevention

Screening for Premalignant Lesions

Like cervix cancer, high-grade anal intraepithelial neoplasia (AIN) may be a precursor to anal cancer [8]. Treatment of high-grade AIN can prevent the development of anal cancer, especially in high-risk patients such as MSM and people living with HIV (PLWH) [20]. High-grade AIN can be identified by digital rectal examination, high-resolution anoscopy, biopsy, cytology, and HPV testing. However, routine screening for AIN in high-risk individuals such as MSM or PLWH is controversial because there is a lack of randomized controlled trials indicating that these screening programs are effective in reducing the incidence and mortality of anal cancer [21–23]. Recent systematic reviews and meta-analyses have suggested that anal cytology is effective in the detection of AIN [24, 25]. Although further evaluation of efficacy and cost-effectiveness is needed, screening for anal cancer in high-risk individuals is acceptable and feasible.

HPV Immunization

Considering that most anal cancers are caused by the HPV, HPV vaccination can prevent the development of anal cancer. As mentioned above, anal cancer, like cervical cancer, is preceded by high-grade AIN [20]. Studies on the effectiveness of HPV immunization in MSM reported that the rate of high-grade AIN related to HPV infection (subtype 6, 11, 16, or 18) and the corresponding risks of persistent anal infection with HPV (subtype 6, 11, 16, or 18) were reduced by more than 50% in the intention-to-treat analysis and 74% in the per protocol analysis [26]. There are three commercially available HPV vaccines (Table 1). To prevent high-risk HPV 16 and 18 infections, all three vaccines have a similar good efficacy of more than 80% [26–29]. The Advisory Committee on Immunization Practices recommends routine use of the 9-valent vaccine in children aged 11 and 12 years and catch-up vaccination for individuals up to age 26 who have not previously been vaccinated [30]. The Korea Centers for Disease Control and Prevention also recommended the bi- or quadrivalent vaccine in children aged 9–14 years, as well as catch-up vaccination for people up to 26 years of age who have not been vaccinated previously [31].

Table 1 Human papillomavirus vaccines [1]

Vaccine	HPV type	Administration interval (months)
Bivalent (Cervarix)	16, 18	0, 1, 6
Quadrivalent (Gardasil)	6, 11, 16, 18	0, 2, 6
Nonavalent (Gardasil 9)	6, 11, 16, 18, 31, 33, 45, 52, 58	0, 2, 6

Conclusion

Although anal cancer is a rare malignancy, the incidence of anal cancer is increasing, which is related to an increase in the incidence of HPV infection, particularly subtypes 16 and 18, and to the increased number of patients with HIV/HPV coinfection due to a longer survival period in HIV-infected patients. Risk factors for anal cancer such as sexual activity with more than ten sexual partners, anal receptive intercourse, STD, and HIV infection are associated with HPV infection; other important risk factors include chronic immunosuppression and smoking. There are three types of HPV vaccination, bivalent, quadrivalent, and nonavalent, and these can reduce the risk of anal cancer in high-risk populations.

References

1. Nelson VM, Benson AB 3rd. Epidemiology of anal canal cancer. Surg Oncol Clin N Am. 2017;26(1):9–15.
2. Hong S, Won YJ, Lee JJ, Jung KW, Kong HJ, Im JS, et al. Cancer statistics in Korea: incidence, mortality, survival, and prevalence in 2018. Cancer Res Treat. 2021;53(2):301–15.
3. Korea Central Cancer Registry, National Cancer Center. Annual report of cancer statistics in Korea in 2018. Ministry of Health and Welfare, 2020.

4. Deshmukh AA, Suk R, Shiels MS, Sonawane K, Nyitray AG, Liu Y, et al. Recent trends in squamous cell carcinoma of the anus incidence and mortality in the United States, 2001-2015. J Natl Cancer Inst. 2020;112(8):829–38.
5. Brewster DH, Bhatti LA. Increasing incidence of squamous cell carcinoma of the anus in Scotland, 1975-2002. Br J Cancer. 2006;95(1):87–90.
6. Grulich AE, Poynten IM, Machalek DA, Jin F, Templeton DJ, Hillman RJ. The epidemiology of anal cancer. Sex Health. 2012;9(6):504–8.
7. Frisch M, Glimelius B, van den Brule AJ, Wohlfahrt J, Meijer CJ, Walboomers JM, et al. Sexually transmitted infection as a cause of anal cancer. N Engl J Med. 1997;337(19):1350–8.
8. Fenger C. Anal neoplasia and its precursors: facts and controversies. Semin Diagn Pathol. 1991;8(3):190–201.
9. Machalek DA, Poynten M, Jin F, Fairley CK, Farnsworth A, Garland SM, et al. Anal human papillomavirus infection and associated neoplastic lesions in men who have sex with men: a systematic review and meta-analysis. Lancet Oncol. 2012;13(5):487–500.
10. Williams GR, Lu QL, Love SB, Talbot IC, Northover JM. Properties of HPV-positive and HPV-negative anal carcinomas. J Pathol. 1996;180(4):378–82.
11. Lim ST, Levine AM. Non-AIDS-defining cancers and HIV infection. Curr Infect Dis Rep. 2005;7(3):227–34.
12. Crum-Cianflone NF, Hullsiek KH, Marconi VC, Ganesan A, Weintrob A, Barthel RV, et al. Anal cancers among HIV-infected persons: HAART is not slowing rising incidence. AIDS. 2010;24(4):535–43.
13. Patel P, Hanson DL, Sullivan PS, Novak RM, Moorman AC, Tong TC, et al. Incidence of types of cancer among HIV-infected persons compared with the general population in the United States, 1992-2003. Ann Intern Med. 2008;148(10):728–36.
14. Silverberg MJ, Lau B, Justice AC, Engels E, Gill MJ, Goedert JJ, et al. Risk of anal cancer in HIV-infected and HIV-uninfected individuals in North America. Clin Infect Dis. 2012;54(7):1026–34.
15. Stier EA, Sebring MC, Mendez AE, Ba FS, Trimble DD, Chiao EY. Prevalence of anal human papillomavirus infection and anal HPV-related disorders in women: a systematic review. Am J Obstet Gynecol. 2015;213(3):278–309.
16. Patel HS, Silver AR, Northover JM. Anal cancer in renal transplant patients. Int J Color Dis. 2007;22(1):1–5.
17. Sillman FH, Sedlis A. Anogenital papillomavirus infection and neoplasia in immunodeficient women: an update. Dermatol Clin. 1991;9(2):353–69.
18. Holly EA, Whittemore AS, Aston DA, Ahn DK, Nickoloff BJ, Kristiansen JJ. Anal cancer incidence: genital warts, anal fissure or fistula, hemorrhoids, and smoking. J Natl Cancer Inst. 1989;81(22):1726–31.
19. Daling JR, Weiss NS, Hislop TG, Maden C, Coates RJ, Sherman KJ, et al. Sexual practices, sexually transmitted diseases, and the incidence of anal cancer. N Engl J Med. 1987;317(16):973–7.
20. Gautier M, Brochard C, Lion A, Henno S, Mallet AL, Bodere A, et al. High-grade anal intraepithelial neoplasia: progression to invasive cancer is not a certainty. Dig Liver Dis. 2016;48(7):806–11.
21. Barroso LF. Anal cancer screening. Lancet Oncol. 2012;13(7):e278–9; author reply e80.
22. Palefsky J, Berry JM, Jay N. Anal cancer screening. Lancet Oncol. 2012;13(7):e279–80; author rreply e80.
23. Roark R. The need for anal dysplasia screening and treatment programs for HIV-infected men who have sex with men: a review of the literature. J Assoc Nurses AIDS Care. 2011;22(6):433–43.
24. Chen CC, Chou YY. Predictive value of the anal cytology for detecting anal intraepithelial neoplasia or worse: a systematic review and meta-analysis. Diagn Cytopathol. 2019;47(4):307–14.
25. Gonçalves JCN, Macedo ACL, Madeira K, Bavaresco DV, Dondossola ER, Grande AJ, et al. Accuracy of anal cytology for diagnostic of precursor lesions of anal cancer: systematic review and meta-analysis. Dis Colon Rectum. 2019;62(1):112–20.
26. Palefsky JM, Giuliano AR, Goldstone S, Moreira ED Jr, Aranda C, Jessen H, et al. HPV vaccine against anal HPV infection and anal intraepithelial neoplasia. N Engl J Med. 2011;365(17):1576–85.
27. Giuliano AR, Palefsky JM, Goldstone S, Moreira ED Jr, Penny ME, Aranda C, et al. Efficacy of quadrivalent HPV vaccine against HPV infection and disease in males. N Engl J Med. 2011;364(5):401–11.
28. Joura EA, Giuliano AR, Iversen OE, Bouchard C, Mao C, Mehlsen J, et al. A 9-valent HPV vaccine against infection and intraepithelial neoplasia in women. N Engl J Med. 2015;372(8):711–23.
29. Kreimer AR, González P, Katki HA, Porras C, Schiffman M, Rodriguez AC, et al. Efficacy of a bivalent HPV 16/18 vaccine against anal HPV 16/18 infection among young women: a nested analysis within the Costa Rica vaccine trial. Lancet Oncol. 2011;12(9):862–70.
30. Meites E, Szilagyi PG, Chesson HW, Unger ER, Romero JR, Markowitz LE. Human papillomavirus vaccination for adults: updated recommendations of the advisory committee on immunization practices. MMWR Morb Mortal Wkly Rep. 2019;68(32):698–702.
31. https://nip.kdca.go.kr/irgd/introduce.do?MnLv1=2&MnLv2=14

Epidemiology and Prevention. I-2. Pathologic and Molecular Characteristics of Anal Cancer

Key Points

- Anal cancer is a rare tumor, with squamous cell carcinoma (SCC) being the most frequent histology corresponding to 80% of all cases.
- Human papillomavirus (HPV) infection plays a key role in the development of anal cancer, encoding E5, E6, and E7.
- There are two subtypes of anal adenocarcinoma: mucosal and extramucosal.

Introduction

The anal canal can be divided into thirds. The upper zone is lined by the columnar rectal epithelium; the middle third is lined by the transitional epithelium; and the lower third is lined by the stratified squamous epithelium. Carcinomas of the anal canal may have typical glandular or squamous differentiation patterns that recapitulate the normal epithelium of the upper and lower thirds, respectively. An additional differentiation pattern of squamous cell carcinomas (SCCs), termed basaloid, is present in tumors populated by immature cells derived from the basal layer of the transitional epithelium [1]. The World Health Organization (WHO) classified anal canal tumors into three main groups: epithelial, mesenchymal, and secondary tumors. Epithelial tumors were subdivided into malignant and premalignant lesions. Although cancer of the anal canal is rare, a variety of malignant neoplasms involve tumors in this location. Almost all of these are SCC. Other rare anal canal neoplasms include adenocarcinoma, neuroendocrine tumors, malignant melanoma, lymphomas, and various mesenchymal tumors [2].

Human Papillomavirus Infection

Evidence indicates an association between oncogenic HPV infection with premalignant and malignant lesions of the genital tract, including the anus [3]. Currently, 88% of anal SCC tumor samples are usually positive for HPV, with different rates depending on geographical location [4]. HPV16 infection is the most common, present in 86% of cases. In some cases, co-infection was found with multiple types of HPV [5]. HPV is a non-enveloped virus with circular double-stranded DNA, containing a genome of around 8000 base pairs [3]. HPV can remain in the nuclei of basal epithelial cells for decades after initial infection of the mucosa, which usually occurs through sexual contact [6]. There are more than 240 types described, and the alpha human papillomavirus is generally related to mucosal infection [7]. High-risk HPV genotypes (16 and 18) encode at least three oncoproteins with stimulatory properties: E5, E6, and E7. Protein E7 interacts with the Rb protein (pRb), and E6 is able to bind and inactivate P53 [8].

Kyu Yeoun Won is the lead author of this chapter.

H. J. Chun et al., *Gastrointestinal Cancer*, https://doi.org/10.1007/978-981-99-0815-8_42

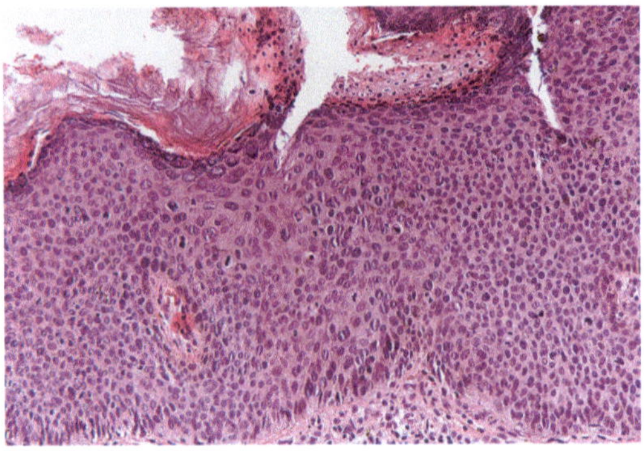

Fig. 1 The histological findings of HSIL consist of a thickened proliferating epithelium containing atypical cells showing abnormal nuclear polarity, nuclear pleomorphism, and high nuclear hyperchromatism: cytoplasmic ratio and increased mitotic activity

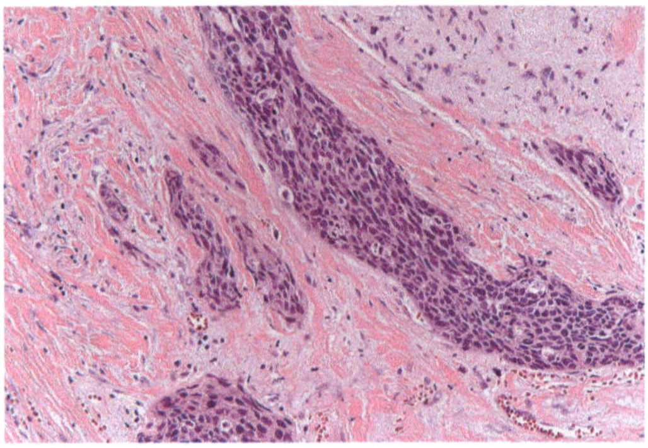

Fig. 2 The basaloid pattern with a peripheral palisade revealed infiltrating nests of hyperchromatic cells that were delimited from the adjacent stroma by hyperchromatic neoplastic nuclei arranged in the peripheral palisade. Keratin pearl formation was absent

Anal Squamous Dysplasia

Low-grade squamous intraepithelial lesion (LSIL) includes mild dysplasia and condyloma acuminatum. Histologically, LSIL shows cytologic atypia and mitotic figures only in the lower third of the epithelium and is associated with koilocytotic atypia.

High-grade squamous intraepithelial lesion (HSIL) includes moderate dysplasia, severe dysplasia, carcinoma in situ, and Bowen disease. Microscopically, HSIL reveals the involvement of two-thirds or more of the squamous epithelium by marked cytological atypia, mitotic figures in the upper two-thirds of the epithelium, atypical mitotic figures, and loss of nuclear polarity (Fig. 1). p16 immunohistochemistry is characteristically diffusely positive and can distinguish HSIL from reactive changes [9].

Anal Squamous Cell Carcinoma

Anal SCC is a malignant epithelial tumor characterized by origin in the anal mucosa, keratin production, intercellular bridges, and frequent HPV infection. This is the most common histology of anal cancer, corresponding to 80% [10]. Tumors located in the anal canal develop predominantly in the transformation zone between the squamous and columnar epithelium of the anal canal [11]. Cells may have large pale eosinophilic squamous cells with or without areas of keratinization. Another pattern is that of tumor-cell islands with prominent palisading of nuclei. Cells can constitute tumor nests and differentiated tumors can present with peripheral palisading or central keratinization [12]. Basaloid SCC refers to a pattern characterized by marked hyperchromasia, scant cytoplasm, and a peripheral palisade of tumor cells, which was previously called cloacogenic carcinoma [13] (Fig. 2). Verrucous carcinoma (VC) is a subtype of SCC. VC displays exophytic and endophytic growth of bulbous fronds of thickened epithelium with a pushing interface. VC lacks the HPV cytopathic effect and severe cytological atypia. In small biopsies, the definitive diagnosis of VC is often impossible and can only be suggested based on clinical information. VC is locally destructive but does not metastasize. In some cases, the areas of unequivocal conventional SCC arise in VC. These cases can metastasize and should be diagnosed as conventional SCC [14].

Molecular Pathology of Anal SCC

Frequent mutations and genomic alterations have been identified in the PIK3CA/AKT/mTOR pathway, most commonly in *PIK3CA*. Overall, the burden of tumor mutations is low [15]. Loss-of-function mutations in *TP53* and *CDKN2A* were significantly enhanced in HPV-negative cases [16].

Anal Adenocarcinoma

This tumor can originate in the mucosa, the anal glands, or fistulas of the anal canal and may appear near the anal duct as a small pedunculated or ulcerated lesion or produce a submucosal mass [12]. An association with Paget's disease and Crohn's disease is described (Fig. 3). Generally, adenocarcinomas associated with congenital or acquired fistulae are mucin-producing. Anal adenocarcinoma is an adenocarcinoma that arises in the glandular epithelium of the anal canal (Fig. 4a, b). There are two subtypes: mucosal and extramucosal. The former arises in the luminal mucosa and is of intestinal type; the latter may be associated with anal gland, a preexisting anal fistula, or other nonfistulating glandular structures of the anal canal (acquired or congenital malformations or embryological remnants) and may be of anal gland type, mucinous type, or intestinal type. Mucosal-type anal adenocarcinomas arise within the luminal mucosa and typically have histopathological characteristics indistinguishable from those of rectal adenocarcinoma. Extramucosal-type anal canal adenocarcinomas, by definition, lack a luminal in situ component, although they can affect the surface mucosa by erosion, colonization, or pagetoid extension:

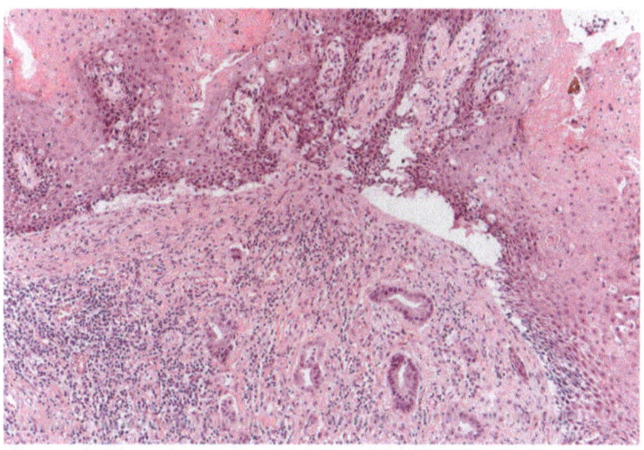

Fig. 3 Atypical vacuolated cells (Paget's cells) are visible in the anal squamous epithelium. Adenocarcinoma is also visible in the subepithelium

1. Anal gland adenocarcinoma: Grossly, this forms a firm infiltrative mass, typically centered on the wall of the anorectal area, 2–5 cm in greatest dimension [17]. Microscopically, haphazardly dispersed glands with cuboidal cells and scant mucin. Tumor cells characteristically express CK7 and MUC5AC and do not express CK20 or CDX2 [18]. The main differential diagnoses include metastases from sites such as to the gynecological tract and breast.
2. Fistula-associated adenocarcinoma: Most of these tumors are mucinous, grossly and mor-

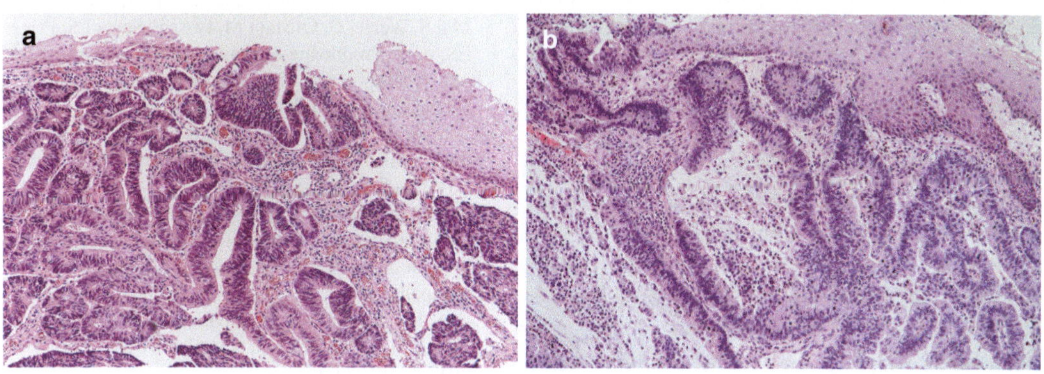

Fig. 4 (**a**) The anal adenocarcinoma was composed of small acini and tubules with limited mucin production. Overlying normal squamous epithelium is seen. (**b**) Another case of adenocarcinoma shows abundant mucin production. Overlying normal squamous epithelium is seen

phologically resembling ordinary colorectal-type mucinous adenocarcinoma.

3. Extramucosal anal canal adenocarcinoma, nonanal gland type and nonfistula-associated: newly recognized group of tumors that may be histogenetically related to other nonfistulating intramural glandular structures including acquired or congenital malformations or embryological remnants.

Molecular Pathology of Anal Adenocarcinoma

A recent study observed rates of *KRAS* and *NRAS* mutations in anal canal adenocarcinoma of 47% and 6%, respectively. Microsatellite instability (MSI) was observed in only 1 of 48 intestinal-type tumors and 0 of 26 anal gland/transitional-type tumors [19].

Other Tumors in the Anal Canal

Melanoma

Anal melanomas are a rare disease and account for 1% of anal and perianal lesions [12]. Two-thirds are found as pigmented lesions, usually ulcerated and bleeding. Similar to melanomas that arise in other mucous membranes, they are generally of the acral lentiginous type. Retrospective studies have reported a poor prognosis, especially in patients with lymph node involvement or metastasis at diagnosis [2].

Neuroendocrine Tumors

Anal neuroendocrine tumors are unusual and account for 1% of all anal cancers [20]. Small-cell anal carcinoma has a poor prognosis and generally begins in the upper part of the anal canal, grows rapidly, and promotes metastasis. Histologically, it may be confused with SCC due to basal features, but immunohistochemistry is an important tool for differential diagnosis [12].

Mesenchymal Tumors

Uncommonly lipomas, hemangiomas, leiomyomas and leiomyosarcomas, rhabdomyosarcomas, granular cell tumors, and Kaposi sarcoma may be located in the anal and perianal region [12].

Conclusion

Anal cancer is a rare tumor. HPV encoding E5, E6, and E7 plays a key role in the development of anal cancer. SCC is the most common subtype of anal cancer, accounting for 80% of all cases. Anal adenocarcinoma is an adenocarcinoma that arises in the glandular epithelium of the anal canal. There are two subtypes: mucosal and extramucosal. Anal melanomas are a rare disease and account for 1% of anal and perianal lesions.

References

1. Kumar V, Abbas AK, Aster JC. Robbins and Cotran pathologic basis of disease, 9th ed. 2014. 815 p.
2. Hoff PM, Coudry R, Moniz CM. Pathology of anal cancer. Surg Oncol Clin N Am. 2017;26(1):57–71.
3. Ostrbenk A, Kocjan BJ, Hosnjak L, Li J, Deng Q, Sterbenc A, et al. Identification of a novel human papillomavirus, type HPV199, isolated from a nasopharynx and Anal Canal, and complete genomic characterization of papillomavirus species Gamma-12. PLoS One. 2015;10(9):e0138628.
4. Alemany L, Saunier M, Alvarado-Cabrero I, Quiros B, Salmeron J, Shin HR, et al. Human papillomavirus DNA prevalence and type distribution in anal carcinomas worldwide. Int J Cancer. 2015;136(1):98–107.
5. Mai S, Welzel G, Ottstadt M, Lohr F, Severa S, Prigge ES, et al. Prognostic relevance of HPV infection and p16 overexpression in squamous cell anal cancer. Int J Radiat Oncol Biol Phys. 2015;93(4):819–27.
6. Hellner K, Munger K. Human papillomaviruses as therapeutic targets in human cancer. J Clin Oncol. 2011;29(13):1785–94.
7. Egawa N, Egawa K, Griffin H, Doorbar J. Human papillomaviruses; epithelial tropisms, and the development of neoplasia. Viruses. 2015;7(7):3863–90.
8. Klingelhutz AJ, Roman A. Cellular transformation by human papillomaviruses: lessons learned by comparing high- and low-risk viruses. Virology. 2012;424(2):77–98.
9. Darragh TM, Colgan TJ, Cox JT, Heller DS, Henry MR, Luff RD, et al. The lower anogenital squamous terminology standardization proj-

ect for HPV-associated lesions: background and consensus recommendations from the College of American Pathologists and the American Society for Colposcopy and Cervical Pathology. Arch Pathol Lab Med. 2012;136(10):1266–97.
10. Flejou JF. An update on anal neoplasia. Histopathology. 2015;66(1):147–60.
11. Leeds IL, Fang SH. Anal cancer and intraepithelial neoplasia screening: a review. World J Gastrointest Surg. 2016;8(1):41–51.
12. Fenoglio-Preiser C, Stemmermann G, Lantz P. Gastrointestinal pathology: an atlas and text. 2008. 1067–97 p.
13. Graham RP, Arnold CA, Naini BV, Lam-Himlin DM. Basaloid squamous cell carcinoma of the anus revisited. Am J Surg Pathol. 2016;40(3):354–60.
14. Zidar N, Langner C, Odar K, Hosnjak L, Kamaradova K, Daum O, et al. Anal verrucous carcinoma is not related to infection with human papillomaviruses and should be distinguished from giant condyloma (Buschke-Lowenstein tumour). Histopathology. 2017;70(6):938–45.
15. Cacheux W, Dangles-Marie V, Rouleau E, Lazartigues J, Girard E, Briaux A, et al. Exome sequencing reveals aberrant signalling pathways as hallmark of treatment-naive anal squamous cell carcinoma. Oncotarget. 2018;9(1):464–76.
16. Chung JH, Sanford E, Johnson A, Klempner SJ, Schrock AB, Palma NA, et al. Comprehensive genomic profiling of anal squamous cell carcinoma reveals distinct genomically defined classes. Ann Oncol. 2016;27(7):1336–41.
17. Lisovsky M, Patel K, Cymes K, Chase D, Bhuiya T, Morgenstern N. Immunophenotypic characterization of anal gland carcinoma: loss of p63 and cytokeratin 5/6. Arch Pathol Lab Med. 2007;131(8):1304–11.
18. Hobbs CM, Lowry MA, Owen D, Sobin LH. Anal gland carcinoma. Cancer. 2001;92(8):2045–9.
19. Herfs M, Roncarati P, Koopmansch B, Peulen O, Bruyere D, Lebeau A, et al. A dualistic model of primary anal canal adenocarcinoma with distinct cellular origins, etiologies, inflammatory microenvironments and mutational signatures: implications for personalised medicine. Br J Cancer. 2018;118(10):1302–12.
20. Lee RT, Ferreira J, Friedman K, Moss SF. A rare cause of constipation: obstructing small cell neuroendocrine carcinoma of the anal canal. Int J Color Dis. 2015;30(9):1291–2.

Staging and Treatment. II-1. Staging and Prognosis

Key Points

- Diagnostic workup should include digital rectal examination, inguinal lymph node evaluation, anoscopy or endoscopy with biopsy, and imaging studies such as chest/abdomen CT, pelvis CT or MRI, and PET/CT (if available).
- The prognosis of anal carcinoma (cancer) is related to the size of the primary tumor and the presence of lymph node metastases (metastasis).
- Recent data suggested that HPV DNA load and p16 expression would affect overall survival and disease-specific survival.

Introduction

Cancer of the anal region is relatively rare in gastrointestinal tract malignancy. However, the worldwide incidence of anal cancer has increased [1, 2]. Because current guidelines do not recommend surgical treatment as a first therapeutic option, the staging of anal cancer is based on clinical staging by physical examination and radiological imaging. In this chapter, we will discuss the diagnostic workup, staging, and prognosis of anal cancer.

Hyeon Jeong Goong is the lead author of this chapter.

Staging and Workup of Anal Cancer

In patients with a clinical suspicion of anal cancer, complete medical history taking should be documented, including relevant symptoms, medical conditions, and comorbidity. Physical examination is necessary and consists of digital rectal examination and gynecological examination. Digital rectal examination enables the detection of anal/perianal lesions and regional lymph nodes, including the inguinal area. Gynecological examination is performed to assess the status of vaginal involvement and human papillomavirus (HPV) status. It is recommended to confirm the human immunodeficiency virus (HIV)/HPV status related to the etiology and prognosis. Anoscopy, proctoscopy, or colonoscopy are recommended for biopsy-proven histologic confirmation. In western guidelines, colonoscopy is not essential because synchronous lesions in the proximal colon are not reported in anal squamous cell carcinoma [3]. After confirmation of histological differentiation, an accurate staging is required to estab-

H. J. Chun et al., *Gastrointestinal Cancer*, https://doi.org/10.1007/978-981-99-0815-8_43

lish a therapeutic plan. The imaging studies to be performed include chest/abdomen/pelvis computed tomography (CT) and/or pelvis magnetic resonance imaging (MRI) and are used to investigate the tumor size, local extension, the presence of regional/distant lymph node metastasis, and distant metastasis. An FDG-PET/CT scan can also be considered for staging and planning radiation therapy. In a previous study, the sensitivity and specificity of PET/CT to detect lymph node involvement were 31%–100% and 53%–98%, respectively [4, 5]. Additionally, the PET/CT scan findings changed the initial clinical stage assessed by either CT or MRI in 5.1–42% of patients [5–7]. In addition, due to the characteristics of FDG-avid properties of most anal cancer, PET/CT scan may be useful for planning radiation therapy by defining the metabolically active tumor sites [8]. Endoscopic ultrasound may be considered to determine the depth of tumor invasion but is not mandatory due to its operator dependency and small field of view. To assess lymph node status that is not confirmatory on CT or MRI, ultrasonography-guided fine needle aspiration may be useful to evaluate palpable inguinal lymph node.

The description of tumor status associated with the treatment plan and prognosis is usually based on the TNM stage with an assessment of size and of adjacent organ involvement (T stage), regional lymph no involvement (N stage), and metastatic spread (M stage). The TNM staging suggested by the eighth edition of the AJCC for anal cancer is summarized in Table 1 [9].

Table 1 American Joint Committee on Cancer (AJCC) TNM staging classification for anal cancer

Definitions for T, N, M	
T	**Primary tumor**
Tx	Primary tumor not assessed
T0	No evidence of primary tumor
T1	High-grade squamous intraepithelial lesion (previously termed carcinoma in situ, Bowen disease, anal intraepithelial neoplasia II–III, high-grade anal intraepithelial neoplasia)
T1	Tumor ≤2 cm (tumor 2 cm or less)
T2	Tumor <2 cm and ≤5 cm (tumor more than 2 cm but not more than 5 cm)
T3	Tumor <5 cm (tumor more than 5 cm)
T4	Tumor of any size invades adjacent organs such as the vagina, urethra, bladder (and 삭제)
N	**Regional lymph nodes**
Nx	Regional lymph nodes not assessed (cannot be assessed)
N0	No regional lymph node metastasis
N1	Metastasis in inguinal, mesorectal, internal, or external iliac nodes
N1a	Metastasis in inguinal, mesorectal, or internal iliac lymph nodes
N1b	Metastasis in external iliac lymph nodes
N1c	Metastasis in external iliac with any N1a nodes
M	**Distant metastasis**
M0	No distant metastasis
M1	Distant metastasis

Staging system for anal cancer			
Stage	**T**	**N**	**M**
0	Tis	N0	M0
I	T1	N0	M0
IIA	T2	N0	M0
IIB	T3	N0	M0
IIIA	T1–2	N1	M0
IIIB	T4	N0	M0
IIIC	T3–4	N1	M0
IV	Any T	Any N	M1

Adapted from the eighth Edition (2017) American Joint Committee on Cancer (AJCC) TNM Staging system [7]

Prognosis of Anal Cancer

According to the Surveillance, Epidemiology, and End Results (SEER) Cancer Stat Facts of anal cancer, 47.1% of patients are diagnosed at the local stage with a 5-year relative survival of 81.9%, 33% of patients at the regional stage with a 5-year relative survival of 65.5%, and 13% of patients at the distant stage with a 5-year relative survival of 34.5% [10]. The overall 5-year relative survival was 68.7% based on SEER 2011–2017 data, with an increase from 55.94 to 70.76% during the period from 1975 to 2013. Furthermore, in global statistics for 36 cancers in 185 countries, the death rate of anal cancer among all cancer sites was 0.2% [11]. According to Korean data from the Korean Central Cancer Registry, in the period 1993–2015, the overall 5-year relative survival rate was 66.5%, with 76.2% in the local stage, 64.9% in the regional stage, and 35% in the distant stage [12]. The 5-year survival of patients treated with chemoradiation therapy was 76.4%. In all histological types of anal cancer, the 5-year relative survival rate increased from 39.7 to 66.5% with better staging and advanced radiation therapy techniques. The survival rate was higher in women and in patients aged <40 years.

The prognosis of anal carcinoma is related to the size of the primary tumor and the presence of lymph node metastases. Previous studies reported that lymph node involvement, male sex, and tumor size were independent prognostic factors [13–16]. Another prognostic factor recently suggested is the HPV DNA load and p16 expression. In an analysis of 143 patients with stage I to III anal cancer, p16 positivity was an independent prognostic factor for overall survival (OS) and disease-specific survival [17]. Additionally, in a meta-analysis of 16 studies including 1724 patients with anal cancer, HPV DNA positivity, $p16^{INK4a}$ positivity, and combined HPV DNA/$p16^{INK4a}$ positivity showed better OS compared to HPV DNA/$p16^{INK4a}$ negativity (hazard ratio [HR] 0.54, 95% confidence interval [CI], 0.33–0.89; HR 0.37, 95% CI 0.24–0.57; HR 0.36, 95% CI 0.22–0.58, respectively) [18].

Conclusion

According to available studies, most patients with anal cancer are diagnosed at an early stage. The prognosis of anal cancer is related to the T stage and the N stage of the primary tumor. Therefore, accurate TNM staging at diagnosis is essential for predicting prognosis and the therapeutic strategy.

References

1. Islami F, Ferlay J, Lortet-Tieulent J, Bray F, Jemal A. International trends in anal cancer incidence rates. Int J Epidemiol. 2017;46:924–38.
2. Park HC, Jung KW, Kim BW, Shin A, Won YJ, Oh JH, et al. Characteristics and survival of Korean anal cancer from the Korea central cancer registry data. Ann Coloproctol. 2013;29:182–5.
3. Rao S, Guren MG, Khan K, Brown G, Renehan AG, Steigen SE, et al. Anal cancer: ESMO clinical practice guidelines for diagnosis, treatment and follow-up. Ann Oncol. 2021;32:1087–100.
4. Caldarella C, Annunziata S, Treglia G, Sadeghi R, Ayati N, Giovanella L. Diagnostic performance of positron emission tomography/computed tomography using fluorine-18 fluorodeoxyglucose in detecting locoregional nodal involvement in patients with anal canal cancer: a systematic review and meta-analysis. ScientificWorldJournal. 2014;2014:196068.
5. Mahmud A, Poon R, Jonker D. PET imaging in anal canal cancer: a systematic review and meta-analysis. Br J Radiol. 2017;90:20170370.
6. Bhuva NJ, Glynne-Jones R, Sonoda L, Wong WL, Harrison MK. To PET or not to PET? That is the question. Staging in anal cancer. Ann Oncol. 2012;23:2078–82.
7. Jones M, Hruby G, Solomon M, Rutherford N, Martin J. The role of FDG-PET in the initial staging and response assessment of anal cancer: a systematic review and meta-analysis. Ann Surg Oncol. 2015;22:3574–81.
8. Albertsson P, Alverbratt C, Liljegren A, Bjorkander E, Strandell A, Samuelsson O, et al. Positron emission tomography and computed tomographic (PET/CT) imaging for radiation therapy planning in anal cancer: a systematic review and meta-analysis. Crit Rev Oncol Hematol. 2018;126:6–12.
9. Welton ML, Steele SR, Goodman KA, et al. Anus. In: Amin MB, editor. AJCC cancer staging manual. 8th ed.: Springer; 2017.
10. Anonymous. SEER cancer stat facts: anal cancer. 2019. https://seer.cancer.gov/statfacts/html/anus.html.
11. Bray F, Ferlay J, Soerjomataram I, Siegel RL, Torre LA, Jemal A. Global cancer statistics 2018:

GLOBOCAN estimates of incidence and mortality worldwide for 36 cancers in 185 countries. CA Cancer J Clin. 2018;68:394–424.
12. Hur H, Jung K-W, Kim B-W, Oh C-M, Won Y-J, Oh JH, et al. Long-term oncologic outcome and its relevant factors in anal cancer in Korea: a nationwide data analysis. Ann Coloproctol. 2020;36:35–40.
13. Bartelink H, Roelofsen F, Eschwege F, Rougier P, Bosset JF, Gonzalez DG, et al. Concomitant radiotherapy and chemotherapy is superior to radiotherapy alone in the treatment of locally advanced anal cancer: results of a phase III randomized trial of the European Organization for Research and Treatment of Cancer Radiotherapy and Gastrointestinal Cooperative Groups. J Clin Oncol. 1997;15:2040–9.
14. Ajani JA, Winter KA, Gunderson LL, Pedersen J, Benson AB 3rd, Thomas CR Jr, et al. Prognostic factors derived from a prospective database dictate clinical biology of anal cancer: the intergroup trial (RTOG 98-11). Cancer. 2010;116:4007–13.
15. Glynne-Jones R, Sebag-Montefiore D, Adams R, Gollins S, Harrison M, Meadows HM, et al. Prognostic factors for recurrence and survival in anal cancer. Cancer. 2013;119:748–55.
16. Bilimoria KY, Bentrem DJ, Rock CE, Stewart AK, Ko CY, Halverson A. Outcomes and prognostic factors for squamous-cell carcinoma of the anal canal: analysis of patients from the National Cancer Data Base. Dis Colon Rectum. 2009;52:624–31.
17. Serup-Hansen E, Linnemann D, Skovrider-Ruminski W, Høgdall E, Geertsen PF, Havsteen H. Human papillomavirus genotyping and p16 expression as prognostic factors for patients with American Joint Committee on cancer stages I to III carcinoma of the anal canal. J Clin Oncol. 2014;32:1812–7.
18. Urbute A, Rasmussen CL, Belmonte F, Obermueller T, Prigge E-S, Arbyn M, et al. Prognostic significance of HPV DNA and $p16^{INK4a}$ in anal cancer: a systematic review and meta-analysis. Cancer Epidemiol Biomark Prev. 2020;29:703.

Staging and Treatment. II-2. Overview of Treatment: According to the Tumor Stage

Key Points

- Treatment of anal cancer differs dramatically from that of adenocarcinomas of the lower rectum.
- Radiotherapy (RT) with concomitant 5-fluoruracil (5-FU) and mitomycin C is recommended as standard of care for patients with localized squamous cell carcinoma of the anus (SCCA). Surgery is pursued only as salvage therapy in the setting of residual or recurrent disease.
- Chemoradiotherapy (CRT) for locally advanced anal cancer should be administered with an RT dose of >50 Gy; the optimal dose for different tumor stages is not known.
- Capecitabine can be used as an alternative to 5-FU in combination with mitomycin C and RT.
- Neoadjuvant or adjuvant chemotherapy is generally not recommended.
- Pre-CRT colostomy should be considered in patients with locally advanced anal cancers with (or expected) anorectal pain or fecal incontinence and perianal fistula. Patients should be informed about the possibility that a colostomy is permanent.
- Salvage surgery should be considered in patients with local residual or recurrent disease after CRT.
- The involvement of the anal sphincter complex requires exenterative surgery, and imaging evaluation should include a thorough evaluation of the pelvic compartments to enable surgical planning.
- The mainstay of salvage surgery is abdominoperineal excision (APE), but more radical exenterative operations can be considered to achieve an R0 resection.
- APE for recurrent anal cancer is a different operation from that used for rectal cancer. In almost all cases, perineal reconstruction using musculocutaneous flaps should be considered.

Jong Wook Kim is the lead author of this chapter.

H. J. Chun et al., *Gastrointestinal Cancer*, https://doi.org/10.1007/978-981-99-0815-8_44

Introduction

Carcinoma of the anal canal is a rare malignancy, although its incidence is steadily increasing. Anal cancer is a rare disease that accounts for <1% of all new cancer diagnoses and <3% of gastrointestinal tumors. The most common histological subtype is squamous cell carcinoma of the anus (SCCA) with an annual incidence of 0.5–2.0 in 100,000 [1]. The development of anal cancer is a multifocal process largely associated with human papillomavirus (HPV) infection. Treatment of anal cancer differs by disease stage and patient's physical condition. In this chapter, we review different treatment options according to the stage of the disease.

Management of Local/Locoregional Disease

Initial Management of Local and Locoregional Diseases

The primary objective of treatment is to achieve cure with locoregional control, preservation of anal function, and the best possible quality of life. Treatment of anal cancer differs dramatically from that of adenocarcinomas of the lower rectum. Combinations of mitomycin C (MMC) and 5-fluorouracil (5-FU)-based chemoradiotherapy (CRT) have been established as the standard of care, leading to complete tumor regression in 80–90% of patients, with locoregional failures (LRF) of ~15%; other cytotoxic agents (mainly cisplatin) can be considered, if clinically indicated [2, 3].

A multidisciplinary approach is mandatory, involving radiation oncologists, medical oncologists, surgeons, radiologists, and pathologists. Concurrent chemoradiation therapy with a doublet chemotherapy regimen is a standard treatment regimen and is curative when appropriate [4]. Surgery is pursued only as salvage therapy in the setting of residual or recurrent disease [4], and the role of surgery as a salvage treatment is accepted [5].

Chemoradiotherapy

Early randomized controlled European studies have shown that synchronous CRT with 5-FU and MMC as a primary treatment modality is superior to RT alone [6, 7]. In a phase III study comparing 5-FU with 5-FU and MMC, both in combination with RT, the superiority of the combination of MMC and 5-FU was confirmed [8].

The second generation of randomized studies investigated the role of cisplatin to replace MMC in combination with 5-FU and RT [9–11]. In these studies, cisplatin and 5-FU were also used before or after CRT as neoadjuvant or maintenance treatment, respectively. The results of these studies found that cisplatin in combination with 5-FU infusion and RT did not improve complete response rates or disease-free survival (DFS) compared to MMC. Induction chemotherapy (ChT) or maintenance ChT did not improve the outcomes [9–11]. A proposed treatment algorithm for the management of localized stage I–III anal cancer is shown in Fig. 1 [5].

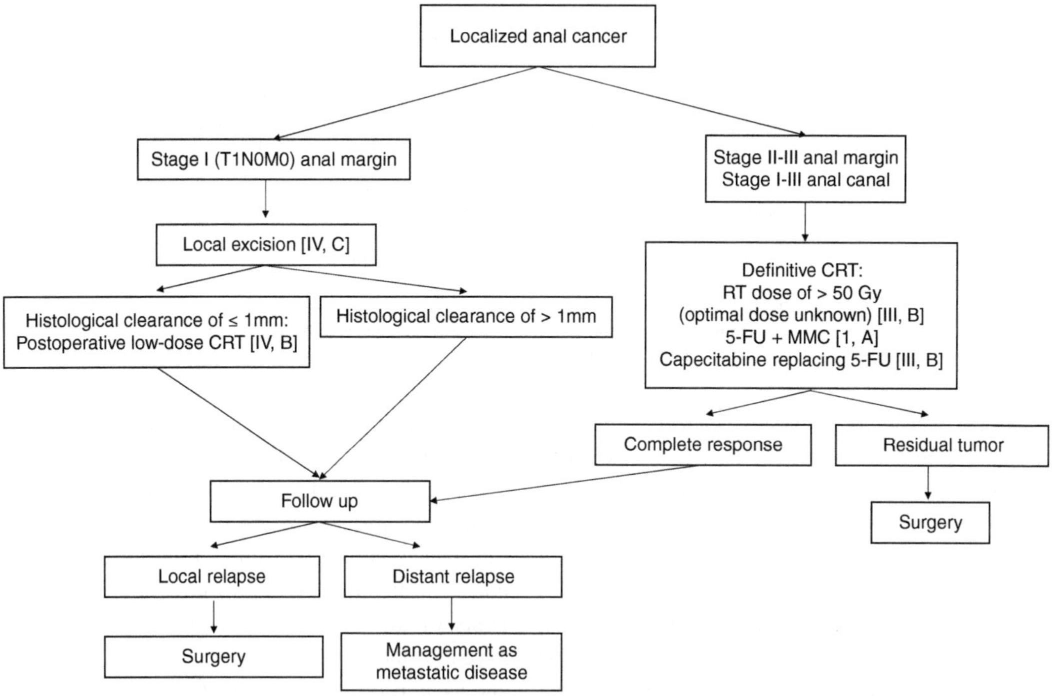

Fig. 1 Treatment algorithm for localized anal cancer (adapted from Rao et al. [12]). *5-FU* 5-fluorouracil, *CRT* chemoradiotherapy, *M* metastasis, *N* node, *MMC* mitomycin C, *RT* radiotherapy, *T* tumor. [a] The optimum timepoint to assess clinical tumor response after CRT is 26 weeks. [b] In cases where surgery cannot be performed

Role of the Surgeon in Locoregional Anal Canal Cancer

Although 80% of patients with anal cancer are initially treated with CRT, the anal cancer surgeon should provide input into the treatment of most patients. Approximately 10–20% of patients with anal cancer will require a pretreatment colostomy. The two main indications are anorectal pain and fecal incontinence or anticipated fecal incontinence during CRT. Unlike upper rectal cancers, large bowel obstruction is rare for anal cancer. Although closure or reversal of colostomy is documented in the literature, it should only be indicated if the anorectum is functionally intact. Fecal incontinence or anal stenosis often persists due to the high dose of RT to the anal sphincters. Patients should be informed of the high probability that their pretreatment colostomy will be permanent.

Up to a quarter of patients may have a perianal fistula at the time of anal cancer diagnosis. The fistula may be long-lasting, as it may be a malignant fistula. Such fistulae are at high risk for local sepsis during CRT, which may require a treatment gap of >5 days. The presence of a fistula before treatment should be documented and a seton should be placed to secure drainage. The seton may need to remain in situ (with 6-monthly changes) for up to 18 months to allow the RT changes to completely settle before the definitive fistulotomy.

Although radical abdominoperineal excision (APE) has been replaced by CRT as primary treatment for most anal cancers [13], there are a number of uncommon scenarios in which there are relative indications for APE as primary treatment. These include the following: (1) where there has been previous pelvic RT and curative RT cannot be given, (2) histology of anal adenocarcinoma or adenosquamous carcinoma where complete response to RT is less likely than for SCCA, (3) the setting of SCCA in a transplant patient on immunosuppressants where there may be doubt that the patient will complete CRT uninterrupted, and (4) an exceptional patient who refuses CRT.

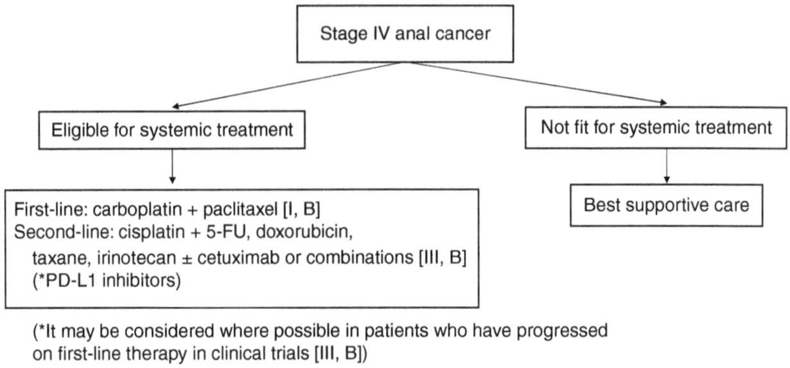

Fig. 2 Treatment algorithm for advanced anal cancer (adapted from Rao et al. [12]). *5-FU* 5-fluorouracil, *BSC* best supportive care, *PD-1* programmed cell death protein 1, *PD-L1* programmed death-ligand 1

Local excision of early-stage cancers in the anal canal is contraindicated [5]. This is associated with an unacceptably high proportion of margin-positive resections and, if followed by CRT, is associated with considerable morbidity to the anal sphincter [14]. Piecemeal resections (anywhere in the anorectum) are strongly discouraged, as it makes the assessment of resection margins in the specimen impossible. The only exception is local excision, usually as a biopsy, of very early cancers in the form of superficial invasive SCCA (SISCCA).

Postoperative CRT

Postoperative CRT should be considered for all patients that have undergone local excision of a cancer in the anal canal, for patients with local excision of an anal margin cancer with a histological margin of 1 mm, for patients who have undergone excision where piecemeal histological assessment and completeness of excision cannot be guaranteed, and in those patients considered at risk of pelvic node involvement [5]. Other indications include rare cases where radical surgery has been performed as primary treatment but the resection margin is involved. Re-excision for a histological positive or close (1 mm) margin is not recommended.

Management of Advanced/Metastatic Disease

Approximately 10–20% of patients experience distant relapse and ~10% present with de novo metastatic disease [7, 15]. Twenty percent of patients develop local failures after CRT, and salvage surgery is only feasible for a proportion of such patients [7, 15, 16]. The common sites of metastatic spread are the para-aortic nodes and the liver, whereas the lungs, bones, peritoneum, and skin are involved less frequently. The prognosis of all metastatic patients is poor with a 5-year relative survival rate of 30%. Figure 2 shows a proposed treatment algorithm for the treatment of stage IV anal cancer [5].

Conclusion

The treatment approach to anal cancer has evolved significantly in recent decades and serves as a model for organ preservation therapy, transitioning from radical surgery to a nonsurgical approach of definitive chemoradiotherapy with 5-FU and MMC. This leads to preservation of anorectal function in most patients. Anal cancer has a low propensity to metastatic spread, making local–regional control of paramount importance. Randomized trials have demonstrated the superiority of 5-FU and MMC chemoradiotherapy over radiation therapy alone, radiation with concurrent 5-FU, as well as induction cisplatin/5-FU alone followed by concurrent radiation therapy using the same regimen. Furthermore, randomized trials have failed to demonstrate a definitive benefit for radiation dose escalation or superiority when substituting cisplatin for MMC. Current investigations include the use of novel cytotoxic and inhibitor-targeted agents, including the epidermal growth factor receptor (EGFR), in efforts to improve outcomes in patients with more advanced disease.

References

1. Islami F, Ferlay J, Lortet-Tieulent J, Bray F, Jemal A. International trends in anal cancer incidence rates. Int J Epidemiol. 2017;46:924–38.
2. Glynne-Jones R, Nilsson PJ, Aschele C, Goh V, Peiffert D, Cervantes A, et al. Anal cancer: ESMO-ESSO-ESTRO clinical practice guidelines for diagnosis, treatment and follow-up. Eur J Surg Oncol. 2014;40:1165–76.
3. Nigro ND, Vaitkevicius VK, Considine B Jr. Combined therapy for cancer of the anal canal: a preliminary report. Dis Colon Rectum. 1974;17:354–6.
4. Ahmed S, Eng C. Optimal treatment strategies for anal cancer. Curr Treat Options Oncol. 2014;15:443–55.
5. Rao S, Guren MG, Khan K, Brown G, Renehan AG, Steigen SE, et al. Anal cancer: ESMO clinical practice guidelines for diagnosis, treatment and follow-up. Ann Oncol. 2021;32:1087–100.
6. Anonymous. Epidermoid anal cancer: results from the UKCCCR randomised trial of radiotherapy alone versus radiotherapy, 5-fluorouracil, and mitomycin. UKCCCR Anal Cancer Trial Working Party. UK Co-ordinating Committee on Cancer Research. Lancet. 1996;348:1049–54.
7. Bartelink H, Roelofsen F, Eschwege F, Rougier P, Bosset JF, Gonzalez DG, et al. Concomitant radiotherapy and chemotherapy is superior to radiotherapy alone in the treatment of locally advanced anal cancer: results of a phase III randomized trial of the European Organization for Research and Treatment of Cancer Radiotherapy and Gastrointestinal Cooperative Groups. J Clin Oncol. 1997;15:2040–9.
8. Flam M, John M, Pajak TF, Petrelli N, Myerson R, Doggett S, et al. Role of mitomycin in combination with fluorouracil and radiotherapy, and of salvage chemoradiation in the definitive nonsurgical treatment of epidermoid carcinoma of the anal canal: results of a phase III randomized intergroup study. J Clin Oncol. 1996;14:2527–39.
9. Ajani JA, Winter KA, Gunderson LL, Pedersen J, Benson AB 3rd, Thomas CR Jr, et al. Fluorouracil, mitomycin, and radiotherapy vs fluorouracil, cisplatin, and radiotherapy for carcinoma of the anal canal: a randomized controlled trial. JAMA. 2008;299:1914–21.
10. James RD, Glynne-Jones R, Meadows HM, Cunningham D, Myint AS, Saunders MP, et al. Mitomycin or cisplatin chemoradiation with or without maintenance chemotherapy for treatment of squamous-cell carcinoma of the anus (ACT II): a randomised, phase 3, open-label, 2 x 2 factorial trial. Lancet Oncol. 2013;14:516–24.
11. Peiffert D, Tournier-Rangeard L, Gerard JP, Lemanski C, Francois E, Giovannini M, et al. Induction chemotherapy and dose intensification of the radiation boost in locally advanced anal canal carcinoma: final analysis of the randomized UNICANCER ACCORD 03 trial. J Clin Oncol. 2012;30:1941–8.
12. Rao S, Guren MG, Khan K, Brown G, Renehan AG, Stegen SE, et al. Anal cancer: ESMO clinical practice guidelines for diagnosis, treatment and follow-up. Ann Oncol. 2021;32(9):1087–100.
13. Downing A, Morris EJ, Aravani A, Finan PJ, Lawton S, Thomas JD, et al. The effect of the UK Coordinating Centre for Cancer Research Anal Cancer Trial (ACT1) on population-based treatment and survival for squamous cell cancer of the anus. Clin Oncol (R Coll Radiol). 2015;27:708–12.
14. Renehan AG, Muirhead R, Sebag-Montefiore D. Limitations of the National Cancer Data Base to evaluate early-stage anal cancer treatment outcomes. JAMA Surg. 2018;153:691.
15. Northover J, Glynne-Jones R, Sebag-Montefiore D, James R, Meadows H, Wan S, et al. Chemoradiation for the treatment of epidermoid anal cancer: 13-year follow-up of the first randomised UKCCCR Anal Cancer Trial (ACT I). Br J Cancer. 2010;102:1123–8.
16. Renehan AG, Saunders MP, Schofield PF, O'Dwyer ST. Patterns of local disease failure and outcome after salvage surgery in patients with anal cancer. Br J Surg. 2005;92:605–14.

Staging and Treatment. II-3. Definitive Chemoradiotherapy for Anal Cancer

Key Points

- Definitive chemoradiotherapy is a standard treatment for locoregional disease of anal cancer, which allows preservation of the anal sphincter.
- The concurrent use of 5-fluorouracil plus mitomycin C is a standard chemotherapy regimen.
- The radiation field encompasses the pelvis from the lumbosacral junction to the inguinal lymph nodes and the anus. Elective nodal irradiation should be performed because anal cancer frequently metastasizes to the regional nodal area.

Introduction

In the past, abdominoperineal resection was performed routinely for anal cancer [1]. Abdominoperineal resection required removal of the anorectum with the creation of a permanent colostomy. Critical issues in the care of patients with anal cancer include not only local control and survival but also organ preservation. Therefore, external beam radiotherapy with concurrent chemotherapy has replaced surgery as the first-line therapy since its introduction by Nigro et al. [2]. Currently, 5-fluorouracil (5-FU) plus mitomycin C (MMC)-based concurrent chemoradiotherapy is the standard of care for anal cancer treatment.

Chemoradiotherapy Versus Radiation Therapy Alone: ACT I and EORTC

The 1996 UK Coordinating Committee on Cancer Research Anal Cancer Trial 1 (ACT 1) randomized 585 patients at any stage to radiotherapy with or without 5-FU/MMC. Although the 3-year overall survival (OS) was similar (65% in the chemoradiotherapy group vs. 58% in the radiotherapy group, $p = 0.86$), the 3-year local failure rates (39% vs. 61%, $p < 0.001$) and the 3-year cancer-specific survival rates (72% vs. 61%, $p = 0.02$) were significantly improved in the chemoradiotherapy group [3, 4]. The 1997 European Organization for Research and Treatment of Cancer (EORTC) trial randomized 110 patients with locally advanced anal cancer (T3–4 or N1–3) to radiotherapy with or without 5-FU/MMC [5]. Although OS was similar, chemoradiotherapy was associated with a 26% higher pathologic remission rate (80% vs. 54%), an 18% higher locoregional control rate at 5 years ($p = 0.02$), and a 32% higher colostomy-free rate ($p = 0.002$). ACT1 and EORTC trials in the late 1990s supported the addition of concurrent chemotherapy to radiotherapy based on supe-

Hwa Kyung Byun and Woong Sub Koom are the lead authors of this chapter.

H. J. Chun et al., *Gastrointestinal Cancer*, https://doi.org/10.1007/978-981-99-0815-8_45

rior locoregional control, colostomy-free survival, and disease-specific survival.

Omission of Mitomycin C: RTOG 87-04/ECOG 1289

The need for MMC in definitive treatment of anal cancer was questioned because MMC is associated with renal, pulmonary, and bone marrow toxicity. The Radiation Therapy Oncology Group (RTOG) 87-04/Eastern Cooperative Oncology Group (ECOG) 1289 trial randomly assigned 310 patients with anal cancer at any stage to radiation with 5-FU alone or 5-FU/MMC [6]. Patients who received 5-FU/MMC had significantly better 4-year disease-free survival rates (73% vs. 51%; $p = 0.0003$) and 4-year colostomy-free survival rates (71% vs. 59%; $p = 0.014$), but complete pathologic response rates and OS were not significantly different between the groups. Grade 4 and 5 toxicities were more common in the MMC group (23% vs. 7%; $p < 0.001$). Based on the results, MMC has remained a standard chemotherapy regimen in combination with 5-FU, despite greater toxicity.

Replacing Mitomycin with Cisplatin: RTOG 98-11 and ACT II

Because early studies using cisplatin as a combined chemotherapy regimen showed promising results in anal cancer, cisplatin was evaluated as a replacement for MMC [7, 8]. The RTOG 98-11 study randomized 682 patients with anal cancer (T2–4 and any N) to either radiation with 5-FU/MMC or induction chemotherapy with 5-FU/cisplatin followed by chemoradiotherapy with 5-FU/cisplatin [9, 10]. The MMC group had better 5-year disease-free survival (68% vs. 58%, $p = 0.006$) and 5-year OS (78% vs. 71%; $p = 0.026$) than the cisplatin group. The ACT II trial investigated whether replacing MMC with cisplatin and whether maintenance chemotherapy improve outcomes [11]. In this study, 940 patients were randomized in a 2 × 2 fashion to 5-FU/MMC vs. 5-FU/cisplatin and observation vs. maintenance chemotherapy with 5-FU/cisplatin. The complete response rates at 26 weeks were similar in the MMC and the cisplatin groups (91% vs. 90%; $p = 0.64$). The 3-year progression-free survival rates were similar in the maintenance and the observation groups (74% vs. 73%; $p = 0.70$). Based on these trials, 5-FU with MMC remains the preferred standard of care, but 5-FU with cisplatin could be considered a reasonable approach.

Principle of Radiation Therapy

Because anal cancer frequently metastasizes to regional nodal area, elective regional nodal irradiation should be performed. The at-risk nodal area includes the mesorectal, presacral, internal and external iliac, and inguinal nodes. Initially, the radiation field commonly encompasses the pelvis from the lumbosacral junction, inguinal lymph nodes, and anus (Fig. 1). The upper border is reduced to the lower end of the sacroiliac joints after 30.6–36 Gy to reduce the risk of radiation enteritis. A further field reduction is made after 45 Gy so that a boost dose can be administered to the primary tumor and metastatic nodes to the total dose of 54–59.4 Gy. It may not be possible to deliver more than about 50.4 Gy to abnormal nodes in the pelvis if these lie adjacent to the small bowel; in many cases, these doses are sufficient to achieve disease control [12].

The optimal radiation dose has not yet been determined. The prescribed dose varies by tumor size and risk of microscopic spread in the nodal area. The NCCN guidelines recommend a “shrinking field technique.” The low-risk elective nodal area is prescribed at 30.6 Gy in 1.8 Gy per fraction. The elective high-risk nodal area is sequentially prescribed an additional 14.4 Gy in 1.8 Gy per fraction for a total dose of 45 Gy. Finally, for T1–2 lesions with residual disease after 45 Gy, T3–4 lesions, or metastatic lymph nodes, an additional 5.4–14.4 Gy in 1.8–2 Gy per fraction is sequentially prescribed for a total dose of 50.4–59.4 Gy. Concurrent chemotherapy (typically 5-FU/MMC) is administered in the first and fifth weeks of radiotherapy [13].

The primary tumor should be indicated by a radio-opaque marker during simulation. Complementary imaging studies, such as magnetic resonance imaging (MRI) or positron emission

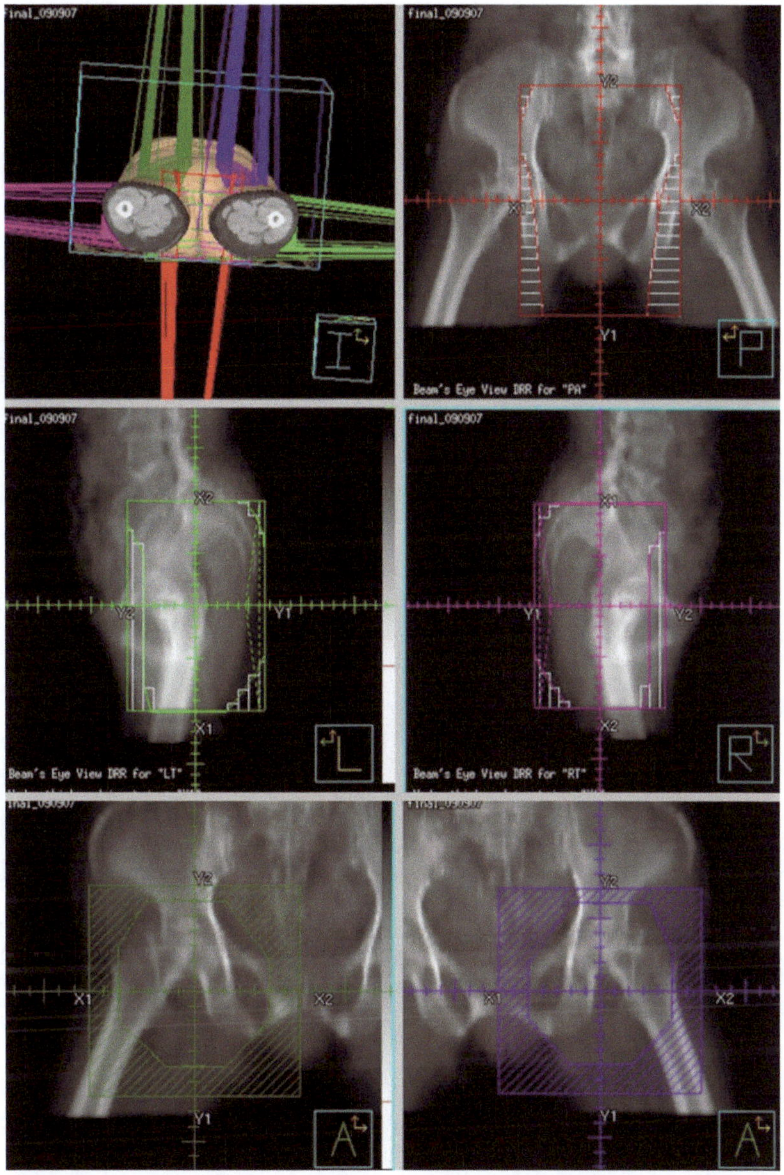

Fig. 1 An example of treatment field of the three-dimensional radiotherapy. This is an initial radiation field encompassing the pelvis from lumbosacral junction, inguinal lymph nodes, and anus

tomography- computed tomography (PET-CT), can be electronically fused to the radiotherapy planning CT scan for better target delineation

Intensity-Modulated Radiation Therapy: RTOG 05-29

Intensity-modulated radiation therapy (IMRT) has facilitated the delivery of more conformal doses to the tumor while reduced doses to the surrounding normal organs at risk (Fig. 2) [14]. The RTOG 05-29 study prospectively evaluated the dose-painted IMRT and the concurrent 5FU/MMC [15]. Patients with T2N0 disease received doses of 42 Gy to elective nodal area and 50.4 Gy to anal tumors in 28 fractions, and patients with T3-4N0-3 disease received 45 Gy to elective nodal area and 50.4 Gy to metastatic nodes <3 cm or 54 Gy to metastatic nodes >3 cm and 54 Gy to anal tumors in 30 fractions. IMRT significantly reduced acute grade 2+ hematologic toxicities

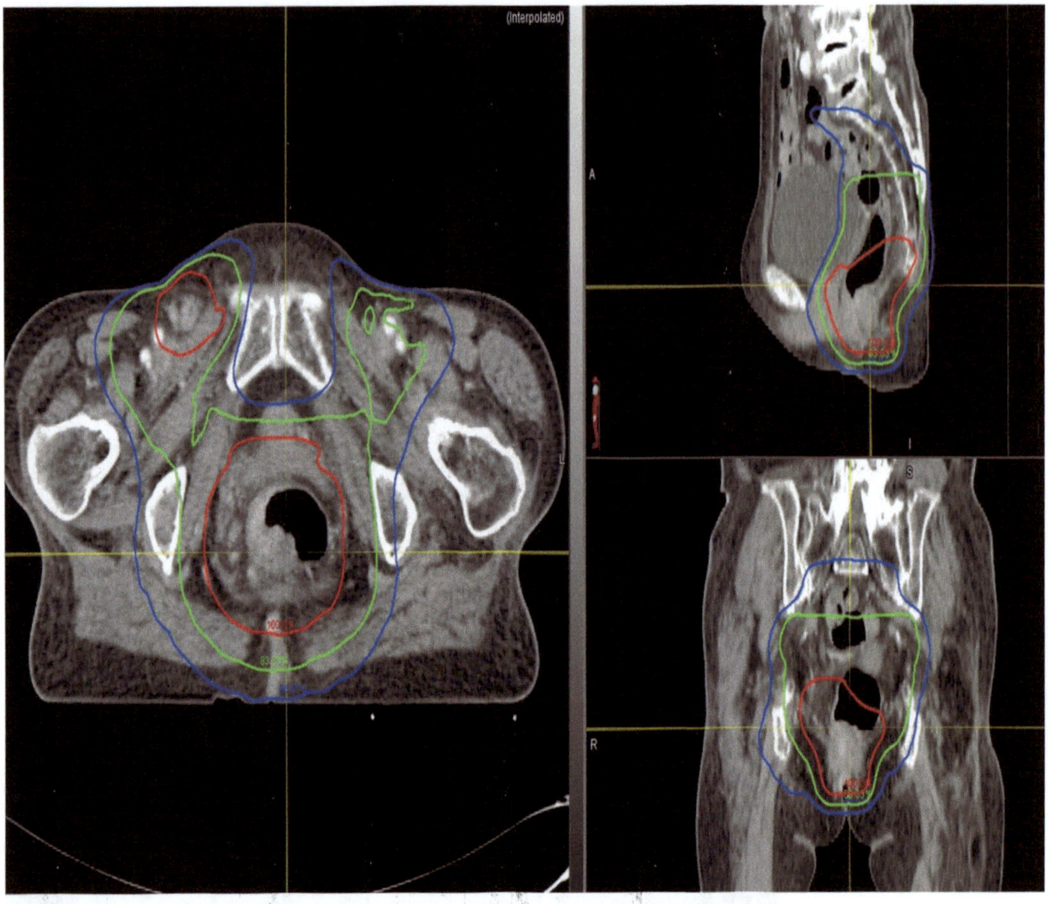

Fig. 2 An example of radiation dose distribution of the intensity-modulated radiation therapy. Shrinking field radiation therapy was applied for this case. Red, green, and blue lines represent isodose lines of 54 Gy, 45 Gy, and 36 Gy, respectively, with 1.8 Gy fraction dose

(73% vs. 85%, $p = 0.032$), acute grade 3+ gastrointestinal toxicities (21% vs. 36%, $p = 0.008$), and acute grade 3+ dermatologic toxicities (23% vs. 49%, $p < 0.001$) compared to the radiation with 5-FU/MMC arm in the RTOG 98-11 trial [10, 15].

Side Effects

Pelvic irradiation can cause acute and late toxicity, including hematological, dermatological, genitourinary, and gastrointestinal toxicities. Perineal dermatitis, anoproctitis, and decreased blood cell counts are common acute toxicities. Late toxicity includes altered bowel, urinary, and sexual function, impacting on the long-term quality of life. Female patients should be considered for vaginal dilators and advised of the symptoms of vaginal stenosis. Patients should be informed about infertility risks and provided with information on sperm banking (male patients), oocyte, egg or ovarian tissue banking, and ovary transposition (female patients) prior to treatment [13].

Timing to Assess Clinical Response

Full regression of anal cancer often takes weeks to months after the completion of chemoradiotherapy. Early evaluation could lead to some patients having unnecessary surgery. A post hoc analysis of the ACT II study suggested that a clinical complete response may deferred to later than 26 weeks [16]. Complete response was achieved in 52% of patients at week 11 after treatment, in 71% at week 18, and in 78% at week 26.

Summary and Conclusion

Definitive chemoradiotherapy is a standard treatment of all locoregional diseases of anal cancer. Definitive chemoradiotherapy yields good oncologic outcomes while allowing anal sphincter preservation. The concurrent use of 5-FU/MMC is a standard chemotherapy regimen, which was established based on superior local control, colostomy-free survival, and disease-specific survival over other regimens. The radiation field commonly encompasses the pelvis from the lumbosacral junction, inguinal lymph nodes, and anus. Elective nodal irradiation includes at-risk nodal area such as mesorectal, presacral, the internal and external iliac, and inguinal nodes. A total prescribed dose of 50.4–59.4 Gy is administered to the tumor and metastatic nodes, and a lower dose of 30.6 Gy–45 Gy is administered to the nodal area depending on the risk of harboring metastases. An advanced radiation delivery technique, such as IMRT, is preferred to reduce toxicity.

References

1. Schraut WH, Wang CH, Dawson PJ, Block GE. Depth of invasion, location, and size of cancer of the anus dictate operative treatment. Cancer. 1983;51:1291–6.
2. Nigro ND, Seydel HG, Considine B, Vaitkevicius VK, Leichman L, Kinzie JJ. Combined preoperative radiation and chemotherapy for squamous cell carcinoma of the anal canal. Cancer. 1983;51:1826–9.
3. Epidermoid anal cancer: results from the UKCCCR randomised trial of radiotherapy alone versus radiotherapy, 5-fluorouracil, and mitomycin. UKCCCR Anal Cancer Trial Working Party. UK Co-ordinating Committee on Cancer Research. Lancet. 1996;348:1049–54.
4. Northover J, Glynne-Jones R, Sebag-Montefiore D, James R, Meadows H, Wan S, et al. Chemoradiation for the treatment of epidermoid anal cancer: 13-year follow-up of the first randomised UKCCCR Anal Cancer Trial (ACT I). Br J Cancer. 2010;102:1123–8.
5. Bartelink H, Roelofsen F, Eschwege F, Rougier P, Bosset JF, Gonzalez DG, et al. Concomitant radiotherapy and chemotherapy is superior to radiotherapy alone in the treatment of locally advanced anal cancer: results of a phase III randomized trial of the European Organization for Research and Treatment of Cancer Radiotherapy and Gastrointestinal Cooperative Groups. J Clin Oncol. 1997;15:2040–9.
6. Flam M, John M, Pajak TF, Petrelli N, Myerson R, Doggett S, et al. Role of mitomycin in combination with fluorouracil and radiotherapy, and of salvage chemoradiation in the definitive nonsurgical treatment of epidermoid carcinoma of the anal canal: results of a phase III randomized intergroup study. J Clin Oncol. 1996;14:2527–39.
7. Martenson JA, Lipsitz SR, Wagner H Jr, Kaplan EH, Otteman LA, Schuchter LM, et al. Initial results of a phase II trial of high dose radiation therapy, 5-fluorouracil, and cisplatin for patients with anal cancer (E4292): an Eastern Cooperative Oncology Group study. Int J Radiat Oncol Biol Phys. 1996;35:745–9.
8. Rich TA, Ajani JA, Morrison WH, Ota D, Levin B. Chemoradiation therapy for anal cancer: radiation plus continuous infusion of 5-fluorouracil with or without cisplatin. Radiother Oncol. 1993;27:209–15.
9. Ajani JA, Winter KA, Gunderson LL, Pedersen J, Benson AB 3rd, Thomas CR Jr, et al. Fluorouracil, mitomycin, and radiotherapy vs fluorouracil, cisplatin, and radiotherapy for carcinoma of the anal canal: a randomized controlled trial. JAMA. 2008;299:1914–21.
10. Gunderson LL, Winter KA, Ajani JA, Pedersen JE, Moughan J, Benson AB 3rd, et al. Long-term update of US GI intergroup RTOG 98-11 phase III trial for anal carcinoma: survival, relapse, and colostomy failure with concurrent chemoradiation involving fluorouracil/mitomycin versus fluorouracil/cisplatin. J Clin Oncol. 2012;30:4344–51.
11. James RD, Glynne-Jones R, Meadows HM, Cunningham D, Myint AS, Saunders MP, et al. Mitomycin or cisplatin chemoradiation with or without maintenance chemotherapy for treatment of squamous-cell carcinoma of the anus (ACT II): a randomised, phase 3, open-label, 2 × 2 factorial trial. Lancet Oncol. 2013;14:516–24.
12. Halperin EC, Wazer DE, Perez CA, Brady LW. Perez and Brady's principles and practice of radiation oncology. 6th ed. 2019.
13. Nakamori S, Kameyama M, Imaoka S, Furukawa H, Ishikawa O, Sasaki Y, et al. Increased expression of sialyl Lewisx antigen correlates with poor survival in patients with colorectal carcinoma: clinicopathological and immunohistochemical study. Cancer Res. 1993;53:3632–7.
14. Dee EC, Byrne JD, Wo JY. Evolution of the role of radiotherapy for anal cancer. Cancers (Basel). 2021;13:1208.

15. Kachnic LA, Winter K, Myerson RJ, Goodyear MD, Willins J, Esthappan J, et al. RTOG 0529: a phase 2 evaluation of dose-painted intensity modulated radiation therapy in combination with 5-fluorouracil and mitomycin-C for the reduction of acute morbidity in carcinoma of the anal canal. Int J Radiat Oncol Biol Phys. 2013;86:27–33.

16. Glynne-Jones R, Sebag-Montefiore D, Meadows HM, Cunningham D, Begum R, Adab F, et al. Best time to assess complete clinical response after chemoradiotherapy in squamous cell carcinoma of the anus (ACT II): a post-hoc analysis of randomised controlled phase 3 trial. Lancet Oncol. 2017;18:347–56.

Staging and Treatment. II-4. Surgical Treatment

Key Points

- Surgery has a limited role in anal cancer, because the main treatment of anal squamous cell carcinoma is chemoradiotherapy regardless of the location of tumor (anal canal or anal margin).
- Wide local excision can be performed selectively for early superficial anal margin cancer or for the patient who refused a permanent colostomy. It can also be applied to rare anal malignancies such as basal cell carcinoma, perianal Paget's disease, and verrucous carcinoma.
- Abdominoperineal resection is helpful when the disease fails to respond to the curative therapy or has recurred, but it deteriorates the quality of life of patients.
- Inguinal lymph node dissection is not performed routinely. Intermittent colostomy may be helpful for the patient who experiences adverse events of chemoradiotherapy.

Introduction

Before Nigro et al. introduced the combined therapy, surgery had been regarded the only treatment for anal cancer [1]. However, due to the location of the tumor, the options regarding surgical treatment are very limited, unlike those for colorectal cancer, and include wide local excision (WLE) or abdominoperineal resection (APR). In addition, the role of surgery has become narrower as superior outcomes of chemoradiotherapy (CRT) based on 5-fluorouracil and mitomycin C have been demonstrated [2–4].

The prevalence of anal malignancy is rare. A total of 306 patients were diagnosed with anal cancer in Korea in 2018, which represents 0.13% of the total of 243,387 newly diagnosed cancer patients [5]. Squamous cell carcinoma is the most common type among anal cancers, and adenocarcinoma in the anal canal is classified as the advancement or invasion of rectal cancer, which requires strategies for rectal adenocarcinoma: initial surgery or neoadjuvant therapy, including concurrent CRT with or without induction/consolidation chemotherapy (see Part V

Chang Woo Kim is the lead author of this chapter.

H. J. Chun et al., *Gastrointestinal Cancer*, https://doi.org/10.1007/978-981-99-0815-8_46

Colorectal Cancer). Therefore, in this chapter, surgery for squamous cell carcinoma of the anal canal or anal margin and other types of anal cancer that could benefit from surgery will be mainly reviewed.

Wide Local Excision

WLE is a resection of the lesion that ensures proper margins. If gross margins are threatened or uncertain, a fresh frozen section can be helpful. Although WLE yields functional advantages by saving the anus, the achievement of radical or curative resection (i.e., complete removal of the tumor and potential metastatic lesions) is questionable in advanced diseases. Therefore, WLE has been applied to only locoregional disease in the anal margin/peripheral area.

Recent National Comprehensive Cancer Network (NCCN) guidelines (Version 2.2021) suggest that all anal canal cancers and advanced perianal cancers greater than T1–2N0 should be treated first with CRT [6]. The guidelines recommended that WLE should be performed with ≤3 mm of the basement membrane invasion with a maximal horizontal spread of ≤7 mm in superficially invasive squamous cell carcinoma. In T1N0 or selective T2N0 perianal cancer, at least 1-cm margins were recommended. European guidelines, which were published around the same time, suggested WLE only for stage 1 anal margin cancer [7]. Similarly, to NCCN, the European Society for Medical Oncology (ESMO) did not recommend WLE for stage 2–3 anal margin or stage 1–3 anal canal cancers. Table 1 shows the results of surgery for anal cancer between the 1950s and 1980s [8–11]. Because there were no randomized controlled trials comparing the outcomes of WLE and APR for anal cancer, even the higher survival rates in the WLE group than in the APR group should be carefully interpreted.

In contrast, some rare anal malignancies can benefit from WLE: basal cell carcinoma, perianal Paget's disease, and verrucous carcinoma. Paterson et al. reported on data collected from 19 patients with basal cell carcinoma for 20 years [12]. Seventeen patients underwent WLE, and no local recurrence was found, but seven patients had multiple diseases at other anatomic sites. Perianal Paget's disease and anal verrucous carcinoma are also quite rare with a small number of case series or reports [13, 14]. In these kinds of anal cancers, the closure of the skin defect after WLE should be considered. The multimodal approach that includes dermatology and plastic surgery is mandatory before surgery. If surgery was expected to expand to adjacent organs, urology and gynecology might be necessary. Figure 1 shows the preoperative design of the skin incision, the plan to flap the skin after WLE, the resected specimen, and the complete skin flap for perianal Paget's disease.

Table 1 Results of surgery for anal cancers

Author, year	Location *N*	WLE	5-year survival	APR	5-year survival
Hardy (1969) [8]	Anal canal 23		27%	Most	No data
	Anal margin 18	Most	No data		30.5%
Beahrs (1976) [9]	Anorectal 111	10 (9%)	80%	47 (42.3%)[a]	57.4%
	Anal canal 35	11 (31.4%)	90.9%	33 (94.3%)[a]	66.7%
	Perianal 31	27 (87.1%)	74.2%	0	
Greenall (1985) [10]	Anal margin 48	31 (64.6%)	67.7%	11 (22.9%)	63.6%
Pintor (1989) [11]	Anal canal 145	9 (6.2%)	Crude 87% Cancer-specific 100%	118 (81.4%)	Crude 62% Cancer-specific 65%
	Anal margin 83	55 (66.3%)	Crude 65% Cancer-specific 69%	18 (21.7%)	Crude 36% Cancer-specific 40%

WLE wide local excision, *APR* abdominoperineal resection
[a] Combined with WLE

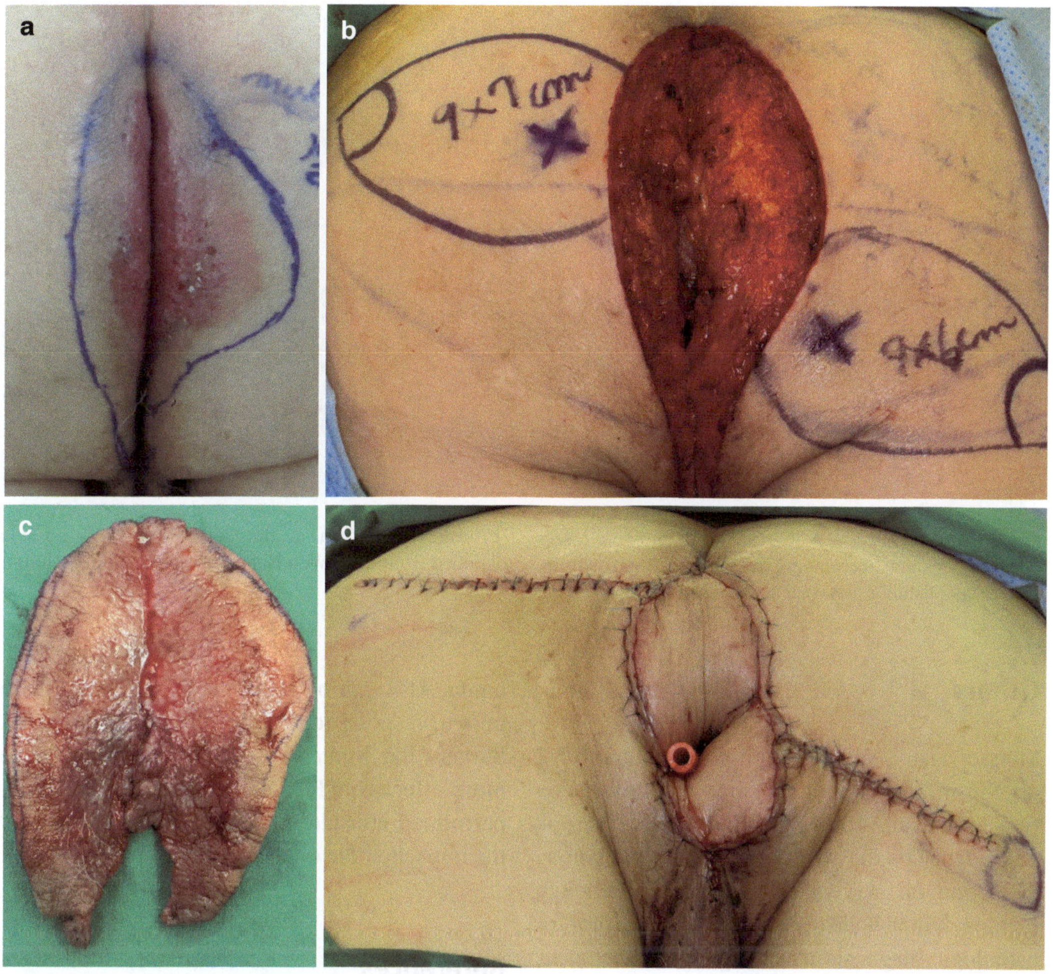

Fig. 1 Wide local excision. (**a**) Perianal Paget's disease: preoperative state. (**b**) After the wide local excision. (**c**) The resected specimen. (**d**) Skin-flap transposition [13]

Abdominoperineal Resection

APR is a more radical method than WLE. It includes sacrificing the anal sphincter and making a permanent colostomy, which deteriorates the quality of life of patients. However, 5-year survival rates for APR were reported as 30–71%, while those for CRT were 56–94% [15, 16]. Although the area of APR has narrowed, it is still helpful for diseases that recurred or showed resistance to curative therapy.

The NCCN guidelines did not recommend APR as the first-line therapeutic option for both anal canal and perianal cancer [6]. It is only considered when a local recurrence is found during surveillance. The ESMO guidelines also suggested WLE or APR for residual tumor after definitive CRT or local relapse [7]. The detailed procedure of APR for anal cancer is similar to that for lower rectal cancer (See Part V Colorectal Cancer), except for reconstruction of the surgical defect. Because combined WLE is often required, a multimodal approach is also needed before surgery. Figure 2 shows resected specimens after APR for anal cancer presenting various clinical characteristics. If a patient refuses a permanent colostomy or has poor performance, WLE could be an alternative option.

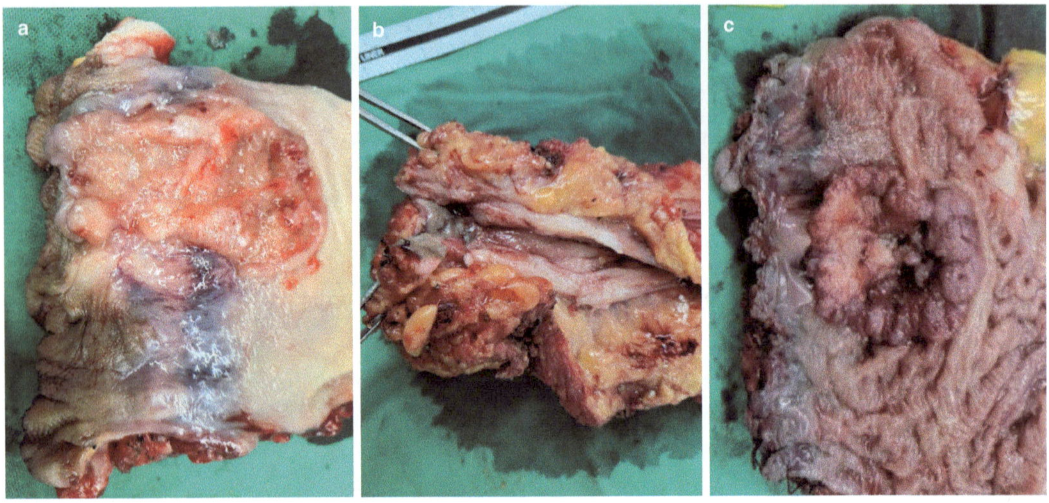

Fig. 2 Surgical specimen after abdominoperineal resection. (**a**) Mucinous carcinoma invading the anal margin. (**b**) Perianal fistula-associated anal canal adenocarcinoma. (**c**) Adenocarcinoma at the dentate line. (Permission obtained from Prof. Woo Ram Kim and Yoon Dae Han)

Others

Metastasis in inguinal lymph nodes refers to N2 or N3 in the American Joint Committee on Cancer (AJCC) staging [17]. However, there is no evidence on the effect of inguinal lymph node dissection on survival improvement. Although inguinal lymph node dissection can be helpful for pathologic diagnosis when inguinal node recurrence is suspected after definitive treatment, the initial suspicious finding of inguinal lymph node metastasis does not require routine inguinal lymph node dissection [6].

Intermittent colostomy or ileostomy can be helpful for patients undergoing CRT and experiencing perianal symptoms: anal pain, bleeding, and fecal incontinence [18]. Surgery does not play a role in miscellaneous anal cancer such as melanoma, Kaposi's sarcoma, and lymphoma.

Conclusion

WLE can be performed selectively for early anal margin cancer or for patients who refuse permanent colostomy. It can also be applied to other anal malignancies such as basal cell carcinoma, perianal Paget's disease, and verrucous carcinoma. APR can be performed when the disease fails to respond to curative therapy or recurred. Surgery has limited roles in anal cancer due to more effective CRT, and it should be carefully performed considering oncologic outcomes and the impact on the quality of life of patients.

References

1. Nigro ND, Vaitkevicius VK, Considine B Jr. Combined therapy for cancer of the anal canal: a preliminary report. Dis Colon Rectum. 1974;17:354–6.
2. Flam M, John M, Pajak TF, Petrelli N, Myerson R, Doggett S, et al. Role of mitomycin in combination with fluorouracil and radiotherapy, and of salvage chemoradiation in the definitive nonsurgical treatment of epidermoid carcinoma of the anal canal: results of a phase III randomized intergroup study. J Clin Oncol. 1996;14:2527–39.
3. Northover J, Glynne-Jones R, Sebag-Montefiore D, James R, Meadows H, Wan S, et al. Chemoradiation for the treatment of epidermoid anal cancer: 13-year follow-up of the first randomised UKCCCR Anal Cancer Trial (ACT I). Br J Cancer. 2010;102:1123–8.
4. Buckstein M, Arens Y, Wisnivesky J, Gaisa M, Goldstone S, Sigel K. A population-based cohort analysis of chemoradiation versus radiation alone for definitive treatment of stage I anal cancer in older patients. Dis Colon Rectum. 2018;61:787–94.
5. Center NC. Annual report of cancer statistics in Korea in 2018. 2021.

6. National Comprehensive Cancer Network. NCCN clinical practice guidelines in oncology: anal carcinoma, version 2.2021. 2021.
7. Rao S, Guren MG, Khan K, Brown G, Renehan AG, Steigen SE, et al. Anal cancer: ESMO clinical practice guidelines for diagnosis, treatment and follow-up(☆). Ann Oncol. 2021;32:1087–100.
8. Hardy KJ, Hughes ES, Cuthbertson AM. Squamous cell carcinoma of the anal canal and anal margin. Aust N Z J Surg. 1969;38:301–5.
9. Beahrs OH, Wilson SM. Carcinoma of the anus. Ann Surg. 1976;184:422–8.
10. Greenall MJ, Quan SH, Stearns MW, Urmacher C, DeCosse JJ. Epidermoid cancer of the anal margin. Pathologic features, treatment, and clinical results. Am J Surg. 1985;149:95–101.
11. Pintor MP, Northover JM, Nicholls RJ. Squamous cell carcinoma of the anus at one hospital from 1948 to 1984. Br J Surg. 1989;76:806–10.
12. Paterson CA, Young-Fadok TM, Dozois RR. Basal cell carcinoma of the perianal region: 20-year experience. Dis Colon Rectum. 1999;42:1200–2.
13. Kim CW, Kim YH, Cho MS, Min BS, Baik SH, Kim NK. Perianal Paget's disease. Ann Coloproctol. 2014;30:241–4.
14. Ehrl D, Rentsch M, Moellhoff N, Wachtel N. Complex microsurgical perineal reconstruction after resection of a giant verrucous carcinoma associated with anal fistulas in Crohn's disease—a unique case report. Int J Color Dis. 2020;35:1337–41.
15. Fuchshuber PR, Rodriguez-Bigas M, Weber T, Petrelli NJ. Anal canal and perianal epidermoid cancers. J Am Coll Surg. 1997;185:494–505.
16. Rousseau DL Jr, Petrelli NJ, Kahlenberg MS. Overview of anal cancer for the surgeon. Surg Oncol Clin N Am. 2004;13:249–62.
17. Anonymous. American Joint Committee on cancer staging manual, 8th ed. https://cancerstaging.org/references-tools/deskreferences/Pages/default.aspx.
18. Renehan AG, O'Dwyer ST. Initial management through the anal cancer multidisciplinary team meeting. Color Dis. 2011;13(Suppl 1):21–8.

Staging and Treatment. II-5. Adjuvant/Palliative Chemotherapy

Key Points

- Although primary treatment for patients with nonmetastatic anal squamous cell carcinoma (SCC) involves concurrent chemoradiation therapy (CCRTx), local excision may also be used. Adjuvant therapy after local excision with inadequate margin is performed by local radiation or re-excision.
- Only 10–20% of patients with anal carcinoma present with extrapelvic metastatic disease, and the most common sites of anal cancer metastasis outside the pelvis are the liver, lung, and extrapelvic lymph nodes.
- For most patients with advanced SCC of the anus, paclitaxel plus carboplatin is the initial chemotherapy regimen with a response rate of 59%.
- Among immune checkpoint inhibitors, nivolumab and pembrolizumab can be used as second-line treatment in advanced anal SCC, with a response rate of 20–24%.

Introduction

The term "anal cancer" usually refers to a squamous cell cancer (SCC) of the anal canal, which represents the majority of cancers arising in the anal region. This chapter will cover adjuvant and palliative chemotherapy of anal SCC.

Although the primary treatment for patients with nonmetastatic anal canal cancer is concurrent chemoradiation therapy (CCRTx), local excision is used in two circumferences. One is for superficially invasive anal cancer, and the other is for T1, N0, well-differentiated perianal cancer or select T2, N0 perianal cancer that does not involve the sphincter. Despite the absence of randomized trials that directly compare upfront CCRTx with surgery, CCRTx has emerged as the preferred treatment method for anal canal SCC because it can cure many patients while preserving the anal sphincter in approximately 70–85%. Local excision may be an option for carefully selected patients with very favorable small (<1 cm) superficially invasive tumors (1 cm) that are completely excised and have 3 mm of invasion of the basement membrane and a maximum

Yehyun Park is the lead author of this chapter.

H. J. Chun et al., *Gastrointestinal Cancer*, https://doi.org/10.1007/978-981-99-0815-8_47

horizontal spread of 7 mm. Such lesions are seen with increasing frequency because anal cancer screening in high-risk populations is becoming more common. Local surgical resection with negative margins may be an adequate treatment. However, local excision has never been compared to radiotherapy (RTx) or CCRTx, which are considered standard of care in this patient population. If this approach is selected, vigilant follow-up is mandatory, with prompt initiation of CCRTx for recurrent disease.

It has been reported that the most common sites of anal cancer metastasis outside the pelvis are the liver, lung, and extrapelvic lymph nodes. Since anal carcinoma is a rare cancer and only 10–20% of patients with anal carcinoma present with extrapelvic metastatic disease, only limited data are available on this population of patients. Despite this fact, evidence indicates that systemic therapy has some benefit in patients with metastatic anal carcinoma. Palliative RTx can be administered with chemotherapy for local control of a bulky symptomatic primary lesion.

Adjuvant Chemotherapy

Because adjuvant therapy after local excision with inadequate margin is local radiation or re-excision, an adjuvant chemotherapy alone is generally not used in anal cancer.

A retrospective study described 17 patients with completely excised invasive anal cancer, 7 of whom met the criteria for classification as superficially invasive lesions [1]. Those with positive margins (≤2 mm for anal canal cancer and <1 cm for perianal cancer) received local radiation, and after a median follow-up of 45 months, no differences were observed in the 5-year OS or 5-year recurrence-free survival rates (87% for the entire cohort) between the superficially invasive and invasive groups.

Palliative Chemotherapy for Metastatic Anal Cancer

The liver is the most frequent site of distant metastases, but the development of distant metastases has been generally infrequent in patients with SCC of the anal canal. In the United Kingdom Coordination Committee on Cancer Research (UKCCCR) trial, distant metastases developed after combined modality therapy in 10% of patients after a median follow-up of 42 months (interquartile range 28–62) [2]. Systemic therapy is the usual approach for the treatment of metastatic SCC. There may be a small subset of patients with isolated liver metastases who will benefit from resection, but the selection criteria are not defined.

The first-line and second-line systemic chemotherapy of anal cancer is described in Table 1, and specific regimens and dosing are described in Table 2.

Table 1 The first-line and second-line systemic chemotherapy of anal cancer

First-line systemic chemotherapy	Second-line systemic chemotherapy
Carboplatin/paclitaxel ± RTx	Nivolumab
FOLFOX ± RTx	Pembrolizumab
FOLFCIS ± RTx	
5-FU/cisplatin (category 2B) ± RTx	
Modified docetaxel/cisplatin/fluorouracil (DCF) (category 2B)	

Table 2 Regimens and dosing of systemic chemotherapy of anal cancer

Carboplatin/paclitaxel	Carboplatin AUC 5 IV day 1 Paclitaxel 175 mg/m^2 IV day 1 Repeat every 21 days or
	Carboplatin AUC 5 IV day 1 Paclitaxel 80 mg/m^2 IV days 1, 8, 15 Repeat every 28 days
5-FU/cisplatin	Cisplatin 60 mg/m^2 day 1 Continuous infusion of 5-FU 1000 mg/m^2/day IV days 1–4 Repeat every 3 weeks or
	Cisplatin 75 mg/m^2 day 1 Continuous 5-FU infusion 750 mg/m^2/day IV days 1–5 Repeat every 4 weeks
FOLFCIS	Cisplatin 40 mg/m^2 IV for 30 min on day 1 Leucovorin 400 mg/m^2 IV day 1 5-FU 400 mg/m^2 IV bolus on day 1, then 1000 mg/m^2/day × 2 days (total 2000 mg/m^2 over 46–48 h) IV continuous infusion Repeat every 2 weeks
mFOLFOX6	Oxaliplatin 85 mg/m^2 IV day 1 Leucovorin 400 mg/m^2 IV day 1 5-FU 400 mg/m^2 IV bolus on day 1, then 1200 mg/m^2/day × 2 days (a total of 24,000 mg/m^2 over 46–48 h) IV continuous infusion Repeat every 2 weeks
Modified DCF	Docetaxel 40 mg/m^2 IV day 1 Cisplatin 40 mg/m^2 IV day 1 Fluorouracil 1200 mg/m^2/day × 2 days (total 2400 mg/m^2 over 46–48 h) Repeat every 2 weeks
Nivolumab	Nivolumab 240 mg IV every 2 weeks Or nivolumab 3 mg/kg IV every 2 weeks Or nivolumab 480 mg IV every 4 weeks
Pembrolizumab	Pembrolizumab 200 mg IV every 3 weeks Or pembrolizumab 2 mg/kg IV every 3 weeks Or pembrolizumab 400 mg IV every 6 weeks

IV intravenously

Paclitaxel plus Carboplatin

For most patients with advanced SCC of the anus, paclitaxel plus carboplatin is the initial chemotherapy regimen.

In the InterAACT trial, 91 patients with previously untreated advanced anal SCC were randomly assigned to carboplatin (area under the curve of concentration × time [AUC] 5 on day 1 every 28 days) plus weekly paclitaxel (80 mg/m^2 on days 1, 8, and 15, every 28 days) or to cisplatin (60 mg/m^2 on day 1, every 21 days) plus 5-fluorouracil (FU) infusion (1000 mg/m^2 per 24 h on days 1 through 4, every 21 days). The primary outcome was the response rate. Carboplatin plus weekly paclitaxel had similar response rates to cisplatin plus 5-FU (59% versus 57%), but had better median overall survival (OS) (20 versus 12.3 months) and a more favorable toxicity profile (serious adverse events in 36% versus 62%) [3].

Whether treatment-related toxicity is improved using weekly paclitaxel in this regimen as compared with other regimens in which both carboplatin and paclitaxel are administered on day 1 every 3 weeks has not been established.

Cisplatin plus Fluorouracil

The most widely published active regimen for the treatment of metastatic disease is cisplatin plus 5-FU. Consensus-based guidelines from the National Comprehensive Cancer Network (NCCN) [4] and the European Society for Medical Oncology (ESMO) [5] recommend cisplatin plus 5-FU as one of the first-line regimens. However, while response rates of up to 60–65% are reported [6], they are seldom sustained. The best outcomes are achieved in patients who undergo multidisciplinary management for their metastatic disease; in one report, median survival for patients who underwent multidisciplinary management was 53 months compared with 17 months for those undergoing palliative systemic chemotherapy alone [7].

Based on the findings of a randomized trial [3], the NCCN recommend this regimen as category 2B reflecting its similar efficacy but high toxicity, when compared with carboplatin/paclitaxel [4].

Docetaxel, Cisplatin, and Fluorouracil

Combinations of docetaxel, cisplatin, and 5-FU (DCF) are effective, but have potentially higher toxicity. In the largest single-arm phase II trial, 66 patients received 6 cycles of standard DCF or 8 cycles of modified DCF (docetaxel 40 mg/m^2 and cisplatin 40 mg/m^2 on day 1 and 1200 mg/m^2 per day of 5-FU infusion for 2 days, every 2 weeks) depending on age and performance status [8]. The primary endpoint, progression-free survival (PFS) at 12 months, was achieved by 47% of the entire cohort, and a similar percentage of patients with standard and modified DCF had disease progression at 12 months (61 versus 60%, respectively); objective response rates (89% vs 83%), complete response rates (42% vs 47%), and median PFS durations (11 months each) were also similar. Grade 3–4 adverse events were more frequent with standard DCF, including febrile neutropenia, anemia, diarrhea, mucositis, nausea, and fatigue. Based on these results, modified DCF is an option for patients with advanced disease, but potential higher toxicity compared to the other regimens should be considered.

Immunotherapy

Patients with metastatic SCC of the anus should strongly consider therapy directed against the programmed cell death receptor 1 (PD-1). Despite the relatively limited experience with this class of agents in anal SCC, it is consistent with the experience of anti-PD-1 therapy in SCC of the head and neck, another human papillomavirus (HPV)-related malignancy.

Anal cancers may be responsive to PD-1/programmed cell death ligand 1 (PD-L1) inhibitors because they often have high PD-L1 expression and/or a high tumor mutational load despite being microsatellite stable (MSS) [9]. Microsatellite instability (MSI) is uncommon in anal cancer, and MSI or mismatch repair (MMR) testing is not required. Promising results with two immune checkpoint inhibitors that target the PD-1 pathway, nivolumab and pembrolizumab, have been reported in advanced anal SCC, and responses to PD-1/PD-L1 inhibitors are 20–24%.

Nivolumab is a monoclonal antibody that targets PD-1. In a small prospective phase II trial conducted in patients with chemorefractory metastatic anal canal SCC, nivolumab was administered at a dose of 3 mg/kg intravenously (IV) every 2 weeks [10]. A median 6 (interquartile range 3–10) cycles were delivered. Among the 37 participants enrolled, there were 9 objective responses (24%) and 2 complete responses, and an additional 17 (46%) had stable disease as the best response. The median PFS was 4.1 months and the median OS was 11.5 months. Although data were very limited ($n = 13$ patients), overexpression of PD-1 and PD-L1 appeared to correlate with responses. The adverse event profile was manageable and consisted of grade 2 pneumonitis, grade 3 anemia in 5%, and grade 3 fatigue, rash, and hypothyroidism in 3% each.

Pembrolizumab, another anti-PD-1 monoclonal antibody, was studied in the phase 1b multicohort KEYNOTE-028 trial, which included 25 patients with PD-L1-positive anal cancer [11]. Pembrolizumab was administered intravenously at a dose of 10 mg/kg every 2 weeks for up to 2 years. Among the 24 with SCC histology, there were 4 confirmed partial responses (overall response rate 17%), and an additional 10 had stable disease as the best response (42%). The most common adverse events related to treatment were diarrhea, fatigue, and nausea.

Conclusion

For most patients with advanced SCC of the anus, paclitaxel plus carboplatin is the initial chemotherapy regimen with a response rate of 59%. Among immune checkpoint inhibitors, nivolumab and pembrolizumab can be used as second-line treatment in advanced anal SCC, with response rate of 20–24%.

References

1. Arana R, Fléjou J-F, Si-Mohamed A, Bauer P, Etienney I. Clinicopathological and virological characteristics of superficially invasive squamous-cell carcinoma of the anus. Color Dis. 2015;17(11):965–72.
2. Epidermoid anal cancer: results from the UKCCCR randomised trial of radiotherapy alone versus radiotherapy, 5-fluorouracil, and mitomycin. UKCCCR Anal Cancer Trial Working Party. UK Co-ordinating Committee on Cancer Research. Lancet. 1996;348(9034):1049–54.
3. Rao S, Sclafani F, Eng C, Adams RA, Guren MG, Sebag-Montefiore D, et al. International rare cancers initiative multicenter randomized phase II trial of cisplatin and fluorouracil versus carboplatin and paclitaxel in advanced anal cancer: InterAAct. J Clin Oncol. 2020;38(22):2510–8.
4. NCCN clinical practice guidelines in oncology. 2021. https://www.nccn.org/professionals/physician_gls.
5. Glynne-Jones R, Nilsson PJ, Aschele C, Goh V, Peiffert D, Cervantes A, et al. Anal cancer: ESMO-ESSO-ESTRO clinical practice guidelines for diagnosis, treatment and follow-up. Ann Oncol. 2014;25 Suppl 3:iii10–20.
6. Evesque L, Benezery K, Follana P, Tuan Falk A, Doyen J, Reure J, et al. Multimodal therapy of squamous cell carcinoma of the anus with distant metastasis: a single-institution experience. Dis Colon Rectum. 2017;60(8):785–91.
7. Eng C, Chang GJ, You YN, Das P, Rodriguez-Bigas M, Xing Y, et al. The role of systemic chemotherapy and multidisciplinary management in improving the overall survival of patients with metastatic squamous cell carcinoma of the anal canal. Oncotarget. 2014;5(22):11133–42.
8. Kim S, François E, André T, Samalin E, Jary M, El Hajbi F, et al. Docetaxel, cisplatin, and fluorouracil chemotherapy for metastatic or unresectable locally recurrent anal squamous cell carcinoma (Epitopes-HPV02): a multicentre, single-arm, phase 2 study. Lancet Oncol. 2018;19(8):1094–106.
9. Salem ME, Puccini A, Grothey A, Raghavan D, Goldberg RM, Xiu J, et al. Landscape of tumor mutation load, mismatch repair deficiency, and PD-L1 expression in a large patient cohort of gastrointestinal cancers. Mol Cancer Res. 2018;16(5):805–12.
10. Morris VK, Salem ME, Nimeiri H, Iqbal S, Singh P, Ciombor K, et al. Nivolumab for previously treated unresectable metastatic anal cancer (NCI9673): a multicentre, single-arm, phase 2 study. Lancet Oncol. 2017;18(4):446–53.
11. Ott PA, Piha-Paul SA, Munster P, Pishvaian MJ, van Brummelen EMJ, Cohen RB, et al. Safety and antitumor activity of the anti-PD-1 antibody pembrolizumab in patients with recurrent carcinoma of the anal canal. Ann Oncol. 2017;28(5):1036–41.

Part VII

Pancreatic Cancer

Epidemiology, Risk Factors, and Prevention

Key Points

- The incidence of pancreatic cancer (PC) varies between regions (highest in Europe and North America, lowest in Africa), and PC is a malignancy with poor survival but has shown improved survival recently.
- There are various risk factors in PC and are divided into modifiable (such as smoking, alcohol, obesity, environment) and nonmodifiable (such as ethnicity, diabetes, chronic pancreatitis, family history, microbiota, genes).
- For prevention of PC, it is helpful to reduce modifiable risk factors, although nonmodifiable risk factors cannot be controlled.

Introduction

Pancreatic cancer (PC) is one of the most lethal malignancies and is the seventh leading cause of cancer-related deaths. The incidence of PC has continually increased and has been ranked the 11th most common cancer in the world (12th most common cancer in men, 11th most common in women). A total of 458,918 new cases were diagnosed causing 432,242 deaths (4.5% of all deaths caused by cancer) in 2018 compared to 196,000 new cases in 1990, and it is estimated that 335,317 new cases will be diagnosed by 2040 [1, 2]. Detecting PC and premalignant lesions, understanding risk factors, and reducing exposures to PC risk factors will help reduce the growing incidence of this disease.

Dong Wook Lee is the lead author of this chapter.

Epidemiology

Incidence

As described above, the past two decades have seen a doubling in the annual global number of patients with newly diagnosed pancreatic cancer. PC is a malignancy in which risk increases with age and is rarely diagnosed younger than 40 years [2]. In the USA, the risk of death caused by PC increases dramatically with age, from <2 deaths per 100,000 person-years for people aged 35–39 years to >90 deaths per 100,000 person-years for individuals aged >80 years [3].

The incidence of PC varies between regions and populations. The incidence age-standardized rate (ASR) was highest in Europe and North America, followed by Oceania, while the lowest rate was observed in Africa (Fig. 1). A small sex-based difference in incidence is observed in PC, whereby PC is more common in males than in females. In males, the incidence of PC is highest in Hungary (13.7 per 100,000), French Guiana (13.0), and Uruguay (12.8), while the lowest rate

H. J. Chun et al., *Gastrointestinal Cancer*, https://doi.org/10.1007/978-981-99-0815-8_48

(https://gco.iarc.fr/today/online-analysis-map?v).

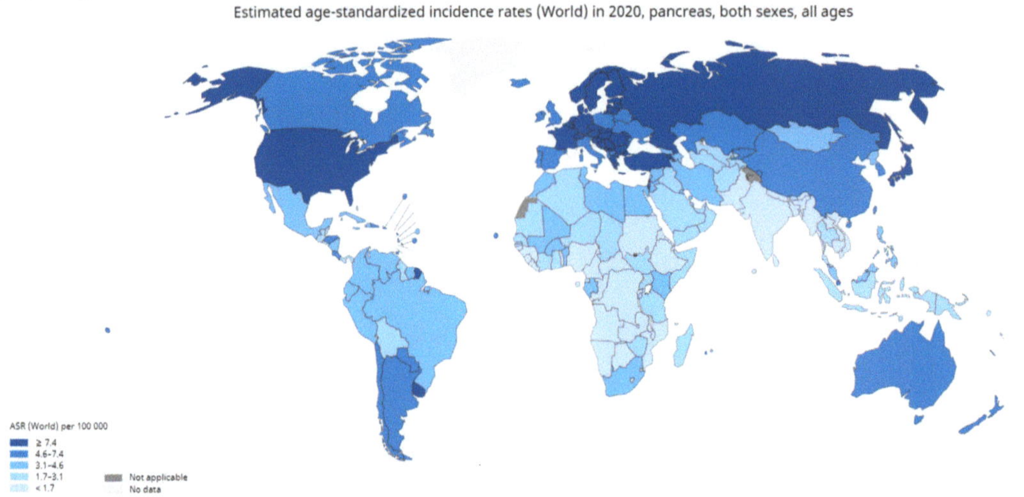

Fig. 1 Estimated age-standardized incidence rates (World) in 2020, pancreas, both sexes, all ages (https://gco.iarc.fr/today/online-analysis-map?v)

is observed in Malawi (0.46) and Botswana (0.82). The countries with the highest incidence of PC in females are Hungary (9.2) and Uruguay (8.9), followed by Japan (8.2) [4].

The reasons for these differences between countries and sexes are not clear. However, it is possible that the environment or exposure to certain risk factors accounts for the geographic variation in the incidence of PC. Recently, potential sex-based differences in the association between smoking and PC incidence were revealed in a Japanese population-based cohort study [5]. In that study, after 5 years of cessation of smoking, the risk of PC became comparable to those who had never smoked in men, while no risk attenuation was observed in women.

Survival

The lowest 5-year overall survival rate (SR) of 9% among all types of malignancies in the USA during 2009 through 2015 and a similar result was observed in European countries in which the mean-age-standardized 5-year SR for patients with PC is the lowest (7%) among 46 types of cancers (the best 10.9% in Croatia and the worst 0% in Malta) [6, 7]. However, the 5-year SR for PC improved from 6% in 2014 to 9% in 2018 globally [1].

Poor SRs are in part attributed to the advanced stage at diagnosis in most cases, with only 20% of patients presenting with resectable stage. In patients receiving surgical resection, the 5-year SR increased up to 25%, and in the USA, the survival rate for stage 1A disease was more than 80% [8]. In Japan, the 5-year SR from 2001 to 2007 was 18.8% for patients with resected PC and 3.1% for unresected PC [9].

According to a recent investigation of recent trends in the stage of newly diagnosed PC, the 5-year SR for PC with stage IA increased from 44.7% in 2004 to 83.7% in 2012, and 10-year survival improved from 36.7% in 2004 to 49.0% in 2007. Moreover, the average age of diagnosis for stage IA and IB patients declined by 3.5 and 5.5 years, respectively. These trends may be attributed to advancements in early diagnosis and early detection [8].

Risk Factors and Prevention

The risk factors for PC have been studied for a long time and have attracted the interest of numerous doctors and researchers. Until now, several risk factors have been demonstrated and can be divided into two categories: modifiable and nonmodifiable risk factors [10].

Modifiable Risk Factors

Smoking

Numerous studies have revealed that smoking is associated with an increased risk of PC [11, 12]. The effects of smoking on the risk of PC were associated with an odds ratio [OR] of 1.74 for current smokes compared with never smokers and the risk highest in smokers of more than 35 cigarettes per day with an OR for PC of 3.0 compared with nonsmokers [3].

Cessation of smoking decreases the risk of PC and the risk after more than 10–20 years of cessation was similar to those of nonsmokers; however, it remains uncertain to prove an association between passive smoking or parental smoking and the risk of PC in a nonsmoking population [13, 14].

Alcohol Intake

According to many studies, the risk of PC increases in heavy drinkers of alcohol compared to low-to-moderate consumers, while there is no significant evidence of interaction between sexes [15, 16]. A recent study found that heavy alcohol drinking was associated with a significant increase in PC risk among current smokers (OR 4.04, 95% confidence interval [CI], 1.58–10.37), while there was no increased risk in nonsmokers (OR 2.01, 95% CI 0.50–8.18). Moreover, increased risk of PC was observed in low-to-moderate drinkers who are current smokers [17]. Thus, there are some investigators who claimed that alcohol is not an independent risk factor for PC, but alcohol should be considered an important risk factor because the association between alcohol and smoking is very close and alcohol is associated with pancreatitis, an established risk factor for PC.

Obesity

According to the American Cancer Society, obesity is an important risk factor for PC compared to a population with a healthy body mass index (18.5–24.9 kg/m^2) [18]. Numerous studies have revealed that obesity is associated with metabolic abnormalities, such as insulin resistance, hyperinsulinemia, and glucose intolerance, which have a close relationship with PC development [19]. Hyperinsulinemia can culminate in an increase in local blood flow and cell division in the pancreas. High concentrations of insulin are capable of activating the insulin-like growth factor 1 (IGF-1) receptor. A recent study proved that IGF-1 promotes cancer cell growth and proliferation by activating the P13K-mTOR and MARK signaling pathway [20].

Dietary Factors

Consumption of red meats (especially cooked at high temperature), cholesterol, fried foods, and other foods containing nitrosamines can increase the risk of PC [21]. Carcinogens in meat and the nitrite of N-nitroso compounds that are used to preserve processed meat are possibly involved in the development of PC [22]. Meanwhile, the intake of folate, cereals, fiber, and fruits has a negative association with PC. Fruits can protect the pancreas against cancer development because vitamin C and other antioxidants can trap free radicals and reactive oxygen molecules, protecting against oxidative damage [23].

Environmental and Occupational Exposures

Several studies have investigated the relationship between environmental/occupational exposure and the risk of PC. Exposure to nickel can increase the risk of PC [24], and the carcinogenic mechanism of nickel includes increasing DNA methylation, inhibiting DNA repair, and inducting apoptosis through the generation of reactive oxygen species [25, 26]. Cadmium is a well-known carcinogen that acts on different steps of carcinogenesis, inhibiting DNA repair and inducing genomic instability. Furthermore, it causes transdifferentiation of pancreatic cells, inhibits DNA repair, and induces or regulates the activity of several oncogenes or tumor suppressor proteins that are expressed in human pancreatic cancer [27, 28]. Conversely, selenium, which is an essential micronutrient, can lower the risk of several cancers, including PC [29]. Selenium can boost p53 activity, leading to DNA repair or apoptosis, and also appears to play a role as an antagonist of cadmium and lead, decreasing the oxidative stress caused by exposure to these components [30, 31].

Nonmodifiable Risk Factors

Ethnicity

There are some differences in the incidence of PC among races. The rates of PC incidence in African Americans are higher than in Caucasians, while the incidence is the lowest in Asian Americans and Pacific Islanders [32]. Differences in the incidence of PC among various races can be attributed to modifiable risk factors including smoking, alcohol consumption, and the dietary factors mentioned above. Studies comparing the oncogene mutations and biomarker immune expression among Chinese, Japanese, and Western populations revealed Asian patients with PC have different expression of *KRAS* and *p53* than in Western populations [33], which may also explain the differences in the survival rates after treatment of PC for different races (better survival in Asian patients than non-Asian).

Diabetes Mellitus

Diabetes mellitus (DM) is not only a risk factor for PC, but is also a consequence of cancer, and many newly diagnosed PC patients report the onset of DM or, for existing DM patients, a worsening of the disease. There are several reports about the association between DM and PC. Long-term DM (more than 3 years) has been associated with an increased risk of PC [34], and many patients with PC report developing DM in the months preceding diagnosis and often observed resolution of DM after PC removal in those with new-onset DM who received surgical resection for their PC [35]. In addition, biomarkers of DM have also been shown to be associated with PC risk, such as fasting glucose, insulin levels, and insulin resistance level in both the European and Chinese populations [36]. Therefore, further studies are needed to investigate whether DM can predict the onset of PC or its use as a marker.

Chronic Pancreatitis

Chronic pancreatitis (CP) can cause recurrent inflammation and damage to the pancreas and lead to the development of PC. In other words, the mechanism underlining the risk of PC in patients with CP may be a multistep oncogenetic sequence, such as ductal epithelial hyperplasia, metaplasia, dysplasia, and *KRAS* gene mutations in patients with CP. Despite this background, fewer than 5% of patients with CP develop PC in the future; thus, CP is a rare cause of PC [37]. More studies are needed to determine the detailed mechanism and correlation between CP and PC.

Family History

Approximately, 5–10% of patients with PC have reported having a family history of PC [38]. Familial PC is defined in most studies as families in which a pair of first-degree relatives (parent, sibling, or child) has been diagnosed with PC. Prospective studies have shown that first-degree relatives of patients with familial PC (individuals with at least two close family members with PC) have a 6.79-fold (95% CI 4.54–9.75) increased risk of PC and it rises to 32-fold higher in relatives with three or more first-degree relatives with PC. Furthermore, the risk is highest among relatives with familial PC in which there is a case of a young patient with PC (age < 50) in the family compared to those without a young patient with PC [39].

Microbiota

A meta-analysis revealed that periodontal disease and tooth loss are associated with a 50–70% increased risk of PC and oral microbiota such as *Porphyromonas gingivalis* and *Aggregatibacter actinomycetemcomitans* are associated with the possibility of development of PC [40]. However, the mechanism of association between microbiota and PC is still unclear, and questions remain as to whether there is a direct causal correlation or whether this reflects a common underlying cause and is therefore not directedly causal.

Helicobacter pylori (H. pylori) has also been associated with PC in some studies, and *H. pylori* colonization enhances the pancreatic carcinogenic activity of N-nitrosamines induced by smoking or dietary sources [41]. However, only CagA-negative strains of *H. pylori* were associated with an increased risk of PC and CagA-positive strains with a lower risk, so more studies are needed to determine strain-specific association [41].

Inherited Genetic Factors

Genetic mutation or variation (so-called germline mutation) is important in increasing the risk of PC, and approximately 10% of patients with PC have a single or multiple genetic predisposition, such as gene variations or alterations [42]. Over the past 15 years, as genomic technology has improved, several germline mutations have been identified to be involved in hereditary forms of PC such as *BRCA1*, *BRCA 2*, *PALB2*, *ATM*, *CDKN2A*, *APC*, *MLH1*, *MSH2*, *MSH6*, *PMS2*, *PRSS1*, and *STK11* [43]. However, these genetic changes explain only 20–25% of the heritability (4–5% of all PC), leaving a high portion of cases that still need to be investigated.

Recently, *BRCA2*-deficient or *PALB2*-deficient cancers have increased sensitivity to PARP inhibitors or mitomycin C, high microsatellite instability PC can be treated with anti-PD1 immunotherapy, and patients with PC with a family history of breast, ovarian, or PC have improved survival when treated with platinum-containing agents [44–46].

Prevention

The best preventive strategy against PC is risk reduction acting on modifiable risk factors such as stopping smoking, low consumption of red meat, frequent intake of fruits and vegetables, and increased physical activity that has been suggested to help reduce the risk of overweight or obesity, which is also associated with PC. Limitations of alcohol consumption are necessary to reduce the risk of PC through the development of pancreatitis.

Nonmodifiable risk factors cannot be controlled, but patients with family history and genetic susceptibility may undergo a screening test for early detection of PC. Early detection of PC has appeared to be a key to reducing mortality and improving SR in PC patients. However, the detection of PC in the general population is not considered effective for detecting PC in an early stage. The International Cancer Screening Consortium for Pancreatic Cancer has agreed that screening be performed as part of a clinical trial or, if not possible, in a center with experience in PC screening [47]. The consensus statements support screening using endoscopic ultrasonography or MRI with less support for CT scanning, which has lower sensitivity [47].

Conclusion

Although several risk factors have been identified, the main etiology is still unclear, and the screening of PC in the general population is not helpful in early detection of PC. These situations have made the PC one of the most lethal malignancies in the world. Moreover, PC has been increasing due to the aging of the global population. However, prevention can be expected by reducing modifiable risk factors, and opportunities for earlier detection of PC could be provided by identifying high-risk individuals and improving diagnostic technologies.

References

1. Bray F, Ferlay J, Soerjomataram I, Siegel RL, Torre LA, Jemal A. Global cancer statistics 2018: GLOBOCAN estimates of incidence and mortality worldwide for 36 cancers in 185 countries. CA Cancer J Clin. 2018;68:394–424.
2. GBD 2017 Pancreatic Cancer Collaborators. The global, regional, and national burden of pancreatic cancer and its attributable risk factors in 195 countries and territories, 1990–2017: a systematic analysis for the Global Burden of Disease Study 2017. Lancet Gastroenterol Hepatol. 2019;4:934–47.
3. Klein AP. Pancreatic cancer epidemiology: understanding the role of lifestyle and inherited risk factors. Nat Rev Gastroenterol Hepatol. 2021;18:493–502.
4. International Agency for Research on Cancer. Cancer Today; 2020. https://gco.iarc.fr/today/online-analysismap?v=2020&mode=population&modepopulation=continents&population=900&populations=900&key=asr&sex=0&cancer=13&type=0&statistic=5&prevalence=0&population_group=0&ages_group%5B%5D=0&ages_group%5B%5D=17&nb_items=10&group_cancer=1&include_nmsc=1&include_nmsc_other=1&projection=natural-earth&color_palette=default&map_scale=quantile&map_nb_colors=5&continent=0&show_ranking=0&rotate=%255B10%252C0%255D.

5. Koyanagi YN, Ito H, Matsuo K, Sugawara Y, Hidaka A, Sawada N, et al. Smoking and pancreatic cancer incidence: a pooled analysis of 10 population-based cohort studies in Japan. Cancer Epidemiol Biomarkers Prev. 2019;28:1370–8.
6. Siegel RL, Miller KD, Jemal A. Cancer statistics, 2020. CA Cancer J Clin. 2020;70:7–30.
7. De Angelis R, Sant M, Coleman MP, Francisci S, Baili P, Pierannunzio D, et al. Cancer survival in Europe 1999–2007 by country and age: results of EUROCARE-5—a population-based study. Lancet Oncol. 2014;15:23–34.
8. Blackford AL, Canto MI, Klein AP, Hruban RH, Goggins M. Recent trends in the incidence and survival of stage 1A pancreatic cancer: a surveillance, epidemiology, and end results analysis. J Natl Cancer Inst. 2020;112:1162–9.
9. Egawa S, Toma H, Ohigashi H, Okusaka T, Nakao A, Hatori T, et al. Japan pancreatic cancer registry; 30th year anniversary: Japan Pancreas Society. Pancreas. 2012;41:985–92.
10. Midha S, Chawla S, Garg PK. Modifiable and non-modifiable risk factors for pancreatic cancer: a review. Cancer Lett. 2016;381:269–77.
11. Rastogi T, Devesa S, Mangtani P, Mathew A, Cooper N, Kao R, et al. Cancer incidence rates among South Asians in four geographic regions: India, Singapore, UK and US. Int J Epidemiol. 2008;37:147–60.
12. Iodice S, Gandini S, Maisonneuve P, Lowenfels AB. Tobacco and the risk of pancreatic cancer: a review and metaanalysis. Langenbecks Arch Surg. 2008;393:535–45.
13. Lynch SM, Vrieling A, Lubin JH, Kraft P, Mendelsohn JB, Hartge P, et al. Cigarette smoking and pancreatic cancer: a pooled analysis from the pancreatic cancer cohort consortium. Am J Epidemiol. 2009;170:403–13.
14. Bao Y, Giovannucci E, Fuchs CS, Michaud DS. Passive smoking and pancreatic cancer in women: a prospective cohort study. Cancer Epidemiol Biomarkers Prev. 2009;18:2292–6.
15. Lucenteforte E, Vecchia CL, Silverman D, Petersen GM, Bracci PM, Ji BT, et al. Alcohol consumption and pancreatic cancer: a pooled analysis in the International Pancreatic Cancer Case-Control Consortium (PanC4). Ann Oncol. 2012;23:374–82.
16. Genkinger JM, Spiegelman D, Anderson KE, Bergkvist L, Bernstein L, van den Brandt PA, et al. Alcohol intake and pancreatic cancer risk: a pooled analysis of fourteen cohort studies. Cancer Epidemiol Biomarkers Prev. 2009;18:765–76.
17. Rahman F, Cotterchio M, Cleary SP, Gallinger S. Association between alcohol consumption and pancreatic cancer risk: a case-control study. PLoS One. 2015;10:e0124489.
18. Calle EE, Rodriguez C, Walker-Thurmond K, Thun MJ. Overweight, obesity, and mortality from cancer in a prospectively studied cohort of U.S. adults. N Engl J Med. 2003;348:1625–38.
19. Jee SH, Ohrr H, Sull JW, Yun JE, Ki M, Samet JM. Fasting serum glucose level and cancer risk in Korean men and women. JAMA. 2005;293:194–202.
20. Valentinis B, Baserga R. IGF-I receptor signalling in transformation and differentiation. Mol Pathol. 2001;54:133–7.
21. Lightsey D. Comment on 'Red and processed meat consumption and risk of pancreatic cancer: meta-analysis of prospective studies'. Br J Cancer. 2012;107:754–5.
22. Beaney AJ, Banim PJR, Luben R, Lentjes MAH, Khaw KT, Hart AR. Higher meat intake is positively associated with higher risk of developing pancreatic cancer in an age-dependent manner and are modified by plasma antioxidants: a prospective cohort study (EPIC-Norfolk) using data from food diaries. Pancreas. 2017;46:672–8.
23. Keum YS, Jeong WS, Kong AN. Chemoprevention by isothiocyanates and their underlying molecular signaling mechanisms. Mutat Res. 2004;555:191–202.
24. Ojajarvi IA, Partanen TJ, Ahlbom A, Boffetta P, Hakulinen T, Nourenkova N, et al. Occupational exposures and pancreatic cancer: a meta-analysis. Occup Environ Med. 2000;57:316–24.
25. Hartwig A, Kruger I, Beyersmann D. Mechanisms in nickel genotoxicity: the significance of interactions with DNA repair. Toxicol Lett. 1994;72:353–8.
26. Ahamed M, Akhtar MJ, Siddiqui MA, Ahmad J, Musarrat J, Al-Khedhairy AA, et al. Oxidative stress mediated apoptosis induced by nickel ferrite nanoparticles in cultured A549 cells. Toxicology. 2011;283:101–8.
27. Candeias S, Pons B, Viau M, Caillat S, Sauvaigo S. Direct inhibition of excision/synthesis DNA repair activities by cadmium: analysis on dedicated biochips. Mutat Res. 2010;694:53–9.
28. Waalkes MP, Cherian MG, Ward JM, Goyer RA. Immunohistochemical evidence of high concentrations of metallothionein in pancreatic hepatocytes induced by cadmium in rats. Toxicol Pathol. 1992;20:323–6.
29. Bardia A, Tleyjeh IM, Cerhan JR, Sood AK, Limburg PJ, Erwin PJ, et al. Efficacy of antioxidant supplementation in reducing primary cancer incidence and mortality: systematic review and meta-analysis. Mayo Clin Proc. 2008;83:23–34.
30. Smith ML, Lancia JK, Mercer TI, Ip C. Selenium compounds regulate p53 by common and distinctive mechanisms. Anticancer Res. 2004;24:1401–8.
31. Fowler BA, Whittaker MH, Lipsky M, Wang G, Chen XQ. Oxidative stress induced by lead, cadmium and arsenic mixtures: 30-day, 90-day, and 180-day drinking water studies in rats: an overview. Biometals. 2004;17:567–8.
32. Rawla P, Sunkara T, Gaduputi V. Epidemiology of pancreatic cancer: global trends, etiology and risk factors. World J Oncol. 2019;10:10–27.
33. Dong M, Nio Y, Tamura K, Song MM, Guo KJ, Guo RX, et al. Ki-ras point mutation and p53 expression in

human pancreatic cancer: a comparative study among Chinese, Japanese, and Western patients. Cancer Epidemiol Biomarkers Prev. 2000;9:279–84.
34. Elena JW, Steplawski E, Yu K, Hartge P, Tobias GS, Brotzman MJ, et al. Diabetes and risk of pancreatic cancer: a pooled analysis from the Pancreatic Cancer Cohort Consortium. Cancer Causes Control. 2013;24:13–25.
35. Chari ST, Leibson CL, Rabe KG, Ransom J, de Andrade M, Petersen GM. Probability of pancreatic cancer following diabetes: a population-based study. Gastroenterology. 2005;129:504–11.
36. Pang Y, Kartsonaki C, Guo Y, Bragg F, Yang L, Bian Z, et al. Diabetes, plasma glucose and incidence of pancreatic cancer: a prospective study of 0.5 million Chinese adults and a meta- analysis of 22 cohort studies. Int J Cancer. 2017;140:1781–8.
37. Yadav D, Lowenfels AB. The epidemiology of pancreatitis and pancreatic cancer. Gastroenterology. 2013;144:1252–61.
38. Jacobs EJ, Chanock SJ, Fuchs CS, Lacroix A, McWilliams RR, Steplowski E, et al. Family history of cancer and risk of pancreatic cancer: a pooled analysis from the Pancreatic Cancer Cohort Consortium (PanScan). Int J Cancer. 2010;127:1421–8.
39. Brune KA, Lau B, Palmisano E, Canto M, Goggins MG, Hruban RH, et al. Importance of age of onset in pancreatic cancer kindreds. J Natl Cancer Inst. 2010;102:109–26.
40. Maisonneuve P, Amar S, Lowenfels AB. Periodontal disease, edentulism, and pancreatic cancer: a meta-analysis. Ann Oncol. 2017;28:985–95.
41. Schulte A, Pandeya N, Fawcett J, Fritschi L, Risch HA, Webb PM, et al. Association between *Helicobacter pylori* and pancreatic cancer risk: a meta- analysis. Cancer Causes Control. 2015;26:1027–35.
42. Ghiorzo P. Genetic predisposition to pancreatic cancer. World J Gastroenterol. 2014;20:10778–89.
43. Solomon S, Das S, Brand R, Whitcomb DC. Inherited pancreatic cancer syndromes. Cancer J. 2012;18:485–91.
44. Villarroel MC, Rajeshkumar NV, Garrido-Laguna I, Jesus-Acosta AD, Kones S, Maitra A, et al. Personalizing cancer treatment in the age of global genomic analyses: PALB2 gene mutations and the response to DNA damaging agents in pancreatic cancer. Mol Cancer Ther. 2011;10:3–8.
45. Le DT, Durham JN, Smith KN, Wang H, Bartlett BR, Aulakh LK, et al. Mismatch repair deficiency predicts response of solid tumors to PD-1 blockade. Science. 2017;357:409–13.
46. Fogelman D, Sugar EA, Oliver G, Shah N, Klein A, Alewine C, et al. Family history as a marker of platinum sensitivity in pancreatic adenocarcinoma. Cancer Chemother Pharmacol. 2015;76:489–98.
47. Goggins M, Overbeek KA, Brand R, Syngal S, Del Chiaro M, Bartsch DK, et al. Management of patients with increased risk for familial pancreatic cancer: updated recommendations from the International Cancer of the Pancreas Screening (CAPS) Consortium. Gut. 2020;69:7–17.

Pathology, Pathogenesis, and Molecular Characteristics

Key Points

- Acinar cells account for 90% of the pancreas, but more than 90% of malignant tumors that occur in the pancreas are pathologically in the form of pancreatic ductal adenocarcinoma (PDAC).
- Histologically, more than 50–90% of cancerous masses are composed of stroma other than cancer cells, called the tumor microenvironment (TME), which is considered an obstacle to anticancer treatment.
- PDAC is caused by the accumulation of various genetic mutations, and mutations commonly found include KRAS, tumor suppressors, and pancreas developmental genes.
- The recent discovery of molecular characteristics based on next-generation sequencing technology provides an opportunity to better understand the pathogenesis of pancreatic cancer and achieve precision medicine.

Introduction

Pancreatic cancer is a malignant neoplasm that occurs in cells that make up the pancreas and includes ductal adenocarcinoma, acinar cell carcinoma, and pancreatic neuroendocrine tumor depending on the pathological findings. The pancreas is made up of acinar cells, neuroendocrine cells, and duct cells. Acinar cells account for 90% of the pancreas, but more than 90% of the malignant tumors that occur in the pancreas are pathologically in the form of adenocarcinoma. This chapter mainly describes the pathology, pathogenesis, and molecular characteristics of pancreatic ductal adenocarcinoma (PDAC).

Jung Hyun Jo and Seungmin Bang are the lead authors of this chapter.

Pathology

Most PDAC arise from progenitor lesions called pancreatic ductal intraepithelial tumors (PanIN), which progress in stages through the acquisition of genetic changes to develop into overt adenocarcinomas [1]. A small number of PDAC arise from cystic tumors such as intraductal papillary mucinous neoplasms (IPMN) [2] (Fig. 1). Histologically, more than 50–90% of cancerous masses are composed of stroma other than cancer cells, called tumor microenvironment (TME) [4]. The main components of TME are cancer-associated fibroblast (CAF) and extracellular matrix (ECM) composed of collagen and hyaluronic acid. In particular, the CAF within the TME is considered an obstacle to anticancer treatment by interfering with the delivery of anticancer drugs and secreting substances that are helpful for cancer cell proliferation [5]. TME is known to play a very important role in

H. J. Chun et al., *Gastrointestinal Cancer*, https://doi.org/10.1007/978-981-99-0815-8_49

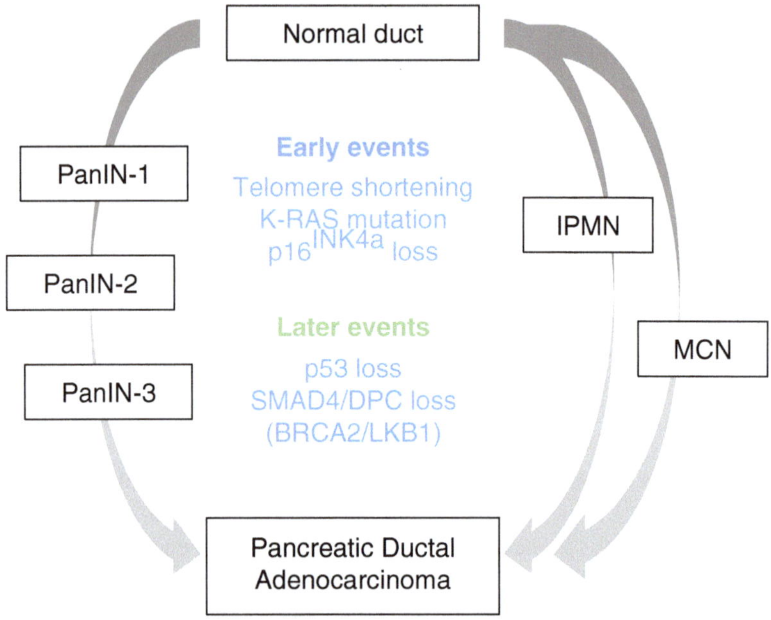

Fig. 1 Developmental model of pancreatic ductal adenocarcinoma. As normal pancreatic duct epithelial cells progress to pancreatic intraepithelial neoplasias (PanIN), a precancerous lesion, Her-2/neu is initially overexpressed, the *KRAS* mutation occurs, and *p16* is inactivated. Inactivation of *p53, DPC4,* and *BRCA2* appears in later stages. Genetic changes documented in PanIN also occur in IPMN and MCN, but these changes do not correlate with specific histological characteristics unlike PanIN (adapted from Hezel et al. [3])

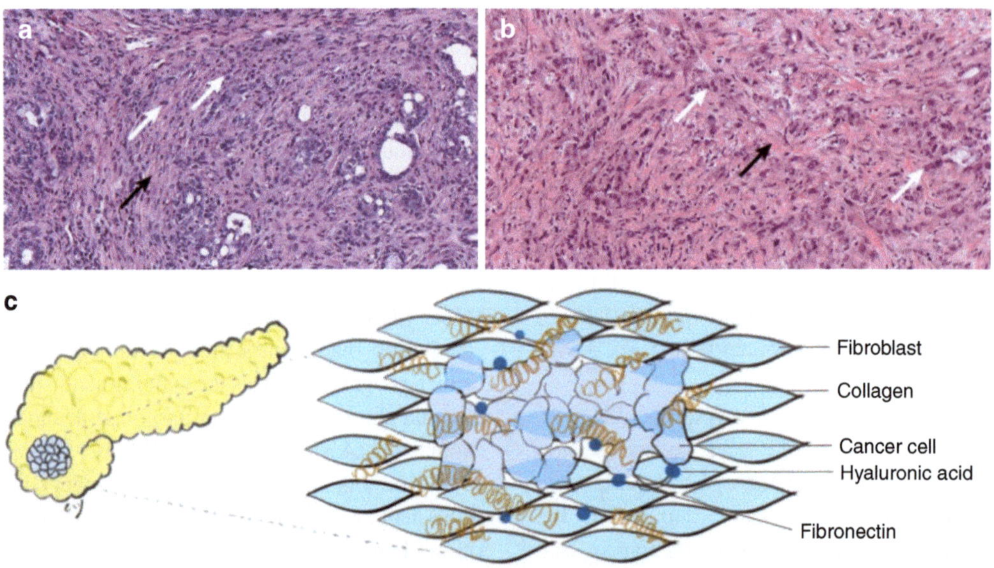

Fig. 2 Histology of the pancreatic cancer stroma and schematic diagram. (**a**, **b**) H&E staining of pancreatic cancer patient tissue. A large amount of fibrotic tissue (black arrow) surrounds pancreatic cancer cells (white arrow). (**c**) Schematic diagram of the tumor microenvironment composed of fibrotic cells and fibrotic tissue surrounding pancreatic cancer cells (adapted from Hosein et al. [4])

the development, progression, and metastasis of cancer, and various studies are ongoing [6] (Fig. 2).

Pathogenesis

PDAC is caused by the accumulation of various genetic mutations, and commonly found mutations include *KRAS*, tumor suppressors, and pancreatic developmental genes [7].

KRAS Mutation

Activating mutations in the KRAS oncogene are found in more than 90% of PDAC [8]. Activation of

KRAS is a mutation that appears early in the carcinogenesis of PDAC and is often found in chronic pancreatitis or PanIN lesions without adenocarcinoma. Point mutations at codon 12 are common, and activation mutations at codons 13 and 61 are rare. The activation mutation maintains 21Kda *KRAS* in a GTP-bound state to continuously activate signaling. In the mouse model, when KRAS is expressed by endogenous KRAS modulators in pancreatic progenitor cells expressing PDX1 or PTF1a, lesions similar to PanIN occur in humans [9]. KRAS signals are transmitted through the RAS-MEK-MAPK and PI3K-AKT pathways and affect cell proliferation, cell viability, and motility [10] (Fig. 3).

RAF activated by KRAS activates MAPK through phosphorylation and MAPK induces an increase in cell proliferative capacity. The PI3K signaling pathway activated by KRAS induces an increase in cell viability and proliferation through downstream proteins such as AKT, p70-S6K, and RAC [11]. Activation of the KRAS downstream protein can also be induced by other genetic mutations. The increase in AKT protein expression is found in 10–20% and BRAF activation mutations are found in 5% [12].

NF-kB, which is involved in the inflammatory response, is also activated by KRAS and affects apoptosis, immune response, angiogenesis, and inflammatory response. Epidermal growth factor (EGF) and the EGF receptor family (EGFR) are located at the top of the KRAS signaling pathway [13]. EGF, transforming growth factor-α (TGF-α), amphiregulin, heparin binding (HB) EGF, betacellulin, and heregulin belong to this ligand. The receptor is HER-1 (EGFR-1), HER-2, HER-3, and HER-4 and is divided into an extracellular domain to which a ligand binds, a hydrophobic cell membrane domain, and an intracellular domain containing tyrosine kinase. Overexpression of these ligands and receptors is found in 10–60% of PDAC, and since the activated signal is transmitted downstream via KRAS, it exhibits an effect similar to the activation mutation of KRAS.

Inactivation of Tumor Suppressor Genes

The inactivation of tumor suppressor genes in the carcinogenesis of PDAC is common, and suppressor genes p16/CDKN2A, p53, and SMAD4/DPC4 are inactivated in more than 50% of cases [8, 14]. Loss of function of the p16/CDKN2A tumor suppressor gene located on chromosome 9p21 is found in more than 95% of PDAC and is

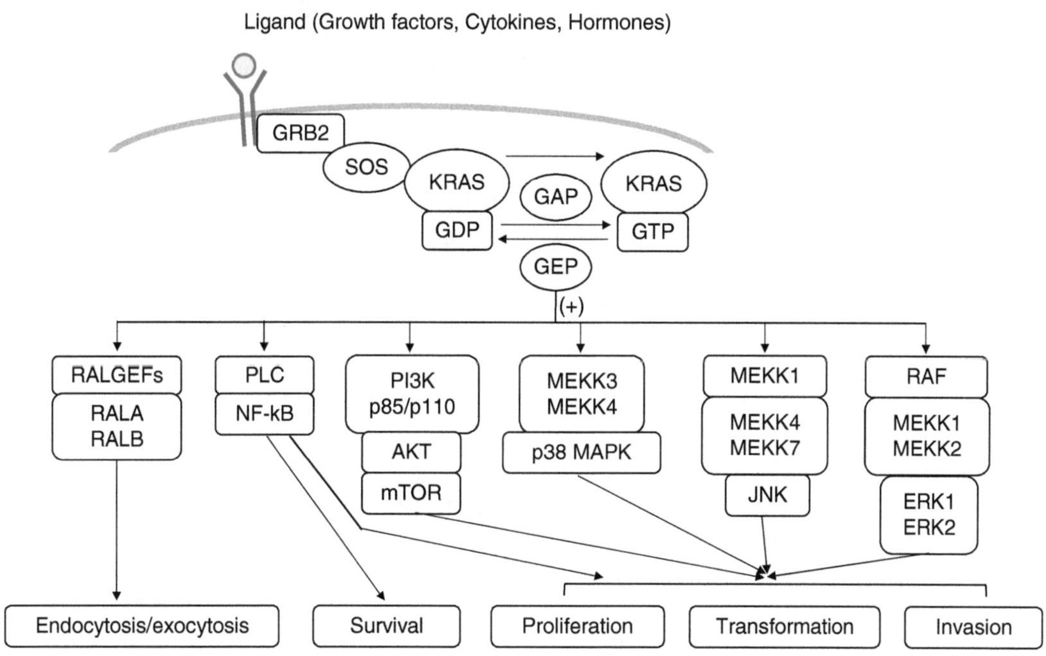

Fig. 3 Schematic image of KRAS activation and downstream pathways (adapted from Buscail et al. [10])

caused by loss of both alleles, point mutations, or regulator hypermethylation [15]. Loss of p16/CDKN2A appears in more advanced lesions after the *KRAS* mutation. In FAMMM syndrome, individuals are born with mutations in this gene in the germline DNA, and the risk of developing multiple melanoma and pancreatic cancer increases 13-fold [16]. The p16/CDKN2A protein inhibits the phosphorylation of the retinoblastoma (RB) protein by cyclin-dependent kinase (CDK) 4 to block entry into the S phase. However, since the risk of pancreatic cancer does not increase in patients with mutations that cannot be inhibited by p16/CDKN2A due to mutations in the CDK4 protein, it is assumed that the function of p16/CDKN2A inhibits carcinogenesis through other mechanisms in addition to the inhibition of CDK4. The p16/CDKN2A gene produces ADP ribosylation factor (ARF) together with CDKN2A, which stabilizes the p53 protein by inhibiting MDM2, which degrades the p53 protein in a ubiquitin-dependent manner. p16/CDKN2A cooperatively induces carcinogenesis with KRAS [15]. Activation of KRAS in epithelial cells without the p16/CDKN2A mutation induces cell death as senescence occurs. The loss of p16/CDKN2A function in KRAS-activated cells helps to overcome apoptosis caused by KRAS activation.

Loss of function due to mutations in the *TP53* tumor suppressor gene appears in 50–75% of PDAC [8]. The p53 mutation is a late change in the cancerous process and is found mainly in PanIN3 lesions that already have alterations in KRAS and p16/CDKN2A.The p53 protein is a tumor suppressor involved in apoptosis, aging, and DNA repair through G1-S and G2-M checkpoint arrest functions and is known as a protein that plays a role as a gatekeeper in cancer development [14]. When DNA damage occurs in cells with p53 mutations, the normal apoptosis process is inhibited, allowing the continuous accumulation of genetic mutations.

Mutations in *SMAD4/DPC4* that mediate transforming growth factor-β (TGFβ) signaling occur in 50% of PDAC due to deletion or point mutation [8]. SMAD4/DPC4 loss of function appears in late PanIN lesions and, thus, is related to advanced lesions as in p53. When TGFβ binds to the serine/threonine kinase receptor, phosphorylation of SMAD2 or SMAD3 occurs. After binding to SMAD4, it moves to the cell nucleus and acts as a transcription factor, regulating cell proliferation, differentiation, death, and migration. TGFβ signaling has two sides: it inhibits epithelial cell growth by inducing the expression of p15/CDKN2B and p21/CIP1 and induces the epithelial-mesenchymal transition (EMT) to induce growth, transformation, and invasiveness in cancer cells [17, 18].

BRCA2 and BRCA1 are autosomally dominant inherited causative genes for hereditary breast and ovarian cancer syndrome and are associated with familial pancreatic cancer [19]. The BRCA gene is involved in the repair of DNA double-strand breaks and cross-links between strands, and the mutation increases the risk of pancreatic cancer by 3.5–10 times [20].

Alterations in Genes of Pancreas Development

It is known that genes involved in pancreatic development play an important role in carcinogenesis. This is supported by the fact that many of the proteins that are abnormally regulated during carcinogenesis also play an important role in development programs. Notch and hedgehog signals are important genes for pancreatic development and are accompanied by significant increases in expression throughout the development of PDAC. The Notch signal inhibits cell differentiation at the developmental stage, and among pancreatic progenitor cells expressing PDX1 and PTF1a, the developmental program operates in cells in which Notch expression is lost, leading to differentiation into endocrine cells and acinar cells [21]. In the carcinogenesis of PDAC, overexpression of Notch signaling-related proteins is frequently observed from the early stage of PanIN lesions, which inhibits the differentiation of cells that are converted into cancer cells [22]. Sonic hedgehog (SHH) is suppressed in the early stages of pancreatic development, so PDX1 transcription factor is expressed in pancreatic progenitor tissue and normal development is induced [23]. In PDAC tissue, overexpression of SHH and PDX1 is common and, like the Notch signal, appears in the early stage of the PanIN lesion [24, 25].

Molecular Characteristics

With the development of research on the mechanisms and genetic changes of PDAC, it has been revealed that there are many genetic factors that affect the development of PDAC. There are gene mutations with high incidence, such as *KRAS, TP53, CDKN2A,* and *SMAD4,* but many genes with low incidence are involved in the development of PDAC. Therefore, to understand the molecular genetic diversity of PDAC, it is necessary not only to understand individual genes but also to approach them individually according to the expression pattern of gene mutations. A study on the classification of PDAC subtypes according to molecular genetic characteristics has been reported. The classification of subtypes is essential for the development of precision medicine, which uses different treatment methods according to molecular genetic characteristics [26].

In the initial classification of molecular genetic subtypes, a method was used to select a set of genes known to be related to PDAC and display the expression pattern of each type of cancer as a heat map through a microarray analysis. Using this approach, Collisson et al. (2011) classified pancreatic cancer into three subtypes: classical, quasimesenchymal (QM), and exocrine-like [27]. In the classical subtype, the expression of epithelial/adhesion-related genes is increased; in the QM subgroup, the expression of mesenchyme-related genes is increased; and in the exocrine-like subtype, the expression of tumor cell-derived digestive enzyme-related genes is relatively high. In the case of the QM subtype, compared to the classical subtype, the survival period was shorter, more sensitive to gemcitabine during chemotherapy, and relatively resistant to erlotinib, showing clinical differences between each subtype.

With the development of new generation sequencing (NGS) technology, studies have been conducted to analyze gene sequences and classify subtypes by whole-exome sequencing of pancreatic cancer cells. PDAC was classified through whole-exome sequencing into four subtypes based on the number of structural variations (SVs), including stable ($SV \leq 50$), scattered ($50 < SV \leq 200$), and unstable ($200 < SV$) subtypes and a locally rearranged subtype in which structural variations occur in only one or two chromosomes [28]. Although the clinical significance of the classification method based on the number of SVs has not yet been fully elucidated, it is known that BRCA mutations in unstable subtypes show a good response to platinum-based chemotherapy.

In 2015, Moffitt et al. profiled PDAC tumors and tissues metastases using microarrays ($n = 206$) and a subset using RNA sequencing [29]. Normal pancreas and TME were excluded based on the fact that most PDAC have a high stromal content that confounds genomic analysis. Researchers divided tumor subtypes into "basal-like" and "classical," and stromal subtypes into "normal" and "activated." The "basal-like" tumor subtype had a worse outcome and the stromal subtypes were also independently prognostic.

Through RNA sequencing and microarray of 261 primary PDAC tissues, Bailey et al. (2016) classified PDAC into the following four subtypes according to the difference in expression of transcription factors related to pancreatic development and regeneration: squamous, pancreatic progenitors, immunogenic, and aberrantly differentiated endocrine exocrine (ADEX) subtype [30]. It was confirmed that there was a difference in the type of mRNA expressed in each group, as well as differences in the major gene programs that affect the development and prognosis of patients. Additionally, when the same patients were classified according to the Collison subtype among existing classifications, squamous showed a QM subtype, ADEX showed exocrine-like, and pancreatic progenitor and immunogenic showed similar patterns and prognosis to the classical type.

Recently, Puleo et al. (2018) reported molecular features of PDAC, including TME gene expression patterns based on 309 PDAC patient samples, and categorized PDAC into five subtypes: pure basal-like, stroma activated, desmoplastic, pure classical, and immune classical [31]. These PDAC subtypes have features of cancers, including immune cells, and were associated with patient outcomes. They also found that the previously reported exocrine-like subtype, called ADEX in a previous study, may result from normal pancreatic acinar cells.

Based on the accumulated data on the molecular characteristics of PDAC, Collison et al. suggested a putative phylotranscriptomic tree of pancreatic cancer [26] (Fig. 4). In the phylotranscriptomic tree, two initial lineages separate PDAC into "squamous" and "classical-pancreatic" subtypes. The "classical-pancreatic" subtype can be divided into the "progenitor" subtype and the "ADEX" subtype, although it is unclear whether the ADEX subtype derives from contamination of the normal epithelium. The "classical-progenitor" subtype is composed of an "immunogenic" subtype and a less immunogenic subtype of the progenitor called a "pure classical progenitor." These four subtypes, squamous, immunogenic progenitor, pure classical progenitor, and exocrine-like (or ADEX), may be called epithelial subtypes, while stromal subtypes have also been subdivided into normal and activated subtypes in a harmonized nomenclature.

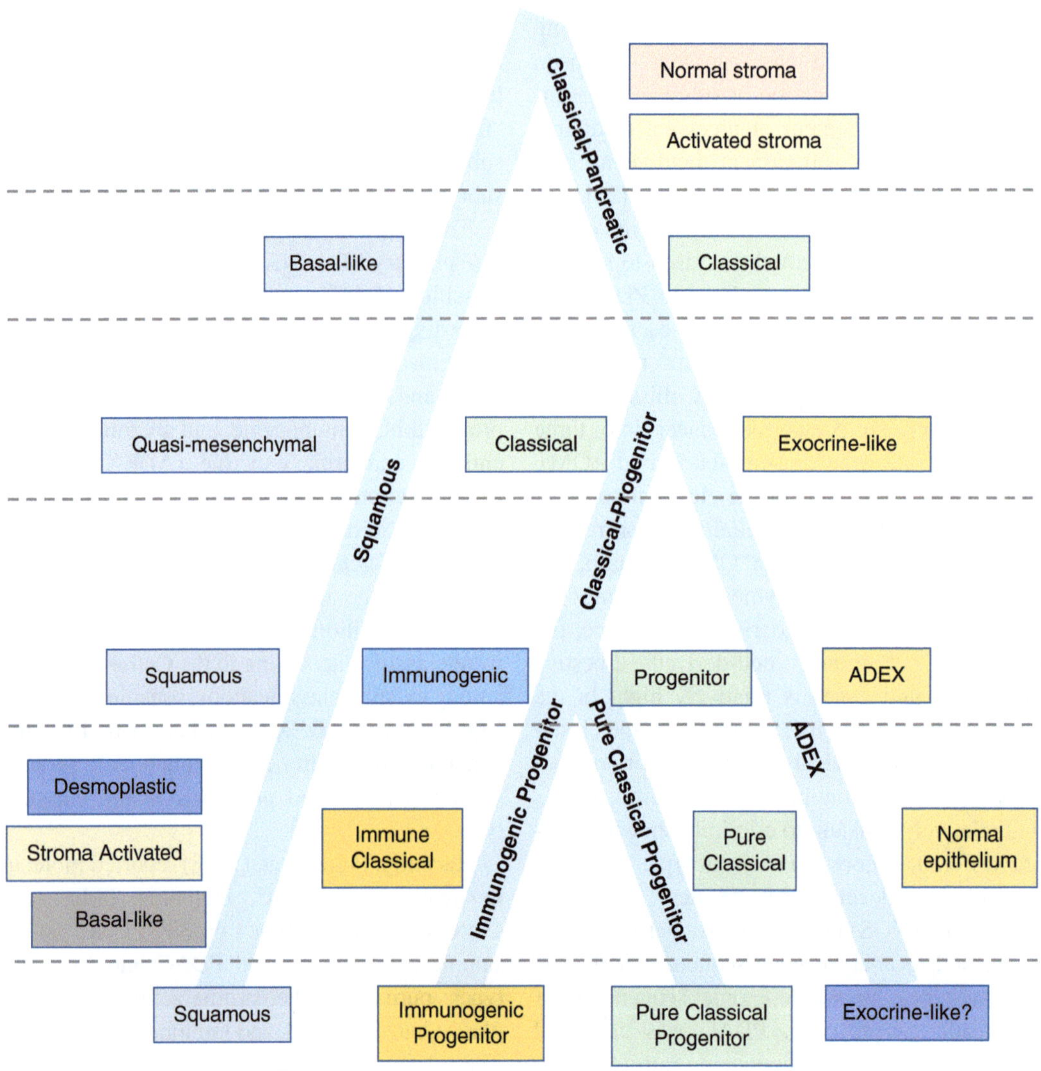

Fig. 4 Molecular classification and phylotranscriptomic tree for pancreatic ductal adenocarcinoma (adapted from Collisson et al. [26])

Conclusion

Pancreatic cancer is a malignant tumor with a poor prognosis. Pathological features, including the tumor microenvironment, are very important for understanding the poor prognosis and therapeutic resistance of pancreatic cancer. Furthermore, the recent discovery of molecular characteristics based on NGS technology provides an opportunity to better understand the pathogenesis of pancreatic cancer and achieve precision medicine. More research is needed to apply these results to the prevention and treatment of pancreatic cancer in real-world clinical practice.

References

1. Hruban RH, Wilentz RE, Goggins M, Offerhaus GJ, Yeo CJ, Kern SE. Pathology of incipient pancreatic cancer. Ann Oncol. 1999;10(Suppl 4):9–11.
2. Scarpa A, Real FX, Luchini C. Genetic unrelatedness of co-occurring pancreatic adenocarcinomas and IPMNs challenges current views of clinical management. Gut. 2018;67:1561–3.
3. Hezel AF, Kimmelman AC, Stanger BZ, Bardeesy N, Depinho RA. Genetics and biology of pancreatic ductal adenocarcinoma. Genes Dev. 2006;20:1218–49.
4. Hosein AN, Brekken RA, Maitra A. Pancreatic cancer stroma: an update on therapeutic targeting strategies. Nat Rev Gastroenterol Hepatol. 2020;17:487–505.
5. Chen X, Song E. Turning foes to friends: targeting cancer-associated fibroblasts. Nat Rev Drug Discov. 2019;18:99–115.
6. Valkenburg KC, de Groot AE, Pienta KJ. Targeting the tumour stroma to improve cancer therapy. Nat Rev Clin Oncol. 2018;15:366–81.
7. Hruban RH, Goggins M, Parsons J, Kern SE. Progression model for pancreatic cancer. Clin Cancer Res. 2000;6:2969–72.
8. Moore PS, Sipos B, Orlandini S, Sorio C, Real FX, Lemoine NR, et al. Genetic profile of 22 pancreatic carcinoma cell lines. Analysis of K-ras, p53, p16 and DPC4/Smad4. Virchows Arch. 2001;439:798–802.
9. Shen R, Wang Q, Cheng S, Liu T, Jiang H, Zhu J, et al. The biological features of PanIN initiated from oncogenic Kras mutation in genetically engineered mouse models. Cancer Lett. 2013;339:135–43.
10. Buscail L, Bournet B, Cordelier P. Role of oncogenic KRAS in the diagnosis, prognosis and treatment of pancreatic cancer. Nat Rev Gastroenterol Hepatol. 2020;17:153–68.
11. Schonleben F, Qiu W, Remotti HE, Hohenberger W, Su GH. PIK3CA, KRAS, and BRAF mutations in intraductal papillary mucinous neoplasm/carcinoma (IPMN/C) of the pancreas. Langenbecks Arch Surg. 2008;393:289–96.
12. Calhoun ES, Jones JB, Ashfaq R, Adsay V, Baker SJ, Valentine V, et al. BRAF and FBXW7 (CDC4, FBW7, AGO, SEL10) mutations in distinct subsets of pancreatic cancer: potential therapeutic targets. Am J Pathol. 2003;163:1255–60.
13. Schlessinger J. Ligand-induced, receptor-mediated dimerization and activation of EGF receptor. Cell. 2002;110:669–72.
14. Jimenez RE, Warshaw AL, Z'Graggen K, Hartwig W, Taylor DZ, Compton CC, et al. Sequential accumulation of K-ras mutations and p53 overexpression in the progression of pancreatic mucinous cystic neoplasms to malignancy. Ann Surg. 1999;230:501–9; discussion 9–11.
15. Moskaluk CA, Hruban RH, Kern SE. p16 and K-ras gene mutations in the intraductal precursors of human pancreatic adenocarcinoma. Cancer Res. 1997;57:2140–3.
16. Lynch HT, Fusaro RM, Lynch JF, Brand R. Pancreatic cancer and the FAMMM syndrome. Fam Cancer. 2008;7:103–12.
17. Platz A, Hansson J, Mansson-Brahme E, Lagerlof B, Linder S, Lundqvist E, et al. Screening of germline mutations in the CDKN2A and CDKN2B genes in Swedish families with hereditary cutaneous melanoma. J Natl Cancer Inst. 1997;89:697–702.
18. Whiteman DC, Milligan A, Welch J, Green AC, Hayward NK. Germline CDKN2A mutations in childhood melanoma. J Natl Cancer Inst. 1997;89:1460.
19. Monnerat C, Chompret A, Kannengiesser C, Avril MF, Janin N, Spatz A, et al. BRCA1, BRCA2, TP53, and CDKN2A germline mutations in patients with breast cancer and cutaneous melanoma. Fam Cancer. 2007;6:453–61.
20. Ferrone CR, Levine DA, Tang LH, Allen PJ, Jarnagin W, Brennan MF, et al. BRCA germline mutations in Jewish patients with pancreatic adenocarcinoma. J Clin Oncol. 2009;27:433–8.
21. Esni F, Ghosh B, Biankin AV, Lin JW, Albert MA, Yu X, et al. Notch inhibits Ptf1 function and acinar cell differentiation in developing mouse and zebrafish pancreas. Development. 2004;131:4213–24.
22. Leach SD. Epithelial differentiation in pancreatic development and neoplasia: new niches for nestin and Notch. J Clin Gastroenterol. 2005;39:S78–82.
23. Morton JP, Mongeau ME, Klimstra DS, Morris JP, Lee YC, Kawaguchi Y, et al. Sonic hedgehog acts at multiple stages during pancreatic tumorigenesis. Proc Natl Acad Sci U S A. 2007;104:5103–8.
24. Ohuchida K, Mizumoto K, Fujita H, Yamaguchi H, Konomi H, Nagai E, et al. Sonic hedgehog is an early developmental marker of intraductal papillary mucinous neoplasms: clinical implications of mRNA levels in pancreatic juice. J Pathol. 2006;210:42–8.
25. Bailey JM, Swanson BJ, Hamada T, Eggers JP, Singh PK, Caffery T, et al. Sonic hedgehog promotes des-

moplasia in pancreatic cancer. Clin Cancer Res. 2008;14:5995–6004.
26. Collisson EA, Bailey P, Chang DK, Biankin AV. Molecular subtypes of pancreatic cancer. Nat Rev Gastroenterol Hepatol. 2019;16:207–20.
27. Collisson EA, Sadanandam A, Olson P, Gibb WJ, Truitt M, Gu SD, et al. Subtypes of pancreatic ductal adenocarcinoma and their differing responses to therapy. Nat Med. 2011;17:500–3.
28. Waddell N, Pajic M, Patch AM, Chang DK, Kassahn KS, Bailey P, et al. Whole genomes redefine the mutational landscape of pancreatic cancer. Nature. 2015;518:495–501.
29. Moffitt RA, Marayati R, Flate EL, Volmar KE, Loeza SG, Hoadley KA, et al. Virtual microdissection identifies distinct tumor- and stroma-specific subtypes of pancreatic ductal adenocarcinoma. Nat Genet. 2015;47:1168–78.
30. Bailey P, Chang DK, Nones K, Johns AL, Patch AM, Gingras MC, et al. Genomic analyses identify molecular subtypes of pancreatic cancer. Nature. 2016;531:47–52.
31. Puleo F, Nicolle R, Blum Y, Cros J, Marisa L, Demetter P, et al. Stratification of pancreatic ductal adenocarcinomas based on tumor and microenvironment features. Gastroenterology. 2018;155:1999–2013.e3.

Clinical Features, Diagnosis, and Staging

Key Points

- The clinical features of pancreatic cancer comprise a triad of abdominal pain, weight loss, and jaundice.
- Decisions about diagnostic management and resectability should involve multidisciplinary consultation at a high-volume center with the use of appropriate imaging studies.
- Computed tomography is the method of choice for the diagnosis and staging of pancreatic cancer.
- In the American Joint Committee on Cancer staging system for pancreatic cancer, T4 is defined when the tumor involves the celiac axis, superior mesenteric artery (SMA), and/or common hepatic artery (CHA), regardless of size.
- Staging of pancreatic cancer is predicated on the identification of four distinct patient groups: resectable, borderline resectable, locally advanced unresectable, and metastases.

Introduction

Pancreatic cancer is the eighth most common cancer and fifth most common cause of cancer-related death in Korea. Pancreatic cancer has a poor prognosis. The 5-year survival rate for pancreatic cancer was only 12.6% in Korea (males 11.9%, female 13.2%) in the period 2014–2018 years. Although early diagnosis of pancreatic cancer is very important for the prognosis of patients, diagnosis is difficult because there are no symptoms in the early stages of pancreatic cancer. In this chapter, the clinical symptoms, diagnosis, and staging of pancreatic cancer are discussed.

Clinical Characteristics

Most patients with pancreatic cancer often experience symptoms as the disease progresses, although in the case of pancreatic head cancer, symptoms develop even in the early stages of the disease. This delayed manifestation of symptoms

Seong-Hun Kim is the lead author of this chapter.

H. J. Chun et al., *Gastrointestinal Cancer*, https://doi.org/10.1007/978-981-99-0815-8_50

often leads to delayed diagnosis [1]. Typical symptoms include abdominal pain, weight loss, and jaundice [2]. Furthermore, floating stool, dyspepsia, nausea, vomiting, and pancreatitis [2] may accompany, and sudden exacerbation of diabetes or onset of diabetes can be indicated [3].

Pain

Pain occurs primarily in the mid-epigastric area (sometimes described as "boring" pain) and manifests itself in pain on the back (due to retroperitoneal invasion of the splanchnic nerve plexus). Pain often exacerbates after eating or lying flat [3].

Jaundice

Jaundice is the first symptom of a patient visiting a hospital. Approximately 50% of patients with jaundice present with obstruction of the extrahepatic bile duct [1]. The first feature is that bilirubin is 2.5–3.0 mg/dL or higher, and jaundice is often associated with pancreatic head cancer. Pruritus is indicated when bilirubin is 6–8 mg/dL or greater [3].

Physical Signs

Gallbladder palpation (Courvoisier's sign), liver enlargement, abdominal mass, and spleen enlargement can also be seen. Migratory superficial thrombophlebitis is also observable. A symptom that occurs in the later stages of the disease is the palpation of the supraclavicular lymph node, which is called Virchow's node. Occasionally, subcutaneous metastases may be palpable in the periumbilical area, which is called Sister Mary Joseph's node [3].

Diagnosis

Imaging

Diagnostic imaging plays an important role in the diagnosis of pancreatic cancer and other abdominal disorders. The most important diagnostic tool is dual-phase contrast-enhanced spiral computed tomography (CT) using the pancreatic cancer protocol [3]. A multidisciplinary approach and appropriate imaging studies are important to determine diagnosis and resectability (Fig. 1) [2].

Ultrasound and Computed Tomography

Transabdominal ultrasound (US) is the most frequently used testing method [1]. In Bipat's meta-analysis, the accuracy of diagnosis was compared with US, CT, and magnetic resonance imaging (MRI), and CT had higher diagnostic sensitivity and specificity [4]. However, CT is not suitable for the screening of pancreatic cancer due to the cost of radiation exposure and the use of contrast media. US is more suitable for screening [4]. In the diagnosis and staging of pancreatic cancer in patients with suspected pancreatic cancer, CT is recommended as a test to assess resectability. The CT criteria for the unresectability of a pancreatic tumor are as follows: (1) distant metastasis, (2) encasement of the celiac axis of the superior mesenteric artery, and/or (3) occlusion of the portal vein or superior mesenteric vein [1] (Fig. 2).

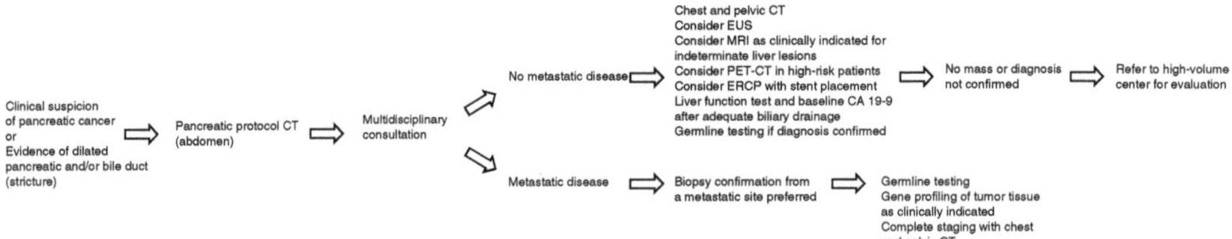

Fig. 1 Clinical presentation and workup guideline of NCCN (Imaging should include a dedicated pancreatic computed tomography of the abdomen or magnetic resonance imaging with contrast)

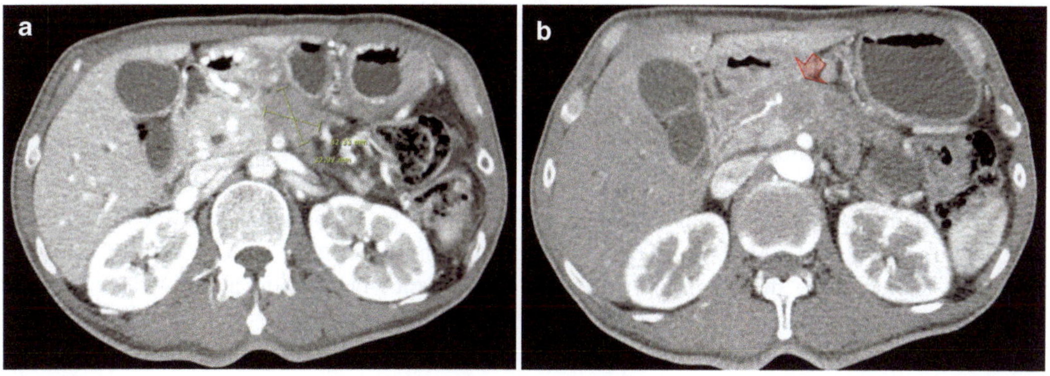

Fig. 2 Pancreatic CT protocol in a patient with pancreatic cancer. (**a**) Portal phase showing a pancreatic cancer measuring 3.6 × 3.3 cm is visible in the body of the pancreas. (**b**) Arterial phase showing that both the celiac trunk and the SMA are encased, and collateral vessels are formed around it

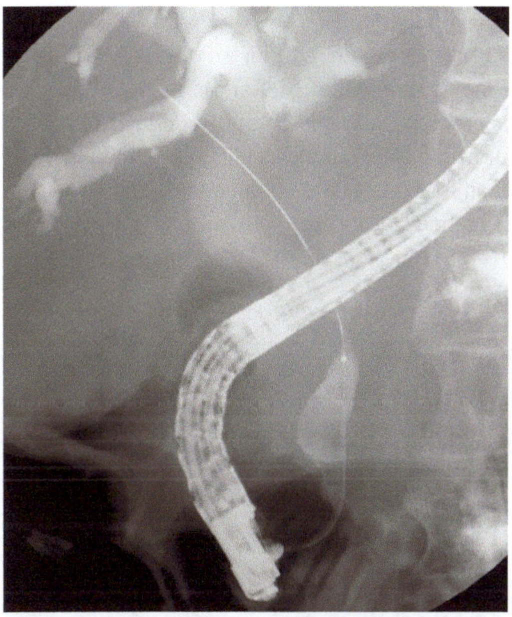

Fig. 3 Endoscopic retrograde cholangiopancreatography of pancreatic cancer with CBD invasion. ERCP showing stricture of the bile duct in a patient with pancreatic cancer

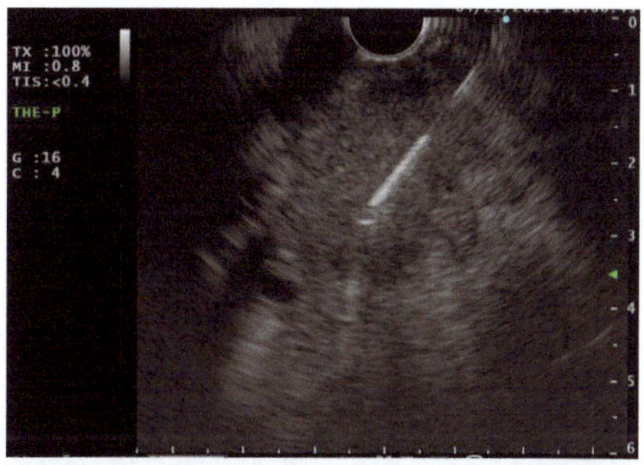

Fig. 4 EUS fine-needle aspiration (FNA)/fine-needle biopsy in pancreatic cancer. EUS image of pancreatic cancer showing the needle during tumor biopsy

Endoscopic Retrograde Cholangiopancreatography

ERCP helps distinguish whether the reason for the narrowing of the pancreaticobiliary tract is benign or malignant. Furthermore, it is useful for the differential diagnosis of tumors in the periampullary region and has the advantage of being able to perform histological examinations (Fig. 3) [1].

Endoscopic Ultrasonography

EUS is the most sensitive test method for the diagnosis of small tumors [1], and the primary site can be confirmed [2]. EUS is recommended when pancreatic cancer is suspected but not clearly diagnosed by CT and MRI [4]. EUS is highly operator-dependent and requires significant technical experience. EUS is a test required for histological diagnosis in patients with non-resectable or borderline resectable cases rather than the test method required for all patients [1]. EUS fine-needle aspiration (FNA)/fine-needle biopsy (FNB) is recommended when pancreatic CT/MRI shows a solid mass and requires pathological confirmation [4] (Fig. 4).

Magnetic Resonance Imaging

Pancreas MRI can be considered for patients with suspected pancreatic cancer if the localized lesion is unknown. Patients with small or isoattenuating pancreatic cancer often do not see the lesion well on CT. In such cases, pancreas MRI has a high detection rate. It is also useful when a differential diagnosis is required [4]. MRI/MRA (magnetic resonance angiography) helps to confirm invasion of blood vessels and, in the case of MRCP, helps to confirm the fluid-containing structure (Fig. 5) [1].

PET-CT

PET-CT provides metabolic information rather than morphological information in a noninvasive test. In the case of pancreatic adenocarcinoma, uptake in the focal region increases. PET/CT is useful for assessing cancer recurrence and for assessing the therapeutic response of neoadjuvant chemotherapy [3]. For PET/CT, tests are considered for patients with suspected metastases after pancreatic CT examination [2].

Serum Tumor Markers

CA 19-9 is not suitable for screening due to false-positive or false-negative results, but CA 19-9 is a valuable adjunct in pancreatic cancer for the diagnosis, prognosis, and monitoring of treatment [1]. A previous study reported sensitivity and specificity for CA 19-9 of 86% and 87%, respectively, using a cutoff value of 37 U/mL [1].

Staging

The American Joint Committee on Cancer (AJCC) staging system for pancreatic cancer is shown in Table 1.

In the eighth edition of the AJCC Cancer Staging manual, the definition of N category has been revised. N1 is currently defined by one to three metastatic nodes and N2 is defined by more than four metastatic lymph nodes. The T category is defined according to size, and T4 no longer includes resectability [2].

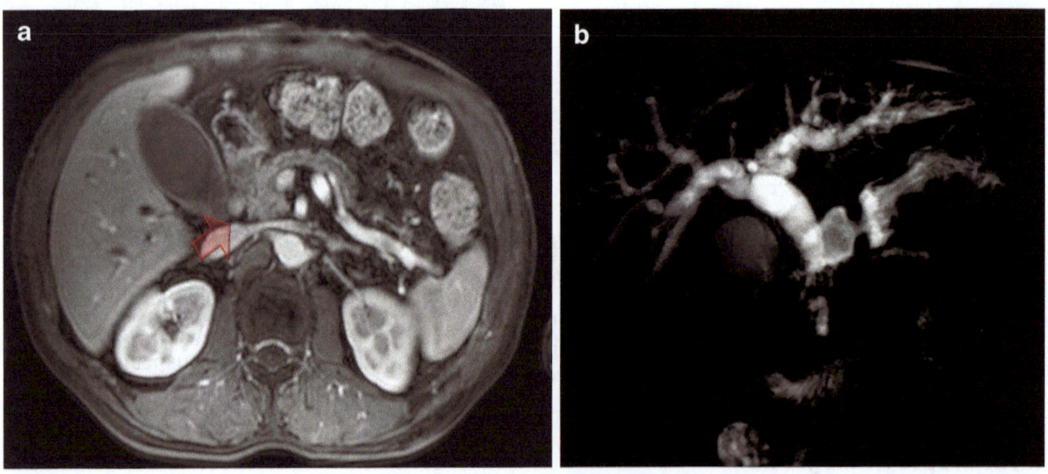

Fig. 5 Pancreas magnetic resonance imaging. Shown is a heterogeneous enhancing mass in an irregular shape with a size of about 3.0 × 1.6 cm near the pancreaticoduodenal groove. These masses narrow the distal CBD and p-duct and induce upward biliary dilation (**a**, **b**)

Table 1 Definitions for T, N, M staging (NCCN Guidelines Version 2.2021) [2]

TNM stages	
Primary tumor (T)	
TX	Primary tumor cannot be assessed
T0	No evidence of primary tumor
Tis	Carcinoma in situ includes: High-grade PanIN (PanIN-3), IPMN with high-grade dysplasia, intraductal tubulopapillary neoplasm with high-grade dysplasia, mucinous cystic neoplasm with high-grade dysplasia
T1	Tumor 2 cm or less
T1a	Tumor 0.5 cm or less
T1b	Tumor greater than 0.5 cm and less than 1 cm
T1c	Tumor greater than 1 cm but no more than 2 cm
T2	Tumor more than 2 cm but no more than 4
T3	Tumor more than 4 cm in greater dimension
T4	Tumor involves celiac axis, superior mesenteric artery, and/or common hepatic artery, regardless of size
Regional LN (N)	
NX	Regional LNs cannot be assessed
N0	No regional LN metastases
N1	Metastases in one to three regional LNs
N2	Metastases in four or more regional LNs
Distant metastasis (M)	
M0	No distant metastasis
M1	Distant metastasis
Stage grouping	
0	Tis N0 M0
IA	T1 N0 M0
IB	T2 N0 M0
IIA	T3 N0 M0
IIB	T1~T3 N1M0
III	T1~T3 N2M0 T4 Any N M0
IV	Any T Any N M1

T stages are classified according to size based on 2 cm and 4 cm (T1, ≤2 cm; T2, >2 cm and ≤4 cm; T3, >4 cm). T4 is defined when the celiac axis and superior mesenteric artery (SMA) and/or common hepatic artery (CHA) are invaded, regardless of tumor size. The stage N is classified by N1 and N2 according to the number of metastasis nodes. At least 12 lymph nodes should be evaluated for an accurate stage N. The stage M is defined by distance metastasis, and the sites with the most metastases are the liver, peritoneal cavity, and lung [4].

Staging is divided into four groups (Table 2). The first group includes those who present with metastatic disease. The second group has locally advanced unresectable diseases but no metastases. The third group is the borderline resectable group where neoadjuvant chemoradiation is recommended. The fourth group is clearly the resectable disease group [3].

Decisions about the possibility for resectability should be made by consensus at multidisciplinary meetings/discussions [2].

Table 2 Criteria defining resectability status at diagnosis (NCCN Guidelines Version 2.2021) [2]

Resectability status	Arterial	Venous
Resectable	• No arterial tumor contact (celiac axis [CA], superior mesenteric artery [SMA], or common hepatic artery [CHA])	• No tumor contact with the superior mesenteric vein [SMV] or portal vein [PV] or ≤180° contact without vein contour irregularity
Borderline resectable	*Pancreatic head/uncinate process:* • Solid tumor contact with CHA without extension to CA or hepatic artery bifurcation allowing for safe and complete resection and reconstruction • Solid tumor contact with the SMA of ≤180° • Solid tumor contact with variant arterial anatomy (e.g., accessory right hepatic artery, replaced right hepatic artery, replaced CHA, and the origin of replaced or accessory artery) and the presence and degree of tumor contacts should be noted if present, as it may affect surgical planning *Pancreatic body/tail:* • Solid tumor contact with the CA of ≤180° • Solid tumor contact with the CA of >180° without involvement of the aorta and with intact and uninvolved gastroduodenal artery, thereby permitting a modified Appleby procedure (some panel members prefer these criteria to be in the locally advanced category)	• Solid tumor contact with the SMV or PV of >180°, contact of ≤180° with contour irregularity of the vein or thrombosis of the vein but with suitable vessel proximal and distal to the site of involvement allowing for safe and complete resection and vein reconstruction • Solid tumor contact with the inferior vena cava (IVC)
Locally advanced	*Pancreatic head/uncinate process:* • Solid tumor contact with SMA > 180° • Solid tumor contact with the CA > 180° *Pancreatic boy/tail:* • Solid tumor contact of >180° with the SMA or CA • Solid tumor contact with the CA and aortic involvement	• Unreconstructible SMV/PV due to tumor involvement or occlusion (can be due to tumor or bland thrombus)

Conclusion

Pancreatic cancer should be suspected if symptoms such as typical epigastric pain, weight loss, and jaundice are present. In particular, if there is newly diagnosed or recently exacerbated diabetes, abdominal CT should be performed to differentiate pancreatic cancer. Pancreatic cancer staging uses the AJCC cancer staging and NCCN guidelines, and a multidisciplinary approach is needed to make treatment decisions for pancreatic cancer.

References

1. Sleisenger and Fordtran's gastrointestinal and liver disease, vol 2, 10th ed. Philadelphia: Elsevier Inc; 2016.
2. NCCN. NCCN guidelines version 2.2021. 2021. Pancreatic adenocarcinoma.
3. Harrison's principles of internal medicine. 20th ed. New York: McGraw-Hill Education; 2018.
4. Korean clinical practice guideline for pancreatic cancer 2021.

Treatment

Key Points

- Surgical resection is the only potentially curative treatment for pancreatic cancer.
- The adjuvant chemotherapy recommended after pancreatic cancer resection is modified FOLFIRINOX (fluorouracil, oxaliplatin, irinotecan, and leucovorin) for patients with good performance status or gemcitabine and capecitabine or gemcitabine alone for patients with poor functional status.
- Combined cytotoxic regimens have improved survival in advanced pancreatic cancer. Current standard first-line regimens for patients with metastatic disease include gemcitabine and albumin-bound paclitaxel or FOLFIRINOX.
- Multidisciplinary management, comprehensive germline testing, and integrative supportive care are recommended.

Introduction

Pancreatic ductal adenocarcinoma (PDAC) is a deadly solid gastrointestinal cancer, and radial surgical resection is essential for long-term survival [1]. But, at the time of diagnosis, resectable PDAC accounts for only approximately 10–20% of all patients, and most patients were classified as advanced stage [2–4]. Cancer recurrence occurs in 70–80% of PDAC patients detected in the early stages after surgery. Depending on the stage of PDAC, treatment options include surgery, chemotherapy, radiation therapy, combined chemotherapy and radiation therapy, and palliative care [5, 6]. Various methods of therapeutic anticancer treatment have been used for decades. Conventional chemotherapy, in particular, has become an important treatment option for individuals who are not candidates for resection. Chemotherapy can be utilized to achieve neoadjuvant, adjuvant, or palliative goals. The purpose of this chapter is to discuss the current state and future of anticancer treatments in PDAC.

Resectable/Borderline Resectable Pancreatic Cancer

Neoadjuvant Therapy

Neoadjuvant treatment has the potential to eliminate occult metastatic disease and increase the number of patients suitable for systemic therapy. A previous study reported the high rate of futile surgery in patients with even radiologically resectable or borderline resectable pancreatic cancer and suggested neoadjuvant treatment in high-risk patients [7]. The National

Hee Seung Lee and Seungmin Bang are the lead authors of this chapter.

H. J. Chun et al., *Gastrointestinal Cancer*, https://doi.org/10.1007/978-981-99-0815-8_51

Comprehensive Cancer Network (NCCN) guideline suggests neoadjuvant treatment for selected patients who appear technically resectable but have poor prognostic characteristics (i.e., markedly elevated carbohydrate antigen (CA) 19–9, large primary tumors, large regional lymph nodes, excessive weight loss, and extreme pain) [8]. The advantages of neoadjuvant therapy include the ability to shrink tumors to enhance the probability of a margin-free resection, select patients with PDAC with more stable disease, and treat micrometastases at an earlier stage [9]. In 58 patients with borderline resectable pancreatic cancer (BRPC), a multi-institutional randomized controlled trial found that individuals receiving neoadjuvant treatment had higher margin-negative resection rates than those undergoing first surgery (82.4% vs 33.3%; $p = 0.01$) [10]. Previous research has indicated that preoperative therapy of BRPC can be successful and well-tolerated [11]. After efficient neoadjuvant therapy, the potential for R0 resection is increased in patients with BRPC, and the survival of patients who received surgical resection is better than that of those who did not [12].

In the phase III PREOPANC study, 236 patients were randomly assigned to undergo neoadjuvant gemcitabine-based chemoradiation followed by surgery or first surgery followed by adjuvant gemcitabine. In the selected subset of 113 patients with BRPC who received neoadjuvant chemoradiotherapy, an overall survival (OS) advantage was observed (17.6 vs 13.2 months; hazard ratio (HR), 0.62 [95% confidence interval (CI), 0.40–0.95]) [13].

The benefit of neoadjuvant treatment in resectable PDAC is being studied. One of the potential limitations of neoadjuvant treatment is the lack of a significant tumor response in most patients [14]. Inadequate tumor response may promote tumor growth, alleviating the possibility of completely resecting the tumor. In Japan, a phase III trial of neoadjuvant gemcitabine with S-1 (Prep-02/JSAP-05) was conducted [15]. Prep-02/JSAP-05 revealed a substantial survival benefit of neoadjuvant chemotherapy, with a median OS of 36.7 vs 26.6 months for initial surgery (HR 0.72, $p = 0.015$). Approximately 80% of the patients who participated in this trial had resectable PDAC at the time of diagnosis. A phase II randomized study of the South West Oncology Group S1505 with 102 patients evaluated modified perioperative FOLFIRINOX or gemcitabine and albumin-bound paclitaxel. There was no difference in OS between the modified FOLFIRINOX and gemcitabine with albumin-bound paclitaxel, with 2-year OS rates of 47% (95% CI, 31–61%) and 48%, respectively (95% CI, 31–63%). The median OS was 22.4 and 23.6 months, respectively [16]. Although there is still controversy about the effectiveness of neoadjuvant therapy for resectable PDAC, some data suggest the potential benefit of neoadjuvant therapy for resectable PDAC with better surgical outcome and PFS [17].

Surgery

The only possible curative therapy for pancreatic cancer is surgical resection. To determine resectability, the main tumor and the involvement of nearby arteries, such as the celiac artery and vein, the portal vein, and the liver artery, must be assessed (Fig. 1) [18]. Only 15–20% of patients

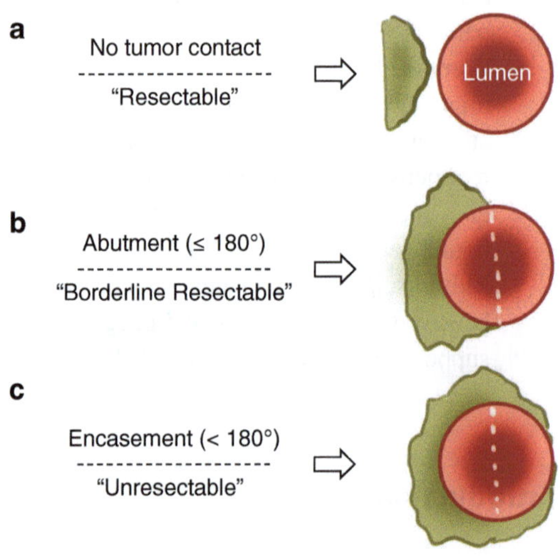

Fig. 1 Tumor and vessel anatomy in patients with pancreatic cancer. Resectable, borderline resectable, and unresectable tumors are considered according to the major peripancreatic venous and arterial involvement of the tumor. (**a**) Resectable, minimal, or no contact with major vessels. (**b**) Borderline resectable, venous, and arterial abutment or venous encasement with arterial abutment. (**c**) Unresectable, venous, and arterial encasement (adapted from Toesca et al. [18])

are considered candidates for surgical resection after a comprehensive evaluation [19]. To remove malignancies in the head and neck of the pancreas, a pancreaticoduodenectomy (the Whipple surgery) is performed. There were no significant differences in the outcomes for different pancreaticoduodenectomy variants, including pylorus-preserving, subtotal stomach-preserving, and minimally invasive procedures [20]. A distal pancreatectomy, which usually involves a splenectomy, is used to remove tumors in the body or tail of the pancreas. Distal tumors are frequently successfully removed laparoscopically.

Adjuvant Therapy

Adjuvant chemotherapy after PDAC resection is modified FOLFIRINOX (fluorouracil, oxaliplatin, irinotecan, leucovorin) for those with good functional status or gemcitabine and capecitabine or gemcitabine alone for those with poor functional status. Adjuvant treatment recommendations are based on numerous major studies conducted over the last two decades [21–23]. The effectiveness of adjuvant chemotherapy in resected PDAC was determined in the CONKO-001 study, which randomized 368 patients who underwent surgical resection of PDAC to receive 6 months of adjuvant gemcitabine or undergo observation. Patients treated with gemcitabine had a higher median OS than those observed (22.8 vs 20.2 months; HR, 0.76 [95% CI, 0.61–0.95]) [22] (Table 1).

The phase III study ESPAC-4 [23] found that the dual-agent treatment outperformed gemcitabine alone in terms of survival. In this study, 730 patients were randomly assigned to gemcitabine + capecitabine, an oral antimetabolite, or gemcitabine alone for 6 months. Compared to gemcitabine alone, combination treatment improved median OS (28.0 vs 25.5 months: HR, 0.82 [95% CI, 0.68–0.98]). In the most recent multicenter PRODIGE-24 trial [21], 493 patients with resected PDAC, a low serum CA 19–9 (180 U/mL), and an excellent performance status (Eastern Cooperative Oncology Group score, 0–1) were randomized to receive 6 months of adjuvant modified FOLFIRINOX or gemcitabine alone. In this trial, both groups achieved better survival compared to previous trials with gemcitabine in the adjuvant setting. Patients treated with modified FOLFIRINOX had an OS of 54 months, compared to 35 months in those receiving gemcitabine (HR, 0.64 [95% CI, 0.48–0.86]).

As a result, modified FOLFIRINOX is suggested as adjuvant treatment in patients with good functional status after surgical excision of PDAC. In general, individuals who are not suitable for modified FOLFIRINOX therapy could be evaluated for gemcitabine/capecitabine or gemcitabine alone [23, 28]. The role of radiation therapy as an adjuvant therapy for resected PDAC is controversial. Previous research did not sup-

Table 1 Key clinical trials evaluating chemotherapy for pancreatic cancer

Trial	Chemotherapy aim	Regimens	No. of patients	Median survival. months
CONKO-001 [22]	Adjuvant	Gemcitabine	368	13.4 vs 6.7 (DFS)
ESPAC-4 [23]	Adjuvant	Gemcitabine and capecitabine	730	28.0 vs 25.5 (OS)
PRODIGE-24 [21]	Adjuvant	mFOLFIRINOX	493	54.5 vs 35 (OS)
PRODIGE [24]	Palliative, first line	FOLFIRINOX	342	11.1 vs 6.8 (OS)
MPACT [25]	Palliative, first line	Gemcitabine and albumin-bound paclitaxel	861	8.5 vs 6.7 (OS)
NAPOLI-1 [26]	Palliative, second line	5-FU/LV and nanoliposomal irinotecan	417	6.2 vs 4.2 (OS)
POLO [27]	Maintenance	Olaparib	154	7.4 vs 3.8 (PFS)

DFS disease-free survival, *OS* overall survival, *PFS* progression-free survival

port adjuvant radiation for PDAC, as no benefit to OS was found [29, 30].

Treatments for Locally Advanced/ Metastatic Pancreatic Cancer

When most individuals with PDAC are diagnosed, the cancer is already at an advanced unresectable stage. As a result, chemotherapy is the main treatment modality for metastatic PDAC [31, 32]. Gemcitabine has been a mainstay of chemotherapy since a major clinical trial comparing it to 5-FU in 1997, and other clinical studies have evaluated innovative regimens for gemcitabine monotherapy [33]. In advanced PDAC, multiagent cytotoxic treatments have increased survival [24–26]. For individuals with metastatic PDAC, current recommended first-line treatments include gemcitabine and albumin-bound paclitaxel or modified FOLFIRINOX [8]. The Metastatic Pancreatic Cancer Study (MPACT) trial of 861 patients with untreated metastatic PDAC found that gemcitabine and albumin-bound paclitaxel outperformed gemcitabine in terms of OS (median survival, 8.5 vs 6.7 months; HR, 0.72 [95% CI, 0.62–0.83]; $p = 0.001$) [25]. The PRODIGE study of 342 patients with untreated metastatic PDAC found that FOLFIRINOX therapy improved OS compared to gemcitabine (11.1 vs 6.8 months; HR, 0.57 [95% CI, 0.45–0.73]; $p = 0.001$) [24] (Table 1). Between two regimens, the median OS (12.1 vs 10.7 months; $p = 0.157$) and PFS (8.4 vs 8.0 months; $p = 0.134$) were not significantly different in retrospective real-world data [34].

The NAPOLI-1 study found that the combination of nanoliposomal irinotecan, fluorouracil, and leucovorin outperformed fluorouracil and leucovorin (median OS 6.1 vs 4.2 months, HR, 0.67 [95% CI, 0.49–0.92]; $p = 0.012$) [26]. These studies were carried out in patients who were not chosen for any specific condition or genetic trait. On the contrary, the POLO (Pancreas Cancer Olaparib Ongoing) study confirmed a genetic biomarker, the germline variant BRCA1/2, which led to the US Food and Drug Administration (FDA) approval of olaparib, a poly(ADP-ribose) polymerase inhibitor [27]. Olaparib or placebo was administered as a maintenance treatment after platinum-based chemotherapy to patients with a germline BRCA1/2 mutation and metastatic PDAC and was approved based on a progression-free survival benefit compared to placebo (7.4 vs 3.8 months; HR, 0.53 [95% CI, 0.35–0.82]; $p = 0.004$). In the POLO trial, there was no difference in OS between the placebo and olaparib groups (HR, 0.83 [95% CI, 0.56–1.22]; $p = 0.35$) [27].

A systematic review of clinical trials that evaluated the efficacy of following gemcitabine therapy in pancreatic cancer indicated that while data are limited, evidence shows that further chemotherapy is superior to optimal supportive care. Fluoropyrimidine-based chemotherapy regimens are acceptable next options for patients with advanced disease who have previously undergone gemcitabine-based treatment. Patients who had previously had fluoropyrimidine-based therapy may be recommended for gemcitabine-based therapy [8].

Novel Therapies for Pancreatic Cancer

In addition to BRCA, a subset of 10–15% of patients with PDAC present DNA damage repair gene mutations. For patients with PDAC associated with impaired DNA damage repair, novel combination techniques involving targeted agents and combinations of immune therapy are being investigated [35, 36].

There is evidence that blocking of PD-1 activity with pembrolizumab may be beneficial in cancers with mismatch repair deficit (dMMR) [37, 38]. dMMR occurs in approximately 1% of individuals with PDAC and is defined by germline or somatic alterations or loss of MMR genes, such as MLH1 and MSH2 [39, 40]. Pembrolizumab is an anti-PD-1 receptor antibody that inhibits its interaction with PD-L1 and PD-L2, releasing the PD-1-mediated suppression of the immune response and improving antitumor immunity. A phase II KEYNOTE-158 study in patients with 27 different advanced cancers of the dMMR, including the pancreas, indicated that pembrolizumab therapy resulted in long-term responses (objective response rate in 34.3% of patients, with 9.9% complete response). There were 22 patients with PDAC who had an objective response rate in 18.2% of cases.

Missense variations of *KRAS* in codon G12C have been identified in 1–2% of patients with PDAC, and early-phase evaluation of the *KRAS* G12C allele-specific inhibitor sotorasib revealed 1 case of partial response (>30% tumor reduction) and stable disease in a cohort of 12 patients with PDAC with this variant [41, 42]. The *KRAS* wild-type PDAC (lack of the KRAS variant) is reported in 6–8% of all PDAC patients and in up to 16–18% of individuals younger than 50 years at diagnosis. Alternative oncogenic drivers are present in this setting, and targeted agents entrectinib and larotrectinib have activity in TRK fusion proteins (1%), and zenocutuzumab (MCLA-128) is active against the NRG-1 fusion (1%) [43–46].

Inhibition of stroma-related signaling pathways is believed to be a promising approach to reduce stromal density and facilitate the access of cytotoxic medications to tumor cells [47, 48]. A cellular matrix component is currently being investigated as a therapeutic intervention target. Human recombinant PH20 hyaluronidase (PEGPH20) enzymatically depletes hyaluronan (which is abundant in the extracellular matrix of human and mouse PDAC tissues) [49], promoting tumor blood vessel reexpansion and increasing gemcitabine concentration inside the tumor [50]. A phase III trial that evaluated PEGPH20 in combination with gemcitabine and nab-paclitaxel in patients with tumors with high hyaluronic acid content found no S compared to gemcitabine alone [51, 52].

Conclusion

Pancreatic cancer can be difficult to treat surgically due to the location of the organ and because the disease has often spread in the body by the time it is diagnosed. Standard treatment for pancreatic cancer usually consists of surgery, chemotherapy, radiation, or combinations of each, depending on the stage of the cancer. With recent advances in the treatment of metastatic pancreatic cancer, new insights into the biology and genetics of pancreatic cancer, such as *KRAS* mutations, tumor metabolism, and tumor immunology, may be useful in the development of novel treatments.

References

1. Ryan DP, Hong TS, Bardeesy N. Pancreatic adenocarcinoma. N Engl J Med. 2014;371:1039–49.
2. Rahib L, Smith BD, Aizenberg R, Rosenzweig AB, Fleshman JM, Matrisian LM. Projecting cancer incidence and deaths to 2030: the unexpected burden of thyroid, liver, and pancreas cancers in the United States. Cancer Res. 2014;74:2913–21.
3. Kamisawa T, Wood LD, Itoi T, Takaori K. Pancreatic cancer. Lancet. 2016;388:73–85.
4. Ferlay J, Soerjomataram I, Dikshit R, Eser S, Mathers C, Rebelo M, et al. Cancer incidence and mortality worldwide: sources, methods and major patterns in GLOBOCAN 2012. Int J Cancer. 2015;136:E359–86.
5. Hartwig W, Werner J, Jäger D, Debus J, Büchler MW. Improvement of surgical results for pancreatic cancer. Lancet Oncol. 2013;14:e476–85.
6. Park W, Chawla A, O'Reilly EM. Pancreatic cancer: a review. JAMA. 2021;326:851–62.
7. Lee HS, An C, Hwang HK, Roh YH, Kang H, Jo JH, et al. Preoperative prediction of futile surgery in patients with radiologically resectable or borderline resectable pancreatic adenocarcinoma. J Gastroenterol Hepatol. 2020;35:499–507.
8. Tempero MA, Malafa MP, Chiorean EG, Czito B, Scaife C, Narang AK, et al. Pancreatic adenocarcinoma, version 1.2019. J Natl Compr Cancer Netw. 2019;17:202–10.
9. Müller PC, Frey MC, Ruzza CM, Nickel F, Jost C, Gwerder C, et al. Neoadjuvant chemotherapy in pancreatic cancer: an appraisal of the current high-level evidence. Pharmacology. 2021;106:143–53.
10. Jang JY, Han Y, Lee H, Kim SW, Kwon W, Lee KH, et al. Oncological benefits of neoadjuvant chemoradiation with gemcitabine versus upfront surgery in patients with borderline resectable pancreatic cancer: a prospective, randomized, open-label, multicenter phase 2/3 trial. Ann Surg. 2018;268:215–22.
11. Christians KK, Tsai S, Mahmoud A, Ritch P, Thomas JP, Wiebe L, et al. Neoadjuvant FOLFIRINOX for borderline resectable pancreas cancer: a new treatment paradigm? Oncologist. 2014;19:266–74.
12. Tinchon C, Hubmann E, Pichler A, Keil F, Pichler M, Rabl H, et al. Safety and efficacy of neoadjuvant FOLFIRINOX treatment in a series of patients with borderline resectable pancreatic ductal adenocarcinoma. Acta Oncol. 2013;52:1231–3.

13. Versteijne E, Suker M, Groothuis K, Akkermans-Vogelaar JM, Besselink MG, Bonsing BA, et al. Preoperative chemoradiotherapy versus immediate surgery for resectable and borderline resectable pancreatic cancer: results of the Dutch randomized phase III PREOPANC trial. J Clin Oncol. 2020;38:1763–73.
14. Sohal DPS, Duong M, Ahmad SA, Gandhi NS, Beg MS, Wang-Gillam A, et al. Efficacy of perioperative chemotherapy for resectable pancreatic adenocarcinoma: a phase 2 randomized clinical trial. JAMA Oncol. 2021;7:421–7.
15. Motoi F, Kosuge T, Ueno H, Yamaue H, Satoi S, Sho M, et al. Randomized phase II/III trial of neoadjuvant chemotherapy with gemcitabine and S-1 versus upfront surgery for resectable pancreatic cancer (Prep-02/JSAP05). Jpn J Clin Oncol. 2019;49:190–4.
16. Ahmad SA, Duong M, Sohal DPS, Gandhi NS, Beg MS, Wang-Gillam A, et al. Surgical outcome results from SWOG S1505: a randomized clinical trial of mFOLFIRINOX versus gemcitabine/nab-paclitaxel for perioperative treatment of resectable pancreatic ductal adenocarcinoma. Ann Surg. 2020;272:481–6.
17. Yoon MS, Lee HS, Kang CM, Lee WJ, Keum J, Sung MJ, et al. Response to neoadjuvant therapy and prognosis in patients with resectable pancreatic cancer: a propensity score matching analysis. Gut Liver. 2022;16(1):118–28.
18. Toesca DAS, Koong AJ, Poultsides GA, Visser BC, Haraldsdottir S, Koong AC, et al. Management of borderline resectable pancreatic cancer. Int J Radiat Oncol Biol Phys. 2018;100:1155–74.
19. Konstantinidis IT, Warshaw AL, Allen JN, Blaszkowsky LS, Castillo CF, Deshpande V, et al. Pancreatic ductal adenocarcinoma: is there a survival difference for R1 resections versus locally advanced unresectable tumors? What is a “true” R0 resection? Ann Surg. 2013;257:731–6.
20. Martin RC 2nd, Scoggins CR, Egnatashvili V, Staley CA, McMasters KM, Kooby DA. Arterial and venous resection for pancreatic adenocarcinoma: operative and long-term outcomes. Arch Surg. 2009;144:154–9.
21. Conroy T, Hammel P, Hebbar M, Ben Abdelghani M, Wei AC, Raoul J-L, et al. FOLFIRINOX or gemcitabine as adjuvant therapy for pancreatic cancer. N Engl J Med. 2018;379:2395–406.
22. Oettle H, Neuhaus P, Hochhaus A, Hartmann JT, Gellert K, Ridwelski K, et al. Adjuvant chemotherapy with gemcitabine and long-term outcomes among patients with resected pancreatic cancer: the CONKO-001 randomized trial. JAMA. 2013;310:1473–81.
23. Neoptolemos JP, Palmer DH, Ghaneh P, Psarelli EE, Valle JW, Halloran CM, et al. Comparison of adjuvant gemcitabine and capecitabine with gemcitabine monotherapy in patients with resected pancreatic cancer (ESPAC-4): a multicentre, open-label, randomised, phase 3 trial. Lancet. 2017;389:1011–24.
24. Conroy T, Desseigne F, Ychou M, Bouché O, Guimbaud R, Bécouarn Y, et al. FOLFIRINOX versus gemcitabine for metastatic pancreatic cancer. N Engl J Med. 2011;364:1817–25.
25. Von Hoff DD, Ervin T, Arena FP, Chiorean EG, Infante J, Moore M, et al. Increased survival in pancreatic cancer with Nab-paclitaxel plus gemcitabine. N Engl J Med. 2013;369:1691–703.
26. Wang-Gillam A, Li CP, Bodoky G, Dean A, Shan YS, Jameson G, et al. Nanoliposomal irinotecan with fluorouracil and folinic acid in metastatic pancreatic cancer after previous gemcitabine-based therapy (NAPOLI-1): a global, randomised, open-label, phase 3 trial. Lancet. 2016;387:545–57.
27. Golan T, Hammel P, Reni M, Van Cutsem E, Macarulla T, Hall MJ, et al. Maintenance Olaparib for germline BRCA-mutated metastatic pancreatic cancer. N Engl J Med. 2019;381:317–27.
28. Neoptolemos JP, Stocken DD, Bassi C, Ghaneh P, Cunningham D, Goldstein D, et al. Adjuvant chemotherapy with fluorouracil plus folinic acid vs gemcitabine following pancreatic cancer resection: a randomized controlled trial. JAMA. 2010;304:1073–81.
29. Klinkenbijl JH, Jeekel J, Sahmoud T, van Pel R, Couvreur ML, Veenhof CH, et al. Adjuvant radiotherapy and 5-fluorouracil after curative resection of cancer of the pancreas and periampullary region: phase III trial of the EORTC gastrointestinal tract cancer cooperative group. Ann Surg. 1999;230:776–82; discussion 82–4.
30. Neoptolemos JP, Stocken DD, Friess H, Bassi C, Dunn JA, Hickey H, et al. A randomized trial of chemoradiotherapy and chemotherapy after resection of pancreatic cancer. N Engl J Med. 2004;350:1200–10.
31. Sohal DPS, Kennedy EB, Khorana A, Copur MS, Crane CH, Garrido-Laguna I, et al. Metastatic pancreatic cancer: ASCO clinical practice guideline update. J Clin Oncol. 2018;36:2545–56.
32. Sohal DP, Mangu PB, Khorana AA, Shah MA, Philip PA, O'Reilly EM, et al. Metastatic pancreatic cancer: American Society of Clinical Oncology clinical practice guideline. J Clin Oncol. 2016;34:2784–96.
33. Burris HA 3rd, Moore MJ, Andersen J, Green MR, Rothenberg ML, Modiano MR, et al. Improvements in survival and clinical benefit with gemcitabine as first-line therapy for patients with advanced pancreas cancer: a randomized trial. J Clin Oncol. 1997;15:2403–13.
34. Cho IR, Kang H, Jo JH, Lee HS, Chung MJ, Park JY, et al. FOLFIRINOX vs gemcitabine/nab-paclitaxel for treatment of metastatic pancreatic cancer: single-center cohort study. World J Gastrointest Oncol. 2020;12:182–94.
35. Park W, Chen J, Chou JF, Varghese AM, Yu KH, Wong W, et al. Genomic methods identify homologous recombination deficiency in pancreas adenocarcinoma and optimize treatment selection. Clin Cancer Res. 2020;26:3239–47.
36. O'Reilly EM, Lee JW, Zalupski M, Capanu M, Park J, Golan T, et al. Randomized, multicenter, phase II

trial of gemcitabine and cisplatin with or without Veliparib in patients with pancreas adenocarcinoma and a germline BRCA/PALB2 mutation. J Clin Oncol. 2020;38:1378–88.
37. Le DT, Durham JN, Smith KN, Wang H, Bartlett BR, Aulakh LK, et al. Mismatch repair deficiency predicts response of solid tumors to PD-1 blockade. Science. 2017;357:409–13.
38. Asaoka Y, Ijichi H, Koike K. PD-1 blockade in tumors with mismatch-repair deficiency. N Engl J Med. 2015;373:1979.
39. Florou V, Nevala-Plagemann C, Barber KE, Mastroianni JN, Cavalieri CC, Garrido-Laguna I. Treatment rechallenge with checkpoint inhibition in patients with mismatch repair-deficient pancreatic cancer after planned treatment interruption JCO Precis Oncol. 2020;4.
40. Hu ZI, Hellmann MD, Wolchok JD, Vyas M, Shia J, Stadler ZK, et al. Acquired resistance to immunotherapy in MMR-D pancreatic cancer. J Immunother Cancer. 2018;6:127.
41. Nollmann FI, Ruess DA. Targeting mutant KRAS in pancreatic cancer: futile or promising? Biomedicine. 2020;8:281.
42. Skoulidis F, Li BT, Dy GK, Price TJ, Falchook GS, Wolf J, et al. Sotorasib for lung cancers with KRAS p.G12C mutation. N Engl J Med. 2021;384:2371–81.
43. Singh RR, O'Reilly EM. New treatment strategies for metastatic pancreatic ductal adenocarcinoma. Drugs. 2020;80:647–69.
44. Drilon A, Laetsch TW, Kummar S, DuBois SG, Lassen UN, Demetri GD, et al. Efficacy of larotrectinib in TRK fusion–positive cancers in adults and children. N Engl J Med. 2018;378:731–9.
45. Heining C, Horak P, Uhrig S, Codo PL, Klink B, Hutter B, et al. NRG1 fusions in KRAS wild-type pancreatic cancer. Cancer Discov. 2018;8:1087–95.
46. Schram AM, O'Reilly EM, O'Kane GM, Goto K, Kim D-W, Neuzillet C, et al. Efficacy and safety of zenocutuzumab in advanced pancreas cancer and other solid tumors harboring NRG1 fusions. J Clin Oncol. 2021;39:3003.
47. DuFort CC, DelGiorno KE, Hingorani SR. Mounting pressure in the microenvironment: fluids, solids, and cells in pancreatic ductal adenocarcinoma. Gastroenterology. 2016;150:1545–57.e2.
48. Ligorio M, Sil S, Malagon-Lopez J, Nieman LT, Misale S, Di Pilato M, et al. Stromal microenvironment shapes the intratumoral architecture of pancreatic cancer. Cell. 2019;178:160–75.e27.
49. Anonymous. PEGPH20 may improve standard-of-care therapy in pancreatic cancer. Cancer Discov. 2018;8:136.
50. Hingorani SR, Zheng L, Bullock AJ, Seery TE, Harris WP, Sigal DS, et al. HALO 202: randomized phase II study of PEGPH20 plus Nab-paclitaxel/gemcitabine versus Nab-paclitaxel/gemcitabine in patients with untreated, metastatic pancreatic ductal adenocarcinoma. J Clin Oncol. 2018;36:359–66.
51. Cutsem EV, Tempero MA, Sigal D, Oh D-Y, Fazio N, Macarulla T, et al. Randomized phase III trial of Pegvorhyaluronidase alfa with Nab-paclitaxel plus gemcitabine for patients with hyaluronan-high metastatic pancreatic adenocarcinoma. J Clin Oncol. 2020;38:3185–94.
52. Hakim N, Patel R, Devoe C, Saif MW. Why HALO 301 failed and implications for treatment of pancreatic cancer. Pancreas (Fairfax). 2019;3:e1–4.

Part VIII

Intrahepatic/Extrahepatic Cholangiocarcinoma

Epidemiology and Etiology

Key Points

- The incidence of cholangiocarcinoma varies according to exposure to risk factors, with the highest incidence in Southeast Asia, particularly in Thailand.
- Most cholangiocarcinomas are tumors of the perihilar (50–60%) or distal (20–30%) regions, while intrahepatic cholangiocarcinomas account for only approximately 20% of all cholangiocarcinomas.
- Classic risk factors for the development of cholangiocarcinoma include primary sclerosing cholangitis, cysts of the biliary duct, hepatolithiasis, and Caroli's disease.

Introduction

Cholangiocarcinomas arise from the epithelium of the bile ducts. Depending on the anatomical location in the biliary tract, cholangiocarcinomas are classified as intrahepatic, perihilar, and distal. The latter two are known as extrahepatic cholangiocarcinomas, with the second-order bile ducts acting as the separation point. Although these cancers are rare in the USA, the incidence of cholangiocarcinoma has increased worldwide since the 1970s, and prevalence rates are high in certain parts of the world [1–4]. The epidemiology and etiology of cholangiocarcinoma will be discussed here.

Jae Hyuck Chang is the lead author of this chapter.

Epidemiology

Cholangiocarcinomas represent the ninth most common GI malignancy and is the second most common liver cancer after hepatocellular carcinoma (HCC). Hepatobiliary malignancies account for 13% of overall cancer-related mortality worldwide. Cholangiocarcinoma accounts for 10–20% of these deaths [5]. The incidence and age-adjusted mortality of cholangiocarcinoma are higher in men than in women [6]. Most cholangiocarcinomas are extrahepatic cholangiocarcinoma, either perihilar (50–60%) or distal (20–30%) tumors, while intrahepatic cholangiocarcinoma accounts for 20% [7].

The typical age of patients with cholangiocarcinoma is between 50 and 70 years of age, with incidence increasing with age [8]. Most patients are diagnosed older than 65 years in western countries. Cholangiocarcinoma is rare before the age of 40 years [6, 9]. However, patients with cholangiocarcinomas that occur in primary sclerosing cholangitis (PSC) and those with choledochal cysts presented almost 20 years earlier [10, 11]. Unlike gallbladder cancer, where women predominate, the incidence of cholangiocarcinoma is slightly higher in men [8]. This may be related to the higher incidence of PSC in men [12].

The incidence of intrahepatic cholangiocarcinoma has been increasing since the 1980s [2, 13–

H. J. Chun et al., *Gastrointestinal Cancer*, https://doi.org/10.1007/978-981-99-0815-8_52

16]. The incidence of perihilar and extrahepatic cholangiocarcinoma had been declining up to the year 2000 [13, 14, 17–22], but more recent reports suggest an increased incidence in the last 20 years [16]. These trends may be explained, in part, by the misclassification of perihilar tumors as intrahepatic. According to the Surveillance, Epidemiology, and End Results (SEER) database in the USA, the age-adjusted incidence rate for intrahepatic cholangiocarcinomas increased between 1990 and 2001, while the incidence rate for perihilar and distal cholangiocarcinomas decreased during this time period.

The global incidence rates for cholangiocarcinoma are heterogeneous. The incidence of cholangiocarcinoma varies according to exposure to risk factors, ranging from 1 to 2 cases per 100,000 inhabitants in Europe and North America with the highest incidence in Southeast Asia. The highest incidence is observed in Thailand (>80/100,000), and the lowest incidence in Australia (0.1/100,000) [9, 23]. In the USA, ethnic differences were observed in the age-adjusted incidence of cholangiocarcinoma, with the highest rates in Asian and Hispanic descendants (3.3/100,000 and 2.8/100,000, respectively) and the lowest in African Americans (2.1/100,000) [6].

Etiology

Several risk factors for cholangiocarcinoma have been recognized (Table 1), although a specific risk factor cannot be identified for many patients [24]. These risk factors are associated with biliary inflammation and cholestasis; however, there are limited studies exploring the association of risk factors with cholangiocarcinoma.

Table 1 Risk factors for cholangiocarcinoma

Primary sclerosing cholangitis
Congenital abnormalities: choledochal cyst, Caroli disease, congenital hepatic fibrosis
Hepatolithiasis, recurrent pyogenic cholangitis
Parasitic biliary infestation with flukes (*Opisthorchis viverrini, Clonorchis sinensis*)
Hepatitis C and B, cirrhosis
Precursors: intraductal papillary neoplasm of the bile ducts, biliary intraepithelial neoplasia
Obesity, diabetes mellitus, and nonalcoholic fatty liver disease
Genetic disorders: Lynch syndrome, BAP1 tumor predisposition syndrome, cystic fibrosis, and multiple biliary papillomatosis
Thorotrast, dioxin
Heavy alcohol consumption

PSC is one of the most common risk factors for cholangiocarcinoma, particularly in the USA and Europe; however, only 10% of cholangiocarcinomas are attributed to PSC. The annual incidence of cholangiocarcinoma in patients with PSC has been estimated to be between 0.6 and 1.5% per year, with a lifetime risk of 5–15% [3, 25–31]. Over one-third of cases of cholangiocarcinoma are detected within 2 years of the initial diagnosis of PSC. A new diagnosis of PSC should raise suspicion of cholangiocarcinoma [3]. Cholangiocarcinomas develop at a significantly younger age (between the ages of 30 and 50) in patients with PSC than in those without PSC. Alcohol consumption has been suggested to increase the risk of cholangiocarcinoma in patients with PSC [27]. Surveillance in patients with PSC is recommended with annual imaging techniques and the serum CA 19.9 level. The association between cholangiocarcinoma and inflammatory bowel disease is controversial and likely influenced by the presence and duration of PSC [6].

Congenital abnormalities of the biliary tree (Caroli disease: a variant of choledochal cyst disease characterized by multiple cystic dilations of the intrahepatic biliary ducts, congenital hepatic fibrosis, and choledochal cysts) account for an approximately 15% risk of malignant change in the adult (average age at diagnosis 34) [32–34]. Patients with Caroli disease and choledochal cysts, in particular types I and IV, have a 50% increased risk of cholangiocarcinoma, with lifetime incidence rates of 6–30%. Cyst excision reduces, but does not eliminate, the risk of developing cholangiocarcinoma [5].

Hepatolithiasis with recurrent pyogenic cholangitis carries a 10% risk of cholangiocarcinoma. Recurrent bacterial cholangitis with biliary-enteric drainage has also been associated with the development of cholangiocarcinoma [35]. Stone disease affecting only the intrahepatic bile ducts is extremely rare in western countries, but it is endemic in certain parts of Southeast Asia. In

Taiwan, 50–70% of patients undergoing cholangiocarcinoma resection have associated hepatolithiasis [36, 37].

Parasitic biliary infestation with flukes (i.e., most common are *Opisthorchis viverrini* and *Clonorchis sinensis*) is a prevalent etiology of cholangiocarcinoma in Asia [38].

Intrahepatic cholangiocarcinoma has been associated with hepatitis C virus (HCV) and hepatitis B virus (HBV) infection and cirrhosis, while perihilar cholangiocarcinoma has been associated only with cirrhosis [4, 6, 39]. Association studies between cholangiocarcinoma and viral hepatitis have shown inconsistencies across continents. In Japan, patients with HCV-related cirrhosis developed cholangiocarcinoma at 3.5% at 10 years [40]. In the USA, intrahepatic cholangiocarcinoma was associated with HCV at adjusted relative risk [RR] 2.55, 95% CI 1.31–4.95 [41]. An association has been suggested between HBV infection and cholangiocarcinoma, but the data are less compelling than for HCV [42–45].

Three precursors, such as intraductal papillary neoplasm of the bile ducts [46], intraductal tubulopapillary neoplasm of the bile ducts [47], and biliary intraepithelial neoplasia [48], are known to progress to invasive cholangiocarcinoma.

Obesity, diabetes mellitus, and nonalcoholic fatty liver disease have been associated with an increased risk of cholangiocarcinoma, but the data are inconsistent [6, 49]. With the increase of these conditions in Western industrialized countries, there is a trend that could explain the increasing incidence of intrahepatic cholangiocarcinomas in these countries.

At least four genetic disorders are associated with an increased risk of cholangiocarcinoma: Lynch syndrome (hereditary nonpolyposis colorectal cancer), BAP1 tumor predisposition syndrome, cystic fibrosis, and a rare inherited disorder called multiple biliary papillomatosis.

Carcinogens such as thorotrast (used as a radiological contrast agent in the past) and dioxins have been associated with an increased risk of cholangiocarcinoma [50]. Heavy alcohol consumption has also been associated with cholangiocarcinoma [6, 39, 49].

Conclusion

Patients with cholangiocarcinoma are generally between the ages of 50 and 70, and the incidence of cholangiocarcinoma has increased in most countries over the past decades. Several risk factors for cholangiocarcinoma have been recognized. However, in many patients, no specific risk factors are identified. The main risk factors vary from region to region. Primary sclerosing cholangitis and choledochal cysts are prevalent in the USA and Europe, and hepatobiliary flukes are prevalent in Southeast Asia.

References

1. Andersen JB, Spee B, Blechacz BR, Avital I, Komuta M, Barbour A, et al. Genomic and genetic characterization of cholangiocarcinoma identifies therapeutic targets for tyrosine kinase inhibitors. Gastroenterology. 2012;142:1021–31.e15.
2. Saha SK, Zhu AX, Fuchs CS, Brooks GA. Forty-year trends in cholangiocarcinoma incidence in the U.S.: intrahepatic disease on the rise. Oncologist. 2016;21:594–9.
3. Boonstra K, Weersma RK, van Erpecum KJ, Rauws EA, Spanier BW, Poen AC, et al. Population-based epidemiology, malignancy risk, and outcome of primary sclerosing cholangitis. Hepatology. 2013;58:2045–55.
4. Palmer WC, Patel T. Are common factors involved in the pathogenesis of primary liver cancers? A meta-analysis of risk factors for intrahepatic cholangiocarcinoma. J Hepatol. 2012;57:69–76.
5. Shaib Y, El-Serag HB. The epidemiology of cholangiocarcinoma. Semin Liver Dis. 2004;24:115–25.
6. Tyson GL, El-Serag HB. Risk factors for cholangiocarcinoma. Hepatology. 2011;54:173–84.
7. Murakami Y, Uemura K, Sudo T, Hashimoto Y, Nakashima A, Kondo N, et al. Prognostic factors after surgical resection for intrahepatic, hilar, and distal cholangiocarcinoma. Ann Surg Oncol. 2011;18:651–8.
8. Van Dyke AL, Shiels MS, Jones GS, Pfeiffer RM, Petrick JL, Beebe-Dimmer JL, et al. Biliary tract cancer incidence and trends in the United States by demographic group, 1999-2013. Cancer. 2019;125:1489–98.
9. Sripa B, Pairojkul C. Cholangiocarcinoma: lessons from Thailand. Curr Opin Gastroenterol. 2008;24:349–56.
10. Vauthey JN, Blumgart LH. Recent advances in the management of cholangiocarcinomas. Semin Liver Dis. 1994;14:109–14.

11. Broomé U, Olsson R, Lööf L, Bodemar G, Hultcrantz R, Danielsson A, et al. Natural history and prognostic factors in 305 Swedish patients with primary sclerosing cholangitis. Gut. 1996;38:610–5.
12. Henson DE, Albores-Saavedra J, Corle D. Carcinoma of the extrahepatic bile ducts. Histologic types, stage of disease, grade, and survival rates. Cancer. 1992;70:1498–501.
13. Patel T. Increasing incidence and mortality of primary intrahepatic cholangiocarcinoma in the United States. Hepatology. 2001;33:1353–7.
14. Shaib YH, Davila JA, McGlynn K, El-Serag HB. Rising incidence of intrahepatic cholangiocarcinoma in the United States: a true increase? J Hepatol. 2004;40:472–7.
15. Banales JM, Cardinale V, Carpino G, Marzioni M, Andersen JB, Invernizzi P, et al. Expert consensus document: cholangiocarcinoma: current knowledge and future perspectives consensus statement from the European Network for the Study of Cholangiocarcinoma (ENS-CCA). Nat Rev Gastroenterol Hepatol. 2016;13:261–80.
16. Florio AA, Ferlay J, Znaor A, Ruggieri D, Alvarez CS, Laversanne M, et al. Global trends in intrahepatic and extrahepatic cholangiocarcinoma incidence from 1993 to 2012. Cancer. 2020;126:2666–78.
17. Jepsen P, Vilstrup H, Tarone RE, Friis S, Sørensen HT. Incidence rates of intra- and extrahepatic cholangiocarcinomas in Denmark from 1978 through 2002. J Natl Cancer Inst. 2007;99:895–7.
18. West J, Wood H, Logan RF, Quinn M, Aithal GP. Trends in the incidence of primary liver and biliary tract cancers in England and Wales 1971-2001. Br J Cancer. 2006;94:1751–8.
19. Rajagopalan V, Daines WP, Grossbard ML, Kozuch P. Gallbladder and biliary tract carcinoma: a comprehensive update, part 1. Oncology (Williston Park). 2004;18:889–96.
20. Khan SA, Taylor-Robinson SD, Toledano MB, Beck A, Elliott P, Thomas HC. Changing international trends in mortality rates for liver, biliary and pancreatic tumours. J Hepatol. 2002;37:806–13.
21. Patel T. Worldwide trends in mortality from biliary tract malignancies. BMC Cancer. 2002;2:10.
22. Welzel TM, McGlynn KA, Hsing AW, O'Brien TR, Pfeiffer RM. Impact of classification of hilar cholangiocarcinomas (Klatskin tumors) on the incidence of intra- and extrahepatic cholangiocarcinoma in the United States. J Natl Cancer Inst. 2006;98:873–5.
23. Khan SA, Emadossadaty S, Ladep NG, Thomas HC, Elliott P, Taylor-Robinson SD, et al. Rising trends in cholangiocarcinoma: is the ICD classification system misleading us? J Hepatol. 2012;56:848–54.
24. Chapman RW. Risk factors for biliary tract carcinogenesis. Ann Oncol. 1999;10(Suppl 4):308–11.
25. Bergquist A, Ekbom A, Olsson R, Kornfeldt D, Lööf L, Danielsson A, et al. Hepatic and extrahepatic malignancies in primary sclerosing cholangitis. J Hepatol. 2002;36:321–7.
26. Lee YM, Kaplan MM. Primary sclerosing cholangitis. N Engl J Med. 1995;332:924–33.
27. Bergquist A, Glaumann H, Persson B, Broomé U. Risk factors and clinical presentation of hepatobiliary carcinoma in patients with primary sclerosing cholangitis: a case-control study. Hepatology. 1998;27:311–6.
28. de Groen PC. Cholangiocarcinoma in primary sclerosing cholangitis: who is at risk and how do we screen? Hepatology. 2000;31:247–8.
29. Burak K, Angulo P, Pasha TM, Egan K, Petz J, Lindor KD. Incidence and risk factors for cholangiocarcinoma in primary sclerosing cholangitis. Am J Gastroenterol. 2004;99:523–6.
30. Claessen MM, Vleggaar FP, Tytgat KM, Siersema PD, van Buuren HR. High lifetime risk of cancer in primary sclerosing cholangitis. J Hepatol. 2009;50:158–64.
31. Chapman MH, Webster GJ, Bannoo S, Johnson GJ, Wittmann J, Pereira SP. Cholangiocarcinoma and dominant strictures in patients with primary sclerosing cholangitis: a 25-year single-centre experience. Eur J Gastroenterol Hepatol. 2012;24:1051–8.
32. Khan SA, Thomas HC, Davidson BR, Taylor-Robinson SD. Cholangiocarcinoma. Lancet. 2005;366:1303–14.
33. Scott J, Shousha S, Thomas HC, Sherlock S. Bile duct carcinoma: a late complication of congenital hepatic fibrosis. Case report and review of literature. Am J Gastroenterol. 1980;73:113–9.
34. Lipsett PA, Pitt HA, Colombani PM, Boitnott JK, Cameron JL. Choledochal cyst disease. A changing pattern of presentation. Ann Surg. 1994;220:644–52.
35. Tocchi A, Mazzoni G, Liotta G, Lepre L, Cassini D, Miccini M. Late development of bile duct cancer in patients who had biliary-enteric drainage for benign disease: a follow-up study of more than 1,000 patients. Ann Surg. 2001;234:210–4.
36. Chen MF. Peripheral cholangiocarcinoma (cholangiocellular carcinoma): clinical features, diagnosis and treatment. J Gastroenterol Hepatol. 1999;14:1144–9.
37. Su CH, Shyr YM, Lui WY, P'Eng FK. Hepatolithiasis associated with cholangiocarcinoma. Br J Surg. 1997;84:969–73.
38. Watanapa P, Watanapa WB. Liver fluke-associated cholangiocarcinoma. Br J Surg. 2002;89:962–70.
39. Shaib YH, El-Serag HB, Nooka AK, Thomas M, Brown TD, Patt YZ, et al. Risk factors for intrahepatic and extrahepatic cholangiocarcinoma: a hospital-based case-control study. Am J Gastroenterol. 2007;102:1016–21.
40. Kobayashi M, Ikeda K, Saitoh S, Suzuki F, Tsubota A, Suzuki Y, et al. Incidence of primary cholangiocellular carcinoma of the liver in Japanese patients with hepatitis C virus-related cirrhosis. Cancer. 2000;88:2471–7.
41. El-Serag HB, Engels EA, Landgren O, Chiao E, Henderson L, Amaratunge HC, et al. Risk of hepatobiliary and pancreatic cancers after hepatitis C virus

infection: a population-based study of U.S. veterans. Hepatology. 2009;49:116–23.
42. Donato F, Gelatti U, Tagger A, Favret M, Ribero ML, Callea F, et al. Intrahepatic cholangiocarcinoma and hepatitis C and B virus infection, alcohol intake, and hepatolithiasis: a case-control study in Italy. Cancer Causes Control. 2001;12:959–64.
43. Chang JS, Tsai CR, Chen LT. Medical risk factors associated with cholangiocarcinoma in Taiwan: a population-based case-control study. PLoS One. 2013;8:e69981.
44. Lee CH, Chang CJ, Lin YJ, Yeh CN, Chen MF, Hsieh SY. Viral hepatitis-associated intrahepatic cholangiocarcinoma shares common disease processes with hepatocellular carcinoma. Br J Cancer. 2009;100:1765–70.
45. Peng NF, Li LQ, Qin X, Guo Y, Peng T, Xiao KY, et al. Evaluation of risk factors and clinicopathologic features for intrahepatic cholangiocarcinoma in southern China: a possible role of hepatitis B virus. Ann Surg Oncol. 2011;18:1258–66.
46. Rocha FG, Lee H, Katabi N, DeMatteo RP, Fong Y, D'Angelica MI, et al. Intraductal papillary neoplasm of the bile duct: a biliary equivalent to intraductal papillary mucinous neoplasm of the pancreas? Hepatology. 2012;56:1352–60.
47. Schlitter AM, Jang KT, Klöppel G, Saka B, Hong SM, Choi H, et al. Intraductal tubulopapillary neoplasms of the bile ducts: clinicopathologic, immunohistochemical, and molecular analysis of 20 cases. Mod Pathol. 2015;28:1249–64.
48. Bickenbach K, Galka E, Roggin KK. Molecular mechanisms of cholangiocarcinogenesis: are biliary intraepithelial neoplasia and intraductal papillary neoplasms of the bile duct precursors to cholangiocarcinoma? Surg Oncol Clin N Am. 2009;18:215–24, vii.
49. Welzel TM, Graubard BI, El-Serag HB, Shaib YH, Hsing AW, Davila JA, et al. Risk factors for intrahepatic and extrahepatic cholangiocarcinoma in the United States: a population-based case-control study. Clin Gastroenterol Hepatol. 2007;5:1221–8.
50. Walker NJ, Crockett PW, Nyska A, Brix AE, Jokinen MP, Sells DM, et al. Dose-additive carcinogenicity of a defined mixture of "dioxin-like compounds". Environ Health Perspect. 2005;113:43–8.

Pathology, Pathogenesis, Clinical Features, and Diagnosis

Key Points

- Genetic mechanisms and pathogenesis of cholangiocarcinoma (CCA) differ considerably by etiology and anatomic location.
- CCA has three predominant macroscopic growth patterns: mass-forming lesions, periductal infiltrating lesions, and intraductal papillary lesions.
- The histopathology of CCA can be classified as small bile duct type and large bile duct type and rare variants.
- Each anatomic subtype of CCA has distinct clinical features and diagnostic approaches.

Introduction

Cholangiocarcinoma (CCA) is a highly lethal adenocarcinoma of the hepatobiliary system, which can be classified as intrahepatic, perihilar, and distal. Each anatomic subtype has distinct genetic aberrations, clinical presentations, and therapeutic approaches. In this chapter, a comprehensive review of pathology, pathogenesis, clinical features, and diagnostic approach of CCA will be provided and discussed.

Genetic and Epigenetic Aberrations

Genetic and Epigenetic Aberrations According to Tumor Location

Extensive genomic and epigenomic studies have shown that the molecular landscapes of CCA differ considerably by etiology, highlighting how cancer subtypes in the same organ may arise through different extrinsic and intrinsic carcinogenic processes [1–3]. The findings also illustrate the importance of conducting these molecular studies in diverse populations, as differences between their genomic and epigenomic profiles point to the need for distinct biomarkers and therapies. Among CCAs, genetic aberrations differ depending on their anatomic locations; for example, *FGFR2* fusions are almost exclusively found in intrahepatic CCA (iCCA), whereas

Dong-Won Ahn is the lead author of this chapter.

H. J. Chun et al., *Gastrointestinal Cancer*, https://doi.org/10.1007/978-981-99-0815-8_53

PRKCA–PRKCB fusions are observed in perihilar CCA (pCCA) and distal CCA (dCCA) [3]. For CCAs of other causes, such as those related to herbal carcinogen aristolochic acid, primary biliary cirrhosis, and choledochal cysts, current knowledge of their molecular landscape is sparse owing to insufficient numbers of samples studied.

Common Mutations and Related Molecular Pathways

According to studies of ~500 fluke-related and non-fluke-related CCAs, some of the most commonly mutated genes (mutation frequencies 10–26%) in CCA include *TP53*, *ARID1A*, *KRAS*, *SMAD4*, *BAP1*, and *APC*, followed by at least another 20 genes with lower mutation frequencies of 1–6% [1–9]. Interestingly, the mutation frequencies of driver genes differ between CCA etiologies. For example, *TP53* and *ARID1A* mutations are highly enriched in fluke-related CCAs, whereas *BAP1*, *IDH1*, and *IDH2* mutations are highly enriched in non-fluke-related CCAs (Table 1). These gene mutations are known to be associated with key cancer-related molecular pathways, such as RAS–RAF–MAPK (e.g., *MAP2K4* and *PTEN*), WNT (e.g., *APC* and *RNF43*), DNA repair (e.g., *BRCA2* and *MSH3*), and epigenetic modulation (e.g., *ARID1A* and *BAP1*). Some of these mutated genes may be related to the same biological pathway, and their mutations are usually mutually exclusive but may occasionally occur in combination. For example, members of the Wnt signaling pathway, including *APC*, *RNF43*, *AXIN1*, and different forms of catenin (*CTNNA2*, *CTNND2*, and *CTNNB1*), were found to be mutated, and, when the mutations occurred in combination, they contributed to a higher percentage of CCAs than mutation of a single gene [2].

Epigenetically, CCA tumors exhibit DNA hypermethylation, and distinct DNA hypermethylation patterns are found that differentiate fluke-related CCA (predominantly in CpG islands) and non-fluke-related CCA (predominantly in CpG island shores) [2]. Integrative analysis of somatic mutations and DNA methylation led to the proposal that fluke-related CCAs are probably caused by early exposure to external carcinogenic agents that induce a chronic inflammatory milieu, which results in genome-wide epigenetic dysregulation that drives tumor development; by contrast, in non-fluke-related CCAs, an initial genetic driver mutation causes tumorigenesis, and epigenetic changes occur during this process [1].

Table 1 Genomic and epigenomic aberrations of CCA

Alteration	Enriched in fluke-related CCA	Enriched in non-fluke-related CCA	Found in both CCA types
Mutations	*ACVR1B*, *ARID1A*, *BRCA1*, *FBXW7*, H3K27me3-associated promoter mutations, *MAP2K4*, *MSH3*, *PTEN*, *SMAD4*, *TP53*	*BAP1*, *IDH1*, *IDH2*	*ACVR2A*, *APC*, *ARID2*, *ASXL1*, *BRAF*, *BRCA1*, *BRCA2*, *CDKN1B*, *CTNNB1*, *ELF3*, *KRAS*, *NCOR1*, *NRAS*, *P4HTM*, *PBRM1*, *PIK3R1*, *RASA1*, *RB1*, *RNF43*, *SF3B1*, *STK11*, *TGFBR2*
Copy number alterations	*ERBB2* amplification	NA	NA
Gene fusions	NA	*FGFR2*, *FGFR3*, *PRKACA*, *PRKACB*	NA
Epigenetic phenotype	CpG island hypermethylation	CpG shore hypermethylation	Hypermethylation

CCA cholangiocarcinoma, *NA* not applicable
Adapted from Brindley et al. [10]

Fluke-Related Cholangiocarcinoma

Generally, this group of CCAs exhibits substantially more somatic mutations than non-fluke-related CCAs [2], probably reflecting their underlying etiology associated with fluke-related chronic inflammation. Inactivating mutations that are more prevalent in this subgroup than in non-fluke-related CCAs include *TP53*, *ARID1A*, *ARID2*, *BRCA1*, and *BRCA2* [1, 2, 8, 11, 12]. Noncoding mutations in promoters associated with H3K7me3 have also been found to be enriched [2]. Copy number analysis also detected more frequent *ERBB2* amplification in fluke-related CCAs, which may have considerable clinical implications, as these tumors may be more sensitive to ERBB2 inhibitor treatment. In addition, the expression of several genes, including *TET1*, encoding a DNA demethylation enzyme, and *EZH2*, encoding a histone methyltransferase, has been found to be aberrant, implying that these genes may have a role in the hypermethylation phenotype in CCA [2]. Another study identified two fluke-related CCA subtypes: the C1 subtype that is enriched with mutations in genes, such as *ECT2*, that lead to mitotic checkpoint defects and the C2 subtype that is related to bile acid metabolism, T cell infiltration, and obesity [11].

Non-fluke-Related Cholangiocarcinoma

Inactivating mutations in *PBRM1*, *BAP1*, *PIK3CA*, and *ELF3* and gain-of-function mutations in *IDH1* and *IDH2* are predominantly found in this group of CCAs [1–5]. Chromosome translocations involving mainly *FGFR* and to a lesser extent *PKARC* represent another key genetic alteration [2, 3, 13, 14]. *FGFR2* translocations in CCAs were first discovered through a clinical sequencing program for advanced CCA and are rarely found in fluke-associated CCA. *PRKACA* and *PRKACB* are part of the cAMP-dependent protein kinase signaling pathway and are enriched in non-fluke-related CCA [3]. Epigenetically, this group of CCAs is dominated by hypermethylation in promoter CpG shores [2], with prevalent C>T and/or G>A substitutions at CpG sites [3]. Of note, the distribution of mutations between non-fluke subtypes seems to vary according to the anatomic site of the CCA; for example, *FGFR2* translocations are exclusively found in iCCAs [3, 11].

Fluke Pathophysiology

Chronic liver fluke infection is associated with numerous hepatobiliary diseases, including inflammation of the gallbladder and bile ducts (cholecystitis and cholangitis, respectively), periductal fibrosis, and, ultimately, CCA. Liver fluke infection is thought to drive CCA via multiple distinct but interacting pathways: mechanical damage to the bile duct epithelium caused by adult flukes grazing on the resident cells, notably cholangiocytes; immunopathology driven by chronic infection-related inflammation; and effects of parasite excretory–secretory molecules, including secreted vesicles, proteins, and small molecules [15]. The interplay of these mechanisms, in addition to a traditional diet in disease-endemic areas that is rich in nitrosamine-containing foods, such as fermented fish contaminated with liver fluke metacercariae, is in keeping with current knowledge of carcinogenesis.

The attachment of liver flukes to the biliary wall results in ulceration and formation of precancerous lesions [16]. This process is accompanied by immune cell infiltration and persistent secretion of inflammatory cytokines, such as interleukin (IL)-6, which is well known as a link between inflammation and carcinogenesis, particularly in liver tissue [17]. Elevated IL-6 levels are strongly associated with advanced and persistent periductal fibrosis in *Opisthorchis viverrini (O. viverrini)* infections, which are thought to contribute to the pathogenesis of fluke-induced CCA [18]. Similar to other helminth infections, flukes induce local recruitment of type 2 macrophages, eosinophils, mast cells, and T cells. Parasite- specific B lymphocyte and T lymphocyte responses occur to a diverse array of antigens [18]; however, despite this robust response, sterile immunity does not develop, and older people living in endemic areas are often heavily infected [19, 20], necessitating a vaccine that induces long-term anti-parasite immunity and protects against the onset of fluke-induced CCA.

The hamster model of liver fluke-induced CCA is a powerful tool for investigating the etiology and immunopathogenesis of fluke-infection-associated liver pathologies. Hamsters infected with *O. viverrini* fed a diet high in nitrosamines develop CCA within 6 months [21]. Soon after flukes arrive in the biliary tree, proliferating cholangiocytes can be detected, highlighting a process of constant wounding and repair that occurs over decades in infected people. *Opisthorchis* spp. secrete several molecular entities that contribute to this process, including a glutathione-dependent prostaglandin synthase that drives formation of precancerous lesions [22], a granulin-like growth factor [23], and extracellular vesicles (EVs) [24], the latter two of which drive cholangiocyte proliferation and IL-6 secretion in vitro. Indeed, *O. viverrini* flukes that had undergone CRISPR–Cas9-induced editing of the granulin gene still colonized the biliary tract of hamsters and developed into adult flukes, but the resulting pathological changes were reduced to biliary hyperplasia and fibrosis [25].

Molecular Biology of Progression and Invasion

CCA cells gradually adopt invasive phenotypes to metastasize, for example, by changing to a mesenchymal-like phenotype, which increases their migratory and invasion capabilities, and eventually deposit at distant sites. Various alterations related to cancer hallmarks occur to gain these invasive properties, including those during the invasion process [26, 27] and in angiogenesis and lymphangiogenesis [28].

An integrated and in-depth understanding of the molecular mechanisms in CCA progression could aid in developing precision therapy for advanced CCA. Several pathways are dysregulated and represent potential therapeutic targets, including the inflammation-related IL-6/JAK/STAT3 pathway [29], estrogen and estrogen receptors [30], epithelial–mesenchymal transition [31], EGFR activating the MAPK/ERK pathway [32], and hepatocyte growth factor/AKT/ERK signaling [33]. Further transcription factors involving morphogenetic signaling pathways, for example, Hedgehog, Wnt, and Notch, as well as microRNAs are dysregulated to support the invasiveness of CCA. The PI3K/AKT/mTOR, HIF1α, and MYC pathways are stimulated to support metabolic shifts in CCA cells [34].

Posttranslational modifications, O-GlcNAcylation and glycosylation, have also been shown to mediate CCA invasiveness (Fig. 1). O-GlcNAcylation is a reversible process, in which a single GlcNAc residue is added to proteins, modulating protein function, stability, and localization with or without coordinating phosphorylation. In human CCA tissues, high levels of O-GlcNAcylation have been observed and are associated with a poor prognosis [35]. Upregulation of O-GlcNAcylation enhances the stability of the structural protein vimentin and increases the nuclear translocation of proteins that activate expression of downstream genes involved in epithelial–mesenchymal transition, cell migration, and invasion [36, 37]. Epidemiological studies have indicated that diabetes mellitus is a risk factor and possibly a promoting factor for CCA [38]. Increased levels of O-GlcNAcylation and STAT3 activation have been reported to be key processes in the aggressiveness of CCA cells enhanced by high glucose levels [39, 40]. Increased initial O-GalNAcylation [41] and terminal fucosylation have been implicated in CCA development in the hamster model and in tissues from inpatients with CCA. Modulation of either process substantially affects the metastatic potential of CCA cells. Upregulation of specific high-mannose *N*- glycans facilitates the progression of highly metastatic CCA cells [42, 43] some of which can be detected in the serum from patients with CCA [44]. The collective evidence suggests that certain glycans and/or enzymes involved in glycan synthesis might serve as new biomarkers and targets to manage CCA metastasis.

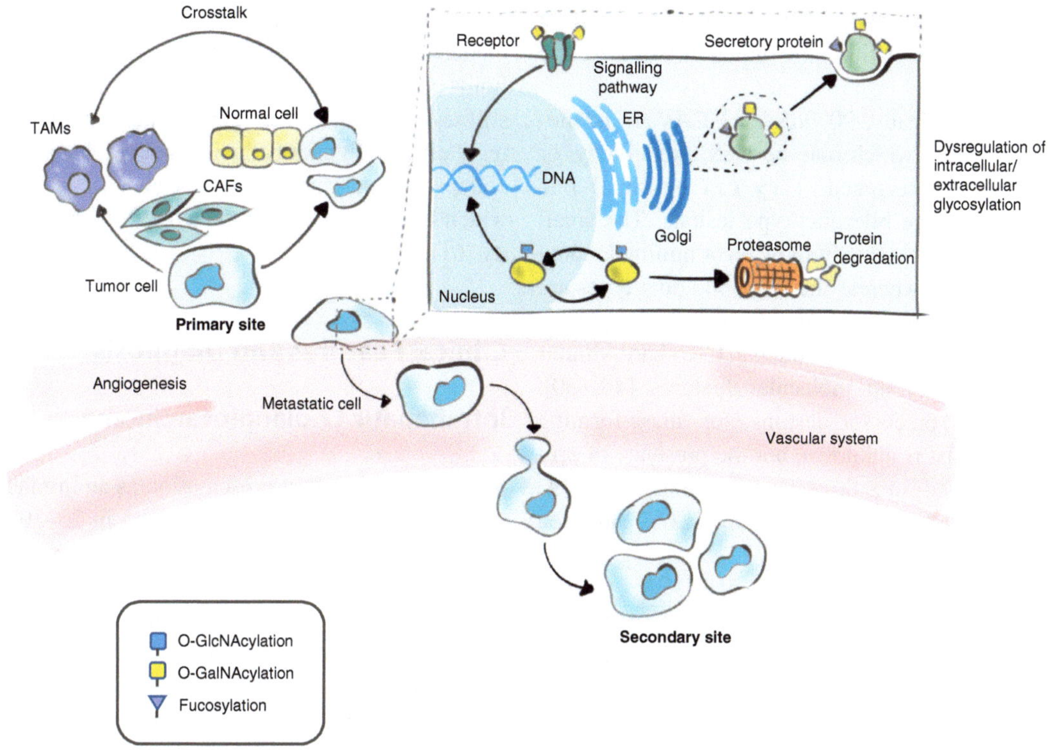

Fig. 1 Cholangiocarcinoma cells gradually adopt invasive phenotypes to metastasize. Several pathways are dysregulated to transform the phenotypes and functions of cholangiocarcinoma cells (CCA). Cancer-associated fibroblasts (CAFs) and tumor-associated macrophages (TAMs) in the tumor microenvironment produce autocrine and paracrine signals that enhance CCA metastasis. The cross talk between CCA cells, CAFs, and TAMs progressively remodels the tumor stroma to facilitate invasion of tumor cells from the primary site to the secondary site. In addition, dysregulation of intracellular O-GlcNAcylation of proteins by adding or removing *N*-acetylglucosamine (GlcNAc) influences function, stability, and localization of several proteins associated with metastasis. Modulation of extracellular glycosylation, for example, fucosylation and O-GalNAcylation of surface glycoproteins or secretory proteins, has an important role in enhancing the metastatic activity of CCA cells. *ER* endoplasmic reticulum (adapted from Brindley et al. [10])

Pathology, Inflammation, and Tumor Microenvironment

CCA has three predominant macroscopic growth patterns: mass-forming lesions, periductal infiltrating lesions, and intraductal papillary lesions. The histopathology may also be classified as small bile duct type (which may derive from septal and interlobular bile ducts, progenitor cells, and possibly hepatocytes), large bile duct type (potentially arising from segmental bile ducts or associated peribiliary glands), and rare variants [45–47]. For iCCA, patients with mass-forming and periductal infiltrating subtypes have the poorest prognosis, whereas those with intraductal papillary lesions have the most favorable outcomes following curative surgical resection [48].

The mass-forming growth pattern is most common in iCCA and is generally seen at presentation as a single, nodular solid mass. Advanced mass-forming iCCA may also have satellite or multifocal tumor growth within the liver. The periductal infiltrating growth pattern of CCA does not form a nodular mass but grows longitudinally along the walls of the large bile ducts and spreads along the portal tracts, resulting in strictures of the affected bile ducts and dilation of the smaller proximal bile ducts. This is the growth pattern most frequently observed in pCCA. The intraductal papillary type of CCA is seen at presentation as a slow-growing polypoid or papillary tumor growing within the lumen of a dilated bile duct [45–47].

Histologically, 90–95% of CCAs are adenocarcinomas, which may be well, moderately, or poorly differentiated. They can be small bile duct- or large bile duct-type lesions. The small bile duct types usually show no or minimal mucin production, whereas the large bile duct types are mucin-producing adenocarcinomas. pCCA, dCCA, and large bile duct iCCA share similar pathological and molecular features [49, 50]. Whether precursor lesions for mass-forming iCCA exist is unknown, but the presence of premalignant dysplastic precursor lesions for pCCA, dCCA, and large bile duct-type iCCA has been established.

Unique rare variants of CCA include intestinal-type CCA, combined hepatocellular carcinoma and CCA (cHCC–CCA), and lymphoepithelioma-like CCA [51, 52]. Cholangiolocellular carcinoma (CLC) is a rare primary liver cancer in which the epithelial component resembles cholangioles (canals of Hering) [52]. It is recommended that CLC is categorized as a histological subtype of well-differentiated iCCA [53].

Unlike conventional HCCs, CCAs frequently have a prominent desmoplastic microenvironment characterized by a dense collagen, fiber-enriched tumor stroma and matricellular proteins (e.g., periostin and tenascin C), an abundance of cancer-associated fibroblasts, and, to a lesser extent, tumor-associated macrophages and varying numbers of innate immune cells [54]. CCAs are also dissimilar to HCC by often being hypovascular [55], although CCAs formed in cirrhosis can display increased vascularity [56].

This evolving and complex desmoplastic tumor microenvironment has a preeminent role in promoting CCA progression, therapeutic resistance, and immunosuppression [57–59]. Cancer-associated myofibroblasts are a major source of secreted stromal components, including multiple growth factors, cytokines, metabolites, extracellular matrix (ECM) proteins, and modifying enzymes that facilitate CCA growth and invasiveness, cell survival, ECM remodeling, and metabolic reprogramming. Indeed, in preclinical models, deletion of cancer-associated fibroblasts limits tumor progression [60]. Stromal matrix stiffness in CCA can trigger signaling pathways regulating malignant behavior and mechanically collapse blood microvessels, causing hypoxia, which limits drug and immune cell bioavailability [61].

Clinical Features and Diagnosis

Intrahepatic Cholangiocarcinoma

iCCA is often seen at presentation as an intrahepatic mass and is incidentally found in 25–30% of patients [62]. Patients with iCCA are often asymptomatic during early disease stages and develop symptoms or signs, such as abdominal pain or less commonly jaundice, during disease progression to an advanced stage. Carbohydrate antigen 19–9 (CA19–9) is the primary serum biomarker used in CCA diagnosis, although it has subpar specificity and can be elevated in various conditions, such as biliary obstruction or pancreatic cancer. Nonetheless, levels of CA19–9 >1000 U/mL are concerning for the presence of metastatic CCA [63]. Imaging modalities used for iCCA diagnosis include conventional ultrasonography, computed tomography (CT), magnetic resonance imaging (MRI), and contrast-enhanced ultrasonography (CEUS). MRI may provide enhanced assessment of the primary mass, whereas CT imaging has superior detection of vascular enhancement and is, therefore, important in determining resectability [64]. In patients with cirrhosis, HCC surveillance may facilitate earlier iCCA diagnosis [65]. However, distinguishing HCC and iCCA can be difficult in this patient population. iCCAs are characterized by an initial arterial contrast enhancement at the tumor periphery and progressive homogeneous contrast enhancement [66, 67]. HCCs are characterized by arterial hyper-enhancement and washout in the portal venous phase or delayed phase. In a cirrhotic liver, gadolinium-enhanced MRI has an increased specificity, but lower sensitivity, for diagnosing HCC and distinguishing it from iCCA when portal venous phase washout rather than conventional delayed phase washout is used [68]. Compared with CT or MRI, CEUS is more likely to misdiagnose iCCA as HCC [69]. In CEUS imaging, iCCAs have an earlier contrast washout from the vascularized portions of the lesions, whereas HCCs have delayed portal venous washout [65]. Hence, CEUS is not reliable as the sole imaging technique to differentiate iCCA from HCC but may be useful in scenarios with inconclusive CT or MRI. Positron emission tomography (PET) scanning is typically not used in the diagnosis of iCCA owing to limited accuracy [70]. 18F-Fluorodeoxyglucose (18F-FDG) PET imaging has reasonable performance in detection of lymph node and distant metastasis and, therefore, may have a role in CCA staging [71]. Histopathological analysis of a biopsy specimen remains the mainstay for confirmation of an iCCA diagnosis. If a patient is eligible for resection, then a biopsy need not be performed.

Perihilar Cholangiocarcinoma and Distal Cholangiocarcinoma

Patients with pCCA and dCCA typically present with painless jaundice owing to underlying biliary obstruction. Following initial CT that may be concerning for pCCA and/or dCCA, a specific type of MRI termed magnetic resonance cholangiopancreatography (MRCP) is employed for CCA detection [72]. The sensitivity and specificity of MRCP to distinguish benign and malignant causes of hilar obstruction are 87% and 85%, respectively [73]. MRCP can also delineate the biliary anatomy before endoscopic intervention with endoscopic retrograde cholangiography (ERC). ERC has a diagnostic and therapeutic role in pCCA and dCCA as it enables detection of malignant strictures and acquisition of biliary brushings for cytology and fluorescence in situ hybridization (FISH) analysis. Biliary cytology or a biopsy sample positive for adenocarcinoma are diagnostic of CCA [74]. However, the sensitivity of biliary cytology for pCCA detection is low (43% according to one meta-analysis [74]). FISH analysis has a higher sensitivity than cytology (65% versus 19% in one series) and similar specificity for detection of CCA [75]. Endoscopic techniques such as cholangioscopy and confocal laser endomicroscopy can be used to visualize indeterminate biliary strictures [76]. However, whether these advanced techniques can improve tissue diagnostic yield through targeted biliary biopsies remains unclear.

Endoscopic ultrasonography (EUS) is useful in the diagnosis and staging of pCCA, as it enables a detailed visual assessment of the extrahepatic bile duct as well as tissue acquisition via fine-needle aspiration (FNA). EUS–FNA has a higher sensitivity for detection of dCCA than detection of pCCA (81% versus 59%) [77]. In addition, EUS-guided tissue acquisition of pCCA is controversial owing to the potential risk of tumor dissemination [78]. PET scanning is typically not utilized in the diagnosis of pCCA owing to limited accuracy [70]. 18F-FDG PET has subpar performance for detection of the primary tumor [70] but may have a role in the assessment of lymph node and distant metastasis [71].

Conclusion

Genetic mechanisms and pathogenesis of CCA differ considerably by etiology and anatomic location. Each anatomic subtype of CCA has distinct clinical features and diagnostic approaches.

References

1. Chan-On W, Nairismagi ML, Ong CK, Lim WK, Dima S, Pairojkul C, et al. Exome sequencing identifies distinct mutational patterns in liver fluke-related and non-infection-related bile duct cancers. Nat Genet. 2013;45:1474–8.
2. Jusakul A, Cutcutache I, Yong CH, Lim JQ, Huang MN, Padmanabhan N, et al. Whole-genome and epigenomic landscapes of etiologically distinct subtypes of cholangiocarcinoma. Cancer Discov. 2017;7:1116–35.
3. Nakamura H, Arai Y, Totoki Y, Shirota T, Elzawahry A, Kato M, et al. Genomic spectra of biliary tract cancer. Nat Genet. 2015;47:1003–10.
4. Farshidfar F, Zheng S, Gingras MC, Newton Y, Shih J, Robertson AG, et al. Integrative genomic analysis

of cholangiocarcinoma identifies distinct IDH-mutant molecular profiles. Cell Rep. 2017;18:2780–94.
5. Jiao Y, Pawlik TM, Anders RA, Selaru FM, Streppel MM, Lucas DJ, et al. Exome sequencing identifies frequent inactivating mutations in BAP1, ARID1A and PBRM1 in intrahepatic cholangiocarcinomas. Nat Genet. 2013;45:1470–3.
6. Liu ZH, Lian BF, Dong QZ, Sun H, Wei JW, Sheng YY, et al. Whole-exome mutational and transcriptional landscapes of combined hepatocellular cholangiocarcinoma and intrahepatic cholangiocarcinoma reveal molecular diversity. Biochim Biophys Acta Mol Basis Dis. 2018;1864:2360–8.
7. Lowery MA, Ptashkin R, Jordan E, Berger MF, Zehir A, Capanu M, et al. Comprehensive molecular profiling of intrahepatic and extrahepatic cholangiocarcinomas: potential targets for intervention. Clin Cancer Res. 2018;24:4154–61.
8. Ong CK, Subimerb C, Pairojkul C, Wongkham S, Cutcutache I, Yu W, et al. Exome sequencing of liver fluke-associated cholangiocarcinoma. Nat Genet. 2012;44:690–3.
9. Zou S, Li J, Zhou H, Frech C, Jiang X, Chu JS, et al. Mutational landscape of intrahepatic cholangiocarcinoma. Nat Commun. 2014;5:5696.
10. Brindley PJ, Bachini M, Ilyas SI, Khan SA, Loukas A, Sirica AE, et al. Cholangiocarcinoma. Nat Rev Dis Primers. 2021;7(1):65.
11. Chaisaingmongkol J, Budhu A, Dang H, Rabibhadana S, Pupacdi B, Kwon SM, et al. Common molecular subtypes among Asian hepatocellular carcinoma and cholangiocarcinoma. Cancer Cell. 2017;32:57–70.e3.
12. Montal R, Sia D, Montironi C, Leow WQ, Esteban-Fabro R, Pinyol R, et al. Molecular classification and therapeutic targets in extrahepatic cholangiocarcinoma. J Hepatol. 2020;73:315–27.
13. Sia D, Losic B, Moeini A, Cabellos L, Hao K, Revill K, et al. Massive parallel sequencing uncovers actionable FGFR2-PPHLN1 fusion and ARAF mutations in intrahepatic cholangiocarcinoma. Nat Commun. 2015;6:6087.
14. Wu YM, Su F, Kalyana-Sundaram S, Khazanov N, Ateeq B, Cao X, et al. Identification of targetable FGFR gene fusions in diverse cancers. Cancer Discov. 2013;3:636–47.
15. Suttiprapa S, Sotillo J, Smout M, Suyapoh W, Chaiyadet S, Tripathi T, et al. Opisthorchis viverrini proteome and host-parasite interactions. Adv Parasitol. 2018;102:45–72.
16. Siripongsakun S, Sapthanakorn W, Mekraksakit P, Vichitpunt S, Chonyuen S, Seetasarn J, et al. Premalignant lesions of cholangiocarcinoma: characteristics on ultrasonography and MRI. Abdom Radiol (NY). 2019;44:2133–46.
17. Wu MY, Yiang GT, Cheng PW, Chu PY, Li CJ. Molecular targets in hepatocarcinogenesis and implications for therapy. J Clin Med. 2018;7(8):213.
18. Sripa B, Mairiang E, Thinkhamrop B, Laha T, Kaewkes S, Sithithaworn P, et al. Advanced periductal fibrosis from infection with the carcinogenic human liver fluke Opisthorchis viverrini correlates with elevated levels of interleukin-6. Hepatology. 2009;50:1273–81.
19. Forrer A, Sayasone S, Vounatsou P, Vonghachack Y, Bouakhasith D, Vogt S, et al. Spatial distribution of, and risk factors for, Opisthorchis viverrini infection in southern Lao PDR. PLoS Negl Trop Dis. 2012;6:e1481.
20. Lun ZR, Gasser RB, Lai DH, Li AX, Zhu XQ, Yu XB, et al. Clonorchiasis: a key foodborne zoonosis in China. Lancet Infect Dis. 2005;5:31–41.
21. Thamavit W, Bhamarapravati N, Sahaphong S, Vajrasthira S, Angsubhakorn S. Effects of dimethylnitrosamine on induction of cholangiocarcinoma in Opisthorchis viverrini-infected Syrian golden hamsters. Cancer Res. 1978;38:4634–9.
22. Pakharukova MY, Zaparina OG, Kovner AV, Mordvinov VA. Inhibition of Opisthorchis felineus glutathione-dependent prostaglandin synthase by resveratrol correlates with attenuation of cholangiocyte neoplasia in a hamster model of opisthorchiasis. Int J Parasitol. 2019;49:963–73.
23. Smout MJ, Sotillo J, Laha T, Papatpremsiri A, Rinaldi G, Pimenta RN, et al. Carcinogenic parasite secretes growth factor that accelerates wound healing and potentially promotes neoplasia. PLoS Pathog. 2015;11:e1005209.
24. Chaiyadet S, Sotillo J, Smout M, Cantacessi C, Jones MK, Johnson MS, et al. Carcinogenic liver fluke secretes extracellular vesicles that promote cholangiocytes to adopt a tumorigenic phenotype. J Infect Dis. 2015;212:1636–45.
25. Arunsan P, Ittiprasert W, Smout MJ, Cochran CJ, Mann VH, Chaiyadet S, et al. Programmed knockout mutation of liver fluke granulin attenuates virulence of infection-induced hepatobiliary morbidity. Elife. 2019;8:e41463.
26. Brivio S, Cadamuro M, Fabris L, Strazzabosco M. Molecular mechanisms driving cholangiocarcinoma invasiveness: an overview. Gene Expr. 2018;18:31–50.
27. Labib PL, Goodchild G, Pereira SP. Molecular pathogenesis of cholangiocarcinoma. BMC Cancer. 2019;19:185.
28. Roy S, Glaser S, Chakraborty S. Inflammation and progression of cholangiocarcinoma: role of angiogenic and lymphangiogenic mechanisms. Front Med (Lausanne). 2019;6:293.
29. Servais FA, Kirchmeyer M, Hamdorf M, Minoungou NWE, Rose-John S, Kreis S, et al. Modulation of the IL-6-signaling pathway in liver cells by miRNAs targeting gp130, JAK1, and/or STAT3. Mol Ther Nucleic Acids. 2019;16:419–33.
30. Alvaro D, Barbaro B, Franchitto A, Onori P, Glaser SS, Alpini G, et al. Estrogens and insulin-like growth factor 1 modulate neoplastic cell growth in human cholangiocarcinoma. Am J Pathol. 2006;169:877–88.
31. Zavadil J, Bottinger EP. TGF-beta and epithelial-to-mesenchymal transitions. Oncogene. 2005;24:5764–74.

32. Claperon A, Mergey M, Nguyen Ho-Bouldoires TH, Vignjevic D, Wendum D, Chretien Y, et al. EGF/EGFR axis contributes to the progression of cholangiocarcinoma through the induction of an epithelial-mesenchymal transition. J Hepatol. 2014;61:325–32.
33. Miyamoto M, Ojima H, Iwasaki M, Shimizu H, Kokubu A, Hiraoka N, et al. Prognostic significance of overexpression of c-Met oncoprotein in cholangiocarcinoma. Br J Cancer. 2011;105:131–8.
34. Pant K, Richard S, Peixoto E, Gradilone SA. Role of glucose metabolism reprogramming in the pathogenesis of cholangiocarcinoma. Front Med (Lausanne). 2020;7:113.
35. Phoomak C, Silsirivanit A, Wongkham C, Sripa B, Puapairoj A, Wongkham S. Overexpression of O-GlcNAc-transferase associates with aggressiveness of mass-forming cholangiocarcinoma. Asian Pac J Cancer Prev. 2012;13 Suppl:101–5.
36. Phoomak C, Vaeteewoottacharn K, Sawanyawisuth K, Seubwai W, Wongkham C, Silsirivanit A, et al. Mechanistic insights of O-GlcNAcylation that promote progression of cholangiocarcinoma cells via nuclear translocation of NF-kappaB. Sci Rep. 2016;6:27853.
37. Phoomak C, Park D, Silsirivanit A, Sawanyawisuth K, Vaeteewoottacharn K, Detarya M, et al. O-GlcNAc-induced nuclear translocation of hnRNP-K is associated with progression and metastasis of cholangiocarcinoma. Mol Oncol. 2019;13:338–57.
38. Saengboonmee C, Seubwai W, Wongkham C, Wongkham S. Diabetes mellitus: possible risk and promoting factors of cholangiocarcinoma: association of diabetes mellitus and cholangiocarcinoma. Cancer Epidemiol. 2015;39:274–8.
39. Phoomak C, Vaeteewoottacharn K, Silsirivanit A, Saengboonmee C, Seubwai W, Sawanyawisuth K, et al. High glucose levels boost the aggressiveness of highly metastatic cholangiocarcinoma cells via O-GlcNAcylation. Sci Rep. 2017;7:43842.
40. Saengboonmee C, Seubwai W, Pairojkul C, Wongkham S. High glucose enhances progression of cholangiocarcinoma cells via STAT3 activation. Sci Rep. 2016;6:18995.
41. Indramanee S, Sawanyawisuth K, Silsirivanit A, Dana P, Phoomak C, Kariya R, et al. Terminal fucose mediates progression of human cholangiocarcinoma through EGF/EGFR activation and the Akt/Erk signaling pathway. Sci Rep. 2019;9:17266.
42. Phoomak C, Silsirivanit A, Park D, Sawanyawisuth K, Vaeteewoottacharn K, Wongkham C, et al. O-GlcNAcylation mediates metastasis of cholangiocarcinoma through FOXO3 and MAN1A1. Oncogene. 2018;37:5648–65.
43. Park DD, Phoomak C, Xu G, Olney LP, Tran KA, Park SS, et al. Metastasis of cholangiocarcinoma is promoted by extended high-mannose glycans. Proc Natl Acad Sci U S A. 2020;117:7633–44.
44. Talabnin K, Talabnin C, Ishihara M, Azadi P. Increased expression of the high-mannose M6N2 and NeuAc3H3N3M3N2F tri-antennary N-glycans in cholangiocarcinoma. Oncol Lett. 2018;15:1030–6.
45. Nakanuma Y, Sato Y, Harada K, Sasaki M, Xu J, Ikeda H. Pathological classification of intrahepatic cholangiocarcinoma based on a new concept. World J Hepatol. 2010;2:419–27.
46. Banales JM, Cardinale V, Carpino G, Marzioni M, Andersen JB, Invernizzi P, et al. Expert consensus document: cholangiocarcinoma: current knowledge and future perspectives consensus statement from the European Network for the Study of Cholangiocarcinoma (ENS-CCA). Nat Rev Gastroenterol Hepatol. 2016;13:261–80.
47. Vijgen S, Terris B, Rubbia-Brandt L. Pathology of intrahepatic cholangiocarcinoma. Hepatobiliary Surg Nutr. 2017;6:22–34.
48. Sirica AE, Dumur CI, Campbell DJ, Almenara JA, Ogunwobi OO, Dewitt JL. Intrahepatic cholangiocarcinoma progression: prognostic factors and basic mechanisms. Clin Gastroenterol Hepatol. 2009;7:S68–78.
49. Bragazzi MC, Ridola L, Safarikia S, Matteo SD, Costantini D, Nevi L, et al. New insights into cholangiocarcinoma: multiple stems and related cell lineages of origin. Ann Gastroenterol. 2018;31:42–55.
50. Akita M, Sofue K, Fujikura K, Otani K, Itoh T, Ajiki T, et al. Histological and molecular characterization of intrahepatic bile duct cancers suggests an expanded definition of perihilar cholangiocarcinoma. HPB (Oxford). 2019;21:226–34.
51. Bae JY, Park YN, Nakanuma Y, Lee WJ, Kim JY, Park C. Intestinal type cholangiocarcinoma of intrahepatic large bile duct associated with hepatolithiasis—a new histologic subtype for further investigation. Hepatogastroenterology. 2002;49:628–30.
52. Brunt E, Aishima S, Clavien PA, Fowler K, Goodman Z, Gores G, et al. cHCC-CCA: consensus terminology for primary liver carcinomas with both hepatocytic and cholangiocytic differentiation. Hepatology. 2018;68:113–26.
53. Balitzer D, Joseph NM, Ferrell L, Shafizadeh N, Jain D, Zhang X, et al. Immunohistochemical and molecular features of cholangiolocellular carcinoma are similar to well-differentiated intrahepatic cholangiocarcinoma. Mod Pathol. 2019;32:1486–94.
54. Brivio S, Cadamuro M, Strazzabosco M, Fabris L. Tumor reactive stroma in cholangiocarcinoma: the fuel behind cancer aggressiveness. World J Hepatol. 2017;9:455–68.
55. Bosmuller H, Pfefferle V, Bittar Z, Scheble V, Horger M, Sipos B, et al. Microvessel density and angiogenesis in primary hepatic malignancies: differential expression of CD31 and VEGFR-2 in hepatocellular carcinoma and intrahepatic cholangiocarcinoma. Pathol Res Pract. 2018;214:1136–41.
56. Xu J, Igarashi S, Sasaki M, Matsubara T, Yoneda N, Kozaka K, et al. Intrahepatic cholangiocarcinomas in cirrhosis are hypervascular in comparison with those in normal livers. Liver Int. 2012;32:1156–64.

57. Cadamuro M, Stecca T, Brivio S, Mariotti V, Fiorotto R, Spirli C, et al. The deleterious interplay between tumor epithelia and stroma in cholangiocarcinoma. Biochim Biophys Acta Mol Basis Dis. 2018;1864:1435–43.
58. Loeuillard E, Conboy CB, Gores GJ, Rizvi S. Immunobiology of cholangiocarcinoma. JHEP Rep. 2019;1:297–311.
59. Vaquero J, Aoudjehane L, Fouassier L. Cancer-associated fibroblasts in cholangiocarcinoma. Curr Opin Gastroenterol. 2020;36:63–9.
60. Affo S, Nair A, Brundu F, Ravichandra A, Bhattacharjee S, Matsuda M, et al. Promotion of cholangiocarcinoma growth by diverse cancer-associated fibroblast subpopulations. Cancer Cell. 2021;39:866–882.e11.
61. Sahai E, Astsaturov I, Cukierman E, DeNardo DG, Egeblad M, Evans RM, et al. A framework for advancing our understanding of cancer-associated fibroblasts. Nat Rev Cancer. 2020;20:174–86.
62. Alvaro D, Bragazzi MC, Benedetti A, Fabris L, Fava G, Invernizzi P, et al. Cholangiocarcinoma in Italy: a national survey on clinical characteristics, diagnostic modalities and treatment. Results from the "Cholangiocarcinoma" Committee of the Italian Association for the study of liver disease. Dig Liver Dis. 2011;43:60–5.
63. Patel AH, Harnois DM, Klee GG, LaRusso NF, Gores GJ. The utility of CA 19-9 in the diagnoses of cholangiocarcinoma in patients without primary sclerosing cholangitis. Am J Gastroenterol. 2000;95:204–7.
64. Kim MJ, Choi JY, Chung YE. Evaluation of biliary malignancies using multidetector-row computed tomography. J Comput Assist Tomogr. 2010;34:496–505.
65. Wildner D, Bernatik T, Greis C, Seitz K, Neurath MF, Strobel D. CEUS in hepatocellular carcinoma and intrahepatic cholangiocellular carcinoma in 320 patients—early or late washout matters: a subanalysis of the DEGUM multicenter trial. Ultraschall Med. 2015;36:132–9.
66. Iavarone M, Piscaglia F, Vavassori S, Galassi M, Sangiovanni A, Venerandi L, et al. Contrast enhanced CT-scan to diagnose intrahepatic cholangiocarcinoma in patients with cirrhosis. J Hepatol. 2013;58:1188–93.
67. Kim SH, Lee CH, Kim BH, Kim WB, Yeom SK, Kim KA, et al. Typical and atypical imaging findings of intrahepatic cholangiocarcinoma using gadolinium ethoxybenzyl diethylenetriamine pentaacetic acid-enhanced magnetic resonance imaging. J Comput Assist Tomogr. 2012;36:704–9.
68. Choi SH, Lee SS, Kim SY, Park SH, Park SH, Kim KM, et al. Intrahepatic cholangiocarcinoma in patients with cirrhosis: differentiation from hepatocellular carcinoma by using gadoxetic acid-enhanced MR imaging and dynamic CT. Radiology. 2017;282:771–81.
69. Vilana R, Forner A, Bianchi L, Garcia-Criado A, Rimola J, de Lope CR, et al. Intrahepatic peripheral cholangiocarcinoma in cirrhosis patients may display a vascular pattern similar to hepatocellular carcinoma on contrast-enhanced ultrasound. Hepatology. 2010;51:2020–9.
70. Petrowsky H, Wildbrett P, Husarik DB, Hany TF, Tam S, Jochum W, et al. Impact of integrated positron emission tomography and computed tomography on staging and management of gallbladder cancer and cholangiocarcinoma. J Hepatol. 2006;45:43–50.
71. Lamarca A, Barriuso J, Chander A, McNamara MG, Hubner RA, ÓReilly D, et al. (18) F-fluorodeoxyglucose positron emission tomography ((18)FDG-PET) for patients with biliary tract cancer: systematic review and meta-analysis. J Hepatol. 2019;71:115–29.
72. Jhaveri KS, Hosseini-Nik H. MRI of cholangiocarcinoma. J Magn Reson Imaging. 2015;42:1165–79.
73. Saluja SS, Sharma R, Pal S, Sahni P, Chattopadhyay TK. Differentiation between benign and malignant hilar obstructions using laboratory and radiological investigations: a prospective study. HPB (Oxford). 2007;9:373–82.
74. Trikudanathan G, Navaneethan U, Njei B, Vargo JJ, Parsi MA. Diagnostic yield of bile duct brushings for cholangiocarcinoma in primary sclerosing cholangitis: a systematic review and meta-analysis. Gastrointest Endosc. 2014;79:783–9.
75. Barr Fritcher EG, Voss JS, Brankley SM, Campion MB, Jenkins SM, Keeney ME, et al. An optimized set of fluorescence in situ hybridization probes for detection of pancreatobiliary tract cancer in cytology brush samples. Gastroenterology. 2015;149:1813–1824.e1.
76. Rizvi S, Eaton J, Yang JD, Chandrasekhara V, Gores GJ. Emerging technologies for the diagnosis of perihilar cholangiocarcinoma. Semin Liver Dis. 2018;38:160–9.
77. Mohamadnejad M, DeWitt JM, Sherman S, LeBlanc JK, Pitt HA, House MG, et al. Role of EUS for preoperative evaluation of cholangiocarcinoma: a large single-center experience. Gastrointest Endosc. 2011;73:71–8.
78. Heimbach JK, Sanchez W, Rosen CB, Gores GJ. Trans-peritoneal fine needle aspiration biopsy of hilar cholangiocarcinoma is associated with disease dissemination. HPB (Oxford). 2011;13:356–60.

Staging and Treatment

Key Points

- Cholangiocarcinoma (CCA) staging is most commonly classified using the TNM staging systems of the American Joint Committee on Cancer (AJCC).
- Intrahepatic, perihilar, and distal CCA are staged independently.
- Complete tumor resection with negative margins is the only curative treatment for CCA.
- Based on evidence from the BILCAP trial, adjuvant capecitabine for 6 months is recommended in patients with resected CCA.
- The combination of gemcitabine plus cisplatin is still considered a standard of care in unresectable disease.
- Targeted therapy and immunotherapy can be considered in selected patients.

Introduction

Cholangiocarcinoma (CCA) staging is most commonly classified using the TNM staging systems of the American Joint Committee on Cancer (AJCC)/Union for International Cancer Control (UICC), which came into effect on January 1, 2018, in its eighth edition. There are separate systems depending on whether the CCA arises primarily from intrahepatic (iCCA), perihilar/hilar (Klatskin) (pCCA), or extrahepatic (distal) bile ducts (dCCA), which all differ in their definitions of tumor stage (T) and in their prognostic stage groupings (Fig. 1a).

Complete tumor resection with negative margins is the only curative treatment for CCA. However, definitive surgery can only be applied to limited patients with well-localized lesions. Patients with CCA often present in the late stages of the disease with nonspecific symptoms, such as painless jaundice, weight loss, or cholangitis. Therefore, the prognosis is poor as these cancers are difficult to diagnose and treat. In advanced cases, the goal of treatment is palliative, and chemotherapy or radiation therapy is considered a standard treatment option.

Jung Won Chun and Sang Myung Woo are the lead authors of this chapter.

H. J. Chun et al., *Gastrointestinal Cancer*, https://doi.org/10.1007/978-981-99-0815-8_54

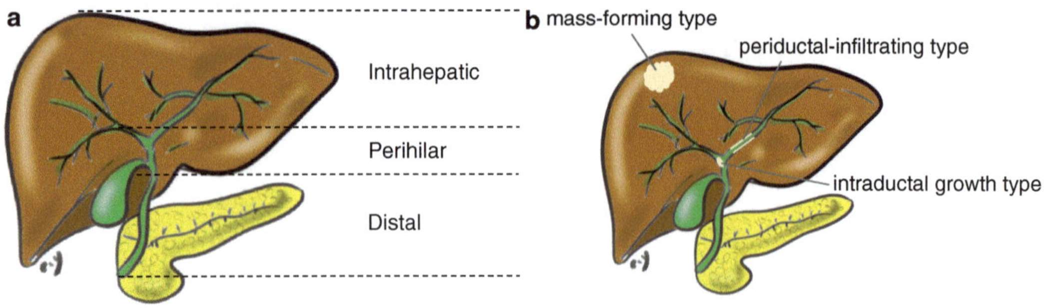

Fig. 1 Anatomic classification of cholangiocarcinoma (Fig. 1a, left panel; Fig. 1b, right panel). Three types of cholangiocarcinoma according to the morphologic classification system proposed by the Liver Cancer Study Group of Japan (adapted from Diagnosis and Management of Cholangiocarcinoma, 2021, springer)

Staging

Intrahepatic Cholangiocarcinoma

The iCCA staining is presented in Table 1. iCCA may arise from microscopic bile in the periphery of the liver to the second-order bile ducts. The Liver Cancer Study Group of Japan (LCSGJ) classifies iCCA into three distinct morphologic subtypes based on gross appearance (Fig. 1b). They are (1) mass formation type, (2) periductal infiltrating type, and (3) intraductal growth type [1]. These growth patterns are shown in differences in risk factors, cell origin, and biological progression [2].

iCCA was previously staged as identical to that of hepatocellular carcinoma in the AJCC staging manual until the seventh Edition. In the AJCC seventh Edition staging manual, the T category was determined by tumor numbers, vascular invasion, and invasion of adjacent organs. Tumor size was excluded because it was not considered a significant prognostic indicator for iCCA. However, size was likely to be associated with survival after several studies and a meta-analysis [3]. And the T stage in the eighth Edition of the AJCC is now classified by tumor size, number of tumors, vascular invasion, extension beyond the visceral peritoneum, and invasion of extrahepatic structures. The revised AJCC eighth Edition incorporates a tumor size cutoff of 5 cm to separate the T1 category into T1a (≤5 cm) and T1b (>5 cm) subgroups. Previous T2a, solitary tumor with vascular invasion, and 2b, multiple tumors, with or without vascular invasion, are combined as T2, indicating an equivalent prognostic value of vascular invasion and tumor mul-

Table 1 Stages of intrahepatic bile duct cancer

AJCC stage	Stage grouping	Stage description[a]
0	Tis	Carcinoma in situ (intraductal tumor)
	N0	No regional lymph node metastasis
	M0	No evidence of distant metastases
IA	T1a	Solitary tumor ≤5 cm without vascular invasion
	N0	No regional lymph node metastasis
	M0	No evidence of distant metastases
IB	T1b	Solitary tumor >5 cm without vascular invasion
	N0	No regional lymph node metastasis
	M0	No evidence of distant metastases
II	T2	Solitary tumor with intrahepatic vascular invasion, **or** there are two or more tumors, with or without vascular invasion
	N0	No regional lymph node metastasis
	M0	No evidence of distant metastases
	T3	Tumor growing through the visceral peritoneum (the outer lining of organs in the abdomen)
IIIA	N0	No regional lymph node metastasis
	M0	No evidence of distant metastases
IIIB	T4	Tumor involving local extrahepatic structures by direct invasion
	N0	No regional lymph node metastasis
	M0	No evidence of distant metastases
	OR	
	Any T	Any size, with or without growing outside the bile duct
	N1	Regional lymph node metastasis present
	M0	No evidence of distant metastases
IV	Any T	Any size, with or without growing outside the bile duct
	Any N	With or without regional lymph node metastasis
	M1	Distant metastasis

tifocality. T3 tumors include any iCCA that perforates the visceral peritoneum. Local direct invasion into the extrahepatic structure, previously T3, is now upgraded to T4, and periductal invasion is removed from the T4 category. T4 tumors are now classified as stage IIIB, whereas they were classified as stage IVA in the seventh Edition. These revisions, mentioned above, were based on detailed pathological analysis of surgical specimens resected from international hepatobiliary centers of excellence [4].

Lymph node metastasis is an important prognostic factor [5]. The principle of the surgical approach to iCCA includes liver resection and regional lymphadenectomy of the liver hilum. The quality of lymph node dissection is also important for optimal tumor staging. Therefore, the eighth Edition of the AJCC recommends harvesting at least six lymph nodes. Regional lymph nodes include areas of the hilar (common bile duct, liver artery, portal vein, and cystic duct), periduodenal, and peripancreatic lymph nodes. These regional lymph node metastases are considered N1 disease, while spreading to extraregional lymph nodes (celiac, periaortic, and pericaval nodes) is considered M1 disease. M1 disease also includes extrahepatic sites, such as the lung, bone, peritoneum, and pleura.

Perihilar Cholangiocarcinoma

Extrahepatic cholangiocarcinoma was divided into pCCA and dCCA due to the different characteristics of the pathology, treatment, and prognosis [6]. pCCA, also known as Klatskin tumor, arises around the bifurcation of the biliary duct proximal to the cystic duct and accounts for 50–60% of all cholangiocarcinomas [7]. The Bismuth–Corlette classification system provides an anatomic description of the tumor location and longitudinal extension of pCCA (Fig. 2) [8]. Type I lesions are limited to the common hepatic duct (CHD) immediately below the confluence of the right and left hepatic ducts; type II tumors involve CHD and extend to the confluence; type III includes type II and extends into the main right hepatic duct (type IIIa) or the left hepatic duct (type IIIb); type IV tumors extend past the confluence involving both the right and left hepatic ducts *or* has multifocal involvement. Although limited due to its failure to characterize the radial extension of cancer cells, it provides a practical manner for surgical oncologists to describe the lesion and, in turn, the anticipated extent of the liver that

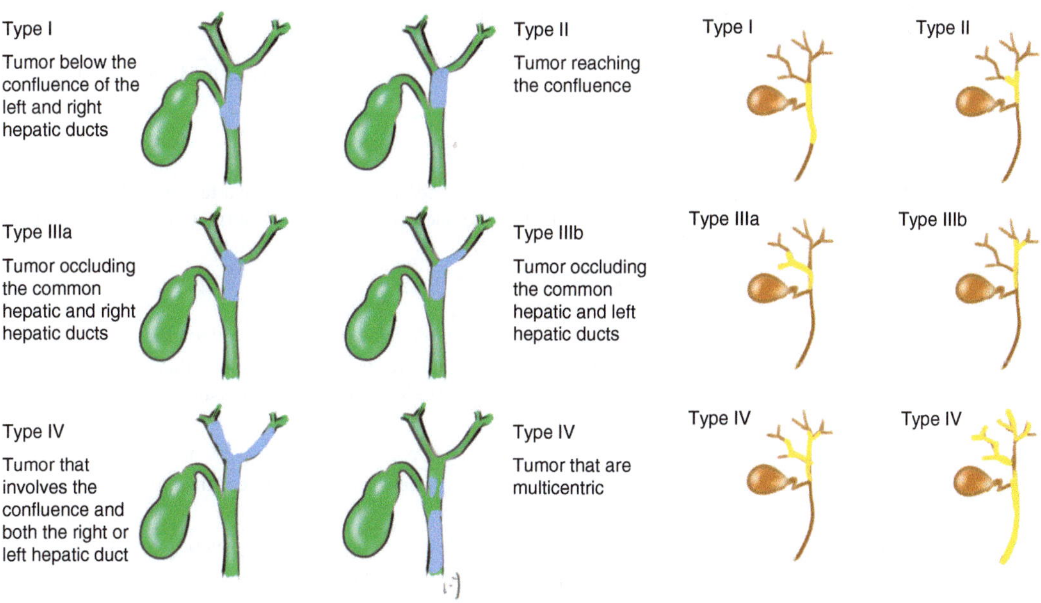

Fig. 2 Bismuth–Corlette classification for perihilar tumors (adapted from UpToDate)

may need to be resected to achieve complete extirpation of the malignancy.

Since the AJCC seventh Edition, pCCA has been recognized as a separate disease from the dCCA. However, histopathological evaluation of surgical specimens, together with preoperative imaging data, is needed to define the correct classification of TNM. The AJCC classification was revised as the eighth Edition of the TNM classification. The major changes in the eighth edition of the AJCC include the incorporation of high-grade intraepithelial biliary neoplasia into carcinoma in situ (Tis) and the elimination of bilateral second-order involvement of the bile duct from T4, in which the T4 stage is no longer related to Bismuth–Corlette type IV (Table 2) [9]. A T1 tumor is confined to the bile duct with extension up to the muscle layer or fibrous tissue. A T2a tumor invades beyond the wall of the bile duct to the surrounding adipose tissue, and a T2b tumor invades the adjacent hepatic parenchyma.

Tumors invading the unilateral branches of the portal vein or hepatic artery are T3 tumors. A T4 tumor is now defined as a tumor that invades the main portal vein and/or the common hepatic artery or its branches bilaterally or grows into other bile ducts on one side (left or right) and a main blood vessel on the other side. T4 tumors are downgraded from stage IVA to stage IIIB.

pCCA frequently metastases to regional lymph node occur in as high as 50% of patients [10, 11]. In the staging of pCCA, the number of

Table 2 Stages of perihilar bile duct cancer

AJCC stage	Stage grouping	Stage description[a]
0	Tis	Carcinoma in situ/high-grade dysplasia
	N0	No regional lymph node metastasis
	M0	No evidence of distant metastases
I	T1	Tumor confined to the bile duct, with extension up to the muscle layer or fibrous tissue layer
	N0	No regional lymph node metastasis
	M0	No evidence of distant metastases
II	T2a or T2b	Tumor invades beyond the wall of the bile duct to surrounding fatty tissue (T2a) or adjacent hepatic parenchyma (T2b)
	N0	No regional lymph node metastasis
	M0	No evidence of distant metastases
IIIA	T3	Tumor invades unilateral branches (left or right) of the main blood vessels (portal vein or hepatic artery)
	N0	No regional lymph node metastasis
	M0	No evidence of distant metastases
	T4	Tumor invades the main portal vein and/or common hepatic artery or its branches bilaterally **or** grows into other bile ducts on one side (left or right) and a main blood vessel on the other side
IIIB	N0	No regional lymph node metastasis
	M0	No evidence of distant metastases
IIIC	Any T	With or without growing outside the bile duct or into nearby blood vessels
	N1	Involves one to three regional lymph nodes, typically involving hilar, cystic duct, common bile duct, hepatic artery, posterior pancreaticoduodenal, and portal vein
	M0	No evidence of distant metastases
IVA	Any T	With or without growing outside the bile duct or into nearby blood vessels
	N2	Involves four or more nearby lymph nodes from the sites described for N1
	M0	No evidence of distant metastases
IVB	Any T	With or without growing outside the bile duct or into nearby blood vessels
	Any N	May or may not have spread to nearby lymph nodes
	M1	Distant metastasis, includes lymph node metastasis distant to the hepatoduodenal ligament

positive lymph nodes is incorporated. The N1 category is defined as metastasis in one to three lymph nodes and is upgraded from IIIB to IIIC. The N2 category (stage IVa) is classified as positive lymph node metastasis in more than three lymph nodes. Previous N2 disease, positive lymph nodes beyond the hepatoduodenal ligament, has become M1 disease (stage IVb) in the eighth Edition. Other common sites of metastasis are the liver, lung bone, peritoneum, brain, and skin.

Distal Extrahepatic Cholangiocarcinoma

Distal bile duct cholangiocarcinoma, located between the entry of the cystic duct and the end of the common bile duct in the ampullary region, compromises approximately 30% of all carcinomas of the bile duct. The seventh Edition of the AJCC used a staging system based on a common anatomic layer, which was described as vague and resulted in wide variations between observers. Instead, the eighth Edition adopted a depth-based approach for DCC, which measured the depth of tumor invasion from the basal lamina of the adjacent normal epithelium to the most deeply infiltrating tumor cells (Table 3). The cutoff values of 5 and 12 mm define the T category as T1, <5 mm; T2, 5–12 mm; and T3, >12 mm. Previously in the T3 category, tumor invasion into adjacent organs such as the pancreas, duodenum, and gallbladder is removed in the eighth Edition. T4 is defined as a tumor invading the celiac axis, the superior mesenteric artery, and/or the common hepatic artery. As in the pCCA, N category is stratified into three tiers based on the number of lymph node metastases (N0, 0; N1, 1–3; N2, >3) unlike the simple evaluation based on the presence of metastatic nodes in the seventh Edition [12]. Regional lymph nodes include the common bile duct and hepatic artery, pancreaticoduodenal nodes, and nodes along the lateral wall of the superior mesenteric artery. Distant metastases to the common site of the liver, lung, and peritoneum are considered M1 disease.

Table 3 Stages of distal bile duct cancer

AJCC stage	Stage grouping	Stage description[a]
0	Tis	Carcinoma in situ/high-grade dysplasia
	N0	No regional lymph node metastasis
	M0	No evidence of distant metastases
I	T1	Tumor invades the bile duct wall with depth <5 mm
	N0	No regional lymph node metastasis
	M0	No evidence of distant metastases
IIA	T2	Tumor invades the bile duct wall with depth 5–12 mm
	N0	No regional lymph node metastasis
	M0	No evidence of distant metastases
	OR	
	T1	Tumor invades the bile duct wall with depth <5 mm
	N1	Involves one to three regional lymph nodes
	M0	No evidence of distant metastases
IIB	T3	Tumor invades the bile duct wall with depth >12 mm
	N0	No regional lymph node metastasis
	M0	No evidence of distant metastases
	OR	
	T2 or T3	Tumor invades 5 mm or more into the bile duct wall
	N1	Involves one to three regional lymph nodes
	M0	No evidence of distant metastases

(continued)

Table 3 (continued)

AJCC stage	Stage grouping	Stage description[a]
IIIA	T1, T2, or T3	Tumor invades into the bile duct wall with any depth
	N2	Involves four or more regional lymph nodes
	M0	No evidence of distant metastases
	T4	Tumor invades to nearby blood vessels (the celiac artery or its branches, the superior mesenteric artery, and/or the common hepatic artery
IIIB	Any N	May or may not have spread to regional lymph nodes
	M0	No evidence of distant metastases
IV	Any T	Tumor has grown to any depth within the bile duct wall, with or without growing into nearby blood vessels
	Any N	May or may not have spread to regional lymph nodes
	M1	Distant metastasis

Treatment

Surgery

The evaluation of the clinical stage based on high-quality imaging allows for the most thorough consideration of resectability and adequate preoperative preparation, where applicable. The definition of resectability depends on the subtype of CCA. However, the presence of metastases and the patient's inability to tolerate a major operation preclude resection for all subtypes. For iCCA, N2 disease and invasion of the main hepatic artery or bilateral hepatic arteries are generally considered unresectable. For pCCA, the presence of N2 disease also excludes resection, in addition to local tumor invasion as follows: (1) bilateral segmental ductal extension, (2) unilateral hepatic atrophy with contralateral bile duct involvement or vascular involvement, and (3) unilateral bile duct involvement with contralateral vascular involvement [13]. Unresectability for dCCA is generally considered to be encapsulation of the hepatic artery or superior mesenteric artery and/or extensive involvement of the portal vein [14].

After determining resectability, surgical treatment of iCCA involves achieving a R0 liver resection and portal lymphadenectomy [15]. Extensive liver resections are usually needed to confirm R0 resection. Similar to the principles of resection for iCCA, surgery for pCCA aims for an R0 resection with adequate biliary drainage, vascular supply, and intrinsic hepatic function. The main surgical procedure is an extended right or left hepatectomy, and often the caudate lobectomy, especially with left-sided tumors. Anatomical proximity to critical vascular structures in pCCA increases the risk of portal venous and hepatic arterial invasion. The surgical management for dCCA does not involve hepatic resection, but is more commonly performed by pancreaticoduodenectomy. Rarely, if the disease is limited to the proximal bile duct, an R0 resection can be achieved with biliary resection and hepaticojejunostomy reconstruction.

The rate, severity, and types of postoperative complications after CCA resection depend on the location of the disease and the extent of surgery, among other factors. The current overall postoperative complication rate is around 40% and postoperative mortality ranges from 0 to 4%. Postoperative liver failure remains the most common cause of mortality after extended hepatectomy [16]. Therefore, a full assessment of the extent of the disease is necessary to ensure complete resection with sufficient functional liver remnant. Patients with borderline or inadequate functional liver remnant can be considered volume optimization strategies, such as portal vein embolization. Biliary drainage prior to operation is also a common selective option to avoid postoperative liver failure. Biliary drainage should be indicated in patients with cholangitis, those undergoing neoadjuvant chemotherapy, and patients undergoing portal vein embolization [13]. However, the routine use of biliary drainage is controversial.

Liver Transplant

Reports on the early experience of liver transplantation for unresectable iCCA and pCCA were disappointing and did not support the use of transplantation [17]. High postoperative mortality and recurrence rates significantly limited the use of LT for CCA. For transplantation to be effective in CCA, there was a clear need for improved patient selection and neoadjuvant therapies to reduce systemic microscopic disease and recurrence rates. Neoadjuvant treatment typically involves chemotherapy (5-fluorouracil [5-FU]) and radiation [18]. The Mayo clinic group published its results in 126 pCCA patients transplanted over an 18-year period using their protocol and demonstrated a 5-year overall survival (OS) of 75% in the highly selected group [19]. Using strict inclusion and exclusion criteria, appropriately selected patients underwent extensive neoadjuvant therapy and then were maintained on capecitabine while waiting for transplantation. Although transplantation appears to provide a significant benefit to the few selected patients with locally advanced pCCA, most CCA patients do not meet the strict eligibility criteria due to disease burden or tumor location.

Adjuvant Therapy

The role of neoadjuvant therapy for CCA is unclear. For locally advanced or metastatic CCA, the ABC-02 trial established cisplatin plus gemcitabine as the optimal regimen [20]. For resectable disease, the current standard of care is surgery (with goal of R0 resection) followed by observation alone. The recently published BILCAP trial showed a trend toward a survival benefit for patients receiving adjuvant capecitabine [21]. A total of 447 patients with biliary tract cancer (BTC) resected with curative intent were randomly assigned to the capecitabine group and to the observation group. Although the study did not reach its primary end point of improving OS in the intention-to-treat analysis, capecitabine was associated with improved OS in the analysis per protocol (53 vs 36 months, $p = 0.028$). Based on evidence from the BILCAP trial, the American Society of Clinical Oncology (ASCO) guidelines recommend adjuvant capecitabine for 6 months in patients with resected BTC [22]. The role of combined chemotherapy and radiation therapy has also been investigated as adjuvant therapy for CCA. The SWOG S0809 trial was a phase II trial that examined the role of adjuvant chemoradiotherapy for extrahepatic CCA and gallbladder cancer (GBC) after complete resection. A nonrandom cohort consisted of patients who received capecitabine and gemcitabine followed by capecitabine concurrent with external-beam radiation [23]. The 2-year survival rate was 65% (67% in R0 resection, 60% in R1 resection) and the median OS was 35 months. The ASCO guidelines incorporated these results and recommended that patients with an R1 resection receive adjuvant chemoradiation [22].

Palliative Chemotherapy

Most biliary tract cancers (BTC) present when at an advanced stage of the disease due to the late onset or absence of symptoms and aggressive tumor biology. Advanced stage describes locally advanced and metastatic disease at presentation and also refers to patients relapsed with local or metastatic disease after surgery. Gemcitabine monotherapy has long been considered standard for the palliative treatment of advanced CCA despite the lack of randomized controlled trials [24]. For patients who receive chemotherapy alone, combination therapy provides the best benefit.

The currently recommended first-line chemotherapy regimen for advanced BTC is derived from the ABC-02 trial that included 410 patients treated with gemcitabine plus cisplatin (Gem-Cis) versus gemcitabine alone. In general, the addition of cisplatin significantly improved survival outcomes: median OS from 8.1 to 11.7 months ($p < 0.001$) and progression-free survival (PFS) from 8 to 5 months ($p < 0.001$) [25]. This combination chemotherapy was also evaluated in Japanese patients, and similar efficacy was confirmed in a randomized multicenter phase II study (BT-22) [26]. The BT22 study demonstrated that Gem-Cis improved median OS compared to gemcitabine alone (11.2 vs 7.7 months).

A second doublet regimen based on gemcitabine is the combination of gemcitabine and S-1, an oral fluoropyrimidine that includes three agents (tegafur, gimeracil, and oteracil). In the Japanese FUGA-BT trial, phase III noninferiority study, gemcitabine plus S1 (Gem-S1) was compared with the standard of care Gem-Cis or patients with advanced or recurrent BTC in terms of OS [27]. Gem-S1 was not inferior to Gem-Cis, with a median OS of 15.1 vs 13.4 months (noninferiority $p = 0.046$) and a median PFS of 6.8 vs 5.8 months, respectively. Other gemcitabine-based doublets have also been evaluated in patients with advanced CCA. Oxaliplatin is an alternative platinum agent to cisplatin, which is less ototoxic and less nephrotoxic.

A recent phase III trial conducted in Korea compared first-line gemcitabine plus oxaliplatin (GEMOX) with a combination of capecitabine and oxaliplatin (XELOX) [28]. In that noninferiority trial, the median PFS for GEMOX and XELOX was 5.3 months and 5.8 months, respectively. There was also no difference in OS (10.6 months vs 10.6 months).

A final gemcitabine-based doublet that was explored in patients with advanced CCA is gemcitabine plus nab-paclitaxel. Sahai et al. reported the results of 74 patients with advanced CCA treated with nab-paclitaxel followed by gemcitabine in their multicenter phase II trial [29]. The regimen was effective, with an objective response rate (ORR), median OS, and PFS of 30%, 12.4 months, and 7.7 months, respectively. Recently, a phase II single-arm trial evaluated a triple regimen of Gem-Cis and nab-paclitaxel for 60 patients with advanced BTC (78% CCA) [30]. The results were impressive, with a median PFS of 11.8 months and a median OS of 19.2 months. This regimen will be further evaluated in a phase III randomized trial (NCT03768414).

In patients with a poor performance status, the benefit of the doublet regimen appeared to be associated with a lower likelihood of treatment effects. For these patients, gemcitabine monotherapy can be considered. Although 5-FU monotherapy showed a low response rate in BTC, leucovorin addition improved response rates (ORR 20–33%) [31–33].

There are few studies in patients with advanced CCA and progression after first-line therapy to evaluate second-line systemic therapy. A systematic review, published in 2014, reported that second-line chemotherapy might benefit selected patients with good performance status [34]. Currently, the FOLFOX regimen (including leucovorin, fluorouracil, and oxaliplatin) is the second-line treatment most used, based on the results of the randomized phase III ABC-06 trial. The trial compared a modified FOLFOX with active symptom control to active symptom control alone. One hundred and sixty-two patients with advanced BTC (72% CCA) were included in this study. A marginal improvement in median OS, from 5.3 months to 6.2 months, while OS rates at 6 and 12 months, showed a clinically significant increase (50.6% and 25.9%, respectively) [35]. In 2021, Yoo et al. reported the results of a randomized phase II study (NIFTY) comparing 5-FU + leucovorin + nanoliposomal irinotecan and 5-FU + leucovorin. The additional benefit of nanoliposomal irinotecan was demonstrated in this study. Of the 174 patients who were assessed for response, the median PFS was significantly better (7.1 vs 1.4 months, $p = 0.0019$) as the median OS (8.6 vs 5.5 months, $p = 0.0349$) and ORR (14.8% vs 5.8%) [36].

Radiotherapy

The role of radiation therapy remains unclear in the treatment of locally advanced but nonmetastatic CCA. Approximately one-half of advanced CCA are confined to the liver, making locoregional therapies such as radiotherapy attractive options [37]. Locoregional therapies have the advantage of averting adverse effects of chemotherapy and provide treatment options for patients unfit for systemic therapy. However, there is no standard of care radiation therapy for patients with advanced CCA due to a paucity of data from randomized trials. Chemoradiotherapy for locally advanced CCA has been considered a possible option according to nonrandomized studies with a median OS between 9 and 21 months [38, 39]. Most studies were carried out in combination with 5-FU, gemcitabine, or cisplatin with a median radiotherapy dose of approximately 50 Gy [39]. Higher biological effective doses could achieve better local control (78% vs 45% after 3 years, $p = 0.03$) and also a survival benefit (not reached vs 27 months, $p = 0.02$) [40]. Modalities for safer dose escalation include the use of stereotactic body radiotherapy (SBRT) and proton beam radiation therapy (PBT). Several prospective and retrospective studies of SBRT led to local control rates of 65–100% in selected patients [41–43]. Another option for dose escalation in unresectable CCA is PBT. Initial studies that included patients treated with palliative intent showed promising results with local control rates of 58–94% with OS 9.6–19.3 months [39].

Targeted Drug Therapy

CCA has a high level of intra- and intertumoral heterogeneity with different genetic alteration profiles. In recent years, advances in whole exome and transcriptome sequencing have shed light on understanding the molecular and epigenomic landscape of CCA, opening the door to customized treatment approaches (Fig. 3) [44]. Currently, the most promising targets are isocitrate dehydrogenase 1/2 (*IDH1/2*) mutants and fusions of the fibroblast growth factor receptor 2 (*FGFR2*) gene mutations, which are the two most common genetic alterations seen in intrahepatic CCA. Mutations in IDH1 and IDH2 were first discovered using NGS and are observed in about 20–25% of iCCA [44, 45]. Ivosidenib (AG-120) is a first-in-class oral small-molecule inhibitor of the mutant IDH1 protein. In the phase III randomized ClarIDHy trial, a significantly longer median PFS was observed in the ivosidenib arm than in the placebo arm (2.7 vs 1.4 months, $p < 0.001$) [46]. In the recently reported mature data, the median OS adjusted for time-adjusted rank preservation structural failure was 10.3 months for ivosidenib and 5.1 months for placebo (HR = 0.49, $p < 0.0001$) [47].

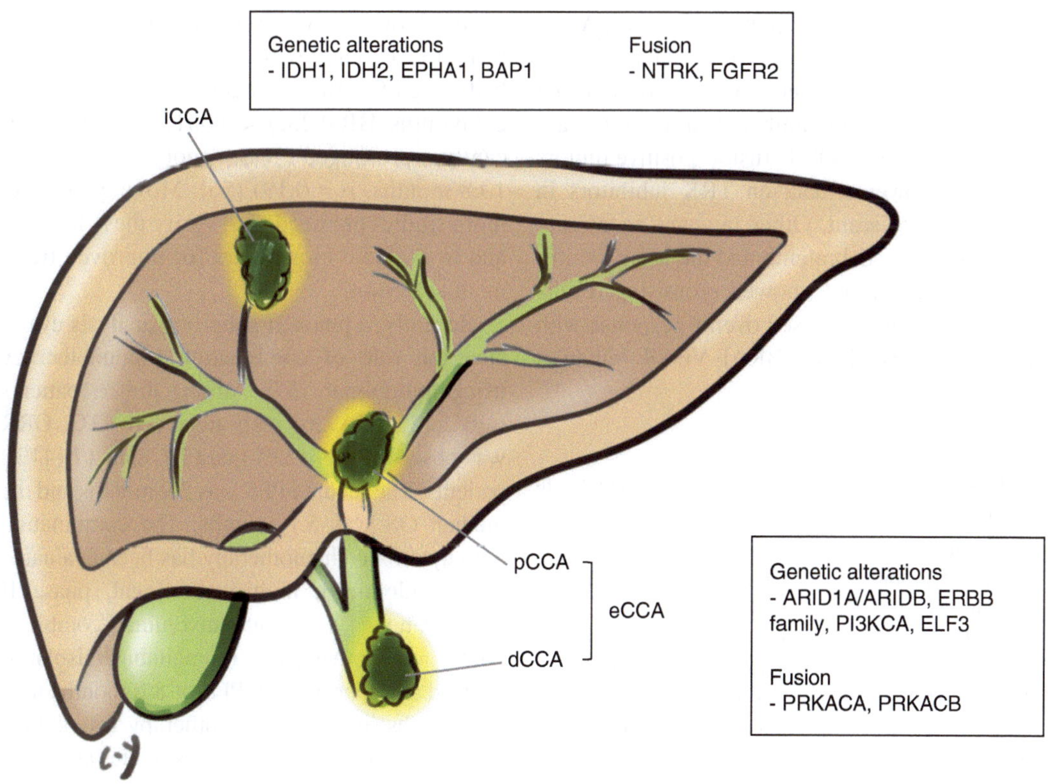

Fig. 3 Representative molecular and epigenomic landscape of cholangiocarcinoma

The second actionable mutation among CCA genes is fusions involving FGFR2, which have been reported in 10–20% of iCCA patients [44]. Based on the results of a phase II study (FIGHT-202), pemigatinib (BGJ398) recently became the first molecularly targeted agent approved by the US Food and Drug Administration to treat CCA patients, specifically for patients with FGFR2 fusion or rearrangement [20]. The pan-FGFR inhibitor infigratinib (BGJ398) was also shown to be effective in a phase II study with CCA patients. The objective response rate was 23.1%, and the median PFS and OS were 7.3 months and 12.2 months, respectively [48, 49]. A phase III clinical trial comparing infigratinib with Gem-Cis is ongoing in the first-line treatment of patients with locally advanced/metastatic CCA and FGFR2 fusion/rearrangement (NCT03773302). Other targeted agents and their corresponding gene mutations are summarized in Table 4.

Neurotrophic tropomyosin receptor kinase (NTRK) gene fusions are rare oncogenic drivers in solid tumors, and the prevalence in CCA has been reported less than 1% [50]. These alterations are actionable since two small-molecule TRK inhibitors (entrectinib and larotrectinib) are clinically active in NTRK fusion-positive tumors [50, 51]. However, data on TRK inhibitors in CCA are very scant. Other targeted agents are BRAF inhibitor dabrafenib and the MEK inhibitor trametinib, which showed promising results of an investigator-assessed overall response with 51% in patients with the BRAF V600E mutation [52].

Table 4 Molecular mutation and targeted therapies in cholangiocarcinomas

NTRK (gene fusion)	Entrectinib, larotrectinib
FGFR1–3 (fusion/rearrangement)	Pemigatinib, infigratinib, futibatinib
IDH1, IDH2	Ivosidenib, enasidenib
HER2	Trastuzumab emtansine
ROS1 (fusion)	Ceritinib, entrectinib
MEK	Selumetinib, trametinib
BRAF	Vemurafenib, dabrafenib
MET	Tivantinib
VEGFR	Ramucirumab

Immunotherapy

Immunotherapy has revolutionized the treatment landscape of many different types of cancer, and studies are currently being explored investigating the role of this strategy in CCA. In 2017, pembrolizumab, a monoclonal antibody directed against the programmed death-1 receptor (PD-1), was approved to treat solid tumors with high microsatellite instability (MSI-H). The phase 1b KEYNOTE-028 trial included 24 patients with PD-L1-positive BTC but negative for MSI-H [53, 54]. The reported ORR was 13% and the median OS and PFS were 6.2 and 1.8 months, respectively. In the larger phase II Keynote-158 trial, ORR was 5.8%, and the median OS and PFS were 7.4 and 2 months [55]. Pembrolizumab provided durable antitumor activity regardless of PD-L1 expression and manageable toxicity. Another PD-1 inhibitor available in CCA is nivolumab. It showed a median PFS of 3.7 months and a median OS of 14.2 months. Interestingly, there appeared to be a correlation between PD-L1 positivity and response. Patients with PD-L1-positive tumors had significantly longer PFS (10.4 vs 2.3 months, HR 0.23, $p < 0.001$) and nonsignificantly prolonged OS (not reached vs 10.8 months, $p = 0.19$) [56]. Moving forward, more studies are needed to verify these findings and to evaluate biomarkers for improved treatment selection.

Recently, a phase II subgroup analysis evaluated the role of combination immunotherapy using ipilimumab [57]. Among the 39 patients (GBC 13, CCA 26) with advanced BTC, ORR was observed in 9 (23%) and DCR in 17 (44%) patients. The median PFS was 2.9 months and the median OS was 5.7 months. The combination with cytotoxic chemotherapy has been evaluated in a randomized, multi-institutional, phase II study. Among 71 patients, nivolumab combined with chemotherapy (gemcitabine/cisplatin) showed a longer median PFS of 8.8 months than 4.1 months in dual immunotherapy (nivolumab and ipilimumab) although OS estimates are pending maturity [58]. A third immune checkpoint inhibitor under evaluation in CCA is the PD-L1 inhibitor durvalumab. In a phase II trial, Oh et al. assessed Gem/cis plus durvalumab and/or CTLA-4 inhibitor tremelimumab in patients with chemo-naïve BTC [59]. The addition of immunotherapy to chemotherapy was tolerable and showed very promising efficacy with ORR 50–73.4%, median PFS 11 to 13 months, and median OS 15–20.7 months.

Conclusion

CCA is an aggressive malignancy with a poor prognosis and is usually categorized by cross-sectional imaging. The TNM staging system of the AJCC eighth Edition is mainly used based on anatomical staging. Surgical intervention combined with adjuvant or neoadjuvant therapies is the only potentially curative treatment option for CCA. Liver transplantation may be considered in highly selected patients. Most patients are diagnosed in an unresectable advanced stage and palliative chemotherapy is considered the main treatment. The combination of cisplatin and gemcitabine has still been the standard treatment for patients in good general condition. Although there is currently no clear evidence on second-line treatment, the FOLFOX regimen is currently used considering the recently published randomized controlled trials. New emerging molecular targeted therapies and immunotherapies are being investigated in various studies and have shown some promise. Research that continuously discovers and applies new targets is needed to improve the prognosis of patients with biliary tract cancer.

References

1. Yamasaki S. Intrahepatic cholangiocarcinoma: macroscopic type and stage classification. J Hepatobiliary Pancreat Surg. 2003;10:288–91.
2. Bagante F, Weiss M, Alexandrescu S, Marques HP, Aldrighetti L, Maithel SK, et al. Long-term outcomes of patients with intraductal growth sub-type of intrahepatic cholangiocarcinoma. HPB (Oxford). 2018;20:1189–97.
3. Mavros MN, Economopoulos KP, Alexiou VG, Pawlik TM. Treatment and prognosis for patients with intrahepatic cholangiocarcinoma: systematic review and meta-analysis. JAMA Surg. 2014;149:565–74.
4. Lee AJ, Chun YS. Intrahepatic cholangiocarcinoma: the AJCC/UICC 8th edition updates. Chin Clin Oncol. 2018;7:6.
5. Lei H-J, Shyr Y-M, Hsia C-Y, Chen M-H, Huang Y-H, Chau G-Y. Surgical management of intrahepatic cholangiocarcinoma: a narrative review. Dig Med Res. 2021;4:4.
6. Zhang W, Yan L-N. Perihilar cholangiocarcinoma: current therapy. World J Gastrointest Pathophysiol. 2014;5:344–54.
7. Klatskin G. Adenocarcinoma of the hepatic duct at its bifurcation within the porta hepatis. An unusual tumor with distinctive clinical and pathological features. Am J Med. 1965;38:241–56.
8. Bismuth H, Corlette MB. Intrahepatic cholangioenteric anastomosis in carcinoma of the hilus of the liver. Surg Gynecol Obstet. 1975;140:170–8.
9. Ebata T, Kosuge T, Hirano S, Unno M, Yamamoto M, Miyazaki M, et al. Proposal to modify the International Union against Cancer staging system for perihilar cholangiocarcinomas. Br J Surg. 2014;101:79–88.
10. Bagante F, Tran T, Spolverato G, Ruzzenente A, Buttner S, Ethun CG, et al. Perihilar cholangiocarcinoma: number of nodes examined and optimal lymph node prognostic scheme. J Am Coll Surg. 2016;222:750–759.e2.
11. Buettner S, van Vugt JLA, Gaspersz MP, Coelen RJS, Roos E, Labeur TA, et al. Survival after resection of perihilar cholangiocarcinoma in patients with lymph node metastases. HPB. 2017;19:735–40.
12. Jun SY, Sung YN, Lee JH, Park KM, Lee YJ, Hong SM. Validation of the eighth American Joint Committee on cancer staging system for distal bile duct carcinoma. Cancer Res Treat. 2019;51:98–111.
13. Mansour JC, Aloia TA, Crane CH, Heimbach JK, Nagino M, Vauthey JN. Hilar cholangiocarcinoma: expert consensus statement. HPB (Oxford). 2015;17:691–9.
14. Sano T, Shimizu Y, Senda Y, Kinoshita T, Nimura Y. Assessing resectability in cholangiocarcinoma. Hepat Oncol. 2014;1:39–51.
15. Khan AS, Dageforde LA. Cholangiocarcinoma. Surg Clin North Am. 2019;99:315–35.
16. Rahbari NN, Garden OJ, Padbury R, Brooke-Smith M, Crawford M, Adam R, et al. Posthepatectomy liver failure: a definition and grading by the International Study Group of Liver Surgery (ISGLS). Surgery. 2011;149:713–24.
17. Meyer CG, Penn I, James L. Liver transplantation for cholangiocarcinoma: results in 207 patients. Transplantation. 2000;69:1633–7.
18. Rea DJ, Heimbach JK, Rosen CB, Haddock MG, Alberts SR, Kremers WK, et al. Liver transplantation with neoadjuvant chemoradiation is more effective than resection for hilar cholangiocarcinoma. Ann Surg. 2005;242:451–61.
19. Rosen CB, Heimbach JK, Gores GJ. Liver transplantation for cholangiocarcinoma. Transpl Int. 2010;23:692–7.
20. Abou-Alfa GK, Sahai V, Hollebecque A, Vaccaro G, Melisi D, Al-Rajabi R, et al. Pemigatinib for previ-

ously treated, locally advanced or metastatic cholangiocarcinoma: a multicentre, open-label, phase 2 study. Lancet Oncol. 2020;21:671–84.
21. Primrose JN, Fox RP, Palmer DH, Malik HZ, Prasad R, Mirza D, et al. Capecitabine compared with observation in resected biliary tract cancer (BILCAP): a randomised, controlled, multicentre, phase 3 study. Lancet Oncol. 2019;20:663–73.
22. Shroff RT, Kennedy EB, Bachini M, Bekaii-Saab T, Crane C, Edeline J, et al. Adjuvant therapy for resected biliary tract cancer: ASCO clinical practice guideline. J Clin Oncol. 2019;37:1015–27.
23. Ben-Josef E, Guthrie KA, El-Khoueiry AB, Corless CL, Zalupski MM, Lowy AM, et al. SWOG S0809: a phase II intergroup trial of adjuvant capecitabine and gemcitabine followed by radiotherapy and concurrent capecitabine in extrahepatic cholangiocarcinoma and gallbladder carcinoma. J Clin Oncol. 2015;33:2617–22.
24. Eckel F, Schmid RM. Chemotherapy in advanced biliary tract carcinoma: a pooled analysis of clinical trials. Br J Cancer. 2007;96:896–902.
25. Valle J, Wasan H, Palmer DH, Cunningham D, Anthoney A, Maraveyas A, et al. Cisplatin plus gemcitabine versus gemcitabine for biliary tract cancer. N Engl J Med. 2010;362:1273–81.
26. Okusaka T, Nakachi K, Fukutomi A, Mizuno N, Ohkawa S, Funakoshi A, et al. Gemcitabine alone or in combination with cisplatin in patients with biliary tract cancer: a comparative multicentre study in Japan. Br J Cancer. 2010;103:469–74.
27. Mizusawa J, Morizane C, Okusaka T, Katayama H, Ishii H, Fukuda H, et al. Randomized phase III study of gemcitabine plus S-1 versus gemcitabine plus cisplatin in advanced biliary tract cancer: Japan Clinical Oncology Group Study (JCOG1113, FUGA-BT). Jpn J Clin Oncol. 2016;46:385–8.
28. Kim ST, Kang JH, Lee J, Lee HW, Oh SY, Jang JS, et al. Capecitabine plus oxaliplatin versus gemcitabine plus oxaliplatin as first-line therapy for advanced biliary tract cancers: a multicenter, open-label, randomized, phase III, noninferiority trial. Ann Oncol. 2019;30:788–95.
29. Sahai V, Catalano PJ, Zalupski MM, Lubner SJ, Menge MR, Nimeiri HS, et al. Nab-paclitaxel and gemcitabine as first-line treatment of advanced or metastatic cholangiocarcinoma: a phase 2 clinical trial. JAMA Oncol. 2018;4:1707–12.
30. Shroff RT, Javle MM, Xiao L, Kaseb AO, Varadhachary GR, Wolff RA, et al. Gemcitabine, cisplatin, and nab-paclitaxel for the treatment of advanced biliary tract cancers: a phase 2 clinical trial. JAMA Oncol. 2019;5:824–30.
31. Chen JS, Jan YY, Lin YC, Wang HM, Chang WC, Liau CT. Weekly 24 h infusion of high-dose 5-fluorouracil and leucovorin in patients with biliary tract carcinomas. Anticancer Drugs. 1998;9:393–7.
32. Choi CW, Choi IK, Seo JH, Kim BS, Kim JS, Kim CD, et al. Effects of 5-fluorouracil and leucovorin in the treatment of pancreatic-biliary tract adenocarcinomas. Am J Clin Oncol. 2000;23:425–8.
33. Takada T, Kato H, Matsushiro T, Nimura Y, Nagakawa T, Nakayama T. Comparison of 5-fluorouracil, doxorubicin and mitomycin C with 5-fluorouracil alone in the treatment of pancreatic-biliary carcinomas. Oncology. 1994;51:396–400.
34. Lamarca A, Hubner RA, David Ryder W, Valle JW. Second-line chemotherapy in advanced biliary cancer: a systematic review. Ann Oncol. 2014;25:2328–38.
35. Lamarca A, Palmer DH, Wasan HS, Ross PJ, Ma YT, Arora A, et al. Second-line FOLFOX chemotherapy versus active symptom control for advanced biliary tract cancer (ABC-06): a phase 3, open-label, randomised, controlled trial. Lancet Oncol. 2021;22:690–701.
36. Yoo C, Kim K-P, Kim I, Kang MJ, Cheon J, Kang BW, et al. Liposomal irinotecan (nal-IRI) in combination with fluorouracil (5-FU) and leucovorin (LV) for patients with metastatic biliary tract cancer (BTC) after progression on gemcitabine plus cisplatin (GemCis): multicenter comparative randomized phase 2b study (NIFTY). J Clin Oncol. 2021;39:4006.
37. Lamarca A, Ross P, Wasan HS, Hubner RA, McNamara MG, Lopes A, et al. Advanced intrahepatic cholangiocarcinoma: post hoc analysis of the ABC-01, -02, and -03 clinical trials. J Natl Cancer Inst. 2020;112:200–10.
38. Valle JW, Borbath I, Khan SA, Huguet F, Gruenberger T, Arnold D. Biliary cancer: ESMO Clinical Practice Guidelines for diagnosis, treatment and follow-up. Ann Oncol. 2016;27:v28–37.
39. Gkika E, Hawkins MA, Grosu A-L, Brunner TB. The evolving role of radiation therapy in the treatment of biliary tract cancer. Front Oncol. 2020;10:604387.
40. Tao R, Krishnan S, Bhosale PR, Javle MM, Aloia TA, Shroff RT, et al. Ablative radiotherapy doses lead to a substantial prolongation of survival in patients with inoperable intrahepatic cholangiocarcinoma: a retrospective dose response analysis. J Clin Oncol. 2016;34:219–26.
41. Gkika E, Hallauer L, Kirste S, Adebahr S, Bartl N, Neeff HP, et al. Stereotactic body radiotherapy (SBRT) for locally advanced intrahepatic and extrahepatic cholangiocarcinoma. BMC Cancer. 2017;17:781.
42. Brunner TB, Blanck O, Lewitzki V, Abbasi-Senger N, Momm F, Riesterer O, et al. Stereotactic body radiotherapy dose and its impact on local control and overall survival of patients for locally advanced intrahepatic and extrahepatic cholangiocarcinoma. Radiother Oncol. 2019;132:42–7.
43. Frakulli R, Buwenge M, Macchia G, Cammelli S, Deodato F, Cilla S, et al. Stereotactic body radiation therapy in cholangiocarcinoma: a systematic review. Br J Radiol. 2019;92:20180688.
44. Valle JW, Lamarca A, Goyal L, Barriuso J, Zhu AX. New horizons for precision medicine in biliary tract cancers. Cancer Discov. 2017;7:943–62.
45. Jusakul A, Cutcutache I, Yong CH, Lim JQ, Huang MN, Padmanabhan N, et al. Whole-genome and epigenomic landscapes of etiologically distinct

subtypes of cholangiocarcinoma. Cancer Discov. 2017;7:1116–35.
46. Abou-Alfa GK, Macarulla T, Javle MM, Kelley RK, Lubner SJ, Adeva J, et al. Ivosidenib in IDH1-mutant, chemotherapy-refractory cholangiocarcinoma (ClarIDHy): a multicentre, randomised, double-blind, placebo-controlled, phase 3 study. Lancet Oncol. 2020;21:796–807.
47. Zhu AX, Macarulla T, Javle MM, Kelley RK, Lubner SJ, Adeva J, et al. Final results from ClarIDHy, a global, phase III, randomized, double-blind study of ivosidenib (IVO) versus placebo (PBO) in patients (pts) with previously treated cholangiocarcinoma (CCA) and an isocitrate dehydrogenase 1 (IDH1) mutation. J Clin Oncol. 2021;39:266.
48. Javle M, Lowery M, Shroff RT, Weiss KH, Springfeld C, Borad MJ, et al. Phase II study of BGJ398 in patients with FGFR-altered advanced cholangiocarcinoma. J Clin Oncol. 2018;36:276–82.
49. Javle MM, Roychowdhury S, Kelley RK, Sadeghi S, Macarulla T, Waldschmidt DT, et al. Final results from a phase II study of infigratinib (BGJ398), an FGFR-selective tyrosine kinase inhibitor, in patients with previously treated advanced cholangiocarcinoma harboring an FGFR2 gene fusion or rearrangement. J Clin Oncol. 2021;39:265.
50. Westphalen CB, Krebs MG, Le Tourneau C, Sokol ES, Maund SL, Wilson TR, et al. Genomic context of NTRK1/2/3 fusion-positive tumours from a large real-world population. NPJ Precis Oncol. 2021;5(1):69.
51. Drilon A, Laetsch TW, Kummar S, DuBois SG, Lassen UN, Demetri GD, et al. Efficacy of larotrectinib in TRK fusion-positive cancers in adults and children. N Engl J Med. 2018;378(8):731–9.
52. Menichincheri M, Ardini E, Magnaghi P, Avanzi N, Banfi P, Bossi R, et al. Discovery of entrectinib: a new 3-aminoindazole as a potent anaplastic lymphoma kinase (ALK), c-ROS oncogene 1 kinase (ROS1), and Pan-tropomyosin receptor kinases (Pan-TRKs) inhibitor. J Med Chem. 2016;59(7):3392–408.
53. Bang Y-J, Ueno M, Malka D, Chung HC, Nagrial A, Kelley RK, et al. Pembrolizumab (pembro) for advanced biliary adenocarcinoma: results from the KEYNOTE-028 (KN028) and KEYNOTE-158 (KN158) basket studies. J Clin Oncol. 2019;37:4079.
54. Piha-Paul SA, Oh DY, Ueno M, Malka D, Chung HC, Nagrial A, et al. Efficacy and safety of pembrolizumab for the treatment of advanced biliary cancer: results from the KEYNOTE-158 and KEYNOTE-028 studies. Int J Cancer. 2020;147:2190–8.
55. Ueno M, Chung HC, Nagrial A, Marabelle A, Kelley RK, Xu L, et al. Pembrolizumab for advanced biliary adenocarcinoma: results from the multicohort, phase II KEYNOTE-158 study. Ann Oncol. 2018;29:viii210.
56. Kim RD, Kim DW, Alese OB, Li D, Shah N, Schell MJ, et al. A phase II study of nivolumab in patients with advanced refractory biliary tract cancers (BTC). J Clin Oncol. 2019;37:4097.
57. Klein O, Kee D, Nagrial A, Markman B, Underhill C, Michael M, et al. Evaluation of combination nivolumab and ipilimumab immunotherapy in patients with advanced biliary tract cancers: subgroup analysis of a phase 2 nonrandomized clinical trial. JAMA Oncol. 2020;6:1405–9.
58. Sahai V, Griffith KA, Beg MS, Shaib WL, Mahalingam D, Zhen DB, et al. A multicenter randomized phase II study of nivolumab in combination with gemcitabine/cisplatin or ipilimumab as first-line therapy for patients with advanced unresectable biliary tract cancer (BilT-01). J Clin Oncol. 2020;38:4582.
59. Oh D-Y, Lee K-H, Lee D-W, Kim TY, Bang J-H, Nam A-R, et al. Phase II study assessing tolerability, efficacy, and biomarkers for durvalumab (D) ± tremelimumab (T) and gemcitabine/cisplatin (GemCis) in chemo-naïve advanced biliary tract cancer (aBTC). J Clin Oncol. 2020;38:4520.

Part IX

Gallbladder Cancer

Epidemiology and Etiology

Key Points

- Gallbladder cancer is known as the most common but aggressive biliary tract cancer.
- Gallbladder cancer ranks 23rd in incidence and is the 20th most deadly cancer worldwide, and the countries with the highest incidence and mortality are located in South America and Asia.
- Gallbladder cancer is one of the few gastrointestinal cancers that is more common in women.
- The etiology of gallbladder cancer is complex and multifactorial: demographic factors, genetics, gallbladder pathology, infection, environmental exposure, anatomical factor, and obesity.

Introduction

The gallbladder is a small, pear-shaped muscular sac located in front of the duodenum and beneath the liver. It temporarily stores the bile that is produced by the liver and aids the digestion of lipids. Gallbladder cancer (GBC) was first described by Maxmillan de Stol in 1777 and has been known as the most common but aggressive biliary cancer with the shortest median survival [1, 2]. In this chapter, we discuss the epidemiology and etiology of GBC.

Epidemiology

Incidence and Mortality

GBC ranks 23rd in terms of cancer incidence and is the 20th most deadly cancer worldwide [3]. In 2020, 115,949 new cases of GBC were diagnosed, representing 0.6% of total cancer deaths, and 84,695 new GBC deaths were reported, representing 0.9% of total cancer deaths [4]. Although the incidence and mortality of GBC are increasing gradually worldwide, the incidence and mortality ranking of GBC among cancers has dropped, as other cancers have increased more rapidly (Fig. 1). Increased cases of cholecystectomy for gallbladder infections and polyps may be a partial explanation for the decrease in the incidence of GBC, but more

Seong Ji Choi and Jai Hoon Yoon are the lead authors of this chapter.

H. J. Chun et al., *Gastrointestinal Cancer*, https://doi.org/10.1007/978-981-99-0815-8_55

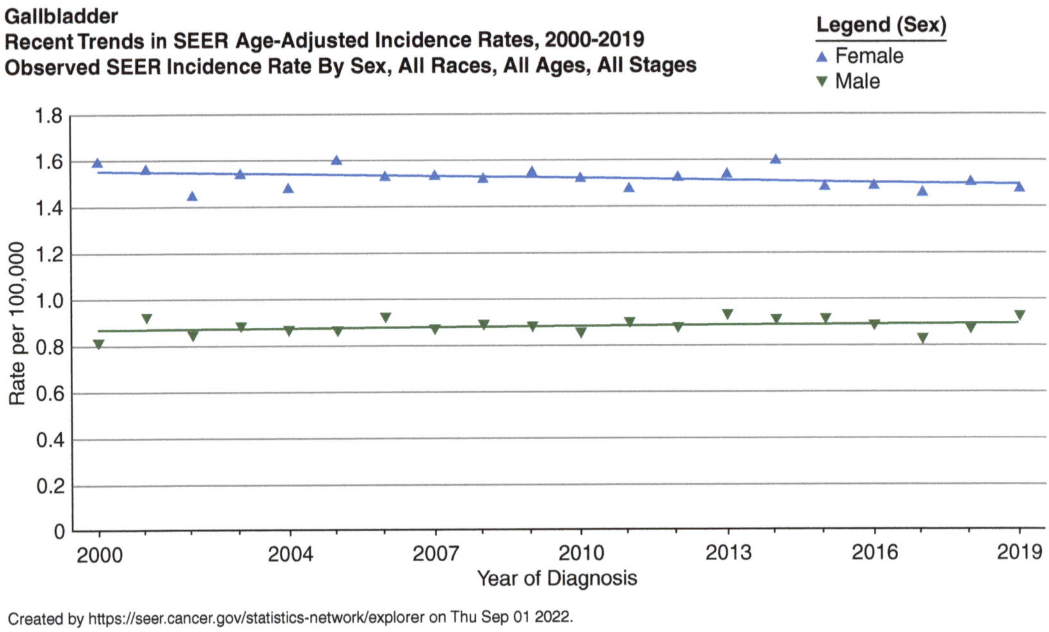

Fig. 1 Recent trends of gallbladder cancer in age-adjusted rates in the USA, 2000–2019

studies are needed to clarify its etiology [5]. However, GBC is a lethal malignancy with an average 5-year survival rate of 28.8% [6]. Although 5-year survival rates range from 2 to 65%, the 5-year survival rate of GBC is relatively low due to the fact that it is often diagnosed in an advanced stage due to its vague symptom or clinical presentation.

Age and Sex

The incidence of GBC tends to increase with age, and most GBC occurs in patients in the sixth and seventh decades of life [7]. Research from the USA showed that age-adjusted incidence rates per 100,000 were 0.2, 1.6, and 4.3 for those aged 20–49 years, 50–64 years, and 65–74 years, respectively [8]. GBC is the 23rd most common cancer in men and the 20th most common cancer in women worldwide. There are only a few gastrointestinal cancers that are more common in women than in men, including anal cancer and GBC. Even after considering the difference in life expectancy between men and women, the cumulative risk of GBC from birth to age 74 is higher in women (0.16%) than in men (0.10%) [3].

Geographical Location

Figure 2 shows the estimated age-standardized incidence rates of GBC worldwide, and the countries with the highest incidence and mortality are in South America and Asia. The top five countries with the highest estimated age-standardized incidence rate per 100,000 include Bolivia (8.5), Chile (5.6), Bangladesh (4.9), Nepal (4.1), and the Republic of Korea (2.9). Top five countries with the highest estimated age-standardized mortality rate per 100,000 are also Bolivia (5.8), Bangladesh (3.9), Chile (3.5), Nepal (3.1), and the Republic of Korea (2.3). Differences in geographical incidence are considered due to differences in environmental exposure and genetic predisposition in relation to carcinogenesis [9]. In addition, countries with a good healthcare system are reported to show a low mortality-to-incidence ratio [10].

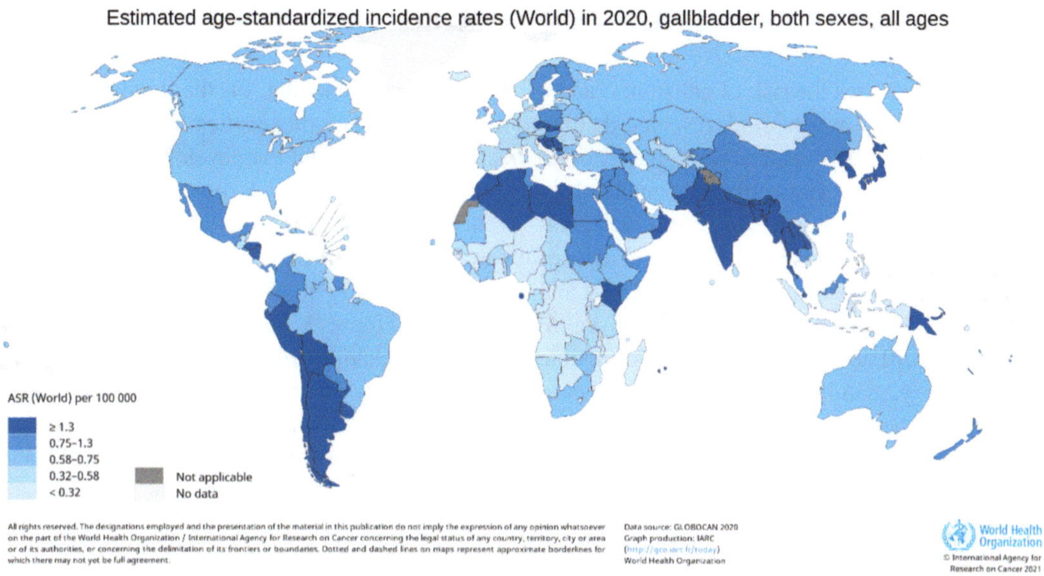

Fig. 2 Global map showing the estimated age-standardized incidence rates of GBC in 2020, gallbladder, both sexes [3]

Etiology

It is difficult to simplify the etiology of GBC because it is complex and multifactorial. Although the carcinogenesis of the gallbladder has not yet been revealed, chronic inflammation is accepted as the most common causative factor for GBC, according to evidence that many other cancers develop from chronic inflammation [11–13]. Many risk factors cause GBC by inducing chronic gallbladder inflammation, and their histopathological and molecular mechanisms have begun to be elucidated [14]. The risk factors for GBC can be categorized into seven groups (Table 1).

Table 1 Etiological factors for gallbladder cancer

Category	Factors
Demography	Advanced age, female sex, geography, ethnicity, low socioeconomic state, obesity
Genetics	Genetic alterations
Gallbladder pathology	Gallstone, gallbladder polyp, porcelain gallbladder, primary sclerosing cholangitis
Infection	*Salmonella*, *Helicobacter*
Environmental exposure	Smoking, alcohol consumption, heavy metals, and drugs
Anatomy	Anomalous pancreaticobiliary duct junction, congenital biliary cyst

Demographic Factors

Advanced age is the most important risk factor for cancer, and GBC is not an exception. It is generally accepted that old people tend to be exposed to a harmful environment and experience a decline in the immune system that aids in the development of cancer [15]. GBC is more common in women worldwide and occurs 2–6 times more often than males [16]. The reason for the difference in incidence between sexes is unclear, but it may be explained by the higher incidence of gallstone, one of the main risk factors for GBC, in females or the higher incidence of GBC in females with multiparity and first pregnancy at an early age [17, 18]. Geographical locations with a high incidence of GBC vary, and with a tendency for higher incidence in indigenous populations, including Mapuche Indians, Native Americans, northern Indian women, Pakistani women, and Korean men [16]. There are several reports that show the association between low socioeconomic status and GBC, and a combination of factors such as malnutrition, micronutrient deficiencies, decreased diet oxidants, poor hygiene, and susceptibility to infection may play a role [19, 20].

Obesity increases the risk of gallstones, and a meta-analysis by Larsson et al. revealed that the risks of GBC are 15% and 66% higher in overweight and obese, respectively, compared to normal-weight individuals [21]. Another meta-analysis by Li et al. assessed the association of overweight and obesity with the risk of GBC, and the risk of GBC increased by 4% for 1 kg/m^2 increase in BMI above 25 kg/m^2 [22]. A possible biological explanation is an increase in the concentration of hormones such as estrogen or insulin in an obese patient [8].

Genetics

As our understanding of the human genome deepens, the role of genetics in GBC has been actively studied, and the development of a high-throughput approach has opened a new era of genetic research. It is widely accepted that GBC carcinogenesis involved multiple alterations in genes, such as *TP53, KRAS, BRAF,* and *PIK3CA* [23, 24]. Figure 3 summarizes the sequential molecular changes in the pathogenesis of gallbladder cancer. Recently, Sharayu et al. revealed that GBC has a strong association with chromosome 7q21.12, which contains the ABCB1 and

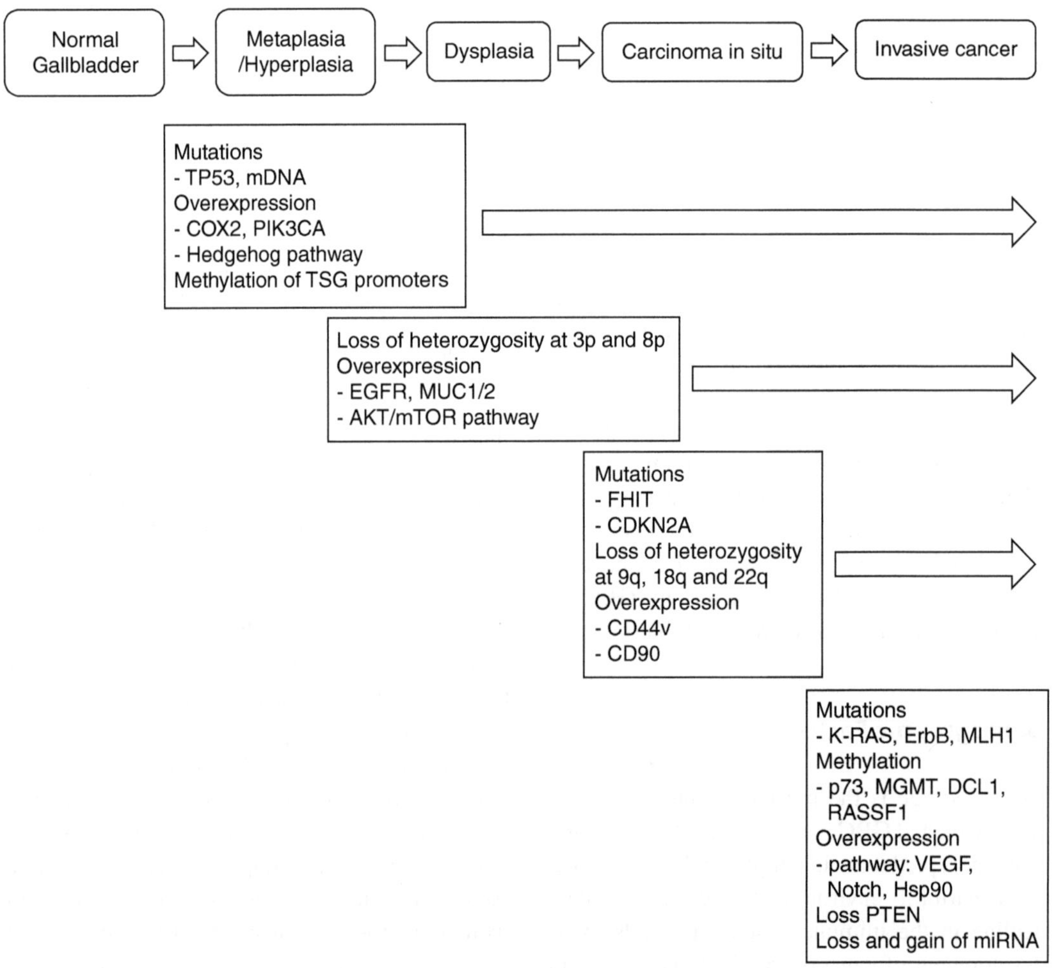

Fig. 3 Sequential morphological and molecular changes in the pathogenesis of gallbladder cancer. *COX-2* cyclooxygenase type II, *TSG* tumor suppressor genes, *MSI* microsatellite instability, *LOH* loss of heterozygosity, *FHIT* fragile histidine triad gene (adapted from Sharma et al. [25], Barreto et al. [26])

ABCB4 ATP binding cassette subfamily B genes, and estimated that their data could explain 23% of the variation in risk of GBC [27].

Gallbladder Pathology

Gallstone

Gallstone (Fig. 4a) is one of the most important risk factors for GBC. A higher incidence of GBC is associated with underlying conditions that cause chronic inflammation of the gallbladder, and 70–90% of GBC cases are accompanied by gallstones [28, 29]. Not only is the presence of gallstone important, but the increase in the size of gallstone also shows a correlation with the risk of GBC (Table 2). Diehl et al. reported that odds ratios (OR) for GBC were 2.4 and 10.1 for the gallstone sized 2.0–2.9 cm and ≥3.0 cm, respectively [35]. Lowenfels et al. also reported that the relative risk for the patients with gallstones ≥3.0 cm was 9.2, compared to patients with gallstones <1.0 cm [36]. Andrea et al. reported that odds ratios (OR) for GBC were 10.1 for the gallstone ≥3.0 cm [37]. Although gallstone is an important risk factor for GBC, the incidence of GBC in patients with gallstones is reported to be 0.59% [38].

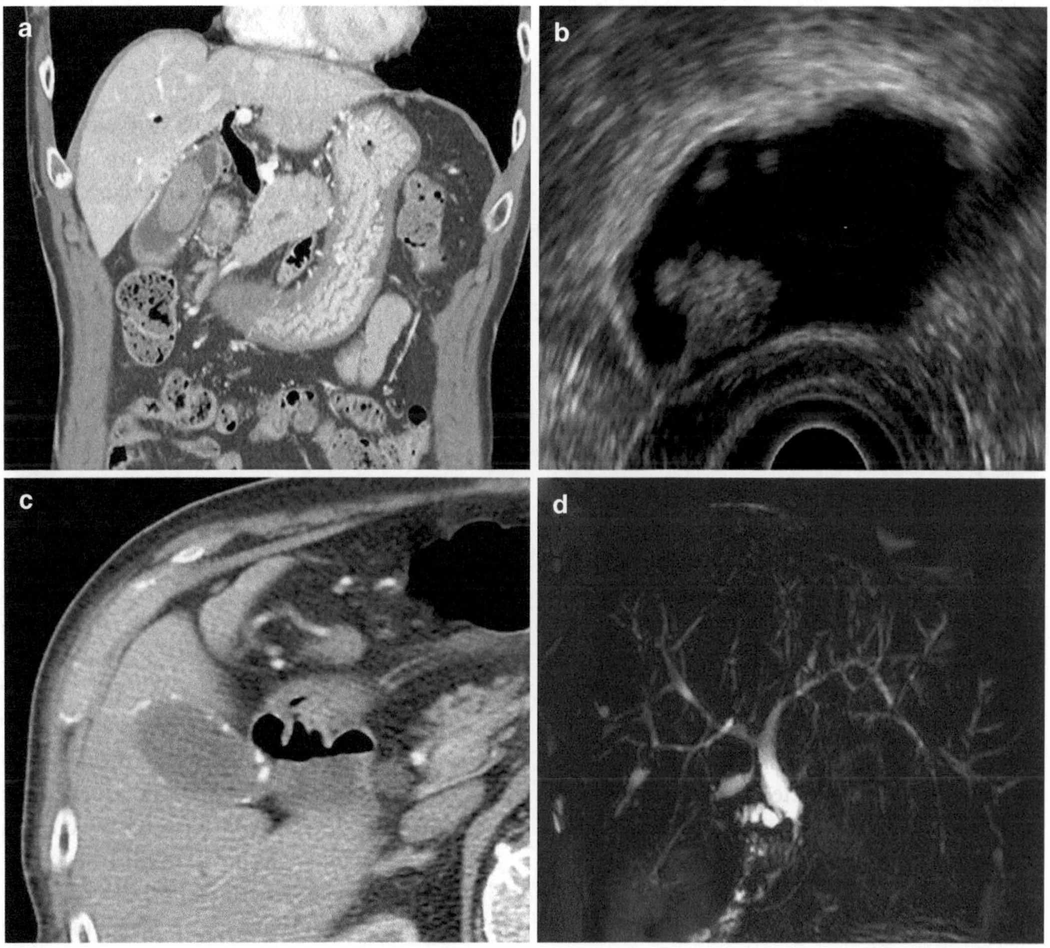

Fig. 4 Images of gallbladder pathology. (**a**) Coronal image of abdominal computed tomography showing a large gallstone in the gallbladder. (**b**) Multiple gallbladder polyps, identified in the image of endoscopic ultrasound. (**c**) Transverse image of abdominal computed tomography showing calcium encrustation on the wall of the gallbladder, suggesting a porcelain gallbladder. (**d**) Image of magnetic resonance cholangiopancreatography showing multiple strictures and beads in the intrahepatic bile duct, suggesting primary sclerosing cholangitis

Table 2 Relative risk of factors related to gallstones for gallbladder cancer [30]

Risk factor	Relative risk	References
Presence of gallstone	3.01–23.8	[29, 31–34]
Size of gallstones		
2.0–2.9 cm	24	[35]
>3.0 cm	9.2–10.1	[36]
Duration of gallstones		
5–19 years of age	4.9	[33]
>20 years	6.0	

Gallbladder Polyp

A gallbladder polyp (Fig. 3b) is a small protrusion of tissue that grows from the lining of the gallbladder and occurs in 1.5–9.9% of the general population. It is usually found incidentally during abdominal imaging studies [39–41]. Gallbladder polyps can be divided into benign and malignant lesion. A benign gallbladder polyp can be classified into neoplastic (ex) cholesterol polyp, adenomyoma, and inflammatory polyp and nonneoplastic (ex) adenoma, fibroma, lipoma, and leiomyoma, and most polyps (up to 90%) are nonneoplastic and are sometimes called pseudopolyps [42].

A benign gallbladder adenoma constitutes about 4% of gallbladder polyps. Unlike colon polyps that follow the adenoma-carcinoma sequence, it is unclear whether GBC develops from gallbladder adenoma [16]. The risk factors for GBC from gallbladder polyps are size (>1 cm), primary sclerosing cholangitis (PSC), sessile morphology, and advanced age (>50 years) [43]. As the size of the gallbladder polyp increases, the incidence of GBC also increases [44, 45]. Malignancy has been reported to be significantly elevated in polyp >1 cm, so cholecystectomy is considered in patients with gallbladder polyp >1 cm [46]. Benign polyps and gallstones are detected in symptomatic patients, but are not associated with asymptomatic patients [39, 47].

Porcelain Gallbladder

The porcelain gallbladder (Fig. 3c) is a rare entity characterized by extensive calcium encrustation of the gallbladder wall and is described as calcified gallbladder, calcifying cholecystitis, and calcarea of chronic cholecystopathia in the literature [48]. Although studies in the mid-1920s suggested a definite correlation between the porcelain gallbladder and GBC, recent studies revealed that the incidence of GBC in the presence of the porcelain gallbladder is 2–6% [49, 50]. The treatment of choice for the porcelain gallbladder is cholecystectomy.

Primary Sclerosing Cholangitis

PSC (Fig. 3d) is a rare cholestatic disease of the liver characterized by progressive chronic inflammation and fibrosis of the bile ducts [51]. Patients with PSC are significantly associated with various malignancies, including cholangiocarcinoma and GBC, and nearly 50% of deaths are due to gastrointestinal cancers [52]. Two cohort studies reported a prevalence of 2.5–3.5% GBC in patients with PSC [53, 54]. Although gallbladder polyps are usually benign, gallbladder polyps in patients with PSC have a higher incidence of dysplastic or malignancy; thus, many guidelines suggest cholecystectomy in patients with gallbladder polyp >8 mm [52, 55].

Infection

Salmonella

It is generally accepted that there is a positive association between GBC and typhoidal *Salmonella typhi* and *S. paratyphi*, and several studies also suggest an association between non-typhoidal *Salmonella* and GBC [56, 57]. Scanu et al. suggested that *Salmonella* could induce cellular transformations, by *TP53* mutations, c-*MYC* amplification, and activation of MAPK and AKT pathways, which resembles the transformation observed in patients with GBC [58]. In endemic areas of *S. typhi*, most chronic carriers contain gallstones, which is an important risk factor for GBC, as previously described [59]. *S. typhi* produces a biofilm that promotes persistent infection of the gallbladder and a typhoid toxin that has carcinogenic potential, thus playing an important role in GBC carcinogenesis [60].

***Helicobacter* (*H. pylori* and *H. bilis*)**

The role of *Helicobacter* spp. in GBC carcinogenesis is still under debate. Kuroki et al. showed hyperproliferation of the biliary epithelium in the *Helicobacter*-infected state [61]. *Helicobacter* spp. have been identified in GBC, but also in extrahepatic cancers and benign biliary tract disease, such as gallstones or chronic cholecystitis [62]. Hassan et al. suggested that *H. pylori* infection aggravates the mucosal lesion of the gallbladder, including mucosal hyperplasia, metaplasia, and lymphoid infiltration that may predispose to the development of GBC [63]. However, the association of *Helicobacter* and GBC was insignificant in a meta-analysis [64].

Environmental Exposure

Different environmental exposures are associated with specific types of cancer. Environmental exposure and lifestyle factors are closely related to the risk factors for GBC that it is sometimes difficult or inability to analyze their individual risks and carcinogenesis mechanism. In addition, the results are often inconsistent among studies. However, increased risks of GBC for smoking were consistently observed and have been accepted generally [65, 66].

Environmental exposures, such as alcohol drinking [67], heavy metals (nickel, cadmium, chromium, lead, arsenic, zinc, etc.) [68, 69], radon [70], aflatoxin [71, 72], and benzene [73], have been suggested as risk factors, but more research is required. Drugs, such as methyldopa [74] and isoniazid [75], have also been suggested.

Anatomical Abnormalities

Anomalous Pancreaticobiliary Duct Junction

Anomalous pancreaticobiliary duct junction (APBDJ) is a congenital malformation in which the junction of the pancreatic duct and the common bile duct occurs outside the duodenal wall and forms a long common channel (>15 mm) [76]. It is commonly associated with various biliary and pancreatic disorders, including choledochal cyst in 80% and biliary tract cancer in 16.1–39.4% [77, 78]. Although there is a variability in the incidence of GBC between different age groups and types of union, GBC was found in 26.5% in patients with APBDJ and in patients aged ≥50 years, while no bile duct and type APBDJ in which the bile duct enters the pancreatic duct showed a higher incidence [78]. Therefore, surgical treatment is generally recommended.

Congenital Biliary Cyst

The congenital biliary cyst represents a rare congenital malformation of the biliary ductal system. It is widely accepted that cholangiocarcinoma is the most common malignancy in congenital biliary cysts, and GBC occurs in 2.5–28% of those with congenital biliary cysts [8]. Lee et al. reported 9.9% of malignant biliary tumors among patients with congenital biliary cysts, and GBC accounts for 44% [79]. Because it is closely associated with APBDJ, it is unclear whether the risk is independent of APBDJ, and a study showed a higher incidence of GBC in patients with APBDJ without dilation of the bile duct [78].

Conclusion

GBC is uncommon, but is the most common cancer among malignant biliary tract malignancies. It is a lethal malignancy with an average 5-year survival rate of 28.8%. GBC is one of the few gastrointestinal cancers that are more common in women, with a cumulative risk of 0.16% in women vs 0.10% in men. There are geographical differences in incidence, probably due to environmental exposure and genetic predisposition. The etiologies of GBC are complex and multifactorial, and we have summarized them in terms of demography, genetics, gallbladder pathology, infection, environmental exposure, and anatomy. Further research on the pathogenesis, clinical characteristics, diagnosis, and treatment of GBC will be discussed in the following chapters.

References

1. Andren-Sandberg A. Diagnosis and management of gallbladder cancer. N Am J Med Sci. 2012;4:293–9.
2. Zhu AX, Hong TS, Hezel AF, Kooby DA. Current management of gallbladder carcinoma. Oncologist. 2010;15:168–81.
3. Ferlay J EM, Lam F, Colombet M, Mery L, Piñeros M, Znaor A, Soerjomataram I, Bray F. Global cancer observatory: cancer today. International Agency for Research on Cancer. https://gco.iarc.fr/today. Accessed 1 Nov 2021.
4. Sung H, Ferlay J, Siegel RL, Laversanne M, Soerjomataram I, Jemal A, et al. Global cancer statistics 2020: GLOBOCAN estimates of incidence and mortality worldwide for 36 cancers in 185 countries. CA Cancer J Clin. 2021;71:209–49.
5. Kim BW, Oh CM, Choi HY, Park JW, Cho H, Ki M. Incidence and overall survival of biliary tract cancers in South Korea from 2006 to 2015: using the National Health Information Database. Gut Liver. 2019;13:104–13.
6. Zhu X, Zhang X, Hu X, Ren H, Wu S, Wu J, et al. Survival analysis of patients with primary gallbladder cancer from 2010 to 2015: a retrospective study based on SEER data. Medicine (Baltimore). 2020;99:e22292.
7. Lai CH, Lau WY. Gallbladder cancer—a comprehensive review. Surgeon. 2008;6:101–10.
8. Rawla P, Sunkara T, Thandra KC, Barsouk A. Epidemiology of gallbladder cancer. Clin Exp Hepatol. 2019;5:93–102.
9. Choi SJ, Kim Y, Jeon J, Gwak HJ, Kim M, Kang K, et al. Association of microbial dysbiosis with gallbladder diseases identified by bile microbiome profiling. J Korean Med Sci. 2021;36:e189.
10. Wang CC, Tsai MC, Wang SC, Peng CM, Lee HL, Chen HY, et al. Favorable gallbladder cancer mortality-to-incidence ratios of countries with good ranking of world's health system and high expenditures on health. BMC Public Health. 2019;19:1025.
11. Li Y, Zhang J, Ma H. Chronic inflammation and gallbladder cancer. Cancer Lett. 2014;345:242–8.
12. Coussens LM, Werb Z. Inflammation and cancer. Nature. 2002;420:860–7.
13. Greten FR, Grivennikov SI. Inflammation and cancer: triggers, mechanisms, and consequences. Immunity. 2019;51:27–41.
14. Liu Z, Kemp TJ, Gao YT, Corbel A, McGee EE, Roa JC, et al. Circulating levels of inflammatory proteins and survival in patients with gallbladder cancer. Sci Rep. 2018;8:5671.
15. Hong H, Wang Q, Li J, Liu H, Meng X, Zhang H. Aging, cancer and immunity. J Cancer. 2019;10:3021–7.
16. Hundal R, Shaffer EA. Gallbladder cancer: epidemiology and outcome. Clin Epidemiol. 2014;6:99–109.
17. Piehler JM, Crichlow RW. Primary carcinoma of the gallbladder. Surg Gynecol Obstet. 1978;147:929–42.
18. Randi G, Franceschi S, La Vecchia C. Gallbladder cancer worldwide: geographical distribution and risk factors. Int J Cancer. 2006;118:1591–602.
19. Serra I, Yamamoto M, Calvo A, Cavada G, Baez S, Endoh K, et al. Association of chili pepper consumption, low socioeconomic status and longstanding gallstones with gallbladder cancer in a Chilean population. Int J Cancer. 2002;102:407–11.
20. Dutta U, Nagi B, Garg PK, Sinha SK, Singh K, Tandon RK. Patients with gallstones develop gallbladder cancer at an earlier age. Eur J Cancer Prev. 2005;14:381–5.
21. Larsson SC, Wolk A. Obesity and the risk of gallbladder cancer: a meta-analysis. Br J Cancer. 2007;96:1457–61.
22. Li ZM, Wu ZX, Han B, Mao YQ, Chen HL, Han SF, et al. The association between BMI and gallbladder cancer risk: a meta-analysis. Oncotarget. 2016;7:43669–79.
23. Javle M, Rashid A, Churi C, Kar S, Zuo M, Eterovic AK, et al. Molecular characterization of gallbladder cancer using somatic mutation profiling. Hum Pathol. 2014;45:701–8.
24. Qu K, Zhang X, Cui R, Liu C. Meta-signature of mutated genes in gallbladder cancer: evidence based high throughput screening assays. Ann Transl Med. 2016;4:229.
25. Sharma A, Sharma KL, Gupta A, Yadav A, Kumar A. Gallbladder cancer epidemiology, pathogenesis and molecular genetics: recent update. World J Gastroenterol. 2017;23:3978–98.
26. Barreto SG, Dutt A, Chaudhary A. A genetic model for gallbladder carcinogenesis and its dissemination. Ann Oncol. 2014;25:1086–97.
27. Mhatre S, Wang Z, Nagrani R, Badwe R, Chiplunkar S, Mittal B, et al. Common genetic variation and risk of gallbladder cancer in India: a case-control genome-wide association study. Lancet Oncol. 2017;18:535–44.
28. Valle JW, Kelley RK, Nervi B, Oh DY, Zhu AX. Biliary tract cancer. Lancet. 2021;397:428–44.
29. Hsing AW, Gao YT, Han TQ, Rashid A, Sakoda LC, Wang BS, et al. Gallstones and the risk of biliary tract cancer: a population-based study in China. Br J Cancer. 2007;97:1577–82.
30. Stinton LM, Shaffer EA. Epidemiology of gallbladder disease: cholelithiasis and cancer. Gut Liver. 2012;6:172–87.
31. Chow WH, Johansen C, Gridley G, Mellemkjaer L, Olsen JH, Fraumeni JF Jr. Gallstones, cholecystectomy and risk of cancers of the liver, biliary tract and pancreas. Br J Cancer. 1999;79:640–4.
32. Ishiguro S, Inoue M, Kurahashi N, Iwasaki M, Sasazuki S, Tsugane S. Risk factors of biliary tract cancer in a large-scale population-based cohort study in Japan (JPHC study); with special focus on cholelithiasis, body mass index, and their effect modification. Cancer Causes Control. 2008;19:33–41.
33. Zatonski WA, La Vecchia C, Przewozniak K, Maisonneuve P, Lowenfels AB, Boyle P. Risk factors

for gallbladder cancer: a Polish case-control study. Int J Cancer. 1992;51:707–11.
34. Khan ZR, Neugut AI, Ahsan H, Chabot JA. Risk factors for biliary tract cancers. Am J Gastroenterol. 1999;94:149–52.
35. Diehl AK. Gallstone size and the risk of gallbladder cancer. JAMA. 1983;250:2323–6.
36. Lowenfels AB, Walker AM, Althaus DP, Townsend G, Domellof L. Gallstone growth, size, and risk of gallbladder cancer: an interracial study. Int J Epidemiol. 1989;18:50–4.
37. Andrea C, Enzo A. Cholesterol gallstones larger than 3 cm appear to be associated with gallbladder cancer: identification of a high risk group of patients that could benefit from preventive cholecystectomy. Ann Surg. 2016;263:e56.
38. Muszynska C, Lundgren L, Lindell G, Andersson R, Nilsson J, Sandstrom P, et al. Predictors of incidental gallbladder cancer in patients undergoing cholecystectomy for benign gallbladder disease: results from a population-based gallstone surgery registry. Surgery. 2017;162:256–63.
39. Jorgensen T, Jensen KH. Polyps in the gallbladder. A prevalence study. Scand J Gastroenterol. 1990;25:281–6.
40. Heyder N, Gunter E, Giedl J, Obenauf A, Hahn EG. [Polypoid lesions of the gallbladder]. Dtsch Med Wochenschr. 1990;115:243–247.
41. Choi YS, Do JH, Seo SW, Lee SE, Oh HC, Min YJ, et al. Prevalence and risk factors of gallbladder polypoid lesions in a healthy population. Yonsei Med J. 2016;57:1370–5.
42. Yang HL, Sun YG, Wang Z. Polypoid lesions of the gallbladder: diagnosis and indications for surgery. Br J Surg. 1992;79:227–9.
43. Lee KF, Wong J, Li JC, Lai PB. Polypoid lesions of the gallbladder. Am J Surg. 2004;188:186–90.
44. Koga A, Watanabe K, Fukuyama T, Takiguchi S, Nakayama F. Diagnosis and operative indications for polypoid lesions of the gallbladder. Arch Surg. 1988;123:26–9.
45. Ishikawa O, Ohhigashi H, Imaoka S, Nakaizumi A, Kitamura T, Sasaki Y, et al. The difference in malignancy between pedunculated and sessile polypoid lesions of the gallbladder. Am J Gastroenterol. 1989;84:1386–90.
46. Okamoto M, Okamoto H, Kitahara F, Kobayashi K, Karikome K, Miura K, et al. Ultrasonographic evidence of association of polyps and stones with gallbladder cancer. Am J Gastroenterol. 1999;94:446–50.
47. Terzi C, Sokmen S, Seckin S, Albayrak L, Ugurlu M. Polypoid lesions of the gallbladder: report of 100 cases with special reference to operative indications. Surgery. 2000;127:622–7.
48. Morimoto M, Matsuo T, Mori N. Management of porcelain gallbladder, its risk factors, and complications: a review. Diagnostics (Basel). 2021;11:1073.
49. Jones MW, Weir CB, Ferguson T. Porcelain gallbladder. Treasure Island: StatPearls; 2021.
50. Khan ZS, Livingston EH, Huerta S. Reassessing the need for prophylactic surgery in patients with porcelain gallbladder: case series and systematic review of the literature. Arch Surg. 2011;146:1143–7.
51. Silveira MG, Lindor KD. Primary sclerosing cholangitis. Can J Gastroenterol. 2008;22:689–98.
52. Fung BM, Lindor KD, Tabibian JH. Cancer risk in primary sclerosing cholangitis: epidemiology, prevention, and surveillance strategies. World J Gastroenterol. 2019;25:659–71.
53. Vazquez-Elizondo G, Mucino-Bermejo J, Mendez-Sanchez N. Gallbladder disease in patients with primary sclerosing cholangitis. Ann Hepatol. 2008;7:182–3.
54. Torabi Sagvand B, Edwards K, Shen B. Frequency, risk factors, and outcome of gallbladder polyps in patients with primary sclerosing cholangitis: a case-control study. Hepatol Commun. 2018;2:1440–5.
55. Karlsen TH, Schrumpf E, Boberg KM. Gallbladder polyps in primary sclerosing cholangitis: not so benign. Curr Opin Gastroenterol. 2008;24:395–9.
56. Iyer P, Barreto SG, Sahoo B, Chandrani P, Ramadwar MR, Shrikhande SV, et al. Non-typhoidal salmonella DNA traces in gallbladder cancer. Infect Agent Cancer. 2016;11:12.
57. Koshiol J, Wozniak A, Cook P, Adaniel C, Acevedo J, Azocar L, et al. Salmonella enterica serovar typhi and gallbladder cancer: a case-control study and meta-analysis. Cancer Med. 2016;5:3310–235.
58. Scanu T, Spaapen RM, Bakker JM, Pratap CB, Wu LE, Hofland I, et al. Salmonella manipulation of host signaling pathways provokes cellular transformation associated with gallbladder carcinoma. Cell Host Microbe. 2015;17:763–74.
59. Crawford RW, Rosales-Reyes R, Ramirez-Aguilar Mde L, Chapa-Azuela O, Alpuche-Aranda C, Gunn JS. Gallstones play a significant role in Salmonella spp. gallbladder colonization and carriage. Proc Natl Acad Sci U S A. 2010;107:4353–8.
60. Di Domenico EG, Cavallo I, Pontone M, Toma L, Ensoli F. Biofilm producing Salmonella typhi: chronic colonization and development of gallbladder cancer. Int J Mol Sci. 2017;18:1887.
61. Kuroki T, Fukuda K, Yamanouchi K, Kitajima T, Matsuzaki S, Tajima Y, et al. Helicobacter pylori accelerates the biliary epithelial cell proliferation activity in hepatolithiasis. Hepatogastroenterology. 2002;49:648–51.
62. de Martel C, Plummer M, Parsonnet J, van Doorn LJ, Franceschi S. Helicobacter species in cancers of the gallbladder and extrahepatic biliary tract. Br J Cancer. 2009;100:194–9.
63. Hassan EH, Gerges SS, El-Atrebi KA, El-Bassyouni HT. The role of H. pylori infection in gall bladder cancer: clinicopathological study. Tumour Biol. 2015;36:7093–8.
64. Cherif S, Bouriat K, Rais H, Elantri S, Amine A. *Helicobacter pylori* and biliary tract cancers: a meta-analysis. Can J Infect Dis Med Microbiol. 2020;2020:9287157.

65. Grainge MJ, West J, Solaymani-Dodaran M, Aithal GP, Card TR. The antecedents of biliary cancer: a primary care case-control study in the United Kingdom. Br J Cancer. 2009;100:178–80.
66. Scott TE, Carroll M, Cogliano FD, Smith BF, Lamorte WW. A case-control assessment of risk factors for gallbladder carcinoma. Dig Dis Sci. 1999;44:1619–25.
67. Ji J, Couto E, Hemminki K. Incidence differences for gallbladder cancer between occupational groups suggest an etiological role for alcohol. Int J Cancer. 2005;116:492–3.
68. Pandey M. Environmental pollutants in gallbladder carcinogenesis. J Surg Oncol. 2006;93:640–3.
69. Chhabra D, Oda K, Jagannath P, Utsunomiya H, Takekoshi S, Nimura Y. Chronic heavy metal exposure and gallbladder cancer risk in India, a comparative study with Japan. Asian Pac J Cancer Prev. 2012;13:187–90.
70. Darby SC, Whitley E, Howe GR, Hutchings SJ, Kusiak RA, Lubin JH, et al. Radon and cancers other than lung cancer in underground miners: a collaborative analysis of 11 studies. J Natl Cancer Inst. 1995;87:378–84.
71. Nogueira L, Foerster C, Groopman J, Egner P, Koshiol J, Ferreccio C, et al. Association of aflatoxin with gallbladder cancer in Chile. JAMA. 2015;313:2075–7.
72. Koshiol J, Gao YT, Dean M, Egner P, Nepal C, Jones K, et al. Association of aflatoxin and gallbladder cancer. Gastroenterology. 2017;153:488–94.e1.
73. Shim KY, Cha SW, Um WH, Chun CG, Jeong SW, Jang JY, et al. Simultaneous occurrence of gallbladder cancer in a laundry couple: association between gallbladder cancer and benzene. Korean J Gastroenterol. 2013;61:107–9.
74. Broden G, Bengtsson L. Biliary carcinoma associated with methyldopa therapy. Acta Chir Scand Suppl. 1980;500:7–12.
75. Lowenfels AB, Norman J. Isoniazid and bile duct cancer. JAMA. 1978;240:434–5.
76. Kamisawa T, Takuma K, Anjiki H, Egawa N, Kurata M, Honda G, et al. Pancreaticobiliary maljunction. Clin Gastroenterol Hepatol. 2009;7:S84–8.
77. Kang CM, Kim KS, Choi JS, Lee WJ, Kim BR. Gallbladder carcinoma associated with anomalous pancreaticobiliary duct junction. Can J Gastroenterol. 2007;21:383–7.
78. Hasumi A, Matsui H, Sugioka A, Uyama I, Komori Y, Fujita J, et al. Precancerous conditions of biliary tract cancer in patients with pancreaticobiliary maljunction: reappraisal of nationwide survey in Japan. J Hepatobiliary Pancreat Surg. 2000;7:551–5.
79. Lee SE, Jang JY, Lee YJ, Choi DW, Lee WJ, Cho BH, et al. Choledochal cyst and associated malignant tumors in adults: a multicenter survey in South Korea. Arch Surg. 2011;146:1178–84.

Pathology, Pathogenesis, Clinical Features, and Diagnosis

Key Points

- The two representative premalignant lesions of GB, BilIN and ICPN, distinguish each other not only by morphologic characteristics but also by pathophysiologic differences.
- The dysplasia-carcinoma sequence is considered the predominant pathway of GB carcinogenesis, while the adenoma-carcinoma sequence is somewhat controversial and shows geographic differences.
- Diagnostic imaging has been the basis for the diagnosis of gallbladder cancer.
- Even with the advancement of diagnostic imaging techniques and biomarkers, many patients with gallbladder cancer are diagnosed intraoperatively at the time of surgical exploration or postoperatively upon examination of a surgically resected specimen.

Introduction

According to the 2019 WHO classification, epithelial gallbladder (GB) tumors are categorized into "benign epithelial tumors and precursors" or "malignant epithelial tumors" (Table 1) [1]. Several terms have been used to describe the overlapping morphological entities of premalignant GB lesions over the years. This has led to varying

Table 1 2019 WHO classification of tumors of the gallbladder and extrahepatic bile ducts

Benign epithelial tumors and precursors
Adenoma
Biliary intraepithelial neoplasia, low or high grade
Intracystic papillary neoplasm with low- or high-grade intraepithelial neoplasia
Intracystic papillary neoplasm with associated invasive carcinoma
Intraductal papillary neoplasm with low- or high-grade intraepithelial neoplasia
Intraductal papillary neoplasm with associated invasive carcinoma
Malignant epithelial tumors
Adenocarcinoma
Adenocarcinoma (biliary/intestinal type)
Clear cell adenocarcinoma
Mucinous cystic neoplasm with associated invasive carcinoma
Mucinous adenocarcinoma
Poorly cohesive carcinoma
Intracystic papillary neoplasm with associated invasive carcinoma
Squamous cell carcinoma
Carcinoma, undifferentiated
Adenosquamous carcinoma
Cholangiocarcinoma
Neuroendocrine tumor (grade 1/2/3)
Neuroendocrine carcinoma (large/small cell)
Mixed neuroendocrine-non-neuroendocrine neoplasm (MiNEN)

Huapyong Kang and Eui Joo Kim are the lead authors of this chapter.

H. J. Chun et al., *Gastrointestinal Cancer*, https://doi.org/10.1007/978-981-99-0815-8_56

Table 2 Analogical intraepithelial premalignant lesions between organs in pancreaticobiliary system

	Mass-forming type	Flat type
Gallbladder	Intracystic papillary neoplasm (ICPN)	Biliary intraepithelial neoplasia (BilIN)
Bile duct	Intraductal papillary neoplasm of the bile duct (IPNB)	Biliary intraepithelial neoplasia (BilIN)
Pancreas	Intraductal papillary mucinous neoplasm (IPMN)	Pancreatic intraepithelial neoplasia (PanIN)

incidence and outcomes for premalignant GB lesions [2]. Thus, a large part of the pathological and clinical characteristics of these lesions are still not clear. In the 2010 WHO classification, the former terms of premalignant GB lesions were recategorized according to their morphological and pathophysiologic characteristics. For the flat microscopic lesion, the previously used term "flat dysplasia" was replaced by "biliary intraepithelial neoplasm (BilIN)." Furthermore, the terms for premalignant exophytic GB neoplasms greater than 1 cm were unified as intracholecystic papillary neoplasms (ICPN). Both BilIN and ICPN have counterparts in other pancreaticobiliary systems (Table 2). A notable change in the WHO classification for 2019 is that the classification system of premalignant lesion changed from a three-tier to a two-tier classification system, with the former low- and intermediate-grade intraepithelial neoplasia or BilIN-1 and BilIN-2, now classified as low-grade, consistent with tumors from other digestive system. Conventional diagnostic imaging modalities for GB cancer showed reliable diagnostic performance, and several new techniques have recently emerged for preoperative imaging and histological diagnosis of GB cancer. In this chapter, the pathology and pathogenesis, as well as the clinical features and diagnosis of GB cancer, will be reviewed.

Pathology

Premalignant Lesion

The two representative premalignant lesions of GB, BilIN and ICPN, distinguish each other not only by morphological characteristics but also by pathophysiological differences.

BilIN, the most common precursor lesion of GB cancer, is defined as microscopic, noninvasive, flat, or (micro)papillary lesions that are confined to the GB lumen [1]. The former terms used as part of the dysplasia-carcinoma sequence "flat dysplasia" and the more recent terms "BilIN-1" and "BilIN-2" are now all replaced by "BilIN, low grade." Furthermore, "BilIN-3" and "carcinoma in situ (CIS)" are now designated "BilIN, high grade" [3]. BilIN is found in the adjacent mucosa in more than 90% of GB cancer [4]. The incidence of low- and high-grade BilIN in resected GB with gallstones in which GB cancer is endemic, 15% and 3.5%, respectively, is higher than in North America, <5% and <0.1%, respectively [1, 5]. Usually, BilINs are incidentally found during microscopic examination and are not grossly visible. The grade of atypia was determined by factors such as the hyperchromicity and morphology of the nuclei, the N:C ratio, the nuclear polarity, and the frequency of mitoses [6]. Immunostaining shows positive cytoplasmic CEA, S100, diffuse nuclear p53, and loss of p16 [7–9]. However, the overlaps in immunostaining results are broad, which excludes their utility in individual cases [1]. Various phenotypes of BilIN are recognized, such as biliary, intestinal, and gastric, while little is revealed about the clinical relevance between them. Although cholecystectomy is curative for high-grade BilIN, there have been limited numbers of cancer recurrences after several years. This indicates that there may be a wide-field cancerization phenomenon in the biliary tract [10].

ICPN is a mass-forming intraluminal-growing noninvasive epithelial neoplasm which can be detected grossly [11]. ICPN recently introduced a unifying terminology, replacing several older terms such as "biliary adenoma," "papillary adenoma," "tubulopapillary adenoma," or "papillomatosis." Due to limited data, the actual incidence of ICPN is unknown. An incidence of less than 1% is reported among resected GB, while in a systematic analysis, 6.4% of invasive GB cancer originated in an ICPN [1, 12]. The frequency is higher in women, and its relationship with stone GB has not been shown to be significant, unlike cancer GB in general. As a GB counterpart to intraductal papillary mucinous neoplasm of the pancreas and intraductal papillary neoplasm of the bile duct, approximately 50% of ICPNs have a papillary architectural pattern [13]. However, ICPNs reveal various growth patterns (papillary, tubular, and tubulopapillary), morphological types, and degrees of atypia. The clinical relevance of different growth patterns is unclear. Four morphologic types of ICPN are recognized: biliary, gastric, intestinal, and oncocytic. The biliary type is the most common morphology found in approximately 50% of ICPNs, with cuboidal cells showing clear to eosinophilic cytoplasm, enlarged nuclei, prominent nucleoli, and typical expression of CK7 and MUC1 [1, 12]. However, ICPNs frequently show heterogeneity in histology and immunochemistry. Regarding degrees of atypia, low-grade ICPNs harbor only mild to moderate atypia, while high-grade ICPNs can exhibit complex architecture, nuclear pleomorphism, and loss of polarity. MUC1 expression is observed in any cell type of high-grade ICPN and could be a marker of high-grade atypia [2]. Invasive carcinoma is found in 55% of ICPNs, in association with extensive high-grade dysplasia, biliary type, and papillary pattern [12]. Noninvasive ICPN shows a good prognosis after cholecystectomy with 78% of the 5-year survival rate. Furthermore, compared to conventional GB cancer, invasive ICPN has a better prognosis with 60% 5-year survival [12].

GB adenoma is also known as a premalignant tumor lesion. After the introduction of ICPN, papillary or tubular adenoma can be classified as ICPN; however, the term "adenoma" has not been used. The association of GB adenoma and invasive malignancy seems very low, reported at 0.14% [14]. In the 2019 WHO classification, pyloric gland adenoma (PGA) has been assigned as a discrete entity from ICPN and other adenomas due to its molecular distinctiveness. PGA is defined as a grossly detectable neoplasm composed of uniform mucinous glands of the pyloric or Brunner gland. PGA shows an increase in beta-catenin expression and a mutation in CTNNB1 in 60%, rather than mutations in TP53 or CDKN2A, which are seen in other types of adenomas [15, 16]. Therefore, it is suggested that the role of PGA in the pathogenesis of GB cancer would be minor [3].

Malignant Lesion

The most common site of origin of GB cancer is the fundus (60%), which is followed by the body and neck (30% and 10%, respectively) [17]. GB cancers generally have the ulcerovegetating macroscopic appearance and can also be infiltrative, papillary, or nodular. However, distinguishing GB cancer from long-lasting cholecystitis is often difficult even by macroscopic examination. Notably, the tumor may not be clearly visible in 10–37% of cases [18]. ICPN-based GB cancer grows into a GB lumen with a papillary or polypoid appearance. *Hyalinizing cholecystitis-associated* cancer often shows a scleroatrophic appearance, sometimes forming a nodularity in a thin-walled GB [19]. Mucinous carcinomas form a more gelatinous tumor [1].

Adenocarcinoma is the most common histological type of GB cancer (>90%) [1]. It is characterized by malignant glands that move unconstrained in a dense desmoplastic stroma [2]. Well-/moderately/poorly differentiated or undifferentiated adenocarcinoma is classified according to its degree of gland formation. Positive for CK7, MUC1, CEA, CA19–9, and CK20 (variable), positivity is a typical immunohistochemical profile of GB adenocarcinoma. The most frequent subtype is pancreatic biliary-type adenocarcinoma, which morphologically and behaviorally resembles pancreatic ductal adenocarcinoma. Unusual subtypes of adenocarcinoma are intestinal-type adenocarcinoma, mucinous adenocarcinoma with >50% of the tumor containing extracellular mucin, clear cell carcinoma, and poorly cohesive carcinoma that shows more aggressive behavior than general GB cancer. Sometimes, pancreatobiliary adenocarcinomas can contain a certain portion of any of the abovementioned unusual adenocarcinoma subtypes, but if the pancreatobiliary type is predominant, it can be categorized as pancreatobiliary-type adenocarcinoma.

Pure squamous cell carcinoma (SCC) of GB is extremely rare (<1% of all biliary malignancy) and generally shows substantial keratinization. A tumor harboring more than 25% of the malignant glandular and squamous component, adenosquamous carcinoma, is also found in GB (~4% of all GB cancer), more frequently than pure SCC [20]. The tumor biology of adenosquamous carcinoma and pure SCC is known to be more aggressive than general GB cancer, which is related to a poor prognosis [20, 21].

Two types of neuroendocrine carcinoma (NEC), small cell and large cell, can rarely arise from GB, which are histologically identical to those that arise in the lung and gastrointestinal tract [22]. NECs are characterized by a high mitotic rate and a high Ki67 index. Differentiation of GB NEC has been reported that almost 90% showed poorly differentiated or undifferentiated tumors [23]. Immunohistochemistry for neuroendocrine markers shows variable positivity, with diffuse staining of synaptophysin and often patchy staining of chromogranin A. Scattered chromogranin A and synaptophysin-positive neuroendocrine cells are commonly observed in ordinary GB adenocarcinoma and should not be diagnosed as neuroendocrine tumor (NET) or NEC. Diffuse overexpression of p53 and diffuse loss of Rb1 are useful to distinguish NEC from grade 3 NET [24]. More than a third of NECs show adenocarcinoma or SCC and are classified as mixed neuroendocrine-non-neuroendocrine neoplasm (MiNEN) [1]. GB NECs are usually diagnosed at an advanced stage and progressed aggressively. Whether the prognosis of GB NEC is poorer than ordinary GB adenocarcinoma is unclear with contradictory results [25, 26].

Pathogenesis

Like other cancers, the pathogenesis of GB cancer is affected by multiple genetic aberrations and environmental factors (Fig. 1). Historically, two different models of GB cancer pathogenesis have been suggested. One is the dysplasia-carcinoma sequence and the other is the adenoma-carcinoma sequence [28].

The dysplasia-carcinoma sequence is considered the predominant pathway of GB carcinogenesis, which starts with chronic inflammation triggered by factors such as gallstone, hyalinizing cholecystitis, or anomalous pancreatobiliary ductal union (APBDU). Metaplasia in the mucosa exposed to chronic inflammation is a very common finding in GB, and cumulated molecular genetic alterations affect oncogenes and the tumor suppressor gene. As a result, it is believed that consecutive emergence of low-grade dysplasia (BilIN, low-grade), CIS (BilIN, high-grade), and invasive carcinoma occurs (Fig. 2) [28]. This sequence is supported by findings that near CIS, dysplasia is commonly found, and more than 80% of invasive GB carcinomas show CIS and dysplasia in the adjacent GB mucosa [28]. Furthermore, the fact that the average age of patients with GB cancer is 15 years older than

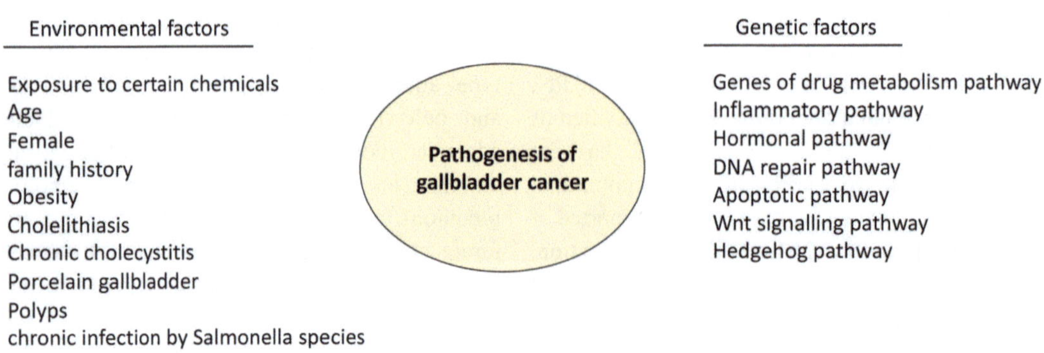

Fig. 1 Schema of factors affecting pathogenesis of GB cancer (Adapted from Mehrotra et al. [27])

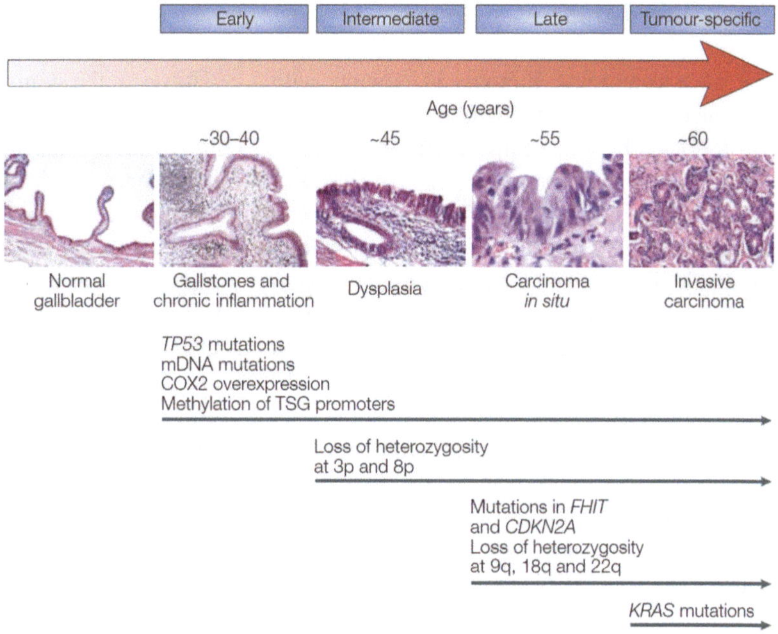

Fig. 2 Dysplasia-carcinoma sequence [4]

that of patients with dysplasia and 5 years older than that of patients with CIS suggests that this sequence from dysplasia to invasive carcinoma takes approximately 10–15 years [29].

Unlike the well-established adenoma-carcinoma sequence in colorectal cancer, GB adenoma to GB cancer pathogenesis is somewhat controversial and less popular than the dysplasia-carcinoma sequence. It was first suggested in 1982, by a study evaluating 1605 cholecystectomy specimens. They found seven adenomas with malignant transformation and adenomatous residue in 19% of invasive carcinomas [30]. The malignant transformation of GB adenoma is more frequent in Eastern countries than Western countries [31]. Therefore, geographical differences could exist in the pathogenesis of GB cancer. Some distinctive molecular changes are suggested for the adenoma-carcinoma sequence, such as overexpression of cyclin D1 and reduced expression of Rb, expression of cyclooxygenase-2, and altered expression of beta-catenin [15, 32, 33]. The size of the adenoma and the age of the patient (older than 50) are believed to be associated with malignant transformation of the adenoma [34]. The actual progression steps and changes in molecular genetics for this sequence need further investigation.

Several molecular alterations have been found in relation to GB cancer. Representatively, they include oncogenes KRAS, HER2, EGFR, BRAF, cyclin D1, and cyclin E; tumor suppressor genes TP53, p16/CDKN2A, p15/CDKN2B, p21/CDKN1A, and FHIT; angiogenic and inflammatory genes COX-2 and VEGF; adhesion molecules CD44 and CD54; mucin proteins MUC-1 and MUC-4; microsatellite instability; and telomeres hTERT [2]. However, the frequencies are different between the demographics and etiology of the patient. For example, Japanese studies showed a higher frequency of KRAS mutations (50–80%) and relatively late onset of TP53 mutations in patients with APBDU-related GB cancer. On the contrary, Chilean studies, where the presence of gallstones is the main etiological factor, showed an early *TP53* mutation and a rare *KRAS* mutation [4]. Therefore, drawing a more accurate map of molecular alteration reflecting demographics, etiology, clinical characteristics, and biological sex is important for the prevention, early detection, and personalized treatment of GB cancer in the future.

Clinical Features

The most common symptoms in patients with GB cancer are abdominal pain, nausea, or vomiting, followed by nonspecific symptoms suggestive of malignant disease such as anorexia, malaise, and weight loss. When GB cancer invades the biliary tree from a direct invasion or a metastatic mass around the region of the hepatoduodenal ligament or porta hepatis, it can cause obstructive jaundice or duodenal obstruction with gastrointestinal obstructive symptoms indicating advanced disease.

On physical examination, distended GB can be palpable as a round mass in the right upper quadrant of the abdomen in patients with jaundice known as the Courvoisier sign. The Courvoisier sign or Courvoisier law was proposed to be associated with malignant biliary obstruction rather than cholelithiasis [35].

However, the symptoms of GB cancer are usually vague and often differ from typical biliary colic. Traditionally, because patients with early GB cancer are silent or have nonspecific symptoms, the preoperative diagnosis rate for GB cancer was only 10–15%, and patients with symptoms suggesting acute cholecystitis showed a better long-term outcome than others who presented otherwise [36]. Even with recent advances in medical imaging modalities such as endoscopic ultrasound, many patients with GB cancer are diagnosed intraoperatively at the time of surgical resection for other reasons such as symptomatic GB stones or postoperatively on histological inspection of the surgically resected GB specimen (Fig. 3).

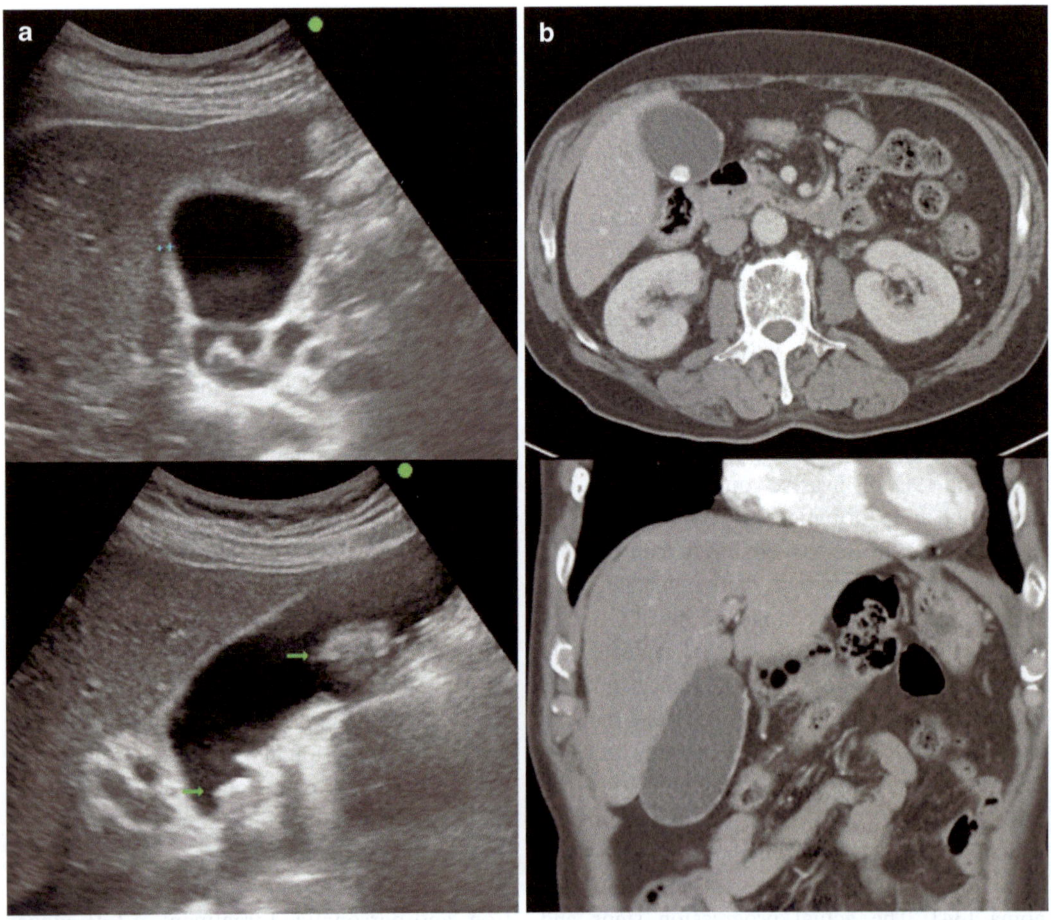

Fig. 3 Diagnostic images of a patient diagnosed with early gallbladder cancer postoperatively (well-differentiated adenocarcinoma confined to mucosa). (**a**) Initial transabdominal ultrasound (TAUS) of the gallbladder with multiple gallbladder stones. (**b**) Computed tomography (CT) scan of the gallbladder with gallbladder stone

Diagnosis

Biomarkers

Cholangiocytes are distributed in a single layer of the biliary tract and have various functions. They secrete bicarbonate and several substances to protect the biliary tract from toxic substances such as bile, bacteria, and other antigens. The most commonly used tumor markers for GB cancer are cancer antigen 19–9 (CA 19–9) and carcinoembryonic antigen (CEA). CA 19–9 and CEA are glycoproteins that are useful for monitoring the progression of GB cancer. However, the sensitivity and specificity of these tests (50–80%) made them poor diagnostic biomarkers [37, 38]. Although these glycoproteins are largely produced in cholangiocarcinoma, they are also elevated in chronic inflammatory diseases that can eventually lead to cholangiocarcinoma or other malignancies such as gastrointestinal or gynecologic malignancies. In clinical practice, these tests may aid in the diagnosis of GB cancer, but translation of the results should be done with caution and should not be used in the diagnosis of GB cancer.

Diagnostic Imaging

Transabdominal ultrasound (TAUS) is one of the first imaging modalities applied to patients with symptoms such as abdominal pain, nausea, vomiting, and abnormal liver function tests.

Because TAUS is a noninvasive imaging technique that does not require any radiation and can be easily accessible at bedside, it is the most frequently performed imaging modality in the diagnosis of GB cancer. GB cancer in TAUS can appear as three distinct morphological types that are exophytic, infiltrative, and polypoid type. The exophytic type appears as a mass of variable echogenicity filling the lumen of the GB, the infiltrative type may appear as irregular focal or diffuse wall thickening of the GB, and the polypoid type appears as an intraluminal fungating mass usually larger than 1 cm in size with fixation to the GB wall. Single lesions, broad bases, and lesions greater than 1 cm are imaging findings known to have malignant potential. Although the sensitivity of TAUS is reported to be 85%, TAUS is largely dependent on the expertise of the operator and the quality of the equipment. Sometimes, combined gallstones may interfere with the visualization of malignant lesions of the GB. Even with recent advances in TAUS equipment with improved high-quality resolutions, still many patients with GB cancer are retrospectively diagnosed to have had indeterminate TAUS findings that were not recognized preoperatively [39].

CT and MRI can be helpful in the diagnosis of GB cancer. The sensitivity of MDCT in the detection of GB cancer is approximately 90% with approximately 85% accuracy in assessing local extent [40, 41]. The morphological types (exophytic, infiltrative, polypoid type) of GB cancers are also valuable in CT and MRI, and the enhancement of GB cancer may show in various patterns (Fig. 4). Although there are limited data on the precision of MRI in the diagnosis of GB cancer, GB cancer can be hyposignal on T1 images and hypersignal or heterogenous on T2 images. With gadolinium enhancement, there may be early irregular enhancement that persists throughout the dynamic study. However, because the feeding vessel of GB is the cystic artery, which is an end artery, the enhancement pattern cannot definitely differentiate GB cancer and inflammatory conditions such as chronic cholecystitis or xanthogranulomatous cholecystitis on CT or MRI. Endoscopic ultrasound (EUS) or intraductal ultrasound (IDUS) can be used for detailed imaging of GB cancer. Because the high-frequency EUS probe can provide high-resolution ultrasound images, EUS or IDUS can visualize the layers of the GB, and it can provide a more detailed structural image to assess the depth of invasion of the GB cancer [42]. The accuracy of EUS in determining the invasion of depth of GB cancer was reported to be ~75 to 100% which can be important for therapeutic decision-making [43]. Recently, with the introduction of artificial intelligence for medical images, diagnostic methods using deep learning techniques for GB lesions are also being tested. In a study on EUS images, the EUS artificial intelligence system learned using EUS images of

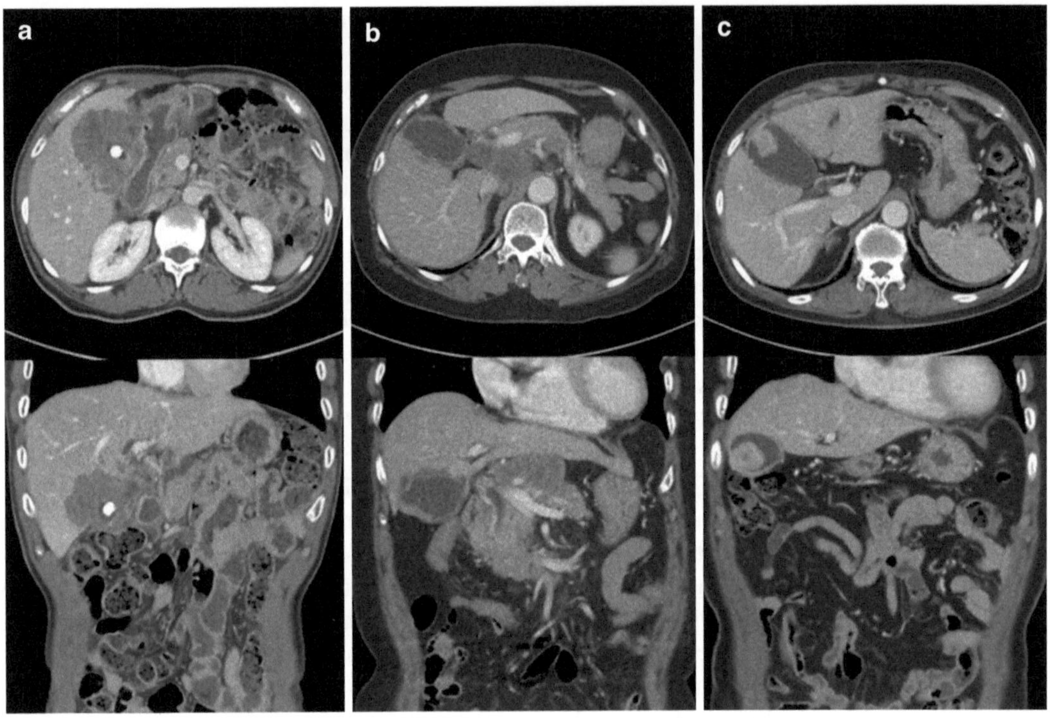

Fig. 4 Images of computed tomography of gallbladder cancer. (**a**) Exophytic-type mass-filling gallbladder lumen. (**b**) Infiltrative-type gallbladder cancer showing irregular wall thickening. (**c**) Polypoid type showing single polyp larger than 1 cm

the GB showed 89.8% precision in differentiation between gallstones and polyps, and the precision of differentiation between neoplasia and nonneoplastic polyps was 74.4% [44]. As the advancement of contrast media has allowed contrast dynamic studies to be performed in the US/EUS, the efficacy of contrast-enhanced harmonic endoscopic ultrasound (CE-EUS) for GB cancer is being investigated [45–47]. Because obtaining GB histology before surgical resection is difficult, diagnostic imaging has been the mainstay of the diagnosis of GB cancer. EUS-guided fine needle aspiration (EUS-FNA) is one of the options that can acquire GB histology with a minimal invasive approach and can be a good candidate for preoperative tissue acquisition. However, there is still scarce evidence to support EUS-FNA for GB cancer, and the risk of bile leakage and peritoneal dissemination of malignancy during the procedure should be carefully interpreted [48–51].

Conclusion

Evidence regarding the pathophysiology and carcinogenesis of GB cancer together with a better understanding of genetic alterations and biomarkers associated with molecular pathogenesis of pancreatobiliary cancers is being accumulated. However, clinically, reaching an era of early diagnosis and prevention of GB cancer still requires further effort. Future research is needed for novel diagnostic modalities, including a preoperative tissue acquisition method and molecular testing.

References

1. WHO Classification of Tumours Editorial Board. WHO classification of tumors: digestive system tumours. 5th ed. Lyon: International Agency for Research on Cancer; 2019.
2. Bal MM, Ramadwar M, Deodhar K, Shrikhande S. Pathology of gallbladder carcinoma: current under-

standing and new perspectives. Pathol Oncol Res. 2015;21:509–25.
3. Gonzalez RS, Raza A, Propst R, Adeyi O, Bateman J, Sopha SC, et al. Recent advances in digestive tract tumors: updates from the 5th edition of the World Health Organization "Blue Book". Arch Pathol Lab Med. 2020;145:607–26.
4. Wistuba II, Gazdar AF. Gallbladder cancer: lessons from a rare tumour. Nat Rev Cancer. 2004;4:695–706.
5. Adsay NV. Neoplastic precursors of the gallbladder and extrahepatic biliary system. Gastroenterol Clin North Am. 2007;36:889–900, vii.
6. Zen Y, Adsay NV, Bardadin K, Colombari R, Ferrell L, Haga H, et al. Biliary intraepithelial neoplasia: an international interobserver agreement study and proposal for diagnostic criteria. Mod Pathol. 2007;20:701–9.
7. Zhao H, Davydova L, Mandich D, Cartun RW, Ligato S. S100A4 protein and mesothelin expression in dysplasia and carcinoma of the extrahepatic bile duct. Am J Clin Pathol. 2007;127:374–9.
8. Wistuba II, Gazdar AF, Roa I, Albores-Saavedra J. p53 protein overexpression in gallbladder carcinoma and its precursor lesions: an immunohistochemical study. Hum Pathol. 1996;27:360–5.
9. Parwani AV, Geradts J, Caspers E, Offerhaus GJ, Yeo CJ, Cameron JL, et al. Immunohistochemical and genetic analysis of non-small cell and small cell gallbladder carcinoma and their precursor lesions. Mod Pathol. 2003;16:299–308.
10. Albores-Saavedra J, Murakata L, Krueger JE, Henson DE. Noninvasive and minimally invasive papillary carcinomas of the extrahepatic bile ducts. Cancer. 2000;89:508–15.
11. Bennett S, Marginean EC, Paquin-Gobeil M, Wasserman J, Weaver J, Mimeault R, et al. Clinical and pathological features of intraductal papillary neoplasm of the biliary tract and gallbladder. HPB (Oxford). 2015;17:811–8.
12. Adsay V, Jang KT, Roa JC, Dursun N, Ohike N, Bagci P, et al. Intracholecystic papillary-tubular neoplasms (ICPN) of the gallbladder (neoplastic polyps, adenomas, and papillary neoplasms that are ≥1.0 cm): clinicopathologic and immunohistochemical analysis of 123 cases. Am J Surg Pathol. 2012;36:1279–301.
13. Klöppel G, Adsay V, Konukiewitz B, Kleeff J, Schlitter AM, Esposito I. Precancerous lesions of the biliary tree. Best Pract Res Clin Gastroenterol. 2013;27:285–97.
14. Lee K-B. Histologic and molecular pathogenesis of gallbladder cancer. Korean J Pancreas Biliary Tract. 2018;23:1–6.
15. Chang HJ, Jee CD, Kim WH. Mutation and altered expression of beta-catenin during gallbladder carcinogenesis. Am J Surg Pathol. 2002;26:758–66.
16. Wistuba II, Miquel JF, Gazdar AF, Albores-Saavedra J. Gallbladder adenomas have molecular abnormalities different from those present in gallbladder carcinomas. Hum Pathol. 1999;30:21–5.
17. Albores-Saavedra J, Alcántra-Vazquez A, Cruz-Ortiz H, Herrera-Goepfert R. The precursor lesions of invasive gallbladder carcinoma. Hyperplasia, atypical hyperplasia and carcinoma in situ. Cancer. 1980;45:919–27.
18. Roa I, Araya JC, Villaseca M, Roa J, de Aretxabala X, Ibacache G. Gallbladder cancer in a high risk area: morphological features and spread patterns. Hepatogastroenterology. 1999;46:1540–6.
19. Patel S, Roa JC, Tapia O, Dursun N, Bagci P, Basturk O, et al. Hyalinizing cholecystitis and associated carcinomas: clinicopathologic analysis of a distinctive variant of cholecystitis with porcelain-like features and accompanying diagnostically challenging carcinomas. Am J Surg Pathol. 2011;35:1104–13.
20. Roa JC, Tapia O, Cakir A, Basturk O, Dursun N, Akdemir D, et al. Squamous cell and adenosquamous carcinomas of the gallbladder: clinicopathological analysis of 34 cases identified in 606 carcinomas. Mod Pathol. 2011;24:1069–78.
21. Chan KM, Yu MC, Lee WC, Jan YY, Chen MF. Adenosquamous/squamous cell carcinoma of the gallbladder. J Surg Oncol. 2007;95:129–34.
22. Henson DE, Albores-Saavedra J, Corle D. Carcinoma of the gallbladder. Histologic types, stage of disease, grade, and survival rates. Cancer. 1992;70:1493–7.
23. Yao JC, Hassan M, Phan A, Dagohoy C, Leary C, Mares JE, et al. One hundred years after "carcinoid": epidemiology of and prognostic factors for neuroendocrine tumors in 35,825 cases in the United States. J Clin Oncol. 2008;26:3063–72.
24. Konukiewitz B, Schlitter AM, Jesinghaus M, Pfister D, Steiger K, Segler A, et al. Somatostatin receptor expression related to TP53 and RB1 alterations in pancreatic and extrapancreatic neuroendocrine neoplasms with a Ki67-index above 20. Mod Pathol. 2017;30:587–98.
25. Yan S, Wang Y, Chen X, Zhang Y, Huang Z, Zhao J, et al. Clinical analysis of 15 cases of gallbladder neuroendocrine carcinoma and comparison with gallbladder adenocarcinoma using a propensity score matching. Cancer Manag Res. 2020;12:1437–46.
26. Do MY, Jang SI, Kang HP, Kim EJ, Lee KJ, Park GE, et al. Comparison of the clinical features and outcomes of gallbladder neuroendocrine carcinoma with those of adenocarcinoma: a propensity score-matched analysis. Cancers (Basel). 2021;13:4713.
27. Mehrotra R, Tulsyan S, Hussain S, Mittal B, Saluja SS, Singh S, et al. Genetic landscape of gallbladder cancer: global overview. Mutat Res Rev Mutat Res. 2018;778:61–71.
28. Roa I, de Aretxabala X, Araya JC, Roa J. Preneoplastic lesions in gallbladder cancer. J Surg Oncol. 2006;93:615–23.
29. Roa I, Araya JC, Villaseca M, De Aretxabala X, Riedemann P, Endoh K, et al. Preneoplastic lesions and gallbladder cancer: an estimate of the period required for progression. Gastroenterology. 1996;111:232–6.

30. Kozuka S, Tsubone N, Yasui A, Hachisuka K. Relation of adenoma to carcinoma in the gallbladder. Cancer. 1982;50:2226–34.
31. Lee SH, Lee DS, You IY, Jeon WJ, Park SM, Youn SJ, et al. Histopathologic analysis of adenoma and adenoma-related lesions of the gallbladder. Korean J Gastroenterol. 2010;55:119–26.
32. Xuan YH, Choi YL, Shin YK, Kook MC, Chae SW, Park SM, et al. An immunohistochemical study of the expression of cell-cycle-regulated proteins p53, cyclin D1, RB, p27, Ki67 and MSH2 in gallbladder carcinoma and its precursor lesions. Histol Histopathol. 2005;20:59–66.
33. Seki S, Kitada T, Sakaguchi H, Hirohashi K, Kinoshita H. Cyclooxygenase-2 expression in the adenoma-carcinoma sequence of human gallbladder. Am J Gastroenterol. 2002;97:2146–7.
34. Boulton RA, Adams DH. Gallbladder polyps: when to wait and when to act. Lancet. 1997;349:817.
35. Fitzgerald JE, White MJ, Lobo DN. Courvoisier's gallbladder: law or sign? World J Surg. 2009;33:886–91.
36. Misra S, Chaturvedi A, Misra NC, Sharma ID. Carcinoma of the gallbladder. Lancet Oncol. 2003;4:167–76.
37. Strom BL, Iliopoulos D, Atkinson B, Herlyn M, West SL, Maislin G, et al. Pathophysiology of tumor progression in human gallbladder: flow cytometry, CEA, and CA 19-9 levels in bile and serum in different stages of gallbladder disease. J Natl Cancer Inst. 1989;81:1575–80.
38. Strom BL, Maislin G, West SL, Atkinson B, Herlyn M, Saul S, et al. Serum CEA and CA 19-9: potential future diagnostic or screening tests for gallbladder cancer? Int J Cancer. 1990;45:821–4.
39. Wibbenmeyer LA, Sharafuddin MJ, Wolverson MK, Heiberg EV, Wade TP, Shields JB. Sonographic diagnosis of unsuspected gallbladder cancer: imaging findings in comparison with benign gallbladder conditions. AJR Am J Roentgenol. 1995;165:1169–74.
40. Kim SJ, Lee JM, Lee JY, Choi JY, Kim SH, Han JK, et al. Accuracy of preoperative T-staging of gallbladder carcinoma using MDCT. AJR Am J Roentgenol. 2008;190:74–80.
41. Yoshimitsu K, Honda H, Shinozaki K, Aibe H, Kuroiwa T, Irie H, et al. Helical CT of the local spread of carcinoma of the gallbladder: evaluation according to the TNM system in patients who underwent surgical resection. AJR Am J Roentgenol. 2002;179:423–8.
42. Fujita N, Noda Y, Kobayashi G, Kimura K, Yago A. Diagnosis of the depth of invasion of gallbladder carcinoma by EUS. Gastrointest Endosc. 1999;50:659–63.
43. Sadamoto Y, Kubo H, Harada N, Tanaka M, Eguchi T, Nawata H. Preoperative diagnosis and staging of gallbladder carcinoma by EUS. Gastrointest Endosc. 2003;58:536–41.
44. Jang SI, Kim YJ, Kim EJ, Kang H, Shon SJ, Seol YJ, et al. Diagnostic performance of endoscopic ultrasound-artificial intelligence using deep learning analysis of gallbladder polypoid lesions. J Gastroenterol Hepatol. 2021;36:3548.
45. Hirooka Y, Naitoh Y, Goto H, Ito A, Hayakawa S, Watanabe Y, et al. Contrast-enhanced endoscopic ultrasonography in gallbladder diseases. Gastrointest Endosc. 1998;48:406–10.
46. Leem G, Chung MJ, Park JY, Bang S, Song SY, Chung JB, et al. Clinical value of contrast-enhanced harmonic endoscopic ultrasonography in the differential diagnosis of pancreatic and gallbladder masses. Clin Endosc. 2018;51:80–8.
47. Hijioka S, Nagashio Y, Ohba A, Maruki Y, Okusaka T. The role of EUS and EUS-FNA in differentiating benign and malignant gallbladder lesions. Diagnostics (Basel). 2021;11:1586.
48. Jacobson BC, Pitman MB, Brugge WR. EUS-guided FNA for the diagnosis of gallbladder masses. Gastrointest Endosc. 2003;57:251–4.
49. Singla V, Agarwal R, Anikhindi SA, Puri P, Kumar M, Ranjan P, et al. Role of EUS-FNA for gallbladder mass lesions with biliary obstruction: a large single-center experience. Endosc Int Open. 2019;7:E1403–9.
50. Wu LM, Jiang XX, Gu HY, Xu X, Zhang W, Lin LH, et al. Endoscopic ultrasound-guided fine-needle aspiration biopsy in the evaluation of bile duct strictures and gallbladder masses: a systematic review and meta-analysis. Eur J Gastroenterol Hepatol. 2011;23:113–20.
51. Varadarajulu S, Eloubeidi MA. Endoscopic ultrasound-guided fine-needle aspiration in the evaluation of gallbladder masses. Endoscopy. 2005;37:751–4.

Staging and Treatment

Key Points

- In the revised eighth edition of the AJCC staging system, T2 gallbladder carcinoma was divided into two groups: tumors on the peritoneal side (T2a) and tumors on the hepatic side (T2b).
- The involvement of the regional lymph nodes is now classified according to the number of positive nodes, rather than based on the anatomic location of the lymph nodes involved.
- For patients with early-stage disease, surgery alone can provide a cure. Unfortunately, fewer than 10% of symptomatic patients and only 20% of patients diagnosed incidentally with cholecystectomy have early-stage gallbladder cancer.
- Palliation goals for advanced gallbladder cancer are relief of pain, jaundice, and intestinal obstruction and prolongation of life.

Introduction

In this chapter, we review the staging and treatment of gallbladder cancer. Several staging systems have been used for gallbladder cancer. Although the staging system developed by Nevin was previously used in Europe [1], the tumor, node, metastasis (TNM) staging system of the combined American Joint Committee on Cancer (AJCC)/Union for International Cancer Control (UICC) is now the preferred classification scheme [2].

For patients with early-stage disease, surgery alone can provide a cure. Unfortunately, fewer than 10% of symptomatic patients and only 20% of patients diagnosed incidentally with cholecystectomy have early-stage gallbladder cancer.

The goals of palliation for advanced gallbladder cancer are relief of pain, jaundice, and bowel obstruction and prolongation of life. Patients experiencing pain from local growth may benefit from radiation therapy with or without concomitant chemotherapy. Although a biliary or intestinal bypass can be considered, percutaneous or endoscopic approaches are generally preferred given the limited median survival in patients with advanced disease (generally less than 6 months).

Staging

In the AJCC staging system, gallbladder cancer is classified into four stages based on the depth of invasion of the gallbladder wall and the extent of spread to surrounding organs and lymph nodes (Fig. 1) [4]. In the eighth revised edition of the AJCC staging system [2], gallbladder car-

---

Min Kyu Jung is the lead author of this chapter.

H. J. Chun et al., *Gastrointestinal Cancer*, https://doi.org/10.1007/978-981-99-0815-8_57

cinoma T2 was divided into two groups: tumors on the peritoneal side (T2a) and tumors on the hepatic side (T2b). This revision was made based on two retrospective studies showing that invasion of the hepatic side has a worse prognosis compared to tumors located on the peritoneal side [5, 6]. However, it is important to note that it can be difficult to determine the exact location of the tumor, which contributes to the difficulty in predicting the prognosis. In the most updated edition, the staging of the lymph nodes was also changed. Regional lymph node involvement is now classified according to the number of positive nodes, rather than based on the anatomic location of the lymph nodes involved (Table 1) [4]. There is also a recommendation that six or more nodes be harvested and evaluated. This change was based on studies that demonstrated that the number of metastatic lymph nodes and the lymph node ratio are more prognostic than the location of metastatic lymph nodes [7–9]. Regional nodes include those along the common bile duct (CBD), the liver artery, the portal vein, and the cystic duct. Nodes beyond the hepatoduodenal ligament (including periaortic, pericaval, superior mesenteric artery, and celiac artery lymph nodes) are extraregional and staged as distant metastases (M1 disease).

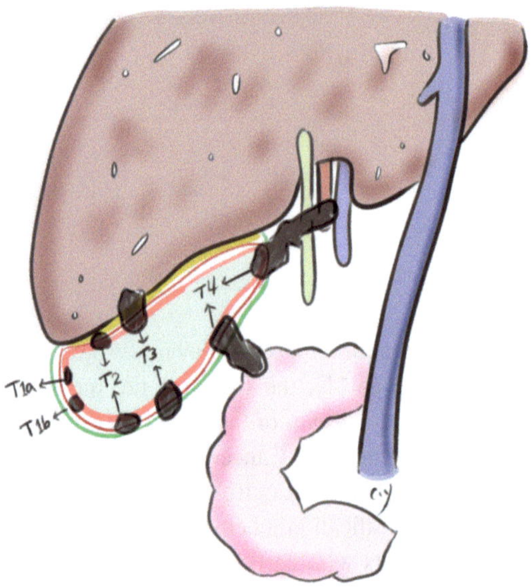

Fig. 1 T staging of gallbladder cancer (adapted from Okumura et al. [3])

Table 1 Staging of gallbladder cancer in AJCC eighth edition [4]

T stage	Primary tumor
Tx	Primary tumor cannot be assessed
T0	No evidence of primary tumor
Tis	Carcinoma in situ
T1	Tumor invades the lamina propria or muscular layer
T1a	Tumor invades the lamina propria
T1b	Tumor invades the muscular layer
T2	Tumor invades the perimuscular connective tissue on the peritoneal side, without involvement of the serosa (visceral peritoneum), or tumor invades the perimuscular connective tissue on the hepatic side, with no extension into the liver
T2a	Tumor invades the perimuscular connective tissue on the peritoneal side, without involvement of the serosa (visceral peritoneum)
T2b	Tumor invades the perimuscular connective tissue on the hepatic side, with no extension into the liver
T3	Tumor perforates the serosa (visceral peritoneum) and/or directly invades the liver and/or other adjacent organ or structure, such as the stomach, duodenum, colon, pancreas, omentum, or extrahepatic bile ducts
T4	Tumor invades main portal vein or hepatic artery or invades two or more extrahepatic organs or structures
N stage	Regional lymph nodes
Nx	Regional lymph nodes cannot be assessed
N0	No regional lymph node metastasis
N1	Metastasis to 1 ~ 3 regional lymph nodes
N2	Metastasis to four or more regional lymph nodes
M stage	Distant metastasis
M0	No distant metastasis
M1	Distant metastasis

Table 1 (continued)

Stage	T	N	M	Description
0	Tis	N0	M0	Cancer in situ
I	T1	N0	M0	Tumor is only in the gallbladder and has not spread
II	T2	N0	M0	Tumor has extended to the perimuscular connective tissue but has not spread elsewhere
IIIA	T3	N0	M0	Tumor has spread beyond the gallbladder but not to nearby arteries or veins. It has not spread to any lymph nodes or other parts of the body
IIIB	T1–3	N1	M0	Tumor of any size has spread to nearby lymph nodes but not to nearby arteries and/or to other parts of the body
IVA	T4	N0 or N1	M0	Tumor has spread to nearby arteries, veins, and/or nearby lymph nodes, but it has not spread to other parts of the body
IVB	Any T	Any N	M1	Any tumor that has spread to other parts of the body
	Any T	N2	M0	Any tumor that has distant lymph node spread, even if it has not spread to distant organs

Treatment

Staging Laparoscopy

Staging laparoscopy is an important method to identify peritoneal implants and nodal disease outside of the hepatoduodenal ligament in patients with proven or suspected gallbladder cancer (Table 2). Gallbladder cancer tends to undergo early nodal involvement in the cystic duct node and choledochal nodes. Spread outside of the hepatoduodenal ligament (including periaortic, pericaval, superior mesenteric artery, and celiac artery lymph nodes) generally means metastatic disease (M1 disease). These nodes should be assessed early during laparoscopy or laparotomy [10].

Staging laparoscopy in this setting is encouraged by the 2014 American Hepato-Pancreato-Biliary Association (AHPBA) consensus statement for gallbladder cancer [11]. It is important to identify patients with unresectable or metastatic disease, given the morbidity of a laparotomy and the limited role of palliative resection in advanced disease.

Incidentally Diagnosed Gallbladder Cancer

Gallbladder cancer is often discovered incidentally during routine cholecystectomy or postoperatively on the final pathology performed for other indications. It accounts for approximately 0.7% of all specimens [12]. In fact, more than half of gallbladder cancers are now diagnosed at the time of cholecystectomy or in a surgical pathology report [12, 13]. The incidental diagnosis of gallbladder cancer has led to earlier detection of cancers and therefore improved oncologic outcomes [14, 15]. Current guidelines for incidentally diagnosed gallbladder cancer recommend resection for T1b, T2, and T3 tumors, unless there is a distant spread on preoperative imaging or poor functional status (Table 2) [11].

Table 2 Surgical principles in the treatment of gallbladder cancer [10]

Surgical principle	Key points
Staging laparoscopy	Highest yield in non-incidentally diagnosed gallbladder cancer, T3 or greater, unfavorable tumor biology, or positive margins after cholecystectomy
Initial exploration	Metastases to celiac axis or aortocaval nodes make further resection futile
Hepatic resection	Standard resection is segments IVB and V, although additional segments may be indicated for R0 resection
Lymphadenectomy	Must include all nodes in the porta hepatis and preferably six or more nodes for complete staging
Bile duct resection	Routine resection is not recommended, but may be necessary for R0 resection in advanced stages
Port-site resection	Routine resection is not recommended, because port-site disease is a marker for disseminated intra-abdominal spread
Extent of resection	T1a tumors: simple cholecystectomy T1b and greater: radical cholecystectomy (hepatic resection + portal lymphadenectomy + cholecystectomy) Surgical morbidity nears 50% and perioperative mortality is approximately 5%

Surgical Treatment to Preoperatively Detected Gallbladder Cancer

In patients with preoperatively detected gallbladder cancer without distant metastases, laparotomy is the treatment of choice, as it allows for extended resections. More recently, current evidence suggests that laparoscopy is feasible with advances in minimally invasive surgery [16, 17].

The status of the cystic duct node in the initial operation is predictive of additional positive nodes in the porta hepatis. However, if the subsequent radical cholecystectomy shows no evidence of residual disease, the disease-free survival of these patients is similar to N0 rather than N1 [18].

For early-stage disease (T1b or T2), patients should undergo radical cholecystectomy with en bloc resection of the adjacent liver parenchyma and hepatoduodenal lymphadenectomy (Fig. 2). Resection of CBD with Roux-en-Y hepaticojejunostomy is not routinely recommended, because it increases morbidity without any survival benefit. However, extrahepatic bile duct resection is necessary if the patient has a positive cystic duct margin on intraoperative frozen section or direct extension [10]. CBD involvement is a marker of decreased survival, even after R0 resection [20].

For later-stage disease (T3 or T4), the extent of resection is debated in the literature. The most important predictors of long-term survival are tumor biology and stage, rather than extent of resection [10, 11].

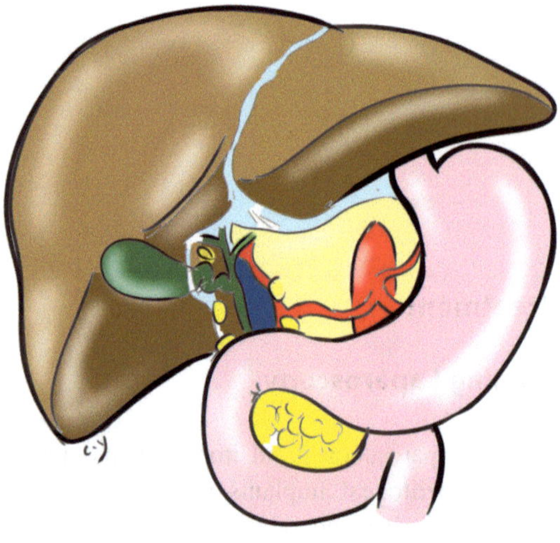

Fig. 2 Extent of radical cholecystectomy (adapted from Qadan et al. [19])

The probability of finding residual disease upon re-resection after incidentally diagnosed gallbladder cancer is dependent on tumor biology. For early-stage disease (T1), the incidence of residual disease in any location was 37.5% [21]. For higher-stage disease (T2 or T3), the incidence jumped from 70 to 80% [21]. Risk factors for residual disease include T3 tumors, perineural invasion, and lymphovascular invasion.

Adjuvant Chemotherapy or Chemoradiotherapy in Resected Gallbladder Cancer

The latest NCCN guidelines recommend consideration of chemotherapy or chemoradiotherapy after resection of gallbladder cancer. However, data are limited and no regimen has emerged as superior in this cohort (no high-quality randomized controlled trials). There are numerous single-center studies, but several large studies offer valuable insight. Decisions about adjuvant therapy should consider individual risks and benefits.

Subsequent to R0 resection, there are data suggesting a survival benefit with the use of adjuvant radiotherapy [22, 23]. Because local regional recurrence was common in patients with pT2 disease or R1 resection for gallbladder cancer, adjuvant chemoradiotherapy prior to progression could be very useful [24]. A National Cancer Data Base analysis of node-positive patients revealed the best overall survival with R0 resection combined with adjuvant chemoradiotherapy [23].

Chemotherapy or Chemoradiotherapy in Unresectable Gallbladder Cancer

The phase 3 trial ABC-02 by Valle et al. supports the use of gemcitabine/cisplatin compared to gemcitabine alone for advanced or metastatic biliary tract cancers, not exclusively gallbladder cancer [25]. The overall survival (OS) difference for the groups was statistically significant (11.7 vs 8.1 months, $p < 0.001$), although both were poor compared to survival after resection [25]. However, gemcitabine/cisplatin offered measurable efficacy in 80% of patients.

Chemotherapy is the traditional therapy for unresectable gallbladder cancer, and no randomized controlled trials have been conducted to examine the role of locoregional therapy (i.e., radiation therapy) for unresectable cancer [26].

Table 3 Targetable genetic mutations in gallbladder cancer [27]

Targetable mutations	Prevalence (%)	Potential agents
EGFR	4–13	Afatinib, erlotinib, cetuximab
HER2/neu amplification	10–16	Trastuzumab, lapatinib, pertuzumab
TP53	4–47	Bevacizumab
ERBB3	0–12	Seribantumab, pertuzumab, trastuzumab
PTEN *PIK3CA*	0–4 6–14	mTOR inhibitors (everolimus)
KRAS	4–13	Trametinib, selumetinib
ARID1A	15	mTOR inhibitors (everolimus), anti-PD-L1 (pembrolizumab) for tumors with microsatellite instability
CDKN2A/B loss	6–19	Palbociclib

Targeted Therapeutic Agents in Gallbladder Cancer

Advanced stage of diagnosis and limited adjuvant chemotherapeutic options have paved the way for targeted therapeutics using next-generation sequencing. Table 3 presents some of the common mutations in gallbladder cancer and the corresponding potential clinical targets [27, 28].

Palliative Therapy

Similar to other biliary cancers, the mainstay of palliative treatment in gallbladder cancer is the maintenance of adequate biliary drainage, nutrition, and local compressive symptoms. Biliary drainage can be achieved by percutaneous catheter placement or endoscopic biliary stents and is ideally performed before initiation of chemotherapy.

Biliary tumors often cause compression of the duodenal or gastric outlet, requiring distal feeding access or gastrojejunal bypass to maintain adequate nutrition. Patients with stage IV gallbladder cancer enrolled in the ABC-02 study derived a modest survival benefit from gemcitabine and cisplatin [25].

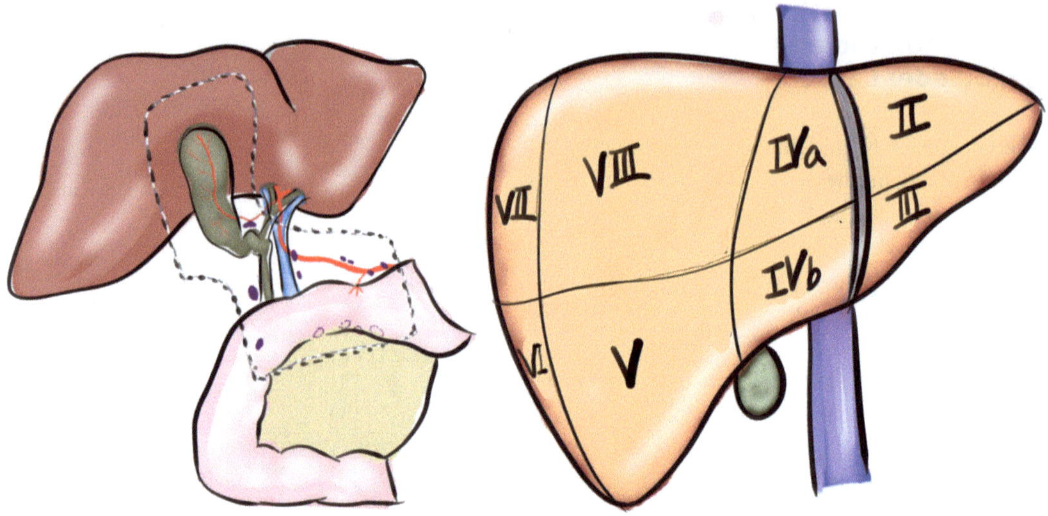

Fig. 3 Lymphatic drainage pattern and of gallbladder and liver segments along the Cantlie line (adapted from Okumura et al. [3])

Conclusion

Gallbladder cancer remains a formidable disease. Surgical management has traditionally been challenging due to the technical difficulties associated with liver resection and biliary reconstruction (Fig. 3). Furthermore, effective cytotoxic agents were limited. However, newer developments in management are leading to significant changes in the prognosis of this disease. Perioperative management for incidentally discovered gallbladder cancer is being better defined based on a more accurate pathological staging. Targeted therapies are also tried with a rapidly evolving landscape. However, much remains undefined in the management of gallbladder cancer, and further studies are urgently needed in this malignancy.

References

1. Nevin JE, Moran TJ, Kay S, King R. Carcinoma of the gallbladder: staging, treatment, and prognosis. Cancer. 1976;37:141–8.
2. Valle JW, Borbath I, Khan SA, Huguet F, Gruenberger T, Arnold D, et al. Biliary cancer: ESMO clinical practice guidelines for diagnosis, treatment and follow-up. Ann Oncol. 2016;27:v28–37.
3. Okumura K, Gogna S, Gachabayov M, Felsenreich DM, McGuirk M, Rojas A, et al. Gallbladder cancer: historical treatment and new management options. World J Gastrointest Oncol. 2021;13:1317–35.
4. Chun YS, Pawlik TM, Vauthey JN. 8th edition of the AJCC cancer staging manual: pancreas and hepatobiliary cancers. Ann Surg Oncol. 2018;25:845–7.
5. Shindoh J, de Aretxabala X, Aloia TA, Roa JC, Roa I, Zimmitti G, et al. Tumor location is a strong predictor of tumor progression and survival in T2 gallbladder cancer: an international multicenter study. Ann Surg. 2015;261:733–9.
6. Lee H, Choi DW, Park JY, Youn S, Kwon W, Heo JS, et al. Surgical strategy for T2 gallbladder cancer according to tumor location. Ann Surg Oncol. 2015;22:2779–86.
7. Liu GJ, Li XH, Chen YX, Sun HD, Zhao GM, Hu SY. Radical lymph node dissection and assessment: impact on gallbladder cancer prognosis. World J Gastroenterol. 2013;19:5150–8.
8. Birnbaum DJ, Vigano L, Russolillo N, Langella S, Ferrero A, Capussotti L. Lymph node metastases in patients undergoing surgery for a gallbladder cancer. Extension of the lymph node dissection and prognostic value of the lymph node ratio. Ann Surg Oncol. 2015;22:811–8.
9. Ito H, Ito K, D'Angelica M, Gonen M, Klimstra D, Allen P, et al. Accurate staging for gallbladder cancer: implications for surgical therapy and pathological assessment. Ann Surg. 2011;254:320–5.
10. D'Angelica M, Dalal KM, DeMatteo RP, Fong Y, Blumgart LH, Jarnagin WR. Analysis of the extent of resection for adenocarcinoma of the gallbladder. Ann Surg Oncol. 2009;16:806–16.

11. Aloia TA, Jarufe N, Javle M, Maithel SK, Roa JC, Adsay V, et al. Gallbladder cancer: expert consensus statement. HPB (Oxford). 2015;17:681–90.
12. Ethun CG, Postlewait LM, Le N, Pawlik TM, Buettner S, Poultsides G, et al. Association of optimal time interval to re-resection for incidental gallbladder cancer with overall survival: a multi-institution analysis from the US extrahepatic biliary malignancy consortium. JAMA Surg. 2017;152:143–9.
13. Shih SP, Schulick RD, Cameron JL, Lillemoe KD, Pitt HA, Choti MA, et al. Gallbladder cancer: the role of laparoscopy and radical resection. Ann Surg. 2007;245:893–901.
14. Hueman MT, Vollmer CM Jr, Pawlik TM. Evolving treatment strategies for gallbladder cancer. Ann Surg Oncol. 2009;16:2101–15.
15. Jensen EH, Abraham A, Habermann EB, Al-Refaie WB, Vickers SM, Virnig BA, et al. A critical analysis of the surgical management of early-stage gallbladder cancer in the United States. J Gastrointest Surg. 2009;13:722–7.
16. Lee SE, Jang JY, Lim CS, Kang MJ, Kim SW. Systematic review on the surgical treatment for T1 gallbladder cancer. World J Gastroenterol. 2011;17:174–80.
17. Pilgrim C, Usatoff V, Evans PM. A review of the surgical strategies for the management of gallbladder carcinoma based on T stage and growth type of the tumour. Eur J Surg Oncol. 2009;35:903–7.
18. Vega EA, Vinuela E, Yamashita S, Sanhueza M, Cavada G, Diaz C, et al. Extended lymphadenectomy is required for incidental gallbladder cancer independent of cystic duct lymph node status. J Gastrointest Surg. 2018;22:43–51.
19. Qadan M, Kingham TP. Technical aspects of gallbladder cancer surgery. Surg Clin North Am. 2016;96:229–45.
20. Nishio H, Ebata T, Yokoyama Y, Igami T, Sugawara G, Nagino M. Gallbladder cancer involving the extrahepatic bile duct is worthy of resection. Ann Surg. 2011;253:953–60.
21. Pawlik TM, Gleisner AL, Vigano L, Kooby DA, Bauer TW, Frilling A, et al. Incidence of finding residual disease for incidental gallbladder carcinoma: implications for re-resection. J Gastrointest Surg. 2007;11:1478–86; discussion 86–7.
22. Mantripragada KC, Hamid F, Shafqat H, Olszewski AJ. Adjuvant therapy for resected gallbladder cancer: analysis of the National Cancer Data Base. J Natl Cancer Inst. 2017;109:djw202.
23. Hoehn RS, Wima K, Ertel AE, Meier A, Ahmad SA, Shah SA, et al. Adjuvant therapy for gallbladder cancer: an analysis of the National Cancer Data Base. J Gastrointest Surg. 2015;19:1794–801.
24. Kim TG. Patterns of initial failure after resection for gallbladder cancer: implications for adjuvant radiotherapy. Radiat Oncol J. 2017;35:359–67.
25. Valle J, Wasan H, Palmer DH, Cunningham D, Anthoney A, Maraveyas A, et al. Cisplatin plus gemcitabine versus gemcitabine for biliary tract cancer. N Engl J Med. 2010;362:1273–81.
26. Verma V, Surkar SM, Brooks ED, Simone CB 2nd, Lin C. Chemoradiotherapy versus chemotherapy alone for unresected nonmetastatic gallbladder cancer: national practice patterns and outcomes. J Natl Compr Cancer Netw. 2018;16:59–65.
27. Jain A, Javle M. Molecular profiling of biliary tract cancer: a target rich disease. J Gastrointest Oncol. 2016;7:797–803.
28. Sicklick JK, Fanta PT, Shimabukuro K, Kurzrock R. Genomics of gallbladder cancer: the case for biomarker-driven clinical trial design. Cancer Metastasis Rev. 2016;35:263–75.

Part X

Gastroenteropancreatic Neuroendocrine Tumor

Classification, Pathology, and Tumor Biology

Key Points

- Neuroendocrine neoplasms are classified according to cell differentiation and proliferation.
- In the pathological diagnosis and classification of gastroenteropancreatic neuroendocrine neoplasms, both histology and immunohistochemistry are important.
- Although the tumor biology of gastroenteropancreatic neuroendocrine neoplasms is complex due to their rarity and heterogeneity, genetic mutations may play a role in tumorigenesis.

Introduction

Gastroenteropancreatic neuroendocrine tumors (GEP-NETs), which originate from the neuroendocrine system of the gastrointestinal tract and pancreas, are very rare and represent heterogeneous biological behavior [1, 2]. GEP-NETs are classified according to their morphology and proliferative activities. With recent advances in the genetics, pathology, and molecular biology of GEP-NETs, the World Health Organization (WHO) classification has made substantial changes in the grading and staging system that guide appropriate therapeutic approaches and better prognostication.

Woo Hyun Paik is the lead author of this chapter.

H. J. Chun et al., *Gastrointestinal Cancer*, https://doi.org/10.1007/978-981-99-0815-8_58

Table 1 WHO classification for gastroenteropancreatic neuroendocrine neoplasms

Classification	Grade	Ki-67 index (%)[a]	Mitotic index (/2mm^2)[b]
Well-differentiated NENs			
NET G1	Low	<3	<2
NET G2	Intermediate	3–20	2–20
NET G3	High	>20	>20
Poorly differentiated NENs			
Small-cell-type NEC	High	>20	>20
Large-cell-type NEC			
MiNEN	Variable	Variable	Variable

NEN neuroendocrine neoplasm, *NET* neuroendocrine tumor, *NEC* neuroendocrine carcinoma, *MiNEN* mixed neuroendocrine-nonneuroendocrine neoplasm

[a] The Ki-67 proliferation index is based on the evaluation of ≥500 cells in regions of higher nuclear labeling. The final grade is determined based on whichever index (mitotic/Ki-67) places the tumor in the highest-grade category

[b] The mitotic index is based on the evaluation of mitoses in 50 high-power fields (0.2 mm^2 each) in area of higher density and is expressed as number of mitoses/2 mm^2

Classification of GEP-NETs

The latest WHO histopathological classification was introduced in 2017 for pancreatic NETs and in 2019 for gastroenteric NETs [3]. According to cell differentiation and proliferation, NETs are classified into five categories: (1) well differentiated, grade 1; (2) well differentiated, grade 2; (3) well differentiated, grade 3; (4) poorly differentiated, grade 3; and (5) mixed neuroendocrine-nonneuroendocrine. The Ki-67 cell proliferation index and mitotic activity indicate cell proliferation activity (Table 1). The grade of the WHO classification usually reflects the malignant potential of NET [4]; however, the histological grade does not always correlate with clinical behavior [5]. A subset of NETs with low histological grade may behave aggressively with rapid growth and distant metastases. In addition to cell differentiation and proliferation, next-generation immunohistochemistry, including lineage-restricted transcription factors and protein correlates of molecular genetic events that reflect the prognosis of NETs, is required [6].

Pathology of GEP-NETs

A histopathological diagnosis with the identification of neuroendocrine markers is required to confirm GEP-NETs. In addition, pathological reports describing cell differentiation and proliferation are also important for the classification of GEP-NETs (Fig. 1).

Histology

Well-differentiated NETs are epithelial neoplasms composed of small cells with relatively uniform round to oval nuclei, inconspicuous nucleoli, and a fine to coarsely granular chromatin pattern described as "salt and pepper" [7]. Cells are arranged with nesting and trabecular patterns [8]. On the contrary, poorly differentiated NETs show a solid "sheetlike" architecture with irregular nuclei, high mitotic characteristics, and less cytoplasmic secretory granules [5]. Both neuroendocrine and nonneuroendocrine components from same clonal origin can be seen in mixed neuroendocrine-nonneuroendocrine neoplasms (MiNENs), in which each component must have at least 30% of the tumor [6, 9]. Both components should be identifiable morphologically and immunohistochemically.

Immunohistochemistry

Traditional general neuroendocrine markers for immunohistochemistry include chromogranin A and synaptophysin, the former being generally

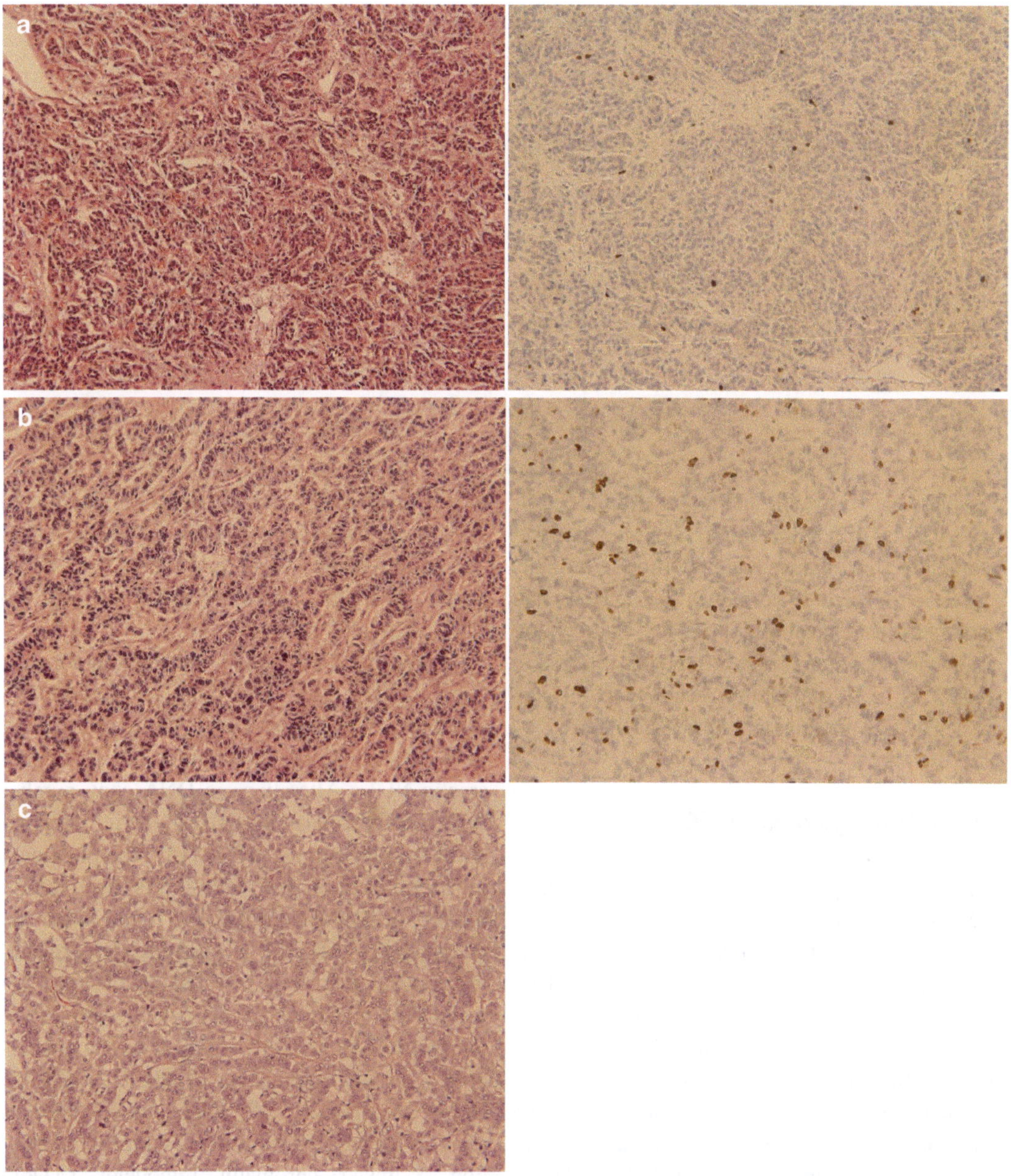

Fig. 1 Microscopic images of neuroendocrine neoplasm according to the WHO classification. (**a**) G1 pancreatic neuroendocrine tumor (H&E staining and Ki-67 immunohistochemistry, ×200), Ki-67 index is positive in 1%; (**b**) G3 well-differentiated pancreatic neuroendocrine carcinoma (H&E staining and Ki-67 immunohistochemistry, ×200), Ki-67 index is positive in 5%; (**c**) G3 poorly differentiated rectal large cell neuroendocrine carcinoma (H&E staining, ×200); (**d**) G3 poorly differentiated ampulla of Vater small cell neuroendocrine carcinoma (H&E staining and Ki-67 immunohistochemistry, ×200), Ki-67 index is positive in 70%

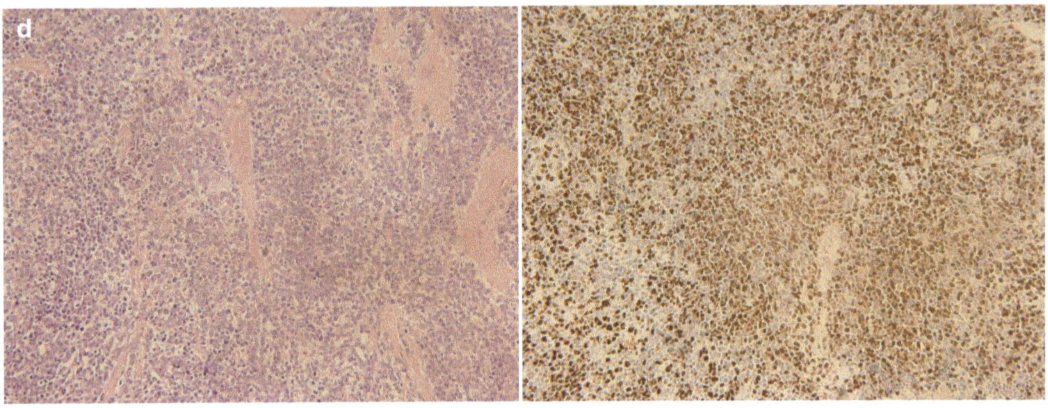

Fig. 1 (continued)

considered more specific and the latter more sensitive [6]. Well-differentiated NETs are positive for neuroendocrine markers and may show a variable expression of peptide hormones [6, 7]. However, immunohistochemical staining for neuroendocrine markers is more limited in poorly differentiated NETs [5]. Chromogranin A and synaptophysin are negative in one-quarter of G3 NETs [6].

Tumor Biology of GEP-NETs

The tumor biology of GEP-NETs is still unclear because of their rarity and heterogeneity. Moreover, different classifications of NETs have made tumor biology research difficult. GEP-NETs are now classified into two distinct categories with different genetic alterations [10]. G3 poorly differentiated neuroendocrine carcinomas are characterized by molecular changes that are commonly detected in conventional adenocarcinomas in the same organ, including *TP53, SMAD4, KRAS,* and *RB* [11–15]. On the contrary, well-differentiated neuroendocrine tumors are defined by different molecular pathways, some of which are common in neuroendocrine cell tumors at other sites, including inherited syndromes [11, 16]. Recently, whole genome sequencing revealed some mutational signatures in GEP-NETs (Fig. 2). Until now, approximately 24 genes have been associated with the tumorigenesis of GEP-NET, and these genes seem to be interconnected with important pathways involved in cell metabolism, chromatin modification, and growth control (Table 2) [17]. Mutations often involve epigenetic regulators rather than oncogenes and tumor suppressor genes that are also affected in other tumors [11].

Pancreatic NETs usually appear sporadically, although they can develop in association with hereditary syndromes. Therefore, genetic mutations may have roles in the tumorigenesis of pancreatic NETs. Alterations in DNA copy number and miRNA are also involved in the tumorigenesis and progression of NETs [18]. The malignant transformation of pancreatic NETs is driven by the progressive accumulation of multiple genetic alterations [19–21]. First, whole exome sequencing of pancreatic NETs revealed that the most frequent gene mutations specify proteins implicated in chromatin remodeling: 44% of the tumors harbored somatic inactivation of *MEN1*, and 43% had inactivation of death domain-associated protein *(DAXX)* or alpha-thalassemia/mental retardation X-linked chromatin remodeler *(ATRX)* mutation [16]. These are closely associated with alternative lengthening of the telomeres *(ALT)* and chromosomal instability (CIN) [22]. CIN is significantly correlated with loss of *DAXX* or *ATRX* and *activation of ALT.* According to previous studies that included a majority of Caucasians, *ALT* was identified in a substantial fraction of pancreatic NETs (48–61%), and unlike this, a lower prevalence (15%) was observed in a small Korean cohort; thus, the prevalence of ALT can vary by ethnicity [23]. A comprehensive molecu-

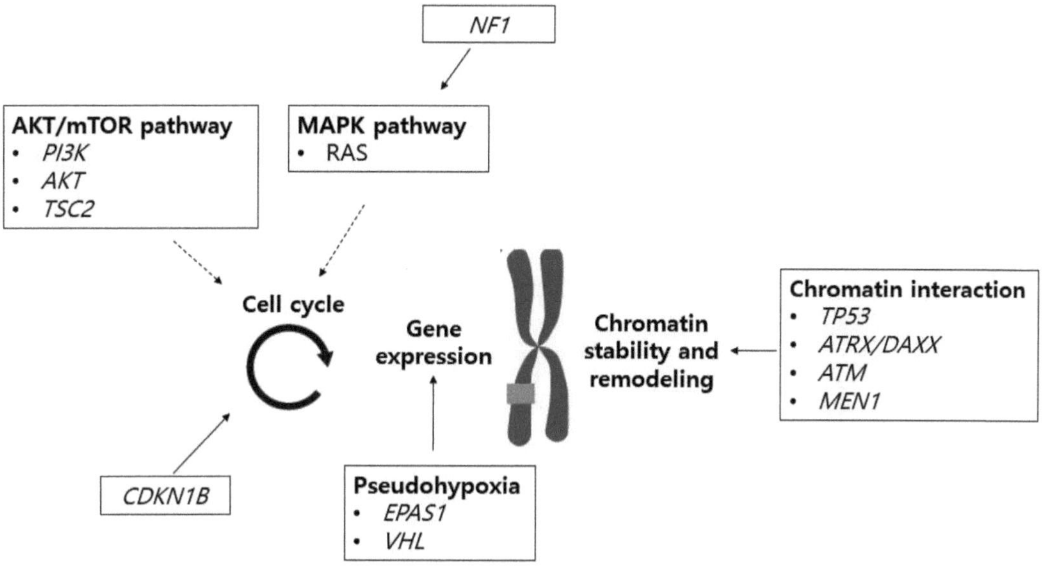

Fig. 2 Gene pathways involved in tumorigenesis of gastroenteropancreatic neuroendocrine tumors [17]

Table 2 Overview of genes involved in pathogenesis of gastroenteropancreatic neuroendocrine tumors [17]

Gene	Gene function	Chronological classification	Involved organ
ATM	Chromatin integrity	Unknown	Pancreas
ATRX	Alternative lengthening of telomeres	Late	Pancreas
CDKN1B	Cell cycle	Unknown	Pancreas, small intestine
DAXX	Alternative lengthening of telomeres	Late	Pancreas
EPAS1	Cell signaling	Early	Duodenum
MEN1	Chromatin modification, DNA repair, transcription, cell division, protein degradation, motility, and adhesion	Early	Pancreas, duodenum, stomach
NF1	Cell signaling	Early	Duodenum
TP53	Chromatin integrity, cell signaling	Unknown	Pancreas
TSC1–2	Cell signaling	Unknown	Pancreas
YY1	Transcriptional regulation	Early	Pancreas

lar analysis of 102 clinically sporadic pancreatic NETs was conducted to define molecular pathology and identify several novel candidate mechanisms that activate mTOR signaling, including novel gene fusion events [24, 25]. This whole genome landscape discovered several frequently mutated genes, including genes of the *DAXX, ATRX, MEN1, mTOR* pathway, and germline variants of *MUTYH* (Fig. 3) [25].

Small intestine NETs are less related to mutational driver events, even in familial cases [26]. High-throughput studies have identified putative driver mutations in *CDKN1B* and *APC* that have been reported in less than 10% of cases [27, 28]. *CDKN1B* encodes the tumor suppressor p27, whose mutation causes cell cycle dysregulation [28]. Recently, *IGF2* was identified as the genetic driver of NET in the small intestine [29]. Chromosomal alterations and epigenetic mutation could be more involved in tumorigenesis of NETs from the small intestine [30]. There are limited data on driver mutations in rectal NETs. Recent whole genome sequencing of 6 liver metastases from rectal NET revealed 11 of 18 somatic mutations, including known tumor-related genes *HSPG2, SERPINF2,* and

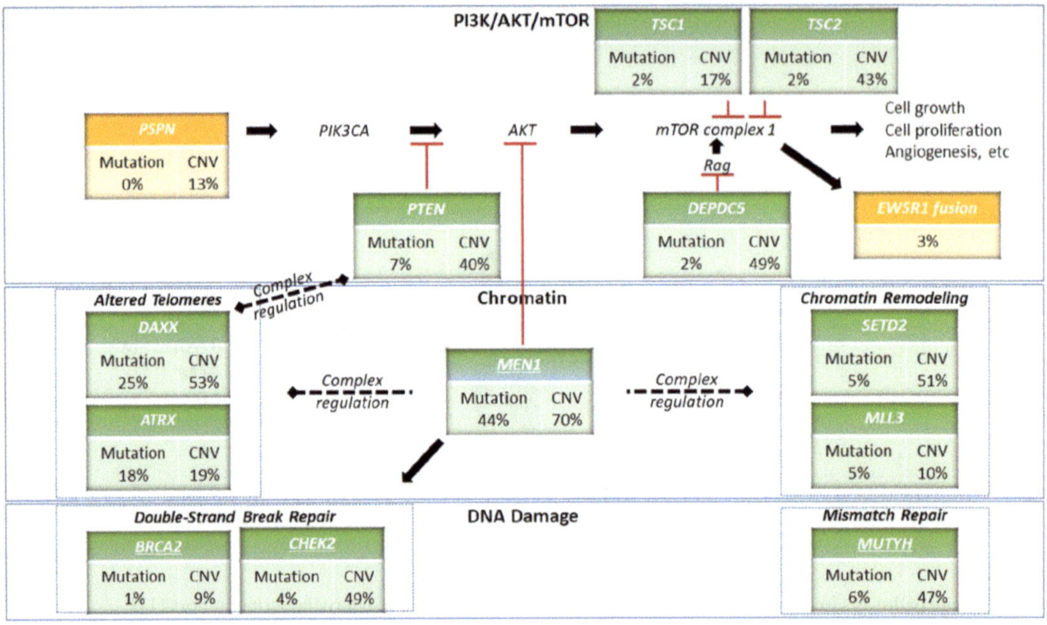

Fig. 3 Core pathways in pancreatic neuroendocrine tumors [11, 25]

SMARCA1 [11, 31]. Repetitive mutations in five genes, including *TP53, PTEN, CDKN2A, FBXW7,* and *AKT1,* have also been reported [32]. There are four types of NETs of the duodenal and ampullary region that have distinct clinical and molecular profiles [33]. The various genetic mutations can occur in the different gastric NETs, including *ATP4A* and *MEN1* in type 1 ECL-cell tumors, *MEN1* in all type 2 tumors and a large number of type 3 tumors, and *CDKN1B* in MEN4 syndrome [11].

Conclusion

Since GEP-NETs are a heterogeneous group, the classification of GEP-NETs is important. In addition to their pathological characteristics, genetic alterations will help to accurately classify prognostic GEP-NETs in the future.

References

1. Toumpanakis CG, Caplin ME. Molecular genetics of gastroenteropancreatic neuroendocrine tumors. Am J Gastroenterol. 2008;103:729–32.
2. Park JK, Paik WH, Lee K, Ryu JK, Lee SH, Kim YT. DAXX/ATRX and MEN1 genes are strong prognostic markers in pancreatic neuroendocrine tumors. Oncotarget. 2017;8:49796–806.
3. Di Mauro A, Scognamiglio G, Aquino G, Cerrone M, Liguori G, Clemente O, et al. Aberrant expression of long non coding RNA HOTAIR and De-regulation of the paralogous 13 HOX genes are strongly associated with aggressive behavior of gastro-entero-pancreatic neuroendocrine tumors. Int J Mol Sci. 2021;22:7049.
4. Paik WH, Lee HS, Lee KJ, Jang SI, Lee WJ, Hwang JH, et al. Malignant potential of small pancreatic neuroendocrine neoplasm and its risk factors: a multicenter nationwide study. Pancreatology. 2021;21:208–14.
5. Oronsky B, Ma PC, Morgensztern D, Carter CA. Nothing but NET: a review of neuroendocrine tumors and carcinomas. Neoplasia. 2017;19:991–1002.
6. Bellizzi AM. Immunohistochemistry in the diagnosis and classification of neuroendocrine neoplasms: what can brown do for you? Hum Pathol. 2020;96:8–33.
7. Borga C, Businello G, Murgioni S, Bergamo F, Martini C, De Carlo E, et al. Treatment personalization in gastrointestinal neuroendocrine tumors. Curr Treat Options in Oncol. 2021;22:29.
8. Klimstra DS, Modlin IR, Coppola D, Lloyd RV, Suster S. The pathologic classification of neuroendocrine tumors: a review of nomenclature, grading, and staging systems. Pancreas. 2010;39:707–12.
9. Frizziero M, Chakrabarty B, Nagy B, Lamarca A, Hubner RA, Valle JW, et al. Mixed neuroendocrine non-neuroendocrine neoplasms: a systematic review

of a controversial and underestimated diagnosis. J Clin Med. 2020;9:273.
10. Rindi G, Klimstra DS, Abedi-Ardekani B, Asa SL, Bosman FT, Brambilla E, et al. A common classification framework for neuroendocrine neoplasms: an International Agency for Research on Cancer (IARC) and World Health Organization (WHO) expert consensus proposal. Mod Pathol. 2018;31:1770–86.
11. Asa SL, La Rosa S, Basturk O, Adsay V, Minnetti M, Grossman AB. Molecular pathology of well-differentiated gastro-entero-pancreatic neuroendocrine tumors. Endocr Pathol. 2021;32:169–91.
12. Maitra A, Tascilar M, Hruban RH, Offerhaus GJ, Albores-Saavedra J. Small cell carcinoma of the gallbladder: a clinicopathologic, immunohistochemical, and molecular pathology study of 12 cases. Am J Surg Pathol. 2001;25:595–601.
13. Takizawa N, Ohishi Y, Hirahashi M, Takahashi S, Nakamura K, Tanaka M, et al. Molecular characteristics of colorectal neuroendocrine carcinoma; similarities with adenocarcinoma rather than neuroendocrine tumor. Hum Pathol. 2015;46:1890–900.
14. Hijioka S, Hosoda W, Matsuo K, Ueno M, Furukawa M, Yoshitomi H, et al. Rb loss and KRAS mutation are predictors of the response to platinum-based chemotherapy in pancreatic neuroendocrine neoplasm with grade 3: a Japanese multicenter pancreatic NEN-G3 study. Clin Cancer Res. 2017;23:4625–32.
15. Yachida S, Vakiani E, White CM, Zhong Y, Saunders T, Morgan R, et al. Small cell and large cell neuroendocrine carcinomas of the pancreas are genetically similar and distinct from well-differentiated pancreatic neuroendocrine tumors. Am J Surg Pathol. 2012;36:173–84.
16. Jiao Y, Shi C, Edil BH, de Wilde RF, Klimstra DS, Maitra A, et al. DAXX/ATRX, MEN1, and mTOR pathway genes are frequently altered in pancreatic neuroendocrine tumors. Science. 2011;331:1199–203.
17. Crona J, Skogseid B. GEP- NETS UPDATE: genetics of neuroendocrine tumors. Eur J Endocrinol. 2016;174:R275–90.
18. Capurso G, Festa S, Valente R, Piciucchi M, Panzuto F, Jensen RT, et al. Molecular pathology and genetics of pancreatic endocrine tumours. J Mol Endocrinol. 2012;49:R37–50.
19. Speel EJ, Richter J, Moch H, Egenter C, Saremaslani P, Rütimann K, et al. Genetic differences in endocrine pancreatic tumor subtypes detected by comparative genomic hybridization. Am J Pathol. 1999;155:1787–94.
20. Zhao J, Moch H, Scheidweiler AF, Baer A, Schäffer AA, Speel EJ, et al. Genomic imbalances in the progression of endocrine pancreatic tumors. Genes Chromosomes Cancer. 2001;32:364–72.
21. Jonkers YM, Claessen SM, Perren A, Schmid S, Komminoth P, Verhofstad AA, et al. Chromosomal instability predicts metastatic disease in patients with insulinomas. Endocr Relat Cancer. 2005;12:435–47.
22. Marinoni I, Kurrer AS, Vassella E, Dettmer M, Rudolph T, Banz V, et al. Loss of DAXX and ATRX are associated with chromosome instability and reduced survival of patients with pancreatic neuroendocrine tumors. Gastroenterology. 2014;146:453–60.e5.
23. Kim JY, Brosnan-Cashman JA, An S, Kim SJ, Song KB, Kim MS, et al. Alternative lengthening of telomeres in primary pancreatic neuroendocrine tumors is associated with aggressive clinical behavior and poor survival. Clin Cancer Res. 2017;23:1598–606.
24. Scarpa A. The landscape of molecular alterations in pancreatic and small intestinal neuroendocrine tumours. Ann Endocrinol (Paris). 2019;80:153–8.
25. Scarpa A, Chang DK, Nones K, Corbo V, Patch AM, Bailey P, et al. Whole-genome landscape of pancreatic neuroendocrine tumours. Nature. 2017;543:65–71.
26. Banck MS, Kanwar R, Kulkarni AA, Boora GK, Metge F, Kipp BR, et al. The genomic landscape of small intestine neuroendocrine tumors. J Clin Invest. 2013;123:2502–8.
27. Alrezk R, Hannah-Shmouni F, Stratakis CA. MEN4 and CDKN1B mutations: the latest of the MEN syndromes. Endocr Relat Cancer. 2017;24:T195–t208.
28. Francis JM, Kiezun A, Ramos AH, Serra S, Pedamallu CS, Qian ZR, et al. Somatic mutation of CDKN1B in small intestine neuroendocrine tumors. Nat Genet. 2013;45:1483–6.
29. Contractor T, Clausen R, Harris GR, Rosenfeld JA, Carpizo DR, Tang L, et al. IGF2 drives formation of ileal neuroendocrine tumors in patients and mice. Endocr Relat Cancer. 2020;27:175–86.
30. Carpizo DR, Harris CR. Genetic drivers of ileal neuroendocrine tumors. Cancers (Basel). 2021;13:5070.
31. Koşaloğlu Z, Zörnig I, Halama N, Kaiser I, Buchhalter I, Grabe N, et al. Identification of immunotherapeutic targets by genomic profiling of rectal NET metastases. Oncoimmunology. 2016;5:e1213931.
32. Park HY, Kwon MJ, Kang HS, Kim YJ, Kim NY, Kim MJ, et al. Targeted next-generation sequencing of well-differentiated rectal, gastric, and appendiceal neuroendocrine tumors to identify potential targets. Hum Pathol. 2019;87:83–94.
33. Vanoli A, La Rosa S, Klersy C, Grillo F, Albarello L, Inzani F, et al. Four neuroendocrine tumor types and neuroendocrine carcinoma of the duodenum: analysis of 203 cases. Neuroendocrinology. 2017;104:112–25.

Multiple Endocrine Neoplasia and Other Inherited Syndromes (MEN-1, VHL, NF-1, Tuberous Sclerosis)

Key Points

- The development of neuroendocrine tumors (NETs) in inherited syndromes is associated with germline mutations that show prominent clinical manifestations.
- Clinicians should distinguish NETs arising from inherited syndromes from sporadic cases.

Introduction

Most neuroendocrine tumors (NETs) are considered sporadic; however, some NETs are related to a heritable group of neoplasms that appear in at least ten genetic syndromes, of which multiple endocrine neoplasia type 1 (MEN-1), von Hippel-Lindau syndrome (VHL), neurofibromatosis type 1 (NF-1), and tuberous sclerosis are representative [1]. The development of NETs in inherited syndrome is associated with germline mutations that show prominent clinical manifestations, and the clinician should differentiate NETs arising from inherited syndrome from sporadic cases through careful history and physical examination, biochemical tests, images, and pathologic results [2]. Up to 10% of pancreatic NETs develop in patients with inherited syndromes that predispose them to cancer [3]. The gastroenteropancreatic NETs in settings of inherited syndrome require different treatment strategies and surveillance and lead to a preclinical diagnosis in family members [4].

MEN-1

Clinical Characteristics

MEN-1 is one of the first described complex autosomal dominantly inherited endocrine tumor syndromes [5]. The prevalence of MEN-1 varies by ethnicity and region, and the estimated prevalence of MEN-1 is 1 to 10 per 100,000 individuals [6]. Typical MEN-1 is defined as a tumor in two of the three main endocrine organs, which in familial MEN-1 includes at least one relative with a tumor in one of the three main endocrine organs [7]. Commonly affected organs are the parathyroid gland, pancreatic islet cells, thymus, and pituitary gland [8]. The organ most frequently affected is the parathyroid gland, which occurs in 95% of cases [9]. Primary hyperparathyroidism is usually the first clinical manifestation observed in MEN-1 patients, typically between 20 and 25 years of age [7, 10], and the clinical penetration of the disease is nearly 100%

Woo Hyun Paik is the lead author of this chapter.

H. J. Chun et al., *Gastrointestinal Cancer*, https://doi.org/10.1007/978-981-99-0815-8_59

by 50 years of age [11]. Pancreaticoduodenal NETs represent the second most common manifestation of MEN-1 with a prevalence of 35% in the 50s [7]. Other endocrine tumors seen in MEN-1 include adrenal cortical tumors, duodenopancreatic neuroendocrine tumors, and rare pheochromocytomas [12].

MEN-4 is a very rare autosomal dominant disease that arises from mutation of a cyclin-dependent kinase inhibitor (*CDKN1B*) on chromosome 12 encoding the p27 protein [2]. The clinical manifestations of MEN-4 are similar to those of MEN-1; however, gastroenteropancreatic NETs are less frequent than in MEN-1 [13].

Genetic and Molecular Characteristics

MEN-1 is caused by germline pathogenic mutation in the *MEN1* tumor suppressor gene encoding for a 610-amino acid protein, menin, located on chromosome 11q13 [5, 14, 15]. Menin is a scaffold protein with more than 40 interacting proteins and thus is involved in various biological functions, including chromatin modification, DNA repair, transcription, cell division, protein degradation, motility, and adhesion [9]. The genetic test for *the* germline mutation *MEN1* is recommended in all patients with clinical suspicion of MEN1 and their first-degree relatives regardless of their symptoms [6, 7, 16]. Classical tumorigenesis of MEN1 depends on a second *MEN1* hit, by a somatic mutation also eliminating the wild-type (WT) allele. However, thymic and duodenal NETs in MEN-1 do not require complete inactivation of *MEN1* [17]. Classical hypermethylation is frequent in NETs; however, methylation patterns are different between MEN-1-related and sporadic pancreatic NETs [18].

Management and Prognosis

Patients with MEN-1 show a shorter life expectancy, and the outcomes of current treatments, which are generally similar to those of the respective tumors that occur in patients without MEN-1, are not as successful due to multiple tumors, which may be larger, more aggressive, and resistant to treatment, and the development of metastases [16]. The timing of surgery for duodenopancreatic NETs that arise from MEN-1 remains controversial, as the germline mutation renders the entire pancreatic parenchyma susceptible to tumorigenesis and the morbidity of postoperative endocrine insufficiency should be balanced against the putative oncologic benefit of any operation [2]. Early resection of NETs in MEN-1 can prevent the development of distant metastases. Organ-sparing resection may be preferred as an initial duodenopancreatic procedure to maintain pancreatic function and delay total pancreatectomy [19]. However, approximately 80% of patients develop metachronous NETs in the duodenopancreatic remnant that may require long-term total pancreatectomy [20]. Therefore, reoperation is often necessary for pancreatic NETs in MEN-1, but reoperations have not been associated with an increase in perioperative morbidity in a recent single-center study [19].

In the Dutch national cohort of MEN-1, most small nonfunctioning pancreatic NETs less than 2 cm in size remained stable at the median follow-up of 3 years; however, germline missense mutations were significantly associated with accelerated growth compared to frameshift and nonsense mutations [21]. These molecular driving events may be used as potential biomarkers in MEN-1.

The prognosis of MEN-1 may be improved by early detection of the tumor before the onset of clinical symptoms. The current MEN-1 guidelines recommend imaging studies annually [16]. Since clinical manifestations of MEN-1 rarely occur below the age of 16 years, routine screening for asymptomatic MEN-1 can be postponed until the age of 16 years [22]. Malignant gastrinoma and foregut carcinoid tumor represent the most common cause of death associated with MEN-1 [23].

VHL

VHL is a highly penetrant autosomal dominant disease and has an incidence of 2.73 per 100,000 people [24, 25]. The most common clinical features are retinal and CNS hemangioblastoma (>70%), pheochromocytoma (10–20%) and renal (up to 60%), pancreatic tumors (35–70%), and endolymphatic sac (10%) [24, 25]. Patients with a family history and CNS hemangioblastoma, pheochromocytoma, or clear cell renal cell carcinoma are diagnosed with VHL. Those without a family history should have two or more CNS hemangioblastoma and a visceral tumor (apart from epididymal and renal cyst) to meet the diagnostic criteria [25].

The prevalence of pancreatic NET and cysts in VHL are 8%–17% and 17%–56%, respectively [25, 26]. Pancreatic cysts, including serous cystadenoma, can be routinely followed without treatment, whereas pancreatic NETs usually require surgical resection. However, differentiation of NET with cyst can be difficult [25]. Likewise, for MEN-1, preservation of pancreatic function must be done with the malignant potential of the NETs in mind.

VHL is a tumor suppressor gene located on chromosome 3p25 and has three exons that encode the VHL protein [27]. Its function involves the oxygen-sensing pathway through hypoxia-inducible factors. The disruption of VHL-protein-mediated degradation of hypoxia-inducible factors contributes to tumor formation by stimulating angiogenesis and proliferation of endothelial cells and pericytes [25, 28].

NF-1

NF-1 is also an autosomal dominant inherited disease caused by mutation of the *NF1* gene on chromosome 17q11; however, approximately half of patients have a de novo mutation [2]. *NF1* is a tumor suppressor gene and encodes a RAS GTPase-activating protein called neurofibromin [29]. Its inactivation led to increased *RAS-MAPK* signaling, causing related diseases collectively known as RASopathies [28, 29]. Clinical manifestations include café-au-lait spots, iris hamartomas and optic gliomas, benign schwannomas, as well as malignant peripheral nerve sheath tumors and pancreatic NET [2]. Pancreatic NETs are not included as part of NF-1 diagnostic criteria, accounting for less than 10% of documented cases [28]. NETs that occur in NF-1 are exclusively duodenopancreatic somatostatinomas, and syndromic somatostatinomas differ from sporadic because they usually secrete less hormones and are less likely to be malignant [30].

Tuberous Sclerosis

Clinical Characteristics

Tuberous sclerosis is a rare hereditary autosomal dominant syndrome caused by a mutation of *TSC1* and *TSC2*, located on chromosomes 9q34 and 16p13.3, respectively [28]. These are tumor suppressor genes and encode the proteins hamartin and tuberin, which involve multiple intracellular signaling pathways that regulate both cell growth and proliferation [31, 32]. Clinical manifestations include multiorgan hamartomas, disabling neurologic features and skin lesions, typically facial angiofibroma, hypomelanocytic macules, ungual fibromas, and shagreen patch [31]. Pancreatic NETs have been reported to be slightly more prevalent in this syndrome, especially those with the *TSC2* mutation [33, 34].

Conclusion

The development of neuroendocrine tumors (NETs) in inherited syndrome is associated with germline mutations. Clinicians should distinguish NETs arising from hereditary syndromes from sporadic cases by not missing the characteristic features of hereditary syndromes (Table 1).

Table 1 Overview of inherited syndrome with NET manifestation

	Gene	NET involved organ	Other manifestation
Multiple endocrine neoplasia type 1	*MEN1*	Parathyroid (95%), gastroenteropancreatic (50%), anterior pituitary (30%), lung and thymus (10%)	Adrenocortical tumor, midfacial angiofibroma, and collagenoma
Multiple endocrine neoplasia type 4	*CDKN1B*	Pituitary and parathyroid (common), gastroenteropancreatic (less common)	
Von Hippel-Lindau syndrome	*VHL*	Adrenal medulla and sympathetic ganglia (15%), pancreas (10%)	Hemangioblastoma of the cerebellum and spinal cord, serous cystadenoma of the pancreas, renal cell carcinoma, aniomata of the retina, endolymphatic sac tumor
Neurofibromatosis type 1	*NF1*	Adrenal medulla (1–5%), pancreas, duodenum	Neurofibroma, café-au-lait spots, iris hamartoma, optic glioma, schwannoma, malignant peripheral nerve sheath tumor
Tuberous sclerosis	*TSC1, TSC2*	Pancreas	Multiorgan hamartoma, skin lesions (typically facial angiofibroma, hypomelanocytic macules, ungual fibromas, and shagreen patch), epilepsy, mental retardation

NET neuroendocrine tumor, *MEN1* odd ratio

References

1. Crona J, Skogseid B. GEP- NETS UPDATE: genetics of neuroendocrine tumors. Eur J Endocrinol. 2016;174:R275–90.
2. Lewis MA. Hereditary syndromes in neuroendocrine tumors. Curr Treat Options Oncol. 2020;21:50.
3. Halfdanarson TR, Rabe KG, Rubin J, Petersen GM. Pancreatic neuroendocrine tumors (PNETs): incidence, prognosis and recent trend toward improved survival. Ann Oncol. 2008;19:1727–33.
4. Ito T, Masui T, Komoto I, Doi R, Osamura RY, Sakurai A, et al. JNETS clinical practice guidelines for gastroenteropancreatic neuroendocrine neoplasms: diagnosis, treatment, and follow-up: a synopsis. J Gastroenterol. 2021;56:1033.
5. Wermer P. Genetic aspects of adenomatosis of endocrine glands. Am J Med. 1954;16:363–71.
6. Niederle B, Selberherr A, Bartsch DK, Brandi ML, Doherty GM, Falconi M, et al. Multiple endocrine neoplasia type 1 and the pancreas: diagnosis and treatment of functioning and non-functioning pancreatic and duodenal neuroendocrine neoplasia within the MEN1 syndrome—an international consensus statement. Neuroendocrinology. 2021;111:609–30.
7. Brandi ML, Gagel RF, Angeli A, Bilezikian JP, Beck-Peccoz P, Bordi C, et al. Guidelines for diagnosis and therapy of MEN type 1 and type 2. J Clin Endocrinol Metab. 2001;86:5658–71.
8. Effraimidis G, Knigge U, Rossing M, Oturai P, Rasmussen ÅK, Feldt-Rasmussen U. Multiple endocrine neoplasia type 1 (MEN-1) and neuroendocrine neoplasms (NENs). Semin Cancer Biol. 2022;79:141–62.
9. Agarwal SK. Multiple endocrine neoplasia type 1. Front Horm Res. 2013;41:1–15.
10. Trump D, Farren B, Wooding C, Pang JT, Besser GM, Buchanan KD, et al. Clinical studies of multiple endocrine neoplasia type 1 (MEN1). QJM. 1996;89:653–69.
11. Machens A, Schaaf L, Karges W, Frank-Raue K, Bartsch DK, Rothmund M, et al. Age-related penetrance of endocrine tumours in multiple endocrine neoplasia type 1 (MEN1): a multicentre study of 258 gene carriers. Clin Endocrinol (Oxf). 2007;67:613–22.
12. Triponez F, Dosseh D, Goudet P, Cougard P, Bauters C, Murat A, et al. Epidemiology data on 108 MEN 1 patients from the GTE with isolated nonfunctioning tumors of the pancreas. Ann Surg. 2006;243:265–72.
13. Frederiksen A, Rossing M, Hermann P, Ejersted C, Thakker RV, Frost M. Clinical features of multiple endocrine neoplasia type 4: novel pathogenic variant and review of published cases. J Clin Endocrinol Metab. 2019;104:3637–46.
14. Chandrasekharappa SC, Guru SC, Manickam P, Olufemi SE, Collins FS, Emmert-Buck MR, et al. Positional cloning of the gene for multiple endocrine neoplasia-type 1. Science. 1997;276:404–7.
15. Agarwal SK, Kester MB, Debelenko LV, Heppner C, Emmert-Buck MR, Skarulis MC, et al. Germline mutations of the MEN1 gene in familial multiple endocrine neoplasia type 1 and related states. Hum Mol Genet. 1997;6:1169–75.
16. Thakker RV, Newey PJ, Walls GV, Bilezikian J, Dralle H, Ebeling PR, et al. Clinical practice guidelines for

multiple endocrine neoplasia type 1 (MEN1). J Clin Endocrinol Metab. 2012;97:2990–3011.
17. Anlauf M, Perren A, Henopp T, Rudolf T, Garbrecht N, Schmitt A, et al. Allelic deletion of the MEN1 gene in duodenal gastrin and somatostatin cell neoplasms and their precursor lesions. Gut. 2007;56:637–44.
18. Tirosh A, Mukherjee S, Lack J, Gara SK, Wang S, Quezado MM, et al. Distinct genome-wide methylation patterns in sporadic and hereditary nonfunctioning pancreatic neuroendocrine tumors. Cancer. 2019;125:1247–57.
19. Albers MB, Manoharan J, Bollmann C, Chlosta MP, Holzer K, Bartsch DK. Results of duodenopancreatic reoperations in multiple endocrine neoplasia type 1. World J Surg. 2019;43:552–8.
20. Lopez CL, Waldmann J, Fendrich V, Langer P, Kann PH, Bartsch DK. Long-term results of surgery for pancreatic neuroendocrine neoplasms in patients with MEN1. Langenbecks Arch Surg. 2011;396:1187–96.
21. Pieterman CRC, de Laat JM, Twisk JWR, van Leeuwaarde RS, de Herder WW, Dreijerink KMA, et al. Long-term natural course of small nonfunctional pancreatic neuroendocrine tumors in MEN1-results from the Dutch MEN1 Study Group. J Clin Endocrinol Metab. 2017;102:3795–805.
22. Manoharan J, Raue F, Lopez CL, Albers MB, Bollmann C, Fendrich V, et al. Is routine screening of young asymptomatic MEN1 patients necessary? World J Surg. 2017;41:2026–32.
23. Goudet P, Murat A, Binquet C, Cardot-Bauters C, Costa A, Ruszniewski P, et al. Risk factors and causes of death in MEN1 disease. A GTE (Groupe d'Etude des Tumeurs Endocrines) cohort study among 758 patients. World J Surg. 2010;34:249–55.
24. Maher ER, Iselius L, Yates JR, Littler M, Benjamin C, Harris R, et al. Von Hippel-Lindau disease: a genetic study. J Med Genet. 1991;28:443–7.
25. Lonser RR, Glenn GM, Walther M, Chew EY, Libutti SK, Linehan WM, et al. von Hippel-Lindau disease. Lancet. 2003;361:2059–67.
26. Libutti SK, Choyke PL, Bartlett DL, Vargas H, Walther M, Lubensky I, et al. Pancreatic neuroendocrine tumors associated with von Hippel Lindau disease: diagnostic and management recommendations. Surgery. 1998;124:1153–9.
27. Latif F, Tory K, Gnarra J, Yao M, Duh FM, Orcutt ML, et al. Identification of the von Hippel-Lindau disease tumor suppressor gene. Science. 1993;260:1317–20.
28. Guilmette JM, Nosé V. Neoplasms of the neuroendocrine pancreas: an update in the classification, definition, and molecular genetic advances. Adv Anat Pathol. 2019;26:13–30.
29. Ratner N, Miller SJ. A RASopathy gene commonly mutated in cancer: the neurofibromatosis type 1 tumour suppressor. Nat Rev Cancer. 2015;15:290–301.
30. Mao C, Shah A, Hanson DJ, Howard JM. Von Recklinghausen's disease associated with duodenal somatostatinoma: contrast of duodenal versus pancreatic somatostatinomas. J Surg Oncol. 1995;59:67–73.
31. Northrup H, Krueger DA. Tuberous sclerosis complex diagnostic criteria update: recommendations of the 2012 international tuberous sclerosis complex consensus conference. Pediatr Neurol. 2013;49:243–54.
32. Dworakowska D, Grossman AB. Are neuroendocrine tumours a feature of tuberous sclerosis? A systematic review. Endocr Relat Cancer. 2009;16:45–58.
33. Arva NC, Pappas JG, Bhatla T, Raetz EA, Macari M, Ginsburg HB, et al. Well-differentiated pancreatic neuroendocrine carcinoma in tuberous sclerosis—case report and review of the literature. Am J Surg Pathol. 2012;36:149–53.
34. Merritt JL 2nd, Davis DM, Pittelkow MR, Babovic-Vuksanovic D. Extensive acrochordons and pancreatic islet-cell tumors in tuberous sclerosis associated with TSC2 mutations. Am J Med Genet A. 2006;140:1669–72.

Gastric NEN. III-1. Epidemiology (Including Risk Factor)/Pathologic and Molecular Characteristics

Key Points

- Gastric neuroendocrine neoplasms (G-NEN) are the most common NEN of the foregut.
- The incidence of G-NEN is steadily increasing in Western countries and in Asia.
- G-NEN is classified into three grades and four subtypes according to characteristics and prognosis.
- Chromogranin A, synaptophysin, and neuron-specific enolase can be used as a molecular and immunohistochemical marker.

Introduction

Gastroenteropancreatic neuroendocrine neoplasms (GEP-NEN) are heterogeneous neoplasms originating from neuroendocrine cells. GEP-NEN can develop anywhere in the gastrointestinal tract and pancreas. Gastric NEN (G-NEN) is the most common NEN of the foregut (thymus, esophagus, lung, stomach, duodenum, and pancreas). G-NEN is generally considered an indolent tumor with a low tendency to metastasize; however, gastric neuroendocrine carcinoma (G-NEC) can progress rapidly once they become metastatic.

Epidemiology of G-NEN

The proportion of G-NEN is relatively low in all GEP-NEN (4–11%) and among all gastric neoplasms (2%) [1–3]. However, the incidence of G-NEN has steadily increased in the last three decades. The estimated annual incidence is 0.4/100,000 people in Western countries [4]. The prevalence reported per 10,000 population was 0.32 for Europe, 0.17 for the United States, and 0.05 for Japan [3]. The increased use of screening endoscopy and better awareness of the disease may be related to the increased incidence and early diagnosis of G-NEN [5–7].

Kwangwoo Nam is the lead author of this chapter.

H. J. Chun et al., *Gastrointestinal Cancer*, https://doi.org/10.1007/978-981-99-0815-8_60

Risk Factor for G-NEN

To date no definitive environmental risk factors have been described about G-NEN [1], but visceral obesity and metabolic syndrome are suggested as potential risk factors for NEN. In a previous study from the United States, diabetes and a family history of cancer increased the risk of G-NEN in women, suggesting that women may have a greater genetic susceptibility to NEN than men [8]. A recent study reported that the risk of GEP-NEN is associated with obesity and the number of metabolic syndrome components (increased waist circumference, high blood pressure, low high-density lipoprotein, high triglycerides, and high fasting plasma glucose), although the proportion of G-NEN is very low (1.4%) [9].

Clinicopathologic Characteristics of G-NEN

Most G-NEN usually arise from subepithelial, histamine-secreting, enterochromaffin-like (ECL) cells, located in the corpus-fundus mucosa [4]. Only a small proportion develop from non-ECL cells of the gastric mucosa. Based on clinical and prognostic characteristics and significance, G-NEN can be classified according to the World Health Organization (WHO) classification (Table 1) [6]. Furthermore, G-NEN is subdivided into four subtypes (Table 2) [5].

Table 1 World Health Organization classification of neuroendocrine neoplasms

	Ki-67 index (%)	Mitotic index
Well-differentiated NENs		
NET G1	<3	<2/10 HPF
NET G2	3–20	2–20/10 HPF
Poorly differentiated NENs		
NEC G3	>20	>20/10 HFP

NEN neuroendocrine neoplasm, *NET* neuroendocrine tumor, *HPF* high-power field, *NEC* neuroendocrine carcinoma
Adapted from Jung et al. [10]

Table 2 Clinicopathological characteristics of gastric neuroendocrine neoplasms

	Gastric NETs/carcinoids			Gastric NECs (poorly differentiated NENs)
	Type 1	Type 2	Type 3	Type 4
Relative frequency	70–80%	5–6%	14–25%	6–8%
Features	Mostly small (<1–2 cm) and multiple	Mostly small (<1–2 cm) and multiple	Solitary often >2 cm	Solitary mostly exulcerated, >2 cm
Associated conditions	CAG	MEN1/ZES	No	No
Histology	Well-differentiated G1	Well-differentiated G1	Well-/moderately differentiated G2	Poorly differentiated G3
Serum gastrin	(Very) high	(Very) high	Normal	(Mostly) normal
Gastric pH	Anacidic	Hyperacidic	Normal	(Mostly) normal
Metastasis	<10%	10–30%	50–100%	80–100%
Tumor-related death	No	<10%	25–30%	≥50%

NET neuroendocrine tumor, *NEC* neuroendocrine carcinoma, *NEN* neuroendocrine neoplasm, *CAG* chronic atrophic gastritis, due to pernicious anemia or *Helicobacter pylori* infection, *MEN1* multiple endocrine neoplasia type1, *ZES* Zollinger-Ellison syndrome
Adapted from Park et al. [5]

Grade

All G-NEN are classified into three proliferative grades, according to WHO 2019 that correlate with malignant potential and prognosis [6, 10]. Grade 1 and 2 NEN correspond to well-differentiated NEN, while grade 3 NEC is poorly differentiated NEN showing a poor prognosis.

Subtypes

Type 1 G-NEN accounts for ~70–80% of G-NEN and is associated with chronic atrophic gastritis (CAG). The absence of gastric acid (achlorhydria, gastric pH >7) is associated with autoimmune CAG that destroys the gastric parietal cells in the body and fundus and stimulates antral G cells to secrete excessive serum gastrin, causing neuroendocrine cell hyperplasia and the development of multifocal polypoid G-NEN. G-NEN lesions are usually small and multiple and have a benign course. Endoscopic resection with regular monitoring is recommended. In general, type 1 G-NEN showed an excellent prognosis with a 5-year survival of almost 100% (90–95%) [6, 11].

Type 2 G-NEN is the least common type of all G-NEN. It is associated with hyperchlorhydria (gastric pH ≤2) underlying gastrinoma with hypergastrinemia in patients with multiple endocrine neoplasia (MEN) type 1. Patients with type 2 G-NEN usually have diarrhea, heartburn, and peptic ulcer, which is commonly associated with Zollinger-Ellison syndrome (ZES). G-NEN in sporadic ZES is rare (<1%). The prognosis for type 2 G-NEN is good with a 5-year survival of 70–90% [6].

Type 3 G-NEN occurs sporadically and is not associated with hypergastrinemia. This type occurs most frequently in men over 50 years of age in the presence of normogastrinemia and normal gastric mucosa. These develop from ECL cells in most cases in the absence of ECL hyperplasia and are not dependent on gastrin. The malignant potential and the chance of metastasis are relatively high compared to type 1 or 2 G-NEN. At diagnosis, tumor presents as a single mass greater than 2 cm, and a high rate of lymph node metastasis (~50–100%) and liver metastasis (22–75%) are reported [10]. Thus, surgical resection is considered in most cases. In some cases, hepatic metastasis can be the initial presentation.

G-NEC is classified as type 4 G-NEN. They are usually of non-ECL cell origin and are gastrin-independent. They occur commonly in males older than 60 years of age. Histologically, they are aggressive NEC grade 3 almost identical to gastric adenocarcinoma. At diagnosis, the tumor presents as a large mass greater than 4 cm, and lymph node and liver metastasis is frequent.

Molecular and Immunohistochemical Characteristics of G-NEN

There were specific markers that can be used to establish the diagnosis and differentiation of G-NEN such as chromogranin, synaptophysin, and neuron-specific enolase (NSE) [12].

Chromogranin A (CgA) is a secreted protein and is used as a biomarker of NEN. CgA has been detected in most neuroendocrine cells and neoplasms. A meta-analysis reported that the sensitivity and specificity are 73% and 95%, respectively, and CgA may have prognostic value in some patients. However, CgA levels are largely affected by liver or kidney disease and the use of proton pump inhibitors; therefore, there are concerns about the precision of the test, and it is recommended that treatment decisions are not based solely on changes in CgA [13].

Synaptophysin is a transmembrane glycoprotein in the membranes of presynaptic vesicles. Synaptophysin is widely distributed in neuroendocrine cells and is a good general marker; however, it is less specific because normal cells, adenomas, and carcinomas of the adrenal cortex can show positivity to synaptophysin.

NSE presents in neurons and neuroendocrine cells and therefore can be used as a marker of NEN. However, NSE is of limited usefulness due to low specificity because there is cross-reactivity in smooth muscle cells, myoepithelial cells, and lymphocytes.

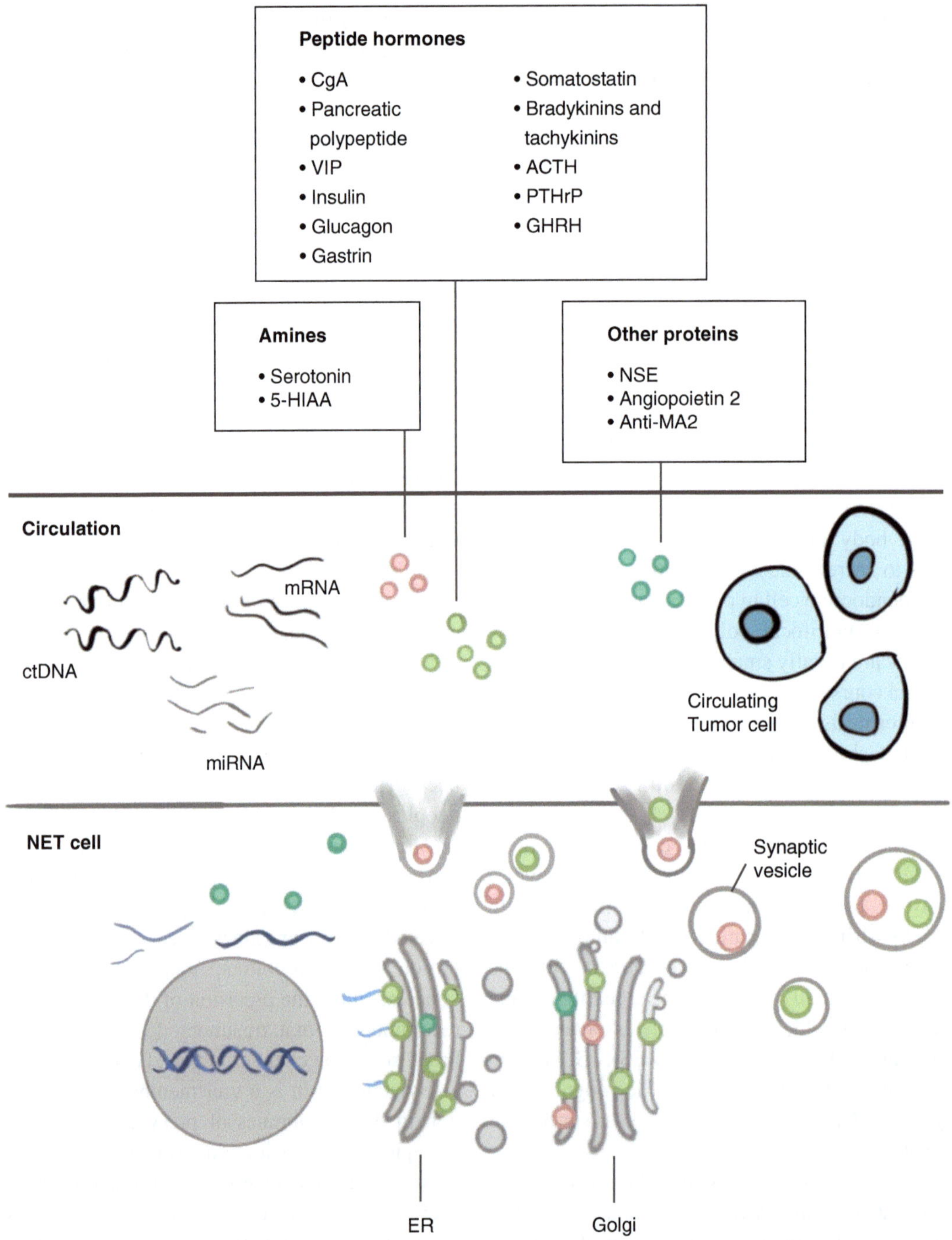

Fig. 1 Common biomarkers for gastroenteropancreatic neuroendocrine neoplasms. (Adapted from Hofland et al. [14])

Other circulating hormones such as serotonin and its metabolites, insulin, glucagon, and gastrin, are potential biomarkers for the diagnosis and surveillance of G-NEN [14] (Fig. 1).

Conclusion

The incidence of G-NEN is not very high but has gradually been increasing with the active application of screening endoscopy. In general, the prognosis for G-NEN is favorable, but grade 3 G-NEC have a poor outcome. CgA, synaptophysin, and NSE can be used as a biomarker of G-NEN but have low specificity.

References

1. Cives M, Strosberg JR. Gastroenteropancreatic neuroendocrine tumors. CA Cancer J Clin. 2018;68:471–87.
2. Dasari A, Shen C, Halperin D, Zhao B, Zhou S, Xu Y, et al. Trends in the incidence, prevalence, and survival outcomes in patients with neuroendocrine tumors in the United States. JAMA Oncol. 2017;3:1335–42.
3. Boyce M, Thomsen L. Gastric neuroendocrine tumors: prevalence in Europe, USA, and Japan, and rationale for treatment with a gastrin/CCK2 receptor antagonist. Scand J Gastroenterol. 2015;50:550–9.
4. Mastracci L, Rindi G, Grillo F, Solcia E, Campora M, Fassan M, et al. Neuroendocrine neoplasms of the esophagus and stomach. Pathologica. 2021;113:5–11.
5. Park MI. Endoscopic treatment for early foregut neuroendocrine tumors. Clin Endosc. 2013;46:450–5.
6. Ahmed M. Gastrointestinal neuroendocrine tumors in 2020. World J Gastrointest Oncol. 2020;12:791–807.
7. Yao JC, Hassan M, Phan A, Dagohoy C, Leary C, Mares JE, et al. One hundred years after "carcinoid": epidemiology of and prognostic factors for neuroendocrine tumors in 35,825 cases in the United States. J Clin Oncol. 2008;26:3063–72.
8. Hassan MM, Phan A, Li D, Dagohoy CG, Leary C, Yao JC. Risk factors associated with neuroendocrine tumors: A U.S.-based case-control study. Int J Cancer. 2008;123:867–73.
9. Santos AP, Santos AC, Castro C, Raposo L, Pereira SS, Torres I, et al. Visceral obesity and metabolic syndrome are associated with well-differentiated gastroenteropancreatic neuroendocrine tumors. Cancers (Basel). 2018;10:293.
10. Jung SW. Endoscopic treatment of gastric and duodenal neuroendocrine tumors: present and future. Korean J Helicobacter Up Gastrointest Res. 2021;21:29–34.
11. Sato Y, Imamura H, Kaizaki Y, Koizumi W, Ishido K, Kurahara K, et al. Management and clinical outcomes of type I gastric carcinoid patients: retrospective, multicenter study in Japan. Dig Endosc. 2014;26:377–84.
12. Chang S, Choi D, Lee SJ, Lee WJ, Park M-h, Kim SW, et al. Neuroendocrine neoplasms of the gastrointestinal tract: classification, pathologic basis, and imaging features. Radiographics. 2007;27:1667–79.
13. National Comprehensive Cancer Network. Neuroendocrine and adrenal tumors. 2021;3
14. Hofland J, Zandee WT, de Herder WW. Role of biomarker tests for diagnosis of neuroendocrine tumours. Nat Rev Endocrinol. 2018;14:656–69.

Gastric NEN. III-2. Staging and Treatment

Key Points

- The American Joint Committee on Cancer (AJCC) TNM system is used most often for GI NET.
- Gastric neuroendocrine neoplasms (NEN)s are subdivided into NEN types I–III, according to measurement of circulating gastrin and gastric pH.
- Treatment of gastric NENs depends on the subtype of the tumor, the degree of differentiation, and the extent of invasion.
- The prognosis for Type I or II is relatively good, but the prognosis for Type III is similar to that for gastric adenocarcinoma.

Introduction

Gastric NENs are biologically different from gastric adenocarcinoma. For gastric NEMs, two staging systems for gastric NENs have been established: the American Joint Committee on Cancer (AJCC) TNM system and the European Neuroendocrine Tumor Society (ENETS) staging system [1, 2]. Treatment and prognosis of gastric NENs vary for different subtypes.

Staging/Treatment/Prognosis

Staging

The AJCC TNM system is most often used for GI NEN. The eighth edition of the AJCC staging system for gastric NENs is suitable only for NEN G1 and G2 and rare well-differentiated G3, which are classified by the WHO 2019 classification (Tables 1 and 2) [1, 2]. Neuroendocrine carcinoma (NEC) and mixed adenoneuroendocrine carcinoma (MANEC), in which at least 30% of tumors consist of neuroendocrine and non-neuroendocrine components, are recommended to be classified according to the gastric carcinoma staging system of the eighth AJCC [1–3].

ENETs, a new classification system for NEMs based on the proliferation index of Ki-67, are used in Europe [3]. Tables 3 and 4 show slight differences between the eighth AJCC and ENETS staging systems [3].

Hee Man Kim is the lead author of this chapter.

H. J. Chun et al., *Gastrointestinal Cancer*, https://doi.org/10.1007/978-981-99-0815-8_61

Table 1 Definition of primary tumor (T), regional lymph node (N), and distant metastasis (M) for gastric NEN [1]

Definitions for TNM	
Primary tumor (T)	
TX	Primary tumor cannot be assessed
T0	No evidence of primary tumor
T1	Lamina propria or submucosa ≤1 cm in size
T2	Muscularis propria or >1 cm in size
T3	Subserosa without penetrating serosa
T4	Perforates the visceral peritoneum (serosa) or other organs or adjacent structures For any T, add (m) for multiple tumors
Regional LN (N)	
Nx	Regional lymph nodes cannot be assessed
N0	No regional lymph node metastasis
N1	Regional lymph node metastasis
Distant metastasis (M)	
M0	No distant metastases
M1	Distant metastasis M1a: metastasis confined to the liver M1b: at least one extrahepatic metastasis M1c: both hepatic and extrahepatic metastases

Table 2 AJCC prognostic stage groups for gastric NEMs [1]

Prognostic stage groups	
Stage I	T1, N0, M0
Stage II	T2 or T3, N0, M0
Stage III	T1 or T2 or T3, N1, M0 T4, N0 or N1, M0
Stage IV	Any T, any N, M1

Treatment

Gastric NENs are subdivided into NEN types I–III, according to the measurement of the circulating gastrin and gastric pH. The clinical characteristics, pathophysiology, aggressiveness, treatment, and prognosis of gastric NENs are different between types. The treatment of gastric NENs depends on the tumor subtype, degree of differentiation, and extent of invasion [4].

Type I: Gastric NENs of type I are generally small, in which regional lymph node metastases are rare [5]. Therefore, endoscopic local excision is recommended in small tumors. Gastric NENs ≤1 cm are treated with endoscopic resection, such as endoscopic polypectomy, endoscopic mucosal resection (EMR), or endoscopic submucosal dissection (ESD) [4]. Gastric NENs 1–2 cm in size and those with submucosal invasion are often treated with endoscopic polypectomy, EMR, or ESD [6]. The guidelines of the National Comprehensive Cancer Network (NCCN) recommend simple surveillance or endoscopic resection for tumors <20 mm in size, and without invasion of the muscularis propria or distant metastases [7]. Gastric NENs >2 cm in size are usually treated with surgical resection or endoscopic resection. For multifocal (≥6) lesions or tumors with features of invasion of the muscularis propria, surgical resection, such as wedge

Table 3 Differences in TNM between the eighth AJCC and ENETS staging systems [3]

NET-AJCC staging classification		**ENETS staging classification**	
T1	Tumor invades the lamina propria or submucosa and ≤1 cm in size	T1	Tumor invades the lamina propria or submucosa and ≤1 cm in size
T2	Tumor invades the muscularis propria or >1 cm in size	T2	Tumor the invades muscularis propria or subserosa or >1 cm in size
T3	Tumor penetrates the subserosa	T3	Tumor the penetrates serosa
T4	Tumor invades the visceral peritoneum (serosal) or other organs or adjacent structures	T4	Tumor invades the adjacent structures
N0	No regional lymph node metastasis	N0	No regional lymph node metastasis
N1	Regional lymph node metastasis	N1	Regional lymph node metastasis
M0	No distant metastasis	M0	No distant metastasis
M1	Distant metastasis	M1	Distant metastasis

Table 4 Different staging between the eighth AJCC and ENETS staging systems [3]

NET-AJCC				ENETS			
Stage	T	N	M	Stage	T	N	M
I	T1	N0	M0	I	T1	N0	M0
II	T2	N0	M0	IIA	T2	N0	M0
	T3	N0	M0	IIB	T3	N0	M0
III	T4	N0	M0	IIIA	T4	N0	M0
	Any T	N1	M0	IIIB	Any T	N1	M0
IV	Any T	Any N	M1	IV	Any T	Any N	M1

resection, is recommended. The ENETS guidelines recommend that surgical resection should be considered only if tumors invade the muscularis propria, or if there is a lymph node or distant metastasis [7]. For recurrent or multifocal type I gastric NENs, antrectomy should be considered as a potential treatment to eliminate the source of gastrin. Somatostatin analogs are considered for patients with recurrent or multifocal type I gastric NEN [7].

Type II: In the NCCN guidelines, the management of type II gastric NENs is similar to type I gastric NENs. However, the ENETS guidelines recommend surgical resection for type II gastric NENs, because they have a higher rate of metastasis than type I [7]. In addition, the gastrinoma should be removed surgically [6]. In patients with gastrinoma, tumor resection increases overall survival [2].

Type III: Type III gastric NENs are treated aggressively with radical gastric resection and D1 and D2 lymph node dissection when the tumor size is ≥2 cm and localized [5]. Type III gastric NENs <2 cm in size can be treated endoscopically with EMR or ESD, or surgical wedge resection [4]. The ENETS guidelines recommend that type III G-NENs be treated as gastric adenocarcinoma [7].

Prognosis

Gastric NENs are identified as small (<1 cm in diameter) and are mainly highly differentiated tumors, but have lymph node metastases in less than 10% of patients [5]. Type I gastric NENs exhibit a 5-year survival of 90–95% [8]. Type II gastric NENs exhibit a 5-year survival of 70–90% [9]. Type III gastric NENs have the worst prognosis of all three ECL cell NENs [10]. The prognosis of Type III gastric NEN is similar to that of gastric adenocarcinomas [4]. The 5-year survival rate of patients is less than 50% [10].

Conclusion

AJCC and ENETS staging systems are available for gastric NEMs. The management and prognosis of gastric NENs depend on the tumor subtype, degree of differentiation, and extent of invasion.

References

1. Woltering E, Bergsland E, Beyer D. Neuroendocrine Tumors of the Stomach. American Joint Committee on Cancer 2017. AJCC cancer staging manual. 8th ed. Springer. 2017. p. 351–359.
2. Amin MB, Edge SB, Greene FL, Byrd DR, Brookland RK, Washington MK, et al. AJCC cancer staging manual. Springer International Publishing; 2018.
3. Couvelard A, Scoazec J-Y. Proposal for a TNM classification of digestive (neuro) endocrine tumors: recommendations of the European Neuroendocrine Tumor Society. Ann Pathol. 2006;2006:413–7.
4. Gluckman CR, Metz DC. Gastric neuroendocrine tumors (carcinoids). Curr Gastroenterol Rep. 2019;21:1–7.
5. Goretzki PE, Mogl MT, Akca A, Pratschke J. Curative and palliative surgery in patients with neuroendocrine tumors of the gastro-entero-pancreatic (GEP) tract. Rev Endocr Metab Disord. 2018;19:169–78.
6. Ahmed M. Gastrointestinal neuroendocrine tumors in 2020. World J Gastrointest Oncol. 2020;12:791.

7. Sato Y, Hashimoto S, Mizuno K-I, Takeuchi M, Terai S. Management of gastric and duodenal neuroendocrine tumors. World J Gastroenterol. 2016;22:6817.
8. Bałdys-Waligórska A, Nowak A. Neuroendocrine neoplasms of the digestive system–current classification and terminology. Nowotwory J Oncol. 2021;71:26–37.
9. Dias AR, Azevedo BC, Alban LBV, Yagi OK, Ramos MFKP, Jacob CE, et al. Gastric neuroendocrine tumor: review and update. ABCD Arq Bras Cir Dig. 2017;30:150–4.
10. Crosby DA, Donohoe CL, Fitzgerald L, Muldoon C, Hayes B, O'Toole D, et al. Gastric neuroendocrinetumours. Dig Surg. 2012;29:331–48.

Lower Gastrointestinal Tract NEN (Small Bowel and Colorectum). IV-1. Epidemiology, Pathology, and Molecular Characteristics

Key Points

- Gastroenteropancreatic neuroendocrine neoplasms (GEP-NENs) are slowly growing rare malignancies arising from the malignant transformation of neuroendocrine cells.
- There is a global increase in the incidence and prevalence of GEP-NENs.
- They can be classified into functioning and nonfunctioning tumors depending on symptoms related to hormones secreted.
- The stage of the disease is the most important factor for survival.

Introduction

Neuroendocrine neoplasms (NENs) are a heterogeneous group of rare malignancies that arise from neuroendocrine cells and are characterized by the ability to produce amines and polypeptides [1]. Gastroenteropancreatic NENs (GEP-NENs) can occur in almost any gastrointestinal tissue and can be grouped into the foregut, midgut, and hindgut origin (Fig. 1), as they share functional characteristics with organs of the same origin. They are rare malignancies that constitute 2% of all malignant tumors of the gastrointestinal tract, but an increase in the reported incidence of GEP-NENs demands global interest, and much remains to be learned about them. GEP-NENs of pancreas and stomach originating from the foregut will be discussed elsewhere, and this chapter will cover other organs of the gastrointestinal tract including the small intestine, appendix, colon, and rectum.

Ji Hyun Kim is the lead author of this chapter.

H. J. Chun et al., *Gastrointestinal Cancer*, https://doi.org/10.1007/978-981-99-0815-8_62

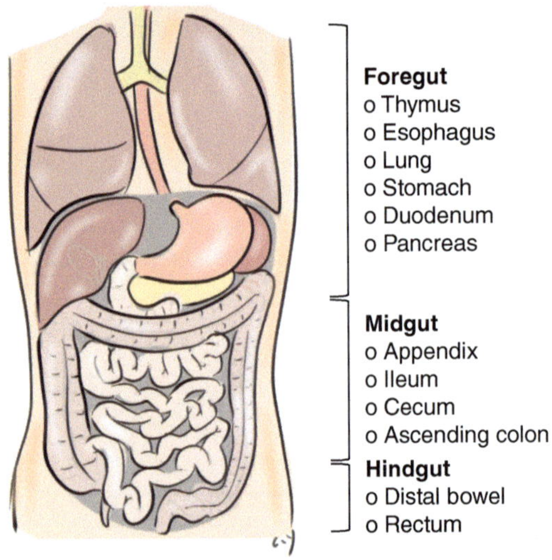

Fig. 1 Neuroendocrine neoplasms grouped by site of organ (adapted from Oronsky et al. [2])

Epidemiology

The incidence and prevalence of NENs have increased in recent decades. Over 40 years, the age-adjusted incidence increased from 1.05/100,000 in 1975 to 5.45/100,000 in 2015 [3], and a similar increase has been reported globally, which could be in part due to increased awareness, advanced imaging, increased use of endoscopy, and early detection of disease [4]. Analysis of the U.S. Surveillance, Epidemiology, and End Results (SEER) database in 2015 identified 43,751 patients with GEP-NENs, among them 48.8% (21,353) were male and 51.2% (22,398) were female. The mean age at diagnosis for all GEP-NEN is 58 years (standard deviation: 15), which is higher compared to data from 1975, and this change is most prominent in localized stages with an increase of 9 years from 40 years ago [3]. The most frequently affected gastrointestinal organs are the rectum (28.64%) and the small intestine (28.08%), followed by the pancreas (16.38%), stomach (9.23%), colon (9.17%), and appendix (8.50%), although the distribution appears to differ with ethnicity. Jejunal and ileal gastrointestinal-NENs are more commonly found in White and African-American patients, while rectal NENs are more frequently found among Asian/Pacific Islanders, American Indian/Alaskan Native, and African-American patients [5]. Most (51.4%) of GEP-NENs are found as localized disease, and approximately 21.9% present with distant metastases. Although genetic alterations have been identified as the cause of malignant transformation in some cases, no identifiable cause is evident, and it is still unknown whether the increase in incidence is due to biological, environmental, or dietary habits [3, 6]. Population-based study from Canada reported the most prevalent sites were small intestine (18.2%) followed by colon (12.9%) and rectum (12.3%). Similar trend was also observed in studies from Asia. In general, there is a growing incidence of gastrointestinal-NENs globally.

Some hereditary syndromes associated with NENs include multiple endocrine neoplasia type 1 (MEN-1), MEN-2, von Hippel-Lindau syndrome, neurofibromatosis, and tuberous sclerosis. As GEP-NENs are slow-growing tumors, the overall survival (OS) duration is comparable to other malignancies. The median OS for all GEP-NENs is reported as 324 months, the best OS is observed in rectal and appendiceal NENs, while the worst OS (67 months) is observed in pancreatic NENs. The reported OS appears to improve with time, mainly due to an increase in the incidence of local stage tumors and the development of chemotherapy agents. Risk factors associated with OS include age, tumor size, tumor grade, and tumor site, but the disease stage was the most important risk factor associated with prognosis [3].

Characteristics

NENs are subdivided into neuroendocrine tumor (NET) and neuroendocrine carcinoma (NEC), according to the most recent World Health Organization (WHO) classification (Table 1). NECs are high grade by definition, and NETs are subdivided into G1, G2, and G3 according to mitotic index and Ki-67 proliferative index. Histologic features depend on the anatomical site and endocrine cell origin, but gastrointestinal NENs have common histopathological features.

Table 1 Classification and grading criteria for neuroendocrine neoplasms (NENs) of the GI tract and hepatobiliary organs

Terminology	Differentiation	Grade	Mitotic rate (mitoses/2 mm^2)	Ki-67 index
NET, G1	Well differentiated	Low	<2	<3%
NET, G2		Intermediate	2–20	3–20%
NET, G3		High	>20	>20%
NEC, small cell type (SCNEC)	Poorly differentiated	High	>20	>20%
NEC, large cell type (LCNEC)			>20	>20%
MiNEN	Well or poorly differentiated	Variable	Variable	Variable

LCNEC large cell neuroendocrine carcinoma, *MiNEN* mixed neuroendocrine non-neuroendocrine neoplasm, *NEC* neuroendocrine carcinoma, *NET* neuroendocrine tumor, *SCNEC* small cell neuroendocrine carcinoma

Macroscopically, they appear as whitish to yellowish solid tumors with nodular or polypoid shape, overlying mucosa is generally intact, and focal ulceration may be present. Microscopically, G1 and G2 NETs have cells possessing round or oval nuclei with "salt and pepper" chromatin and eosinophilic granular cytoplasm with tumor nests in trabecular or sheet-like pattern.

NENs can be divided into functional and nonfunctional tumors depending on secreted peptides and symptoms associated with excessive secretion. The cells have cytoplasmic core granules containing chromogranin A (CgA), synaptophysin, and neuron-specific enolase (NSE). Specific clinical symptoms are related to the type of peptides and amines secreted by different NENs. Typical symptoms include watery diarrhea (caused by release of serotonin), flushing (caused by excessive release of tachykinins and histamine), hypotension, and right-sided heart disease related to hypersecretion of serotonin, and these symptoms usually occur in the presence of hepatic or distant metastases. These symptoms are known as carcinoid syndrome, and diagnosis is supported by an elevated level of 24-h urinary 5-hydroxylindoleacetic acid (5-HIAA) and elevated serum CgA. CgA is released from cytoplasmic chromaffin granules into the blood; thus, serum CgA is increased in both nonfunctioning and functioning NENs, which can be used to monitor tumor burden and treatment response [2]. Foregut tumors have low serotonin (5-HT) content, occasionally secrete adrenocorticotropic hormone (ACTH) or 5-hydroxytryptophan (5-HTP), midgut tumors have high 5-HT content, release serotonin and tachykinins, and rarely secrete 5-HTP, while hindgut tumors rarely contain serotonin, 5-HTP, or ACTH. NENs activate fibroblasts by secreting serotonin, fibroblast growth factor (FGF), platelet-derived growth factor (PDGF), and transforming growth factor β (TGF-β) [4]. Activated fibroblasts cause local and distant fibrosis. Somatostatin receptors and their pathways are involved in the primary regulation of cell proliferation, protein synthesis, and hormone production. Proangiogenic factors such as endothelial growth factor, FGF, and PDGF lead to endothelial proliferation and neovascularization.

Small Intestinal NENs

Small intestinal NENs (SI-NENs) are often multifocal, and more than two-thirds are located in the ileum within 6 cm of the ileocecal valve. They are characteristically well differentiated, but invasive and cause marked fibrotic reactions that can cause intestinal obstruction. Duodenal NENs represent 2–3% of all GEP-NENs, more commonly observed in male patients and often diagnosed incidentally during routine examination. Up to 60% are reported to have metastasized at the time of diagnosis, which is largely affected by tumor size. Duodenal NENs include five types: Gastrinomas secrete excessive gastrin, somatostatinomas secrete excessive somatostatin, gangliocytic paraganglioma, nonfunctioning NENs, and lastly duodenal neuroendocrine carcinomas [1]. Jejunoileal NENs account for up to 28% of all GEP-NENs and most of them are nonfunctioning tumors. They are mostly >2 cm in size and more than 50% are found with metastasis regardless of tumor size. Patients may be asymptomatic or present with symptoms of abdominal pain, obstruction, bleeding, and decreased urination caused by fibrosis of adjacent organs.

Colorectal NENs

A NEN in the appendix is usually found at the tip and is diagnosed incidentally. Up to 90% are found with tumor size <1 cm. Tumor size is associated with metastasis, with tumors <1 cm having less than 10% of metastasis and 5-year survival is 95–100%. Most appendix NENs are well differentiated, and <1% are poorly differentiated G3 tumors. About 70% of colon NENs are located in the right colon, particularly the cecum, and are generally asymptomatic until the size becomes large enough to cause abdominal pain. Some colon NENs are detected during screening colonoscopy. The average size is about 5 cm upon diagnosis accompanied by local or distant metastases, and 5-year survival is 33–42% [4]. There has been a large increase in the incidence of rectal NENs, and Asians and African Americans have a higher incidence and prevalence compared to White patients. Most are asymptomatic and are diagnosed incidentally during screening colonoscopy, but symptoms may include bleeding, pruritus, and change in bowel habits. Endoscopically, they appear as yellowish, round, smooth, sessile polypoid lesions located within 5–10 cm of the anal ridge, and most of them are less than 1 cm in size confined to the submucosa and well differentiated when diagnosed. The 5-year survival rate is 88% but higher survival is observed in localized diseases.

Conclusion

GEP-NENs are rare malignancies, but a continuous increase in incidence and prevalence has been observed globally. They are mostly asymptomatic, nonfunctioning, slow-growing tumors but it can grow rapidly and produce symptoms depending on location, tumor size, and secretion of hormones. They can be diagnosed with endoscopy, biopsy, and imaging studies, and serology of biomarkers can contribute to the differential diagnosis. Prognosis is largely affected by disease stage.

References

1. Modlin IM, Kidd M, Latich I, Zikusoka MN, Shapiro MD. Current status of gastrointestinal carcinoids. Gastroenterology. 2005;128:1717–51.
2. Oronsky B, Ma PC, Morgensztern D, Carter CA. Nothing but NET: a review of neuroendocrine tumors and carcinomas. Neoplasia. 2017;19:991–1002.
3. Xu Z, Wang L, Dai S, Chen M, Li F, Sun J, et al. Epidemiologic trends of and factors associated with overall survival for patients with gastroenteropancreatic neuroendocrine tumors in the United States. JAMA Netw Open. 2021;4:e2124750.
4. Ahmed M. Gastrointestinal neuroendocrine tumors in 2020. World J Gastrointest Oncol. 2020;12:791–807.
5. Yao JC, Hassan M, Phan A, Dagohoy C, Leary C, Mares JE, et al. One hundred years after "carcinoid": epidemiology of and prognostic factors for neuroendocrine tumors in 35,825 cases in the United States. J Clin Oncol. 2008;26:3063–72.
6. Hallet J, Law CH, Cukier M, Saskin R, Liu N, Singh S. Exploring the rising incidence of neuroendocrine tumors: a population-based analysis of epidemiology, metastatic presentation, and outcomes. Cancer. 2015;121:589–97.

Lower Gastrointestinal Tract NEN (Small Bowel and Colorectum). IV-2. Staging and Treatment

Key Points

- In intestinal neuroendocrine tumors (NETs), surgical treatment is performed for radical resection of tumors to reduce the volume of tumors and increase the effectiveness of chemotherapy.
- Among colorectal NET with T1a, endoscopic resection/local resection can be used for the initial treatment. NET with T1b is also performed by local resection or endoscopic resection if there is no evidence of metastasis.
- In unresectable metastatic NETs, somatostatin analogs (octreotide LAR and lanreotide), mTOR inhibitors (everolimus) can be used to treat carcinoid syndrome and inhibition of tumor growth.

Introduction

In intestinal neuroendocrine tumors (NETs), the purpose of surgical treatment is complete radical resection of the tumor. However, in the cases of metastatic or recurrent tumors, the role of surgery is to reduce the volume of tumors and increase the effectiveness of chemotherapy before and after surgery, or to alleviate symptoms caused by tumor hormone secretion [1, 2].

Treatment

Surgical and Endoscopic Management

Small intestine neuroendocrine tumors cause mesenteric metastasis accompanied by fibrosis, which may lead to intestinal obstruction or necrosis. Small intestine neuroendocrine tumors are common in distal ileum. The principles of surgical treatment are mesenteric wedge resection and peripheral lymph node dissection. As the tumor progresses, fibrosis around the tumor progresses, enclosing the blood vessels and intestines, causing intestinal ischemia or intestinal obstruction. For this reason, surgical resection of mesenteric metastases is also recommended for early tumors. Repeat surgery may also be required if mesenteric metastasis remains after surgery [3].

Surgical treatment is sometimes performed for palliative purposes, even if accompanied by distant metastasis or radical resection is impossible. It is performed primarily for the purpose of preventing abdominal symptoms such as intestinal obstruction or necrosis. There have been reports that performing primary tumor and mesenteric lymph node resection increases the survival rate of patients even in neuroendocrine tumors of the intestine with distant unresectable distant metastasis [1]. Resection of primary

Byung Chang Kim is the lead author of this chapter.

H. J. Chun et al., *Gastrointestinal Cancer*, https://doi.org/10.1007/978-981-99-0815-8_63

tumors is performed, and nonsurgical treatment such as ablation or transarterial embolization is sometimes performed for distant metastases such as liver metastases [4].

In neuroendocrine tumors of the appendix, an appendectomy is performed for those with <1 cm, but if it is >2 cm, a right hemicolectomy is required. Even if the size is 1–2 cm, the right hemicolectomy is performed if there is mesoappendix infiltration, resection margin positive, or peripheral lymph node metastases [5].

Among rectal neuroendocrine tumors <1 cm and limited to mucosal and submucosal disease (T1a), endoscopic resection/local resection can be used to remove NETs. Local resection (endoscopic submucosal dissection, transanal surgical resection, and endoscopic microsurgery) can be performed in NETs with 1–2 cm in size and without invasion of surrounding tissues or local metastasis. Endoscopic resection methods include modified mucosal resection (modified EMR) and submucosal dissection. However, if the size is 1–2 cm and there is invasion of surrounding tissue or local metastases, curative resection is performed, including lymph node resection. Similarly, lesions >2 cm in size or invading muscles (T2) undergo curative radical surgery [6–8].

Neuroendocrine tumors in the colon are often found to have progressed more than in the early stages. In the event of invasion of the muscle layer or ≥2 cm, radical bowel resection, including lymph node resection, is performed if there is no other organ metastasis [6–8].

There is no known role for systemic treatment in the adjuvant setting of NETs [8].

Medical Management

Somatostatin Analogs

Somatostatin analogs (SSAs; octreotide and lanreotide) are initial suitable therapy in patients with unresectable metastatic NETs to manage carcinoid syndrome and inhibit tumor growth. The antitumor effects of SSAs were established in the PROMID and CLARINET trials [9, 10]. For symptom control, octreotide (150–250 μg SC TID) or octreotide LAR (20–30 μg intramuscularly) or lanreotide (120 μg subcutaneously, every 4 weeks) was administered to patients with advanced locoregional or distant metastatic NETs. Treatment with octreotide or lanreotide is likely to benefit only those patients who are SSR-positive. The PROMID study showed an antitumor effect of octreotide in advanced neuroendocrine tumor of the midgut [9]. The CLARINET study showed an antitumor effect of lanreotide in advanced, well-differentiated metastatic grade 1 and grade 2 GEP NETs [10].

In general, SSAs are associated with significant improvements in flushing and diarrhea in approximately 75% of patients with carcinoid syndrome. Due to their relatively benign adverse effect profile, SSAs are typically selected as first-line systemic therapy. The long-acting release form of octreotide is used for the chronic treatment of symptoms of carcinoid syndrome [2].

Management of Patients with Negative Somatostatin Receptor Imaging

Most midgut NETs express high levels of somatostatin receptors (SSTR) which are targeted by SSAs. SSTR can be visualized by imaging of the somatostatin receptor. Traditionally, somatostatin receptor scintigraphy (SRS; OctreoScan) has been used to assess SSTR expression. Recently, the ^{68}Ga-dotatate PET scan received US Food and Drug Administration (FDA) approval. Somatostatin receptor PET imaging is recommended as the routine evaluation process in the clinical setting and should be considered the evaluation for SSTR instead of traditional SRS, and/or when a patient with advanced metastatic NETs has a negative OctreoScan. There was a consensus that SSA should be attempted regardless of the results of the somatostatin receptor imaging findings [2].

Role of Mammalian Target of Rapamycin (mTOR) Inhibitors

The mammalian target of rapamycin (mTOR) pathway plays a major role in neuroendocrine tumor (NET) pathogenesis, leading to increased lipid synthesis, protein synthesis, and cellular growth. Upregulation of this pathway is well known in NETs. Everolimus (an mTOR inhibitor) is the preferred treatment for advanced NETs with distant metastasis or advanced locoregional metastasis NETs based on the RADIANT-2 and RADIANT-4 trials [11, 12]. Everolimus was approved by the FDA for the treatment of nonfunctional NETs according to the RADIANT-4 study; this study was conducted for nonfunctional NETs.

Many metastatic midgut NETs (>50% in some studies) secrete serotonin and are associated with the carcinoid syndrome [13]. A trend toward an improvement in everolimus-based PFS was demonstrated in mixed functioning NETs with carcinoid syndrome in the RADIANT-2 study (everolimus+octreotide LAR vs octreotide LAR; HR 0.77, $p = 0.026$, 16.4 vs 11.3 months); however, the study did not meet the prespecified threshold for statistical significance [11]. Despite these results, everolimus should be considered an option for patients with progressive midgut NETs, even if there is a history of carcinoid syndrome [2, 8].

Role of Interferon-α

A phase 3 randomized clinical trial of bevacizumab versus IFN-α showed no evidence of improved PFS with either arm of the study; however, the bevacizumab arm was associated with a higher response rate, longer treatment time, and fewer clinically significant toxicities [14]. IFN-α should generally be considered only if no other option is available to the patient [2].

Choice of Embolization and Peptide Receptor Radiotherapy (PRRT) Therapy

Current transarterial embolic options can be broadly classified into three types: bland embolization, chemoembolization, and radioembolization (also known as selective intrahepatic radiotherapy) [15]. Currently there is no standard-of-care embolization modality and the embolization method is usually determined by institutional preferences. Although radioembolization is generally associated with fewer short-term toxicities than bland or chemoembolization, there have been increased concerns that some patients could develop chronic radioembolization-induced liver disease that was similar to cirrhosis in its radiographic appearance and results in hyperbilirubinemia and portal hypertension [2]. Therefore, patients should be informed of the risks and benefits of each approach.

Patients with advanced midgut NETs were randomly treated with ^{177}Lu-DOTATATE versus high-dose octreotide (60 mg every 4 weeks) in the NETTER-1 trial. ^{177}Lu-DOTATATE is a radiolabeled SSA; peptide receptor radiotherapy (PRRT). In this study, the estimated progression-free survival rate (PFS) at month 20 was 65.2% (95% confidence interval [CI], 50.0–76.8) in the ^{177}Lu-Dotatate group and 10.8% (95% CI, 3.5–23.0) in the control group and the median PFS (primary end point) was 8.4 months in the high-dose octreotide arm and was not yet reached in the ^{177}Lu-DOTATATE arm, translating to a 79% improvement in PFS ($p < 0.00001$) [16].

Management of Refractory Carcinoid Syndrome and Role of Telotristat Ethyl

SSAs (somatostatin analogs; octreotide and lanreotide) are effective in the management of carcinoid syndrome; however, many patients have a suboptimal response or become refractory to SSAs over time [2, 17, 18]. Strategies for the treatment of refractory carcinoid syndrome have included increasing the dose or frequency of SSAs, the addition of short-acting octreotide for breakthrough symptoms, and the initiation of antidiarrheal therapies with loperamide, diphenoxylate-atropine, or other nonspecific medications [2, 8, 19].

The oral serotonin inhibitor telotristat ethyl has been developed for the management of refractory diarrhea in the context of carcinoid syndrome [20]. Telotristat inhibits the enzyme tryptophan hydroxylase, which mediates the rate-limiting step in serotonin biosynthesis. With minimal activity in the central nervous system, it appears to have little effect on the role of serotonin as a neurotransmitter [2]. In the TELESTAR trial, telotristat showed a statistically significant 35% improvement in mean daily bowel movements associated with the 500 mg dose three times daily at week 12 compared to baseline. Furthermore, 5-HIAA levels in urine improved significantly in both treatment groups versus the placebo group: at week 12, mean 5-HIAA levels in urine decreased by 58 mg/24 h in patients receiving the 500 mg dose and 40 mg/24 h with the 250 mg dose; mean 5-HIAA levels in urine increased in the placebo group by 11 mg/24 h at week 12 [2, 21].

Prognosis and Staging

The prognosis of well-differentiated neuroendocrine tumors arising from the small intestine differs depending on the stage of the tumor (Table 1) [22, 23]. However, even in patients with advanced neuroendocrine tumors, including distant metastasis, have a 5-year survival rate of 40%–85%; a 10-year survival rate of 40%–60% [8, 22–25]. Patients with jejunoileal NETs have a relatively poor prognosis, with a 5-year survival rate of 60%, which is poorer than the 5-year survival rate of 72–89% for patients with rectal NETs [23].

The overall prognosis for appendix neuroendocrine tumors is good, and the 10-year survival rate is greater than 98%. Metastasis occurs in less than 1% of tumors between 1–2 cm in size. Therefore, the T classification of the appendiceal NETs was divided by 2 cm, 4 cm, and penetrated the serosal and perforation (Table 2).

The staging of colon and rectal neuroendocrine tumors is used as the same criterion (Table 3), but the prognosis of colonic lesions is worse than that of the rectum. Modlin et al. reported that metastatic lesions were present in 82% of cecal NETs, but only 11%–18% of rectal

Table 1 TNM classification, and stages for neuroendocrine tumors of jejunum and ileum. (NET G1 and G2, and rare well-differentiated G3) (AJCC UICC eighth Edition)

TNM			
T-primary tumor			
TX	Primary tumor cannot be assessed		
T0	No evidence of primary tumor		
T1	Tumor invades mucosa or submucosa and is ≤1 cm		
T2	Tumor invades muscularis propria or size >1 cm		
T3	Invades through the muscularis propria into subserosal tissue without penetration of overlying serosa		
T4	Invades visceral peritoneum (serosa) or other organs or adjacent structures		
	For any T add (m) for multiple tumors		
N-regional lymph nodes			
NX	Regional lymph node status cannot be assessed		
N0	Regional lymph node status cannot be assessed		
N1[a]	Regional lymph node metastasis in <12 nodes		
N2	Large mesenteric masses (>2 cm) and/or extensive nodal deposits (12 or greater), especially those that encase the superior mesenteric vessels		
M-distant metastases (subspecification as in the small bowel)			
MX	Distant metastasis cannot be assessed		
M0	No distant metastases		
M1	Distant metastasis		
M1a	Distant metastasis confined to liver		
M1b	Metastasis in at least one extrahepatic site (e.g., lung, ovary, nonregional lymph node, peritoneum, bone)		
M1c	Both hepatic and extrahepatic metastasis		
Stages AJCC	**T**	**N**	**M**
I	T1	N0	M0
II	T2-3	N0	M0
III	T4	N0	M0
	Any T	N11-2	M0
IV	Any T	Any N	M1

[a]Regional lymph nodes include superior mesenteric and mesenteric nodes; posterior cecal nodes also apply for terminal ileum lesions and 2 cm cutoff for including mesenteric masses in N categorization may be suboptimal [26]

Table 2 TNM classification, and stages for neuroendocrine tumors of appendix. (NET G1 and G2, and rare well-differentiated G3) (AJCC UICC eighth edition)

TNM			
T-primary tumor			
TX	Primary tumor cannot be assessed		
T0	No evidence of primary tumor		
T1	Tumor 2 cm or less in greatest dimension		
T2	Tumor more than 2 cm but less than or equal to 4 cm		
T3	Tumor more than 4 cm or with subserosal invasion or involvement of the mesoappendix		
T4	Tumor perforates the peritoneum or directly invades other adjacent organs or structures (excluding direct mural extension to adjacent subserosal of adjacent bowel), e.g., abdominal wall and skeletal muscle		
	For any T add (m) for multiple tumors		
N-regional lymph nodes			
NX	Regional lymph node status cannot be assessed		
N0	No regional lymph node metastasis		
N1[a]	Regional lymph node metastasis		
M-distant metastases			
MX	Distant metastasis cannot be assessed		
M0	No distant metastases		
M1	Distant metastasis		
M1a	Distant metastasis confined to liver		
M1b	Metastasis in at least one extrahepatic site (e.g., lung, ovary, nonregional lymph node, peritoneum, bone)		
M1c	Both hepatic and extrahepatic metastasis		
Stages AJCC	**T**	**N**	**M**
I	T1	N0	M0
II	T2–3	N0	M0
III	T4	N0	M0
	Any T	N1[a]–2	M0
IV	Any T	Any N	M1

[a] Regional lymph nodes include superior mesenteric and mesenteric nodes; posterior cecal nodes also apply for terminal ileum lesions and 2 cm cutoff for including mesenteric masses in N categorization may be suboptimal [26]

Table 3 TNM classification, and stages for neuroendocrine tumors of colon and rectum. (NET G1 and G2, and rare well-differentiated G3) (AJCC UICC eighth edition)

TNM			
T-primary tumor			
TX	Primary tumor cannot be assessed		
T0	No evidence of primary tumor		
T1	Tumor invades mucosa or submucosa and is ≤2 cm		
T1a	Size <1 cm in greatest dimension		
T1b	Size 1–2 cm in greatest dimension		
T2	Tumor invades muscularis propria or size >2 cm		
T3	Tumor invades subserosa/pericolic/perirectal fat		
T4	Tumor directly invades other organs/structures and/or perforates visceral peritoneum		
For any T add (m) for multiple tumors			
N-regional lymph nodes			
NX	Regional lymph node status cannot be assessed		
N0	Regional lymph node status cannot be assessed		
N1[a]	Regional lymph node metastasis		
M-distant metastases			
MX	Distant metastasis cannot be assessed		
M0	No distant metastases		
M1	Distant metastasis		
M1a	Distant metastasis confined to liver		
M1b	Metastasis in at least one extrahepatic site (e.g., lung, ovary, nonregional lymph node, peritoneum, bone)		
M1c	Both hepatic and extrahepatic metastasis		
Stage grouping			
Stages AJCC	**T**	**N**	**M**
I	T1	N0	M0
IIA	T2	N0	M0
IIB	T3	N0	M0
IIIA	T4	N0	M0
IIIB	Any T	N1[a]	M0
IV	Any T	Any N	M1

[a] Regional lymph nodes include superior mesenteric and mesenteric nodes; posterior cecal nodes also apply for terminal ileum lesions and 2 cm cutoff for including mesenteric masses in N categorization may be suboptimal [26]

NET patients showed metastasis [23]. The prognosis is determined by the stage of the neuroendocrine tumor (Table 3) [8].

Well-known unfavorable risk factors of colorectal NETs are including the size >2 cm, invasion of the muscularis propria, lymphatic invasion, atypical histopathology, presence of >2 mitoses per 10 HPF (more than grade 2) (Table 4), and DNA aneuploidy [8].

Table 4 World Health Organization (WHO) 2019 classification of neuroendocrine tumors

	Mitotic count	Ki-67 index
Neuroendocrine tumor G1	<2 mit/10 HPF	<3%
Neuroendocrine tumor G2	2–20 mit/10 HPF	3–20%
Neuroendocrine tumor G3	>20 mit/10 HPF	>20%

Conclusion

The treatment strategy for intestinal NETs was performed on the basis of stage, such as tumor size and metastasis. Small-sized NETs without metastasis were managed by endoscopic or local resection. The surgical approach could be performed for radical resection and palliative purposes. Somatostatin analogs (octreotide-LAR and lanreotide), mTOR inhibitors (everolimus), embolization, and PRRT therapy, and telotristat ethyl are used for managing the carcinoid syndrome and inhibition of tumor growth in unresectable metastatic NETs. The prognosis of NETs is influenced by tumor staging and grade. Therefore, a precise evaluation should be undertaken before the decision of treatment.

References

1. Howe JR, Cardona K, Fraker DL, Kebebew E, Untch BR, Wang YZ, et al. The surgical management of small bowel neuroendocrine tumors: consensus guidelines of the North American Neuroendocrine Tumor Society. Pancreas. 2017;46:715–31.
2. Strosberg JR, Halfdanarson TR, Bellizzi AM, Chan JA, Dillon JS, Heaney AP, et al. The North American Neuroendocrine Tumor Society consensus guidelines for surveillance and medical management of midgut neuroendocrine tumors. Pancreas. 2017;46:707–14.
3. Akerstrom G, Hellman P, Hessman O, Osmak L. Management of midgut carcinoids. J Surg Oncol. 2005;89:161–9.
4. Gulec SA, Mountcastle TS, Frey D, Cundiff JD, Mathews E, Anthony L, et al. Cytoreductive surgery in patients with advanced-stage carcinoid tumors. Am Surg. 2002;68:667–71; discussion 71–2.
5. Goede AC, Caplin ME, Winslet MC. Carcinoid tumour of the appendix. Br J Surg. 2003;90:1317–22.
6. Anthony LB, Strosberg JR, Klimstra DS, Maples WJ, O'Dorisio TM, Warner RR, et al. The NANETS consensus guidelines for the diagnosis and management of gastrointestinal neuroendocrine tumors (nets): well-differentiated nets of the distal colon and rectum. Pancreas. 2010;39:767–74.
7. Boudreaux JP, Klimstra DS, Hassan MM, Woltering EA, Jensen RT, Goldsmith SJ, et al. The NANETS consensus guideline for the diagnosis and management of neuroendocrine tumors: well-differentiated neuroendocrine tumors of the jejunum, ileum, appendix, and cecum. Pancreas. 2010;39:753–66.
8. Shah MH, Goldner WS, Halfdanarson TR, Bergsland E, Berlin JD, Halperin D, et al. NCCN guidelines insights: neuroendocrine and adrenal Tumors, version 2.2018. J Natl Compr Cancer Netw. 2018;16:693–702.
9. Rinke A, Muller HH, Schade-Brittinger C, Klose KJ, Barth P, Wied M, et al. Placebo-controlled, double-blind, prospective, randomized study on the effect of octreotide LAR in the control of tumor growth in patients with metastatic neuroendocrine midgut tumors: a report from the PROMID study group. J Clin Oncol. 2009;27:4656–63.
10. Caplin ME, Pavel M, Cwikla JB, Phan AT, Raderer M, Sedlackova E, et al. Lanreotide in metastatic enteropancreatic neuroendocrine tumors. N Engl J Med. 2014;371:224–33.
11. Pavel ME, Baudin E, Oberg KE, Hainsworth JD, Voi M, Rouyrre N, et al. Efficacy of everolimus plus octreotide LAR in patients with advanced neuroendocrine tumor and carcinoid syndrome: final overall survival from the randomized, placebo-controlled phase 3 RADIANT-2 study. Ann Oncol. 2017;28:1569–75.
12. Pavel ME, Singh S, Strosberg JR, Bubuteishvili-Pacaud L, Degtyarev E, Neary MP, et al. Health-related quality of life for everolimus versus placebo in patients with advanced, non-functional, well-differentiated gastrointestinal or lung neuroendocrine tumours (RADIANT-4): a multicentre, randomised, double-blind, placebo-controlled, phase 3 trial. Lancet Oncol. 2017;18:1411–22.
13. Strosberg JR, Weber JM, Feldman M, Coppola D, Meredith K, Kvols LK. Prognostic validity of the American Joint Committee on Cancer staging classification for midgut neuroendocrine tumors. J Clin Oncol. 2013;31:420–5.
14. Yao JC, Guthrie KA, Moran C, Strosberg JR, Kulke MH, Chan JA, et al. Phase III prospective randomized comparison trial of depot octreotide plus interferon alfa-2b versus depot octreotide plus bevacizumab in patients with advanced carcinoid tumors: SWOG S0518. J Clin Oncol. 2017;35:1695–703.
15. Kennedy AS. Hepatic-directed therapies in patients with neuroendocrine tumors. Hematol Oncol Clin North Am. 2016;30:193–207.
16. Strosberg J, El-Haddad G, Wolin E, Hendifar A, Yao J, Chasen B, et al. Phase 3 trial of (177)Lu-Dotatate for midgut neuroendocrine tumors. N Engl J Med. 2017;376:125–35.

17. Toumpanakis C, Garland J, Marelli L, Srirajaskanthan R, Soh J, Davies P, et al. Long-term results of patients with malignant carcinoid syndrome receiving octreotide LAR. Aliment Pharmacol Ther. 2009;30:733–40.
18. Ruszniewski P, Ish-Shalom S, Wymenga M, O'Toole D, Arnold R, Tomassetti P, et al. Rapid and sustained relief from the symptoms of carcinoid syndrome: results from an open 6-month study of the 28-day prolonged-release formulation of lanreotide. Neuroendocrinology. 2004;80:244–51.
19. Strosberg J, Weber J, Feldman M, Goldman J, Almhanna K, Kvols L. Above-label doses of octreotide-LAR in patients with metastatic small intestinal carcinoid tumors. Gastrointest Cancer Res. 2013;6:81–5.
20. Pavel M, Horsch D, Caplin M, Ramage J, Seufferlein T, Valle J, et al. Telotristat etiprate for carcinoid syndrome: a single-arm, multicenter trial. J Clin Endocrinol Metab. 2015;100:1511–9.
21. Kulke MH, Horsch D, Caplin ME, Anthony LB, Bergsland E, Oberg K, et al. Telotristat ethyl, a tryptophan hydroxylase inhibitor for the treatment of carcinoid syndrome. J Clin Oncol. 2017;35:14–23.
22. Kim MK, Warner RR, Roayaie S, Harpaz N, Ward SC, Itzkowitz S, et al. Revised staging classification improves outcome prediction for small intestinal neuroendocrine tumors. J Clin Oncol. 2013;31:3776–81.
23. Bosman FT, Carneiro F, Hruban RH, Theise ND. WHO classification of tumours of the digestive system. World Health Organization; 2010.
24. Landerholm K, Zar N, Andersson RE, Falkmer SE, Jarhult J. Survival and prognostic factors in patients with small bowel carcinoid tumour. Br J Surg. 2011;98:1617–24.
25. Jann H, Roll S, Couvelard A, Hentic O, Pavel M, Muller-Nordhorn J, et al. Neuroendocrine tumors of midgut and hindgut origin: tumor-node-metastasis classification determines clinical outcome. Cancer. 2011;117:3332–41.
26. Gonzalez RS, Cates JM, Shi C. Number, not size, of mesenteric tumor deposits affects prognosis of small intestinal well-differentiated neuroendocrine tumors. Mod Pathol. 2018;31:1560–6.

Pancreatic Neuroendocrine Neoplasms. V-1. Epidemiology and Clinical Features

Key Points

- Pancreatic neuroendocrine neoplasms are rare, but their incidence has recently increased.
- The pancreas is the third most common primary site of GEP-NETs in Korea.
- Pancreatic neuroendocrine neoplasms are classified as nonfunctional and functional.
- Most pancreatic neuroendocrine neoplasms are nonfunctional.
- Functional pancreatic neuroendocrine neoplasms secrete hormones that produce unique clinical syndromes.

Introduction

Pancreatic neuroendocrine neoplasms (PNENs) are rare tumors that occur in <1 person per 100,000; however, their incidence has recently increased due to an increase in incidental findings in imaging studies or endoscopy performed for other reasons, leading to the diagnosis of asymptomatic diseases.

Epidemiology

A high prevalence of small PNEN was observed in autopsies [1] and a recent case series reported an incidental histological diagnosis of small

Kyong Joo Lee is the lead author of this chapter.

H. J. Chun et al., *Gastrointestinal Cancer*, https://doi.org/10.1007/978-981-99-0815-8_64

PNEN or microadenomas in 4% of patients who underwent pancreatic resection for conditions other than PNEN [2]. According to Western reports, neuroendocrine tumors in the pancreas account for 1%–10% of all endocrine tumors [3]. In a national registry analysis from Korea, 4951 gastroenteropancreatic neuroendocrine tumors (GEP-NETs) were identified between 2000 and 2009 [4]. The pancreas (8.7%) was the third most common primary site of GEP-NETs. In addition, among the 2345 cases of GEP-NETs surveyed by the Korean Society of Gastrointestinal Cancer in 15 hospitals from 2002–2012, 153 patients were diagnosed with pancreatic neuroendocrine tumors, nonfunctional tumors were common (117 patients, 76.5%), and insulinoma (25 patients, 16.3%) accounted for the majority of functional tumors [5]. Of these patients, 29.4% were asymptomatic and incidentally diagnosed, and 47.7% and 52.3% of these tumors occurred in the head of the pancreas and in the body and tail, respectively. The rates of multiple endocrine neoplasia syndrome were only 1.9%, and there were 98 cases of grade 1 (G1) (64.1%), 37 cases of G2 (24.2%), and 18 cases of G3 tumors (17.7%) according to the 2010 criteria of the World Health Organization (WHO) [5].

PNENs can occur in all age groups, but most cases are diagnosed in the age group 40–60 years. Most PNENs are sporadic but can be associated with hereditary endocrine syndromes. Four inherited disorders have an increased incidence of PNENs, namely: multiple endocrine neoplasia type 1 (MEN1), von Hippel-Lindau disease, von Recklinghausen's disease (neurofibromatosis1), and tuberous sclerosis (Table 1) [6, 7].

The most important inherited disorder is MEN1 because 80–100% of these patients develop nonfunctional PNENs (NF-PNENs), 50–60% develop gastrinomas, 20% develop insulinomas, and 3–5% develop vasoactive intestinal polypeptide-secreting tumors (VIPomas) or glucagonomas. MEN1 accounts for 20–25% of all gastrinomas and 4% of all insulinomas. Most NF-PNENs develop in 10–17% of patients with von Hippel-Lindau disease, 0–10% of patients with neurofibromatosis 1 (primarily duodenal somatostatinomas), and in <1% of patients with tuberous sclerosis [6, 7]. PNENs that develop in patients with genetic syndromes tend to show a relatively good prognosis compared to sporadic cases. Other known risk factors in addition to genetic syndromes include smoking, diabetes, and a history of chronic pancreatitis [8, 9].

Clinical Presentation

Pancreatic neuroendocrine neoplasms (PNENs) are divided into nonfunctional and functional groups based on the properties of the hormones secreted by the neoplasm and their ability to produce a clinical syndrome. Nonfunctional PNENs (NF-PNENs) do not produce a clinical syndrome simply because they do not secrete hormones or because the hormones secreted do not cause specific clinical syndromes. NF-PNENs are discovered incidentally on imaging or are detected as a result of symptoms related to a tumor mass effect. Functional PNENs (F-PNENs) are much less common and present with specific clinical syndromes related to hormonal secretion. The diagnosis of F-PNENs is based on the presence of a clinical syndrome and diagnostic hormonal and functional studies; diagnosis is not based on immunocytochemistry. Both F-PNENs and NF-PNENs may secrete multiple peptides (Table 2) [10].

Table 1 Inherited pancreatic neuroendocrine neoplasms [8]

Syndrome	Prevalence	Gene location	Prevalence of PNENs
Multiple endocrine neoplasia type I	1–10/100,000	11q13	80–100%
Von Hippel-Lindau disease	2–3/100,000	3p25	10–17%
Neurofibromatosis 1	1/4–5000	17q11.2	0–10%
Tuberous sclerosis	1/10,000	9q34	Rare

Table 2 Pancreatic endocrine tumor syndromes [8]

Name of tumor	Hormone	Clinical presentation	Location	Malignant (%)
Gastrinoma (Zollinger-Ellison syndrome)	Gastrin	Abdominal pain Diarrhea Esophageal symptoms	Pancreas: 60% Duodenum: 30% Other: 10%	60–90
Insulinoma	Insulin	Hypoglycemic symptoms	Pancreas: 99–100%	5–15
Glucagonoma	Glucagon	Rash, anemia Diabetes/glucose intolerance Weight loss Thromboembolic disease	Pancreas: 99–100%	60
ViPoma (Verner-Morrison, pancreatic cholera, WDHA)	VIP	Severe watery diarrhea Hypokalemia	Pancreas: 90% Other: 10% (neural, adrenal, peri-ganglionic tissue)	80
Somatostatinoma	Stomatostatin	Diabetes mellitus Cholelithiases Diarrhea Steatorrhea	Pancreas: 56% Duodenum/jejunum: 44%	60
GRFoma	Growth hormone releasing factor	Acromegaly	Pancreas: 30% Lung: 54% Jejunum: 7% Other: 13%	30
ACTHoma (Cushing's syndrome)	ACTH	Cushing's syndrome	Pancreas: 4%–16%	>90
PET causing carcinoid syndrome	Serotonin Tachykinins	Diarrhea Flushing	Pancreas: 100%	60–90
PTHrp-oma	PTHrp	Symptoms due to increased calcium	Pancreas: 100%	80–90

Functional Tumors

Insulinoma

Insulinomas are the most common F-PNENs and comprise 35%–40% of all cases. Patients with F-PNENs present with hypoglycemia due to episodic hyperinsulinemia [11]. Insulinomas occur in 1–4 people per million in the general population and represent 1%–2% of all pancreatic neoplasms [12]. Insulinomas are most commonly present between the ages of 40 and 45 years, with a slight female predominance. Hypoglycemia and hyperinsulinemia develop after fasting in more than 98% of cases. The classical Whipple triad, which includes the following symptoms, helps to diagnose insulinomas: (1) hypoglycemia (plasma glucose <50 mg/dL); (2) hypoglycemic symptoms (weakness, sweating, palpitations, and confusion), and (3) prompt relief of symptoms after glucose administration [13]. In adults with hypoglycemic symptoms or documented hypoglycemia, the gold standard for biochemical diagnosis remains the measurement of plasma glucose, insulin, C-peptide, and proinsulin during a 72-h fast (Table 3). This prolonged fasting test can detect up to 99% of insulinomas [14]. The diagnosis of insulinoma is established using the following criteria: (1) blood glucose ≤40 mg/dL (2.2 mmol/L), (2) insulin ≥6 μU/mL (≥36 pmol/L), (3) C-peptide ≥200 pmol/L, (4) proinsulin ≥5 pmol/L, (5) β-hydroxybutyrate ≤2.7 mmol/L, and (6) absence of sulfonylurea (metabolites) in the plasma or urine [15].

Table 3 Diagnosis of insulinoma [32]

Classical diagnosis	
	Hypoglycemia (plasma glucose <50 mg /dL)
	Hypoglycemic symptoms
	Prompt relief of symptoms following glucose administration
Present consensus	
	At the time of hypoglycemia during a 72-h fasting test:
	5 mIU/L insulin threshold
	0.6 ng/mL C-peptide threshold
	Insulin/C-peptide ratio < 1.0
	20 pmol/L proinsulin cutoff level
	Absence of sulfonylurea (metabolites) in plasma or urine

Gastrinoma

Gastrinomas are the second most common F-PNENs, with an incidence of 0.5–2 per 100,000 people per year [8]. The symptoms of gastrinomas result from hypersecretion of gastrin, which causes refractory peptic ulcer in the stomach and duodenum and secretory diarrhea, referred to as Zollinger-Ellison syndrome (ZES) [16, 17].

Serum gastrin levels should be confirmed to have increased to 200 pg/mL or more when there is a decrease in pH in the stomach (<2) due to elevated gastric acid secretion [18]. Fasting serum gastrin (FSG) is usually the first study performed when a gastrinoma is suspected. It is an ideal screening test, as FSG is elevated in more than 98% of all gastrinomas [19]. FSG levels increase more than tenfold in 40% of patients. If the gastric pH is <2 in these patients, the diagnosis of gastrinoma is confirmed. For the remaining 60% of patients with a less than ten-fold increase in FSG and gastric pH >2, basal acid production and secretin tests should be performed. A BSO level of >15 mEq/hour is indicative of the diagnosis of ZES without prior vagotomy or gastrectomy. The addition of a positive secretin test confirms the diagnosis. Although secretin generally reduces the level of gastrin through the inhibitory feedback loop, secretin stimulation causes an increase in gastrin [20].

Glucagonoma

Glucagonomas are rare even among F-PNENs, with an incidence of 0.01–0.1 per 1,000,000 people per year [15]. Glucagonomas are typically present in the fifth decade of life [21]. Glucagonomas are usually large tumors (>5 cm) that occur in the pancreas and are found primarily in the tail. More than 60% of cases are malignant, and approximately 50%–80% are metastatic at diagnosis. The most common symptom of glucagonoma is dermatitis with migratory necrotic erythema [22]. Other symptoms include glucose intolerance, diarrhea, and deep vein thrombosis. Laboratory findings include anemia (30%–90%) and hypoaminoacidemia (30%–100%). Diagnosis requires serum glucagon levels of >500 pg/mL, although this is not specific to glucagonoma, as other disease entities can cause hyperglucagonemia [23].

VIPoma

VIPomas are detected in 1 million people per year [24]. Symptomatic VIPomas of the pancreas are usually solitary, measure >3 cm in diameter, and occur in the tail of the pancreas in 75% of cases. Vasoactive intestinal peptide (VIP)-secreting tumors have also been found in the bronchus, colon, adrenals, and liver [25]. Seventy to 90% of the cases are malignant and 60%–80% are metastatic on diagnosis.

VIPomas produce a clinical syndrome known as Verner-Morrison syndrome, WDHA syndrome (watery diarrhea, hypokalemia, and achlorhydria), or pancreatic cholera syndrome. Excess VIP produces a large volume of watery diarrhea. The stool volume is greater than 3 L/d in 70%–80% of cases, and diarrhea continues even during fasting, as it is secretory in nature [26].

The diagnosis of VIPoma is suspected in patients with unexplained high-volume secretory diarrhea (>700 mL/day). The diagnosis is established by a serum VIP concentration of >75 pg/mL. Most patients also had clear evidence of a tumor mass in imaging studies.

Somatostatinoma

Somatostatinomas are rare PNENs, occurring in less than one in 40 million people [25]. The mean age at the time of diagnosis of somatostatinoma is 50–55 years, with a roughly equal sex distribution [27]. About half of the cases occur in the pancreas and the other half occur in the duodenum and jejunum. Sixty to 70% of cases are malignant, and pancreatic somatostatinomas are malignant more often than duodenal somatostatinomas. These tumors rarely occur in association with von Hippel-Lindau or MEN1 and in up to 10% of NF1 patients. Most somatostatinomas are found incidentally. The most common symptom of somatostatinomas is due to the tumor mass. True somatostatinoma syndrome is observed in <10% of patients with these tumors.

Somatostatinoma syndrome should be suspected in patients with the classical triad of diabetes or glucose intolerance, cholelithiasis, and diarrhea or steatorrhea. The diagnosis is established by the presence of a fasting plasma somatostatin level exceeding 1000 pg/mL [23]. However, somatostatinoma syndrome is rare and most somatostatinomas are detected as pancreatic or duodenal masses during the evaluation of abdominal pain, jaundice, or weight loss.

Nonfunctional PNENs

Although NF-PNENs secrete several substances such as chromogranin, neuron-specific enolase, pancreatic polypeptide, and ghrelin, they do not exhibit clinical syndromes, unlike F-PNENs [28]. For this reason, they are either discovered incidentally or often present later due to a tumor mass effect, invasion of adjacent structures, or metastatic disease. These symptoms can include abdominal pain, weight loss, anorexia, nausea, and jaundice. Patients may also present with a palpable mass. However, the incidental discovery of these tumors seems to be growing due to the increasing use of computed tomography imaging for other indications.

If the presence of NF-PNEN is suspected, the initial analysis should include serum levels of chromogranin A, which is elevated in 88–100% of cases with a diagnostic sensitivity of 60 to 100% in patients with metastatic disease but <50% in patients with localized disease [29]. Other possible PNEN markers include serum neuron-specific enolase and pancreatic polypeptide, which are elevated in 83%–100% and 63% of PNENs, respectively [30]. Somatostatin receptor scintigraphy, also known as octreotide scan, may also be used in the workup of suspected NF-PNENs [31]. A confirmed diagnosis requires histological analysis.

Conclusion

PNENs are rare tumors, but the incidence is gradually increasing. PNENs are classified into functioning tumors or nonfunctioning tumors. Functioning tumors include insulinoma, gastrinoma, glucagonoma, VIPoma, and somatostatinomas. Nonfunctioning tumors do not produce excess hormones that cause symptoms.

References

1. Kishi S, Sakamoto K, Mori M, Isogawa A, Shiba T. Asymptomatic insulinoma: a case report and autopsy series. Diabetes Res Clin Pract. 2012;98:445–51.
2. Partelli S, Giannone F, Schiavo Lena M, Muffatti F, Andreasi V, Crippa S, et al. Is the real prevalence of pancreatic neuroendocrine tumors underestimated? A retrospective study on a large series of pancreatic specimens. Neuroendocrinology. 2019;109:165–70.
3. Falconi M, Eriksson B, Kaltsas G, Bartsch DK, Capdevila J, Caplin M, et al. ENETS consensus guidelines update for the management of Patients with functional pancreatic neuroendocrine tumors and non-functional pancreatic neuroendocrine tumors. Neuroendocrinology. 2016;103:153–71.
4. Gastrointestinal Pathology Study Group of Korean Society of P, Cho MY, Kim JM, Sohn JH, Kim MJ, Kim KM, et al. Current trends of the incidence and pathological diagnosis of gastroenteropancreatic neuroendocrine tumors (GEP-NETs) in Korea 2000-2009: multicenter study. Cancer Res Treat. 2012;44:157–65.
5. Cho JH, Ryu JK, Song SY, Hwang JH, Lee DK, Woo SM, et al. Prognostic validity of the American Joint Committee on Cancer and the European

Neuroendocrine Tumors Staging Classifications for Pancreatic Neuroendocrine Tumors: a retrospective Nationwide Multicenter study in South Korea. Pancreas. 2016;45:941–6.
6. Alexakis N, Connor S, Ghaneh P, Lombard M, Smart HL, Evans J, et al. Hereditary pancreatic endocrine tumours. Pancreatology. 2004;4:417–33; discussion 34–5.
7. Jensen RT, Berna MJ, Bingham DB, Norton JA. Inherited pancreatic endocrine tumor syndromes: advances in molecular pathogenesis, diagnosis, management, and controversies. Cancer. 2008;113:1807–43.
8. Metz DC, Jensen RT. Gastrointestinal neuroendocrine tumors: pancreatic endocrine tumors. Gastroenterology. 2008;135:1469–92.
9. Leoncini E, Carioli G, La Vecchia C, Boccia S, Rindi G. Risk factors for neuroendocrine neoplasms: a systematic review and meta-analysis. Ann Oncol. 2016;27:68–81.
10. Anderson CW, Bennett JJ. Clinical presentation and diagnosis of pancreatic neuroendocrine tumors. Surg Oncol Clin N Am. 2016;25:363–74.
11. McKenna LR, Edil BH. Update on pancreatic neuroendocrine tumors. Gland Surg. 2014;3:258–75.
12. Oberg K, Eriksson B. Endocrine tumours of the pancreas. Best Pract Res Clin Gastroenterol. 2005;19:753–81.
13. Rostambeigi N, Thompson GB. What should be done in an operating room when an insulinoma cannot be found? Clin Endocrinol. 2009;70:512–5.
14. Service FJ, Natt N. The prolonged fast. J Clin Endocrinol Metab. 2000;85:3973–4.
15. Jensen RT, Cadiot G, Brandi ML, de Herder WW, Kaltsas G, Komminoth P, et al. ENETS consensus guidelines for the management of patients with digestive neuroendocrine neoplasms: functional pancreatic endocrine tumor syndromes. Neuroendocrinology. 2012;95:98–119.
16. Ellison EC, Johnson JA. The Zollinger-Ellison syndrome: a comprehensive review of historical, scientific, and clinical considerations. Curr Probl Surg. 2009;46:13–106.
17. Roy PK, Venzon DJ, Shojamanesh H, Abou-Saif A, Peghini P, Doppman JL, et al. Zollinger-Ellison syndrome. Clinical presentation in 261 patients. Medicine (Baltimore). 2000;79:379–411.
18. Jensen RT, Niederle B, Mitry E, Ramage JK, Steinmuller T, Lewington V, et al. Gastrinoma (duodenal and pancreatic). Neuroendocrinology. 2006;84:173–82.
19. Ito T, Cadiot G, Jensen RT. Diagnosis of Zollinger-Ellison syndrome: increasingly difficult. World J Gastroenterol. 2012;18:5495–503.
20. Mendelson AH, Donowitz M. Catching the zebra: clinical pearls and pitfalls for the successful diagnosis of Zollinger-Ellison syndrome. Dig Dis Sci. 2017;62:2258–65.
21. Wermers RA, Fatourechi V, Wynne AG, Kvols LK, Lloyd RV. The glucagonoma syndrome. Clinical and pathologic features in 21 patients. Medicine (Baltimore). 1996;75:53–63.
22. Kitamura Y, Sato M, Hatamochi A, Yamazaki S. Necrolytic migratory erythema without glucagonoma associated with hepatitis B. Eur J Dermatol. 2005;15:49–51.
23. Ito T, Igarashi H, Jensen RT. Pancreatic neuroendocrine tumors: clinical features, diagnosis and medical treatment: advances. Best Pract Res Clin Gastroenterol. 2012;26:737–53.
24. Dimitriadis GK, Weickert MO, Randeva HS, Kaltsas G, Grossman A. Medical management of secretory syndromes related to gastroenteropancreatic neuroendocrine tumours. Endocr Relat Cancer. 2016;23:R423–36.
25. Grozinsky-Glasberg S, Mazeh H, Gross DJ. Clinical features of pancreatic neuroendocrine tumors. J Hepatobiliary Pancreat Sci. 2015;22:578–85.
26. Grier JF. WDHA (watery diarrhea, hypokalemia, achlorhydria) syndrome: clinical features, diagnosis, and treatment. South Med J. 1995;88:22–4.
27. Harris GJ, Tio F, Cruz AB Jr. Somatostatinoma: a case report and review of the literature. J Surg Oncol. 1987;36:8–16.
28. Li J, Luo G, Fu D, Jin C, Hao S, Yang F, et al. Preoperative diagnosis of nonfunctioning pancreatic neuroendocrine tumors. Med Oncol. 2011;28:1027–31.
29. Taupenot L, Harper KL, O'Connor DT. The chromogranin-secretogranin family. N Engl J Med. 2003;348:1134–49.
30. Panzuto F, Severi C, Cannizzaro R, Falconi M, Angeletti S, Pasquali A, et al. Utility of combined use of plasma levels of chromogranin A and pancreatic polypeptide in the diagnosis of gastrointestinal and pancreatic endocrine tumors. J Endocrinol Investig. 2004;27:6–11.
31. Schillaci O, Spanu A, Scopinaro F, Falchi A, Corleto V, Danieli R, et al. Somatostatin receptor scintigraphy with 111In-pentetreotide in non-functioning gastroenteropancreatic neuroendocrine tumors. Int J Oncol. 2003;23:1687–95.
32. Okabayashi T, Shima Y, Sumiyoshi T, Kozuki A, Ito S, Ogawa Y, et al. Diagnosis and management of insulinoma. World J Gastroenterol. 2013;19:829–37.

Pancreatic Neuroendocrine Neoplasms. V-2. Staging and Treatment

Key Points

- Pancreatic neuroendocrine neoplasm (PNEN) grade and TNM staging are essential to predict prognosis and are considered the most important variables in determining treatment options.
- Surgery is the only curative treatment modality for sporadic PNENs, and resection of the primary tumor in localized, regional, and even metastatic disease can improve patient survival.
- Multiple active systemic treatments including somatostatin analogs, everolimus, and sunitinib for grade 1 and 2 pancreatic neuroendocrine tumors (PNET) are effective in prolonging progression-free survival.
- Chemotherapy is recommended in highly symptomatic and rapidly growing grade 3 pancreatic neuroendocrine carcinomas (PNEC).
- Radiological embolization/radiofrequency ablation and peptide receptor radionuclide therapy (PRRT) are reasonable therapeutic options after the failure of initial medical therapy.

Introduction

The term pancreatic neuroendocrine neoplasm (PNEN) encompasses a diverse set of tumors arising in the pancreas neuroendocrine progenitor cell. PNEN is a rare disease but exhibits a wide spectrum of clinical behavior. Well-differentiated PNENs are referred to as pancreatic neuroendocrine tumors (PNET), while poorly differentiated high-grade PNENs are referred to as pancreatic neuroendocrine carcinomas (PNEC) but exhibit a wide spectrum of clinical behavior that has made classification and treatment difficult. While most PNENs are associated with relatively good survival, there can be significant variability in outcomes based on their biological heterogeneity. In this chapter, the diagnosis and treatment of PNENs will be introduced and described in detail.

Diagnosis

PNEN is often accompanied by various syndromes caused by hormonal hypersecretion at diagnosis, but about 50%–75% of cases are

Sung Ill Jang is the lead author of this chapter.

H. J. Chun et al., *Gastrointestinal Cancer*, https://doi.org/10.1007/978-981-99-0815-8_65

asymptomatic nonfunctional PNENs, which is discovered incidentally. Because it can be characteristically accompanied by various genetic diseases, it is necessary to differentiate it from multiple endocrine neoplasia type 1, which is accompanied by parathyroid hyperplasia, PNENs, pituitary adenoma, and lung/thymic carcinoma.

Diagnosis of Functional PNEN

The diagnosis of Zollinger-Ellison syndrome (ZES) is difficult for the following reasons: the increasing unreliability of commercial gastrin assays, the lack of availability of secretin used to perform secretin provocative tests, and the widespread use of proton pump inhibitors (PPIs) [1]. The diagnosis of ZES can be made by the presence of an inappropriately elevated fasting serum gastrin level associated with hypergastrinemia when gastric acid secretion is present. This diagnosis is achieved by establishing hypergastrinemia when the gastric pH is <2. And an assessment of gastric secretion measuring gastric pH is required. If the FSG level is >ten-fold the normal value and the gastric pH is <2, a diagnosis of ZES is established (40% of all ZES patients). However, in the remaining 60% of patients with ZES, the FSG level is <tenfold elevated with a gastric pH <2 [2]; in these patients, additional tests are needed [3].

The exact criteria for the diagnosis of insulinoma have evolved and varied in different consensus reports and documents [4]. The following diagnostic criteria for insulinoma were proposed: endogenous hyperinsulinism documented by the finding of symptoms, signs, or both, with plasma concentrations of glucose <55 mg/dL (3.0 mmol/L), insulin ≥3.0 μU/mL (18 pmol/L), C-peptide ≥0.6 ng/mL (0.2 nmol/L), and proinsulin ≥5.0 pmol/L. The presence of a plasma β-hydroxybutyrate level of ≤2.7 mmol/L and an increase in plasma glucose of ≥25 mg/dL (1.4 mmol/L) after intravenous glucagon indicates a mediation of the hypoglycemia by insulin.

Diagnosis of Nonfunctional PNEN

Chromogranin A (CgA) and pancreatic polypeptide have been recommended as circulating tumor markers in nonfunctional PNEN. However, the percentage of patients with elevated pancreatic polypeptide levels is lower than that of patients with elevated CgA levels. In patients with nonfunctional PNEN, assessing the CgA level can be useful for the diagnosis of PNEN. Elevated CgA level may be potentially useful for evaluating treatment response, progression, and recurrence at an early stage [5]. CgA can be elevated in both functioning and nonfunctioning PNEN. CgA is more frequently elevated in well-differentiated tumors compared to poorly differentiated PNEN. The effectiveness of PNENs treatment can be associated with a decrease in CgA levels. PPIs can cause false-positive elevation of CgA; however, the levels decrease and normalize after cessation of PPIs. Finally, CgA is currently the biomarker available for the diagnosis of PNEN. It is essential to establish the diagnosis and has some utility in predicting disease recurrence, outcome, and efficacy of therapy. Although evaluation of plasma CgA is necessary for an effective diagnosis and management of PNENs, the standardization of a CgA assay is needed through further studies because of its high rate of false positives resulting from various diseases and conditions.

Imaging Studies

Imaging tests play a very important role in the accurate diagnosis and localization of primary lesions that occur in various regions, confirmation of metastases, staging, and evaluation of treatment response. Radiological examination methods used to diagnose PNEN include barium examination, computed tomography (CT), magnetic resonance imaging (MRI), and angiography. In imaging tests such as CT/MRI, most PNENs are hypervascular masses and show characteristic early contrast enhancement. In addition to these tests, isotope testing is used to diagnose PNEN. In the past, somatostatin receptor scintigraphy (indium-111 octreotide) was mainly used, but the 68-Ga DOTATATE Positron Emission Tomography (PET)/CT test was recently introduced. 68-Ga DOTATATE binds to the somatostatin subtype 2 receptor and has a higher diagnostic accuracy than conventional octreoscan because it identifies lesions with high-resolution PET/CT. However, for inspection, a generator capable of producing 68-Ga DOTATATE with a short half-life must be provided.

Endoscopic ultrasound (EUS) can observe the pancreas with high resolution, so small lesions with a size of 2–3 mm can be identified and histological confirmation can be attempted by performing an additional biopsy. In EUS, an endoscope equipped with a 5- to 10-MHz ultrasonic sensor is inserted up to the stomach or duodenum to photograph the pancreas. It is widely used because it is superior to other imaging methods in the differential diagnosis of pancreatic lesions. In particular, it is useful to differentiate nonfunctional PNEN from pancreatic adenocarcinoma and to identify the location of small tumors (especially insulinomas) <1 cm that are not observed in general imaging tests and are not confirmed by somatostatin receptor scans [6]. Recently, the resolution of CT images has been greatly improved and the detection rate of small tumors has also increased. However, CT still has limitations in detecting pancreatic neuroendocrine tumors <2 cm. The sensitivity of EUS is much higher than that of CT in patients with PNEN who underwent both EUS and CT scans [7]. Through EUS, the anatomical positional relationship between the surrounding blood vessels and the pancreatic duct can be clearly identified, so it can be helpful in determining the extent of resection and the surgical method before surgery. PNEN is a homogeneous hypoechoic lesion in EUS with relatively distinct borders. Early PNEN lesions that are difficult to differentiate from pancreatic adenocarcinoma require additional tests such as endoscopic ultrasound-guided fine-needle aspiration (EUS-FNA) or contrast-enhanced EUS. As a result, the greatest strength of EUS in diagnosing PNEN is that it helps in the differential diagnosis of pancreatic adenocarcinoma that cannot be differentiated by echo pattern through EUS-FNA or biopsy [8].

Staging

Since PNENs often exhibit symptoms through hormone secretion, they are divided into functional and nonfunctional, and the grades are classified according to the degree of cell differentiation [9]. In 2010, the World Health Organization (WHO) renamed the neuroendocrine tumor (NET) as neuroendocrine neoplasm (NEN). NEN was classified into a three-level classification system (G1, G2, G3) based on cell differentiation, mitosis count, and proliferation activity (Ki-67 index). However, there was a difference in response to treatment and survival rates in neuroendocrine tumors with a cell division number corresponding to G2 or a Ki-67 division index of 20% or more, suggesting the need to subdivide the group corresponding to G3 [10]. Furthermore, when G3 was classified according to the Ki-67 cleavage index of 55%, there was a difference in cancer response and survival rate, suggesting the existence of a heterogeneous group in neuroendocrine tumors of G3 [11]. Based on the results of the above study, it is predicted that the response and prognosis to treatment will differ depending on the level of cell differentiation at the Ki-67 cell proliferation index of 20% or more. It is classified into endocrine tumors and poorly differentiated neuroendocrine cancers (Table 1) [12]. Histological grades and various classifications have evolved to attempt to stratify patients into different prognostic groups.

The TNM staging system is used primarily to reflect the prognosis and treatment planning, as well as the WHO grade of the aforementioned pancreatic neuroendocrine tumor. The main stage of TMN is the stage presented by the American Joint Committee on Cancer (AJCC) and the European Neuroendocrine Tumor Society (ENETS) (Table 2) [13, 14]. In the seventh Edition of the AJCC, the T stage was classified according to the size of the tumor of 2 cm, and there was a difference from the ENETS, which classified the tumor

Table 1 World Health Organization 2017 nomenclature and classification for neuroendocrine neoplasms

Nomenclature	Grade	Differentiation	Mitotic count (mitoses/10HPF)	Ki-67 index
NET, grade 1	G1 (low)	Well differentiated	<2	<3%
NET, grade 2	G2 (intermediate)	Well differentiated	2–20	3–20%
NET, grade 3	G3 (high)	Well differentiated	>20	>20%
NEC, grade 3	G3 (high)	Poorly differentiated Small/large cell type	>20	>20%
Mixed neuroendocrine-nonneuroendocrine neoplasm (MiNEN)				

NET Neuroendocrine tumor, *NEC* Neuroendocrine carcinoma high power field

Table 2 The AJCC (eighth ed.) and ENETS staging systems for PNENs

	AJCC	ENETS
T stage		
T1 T2 T3 T4	Tumor limited to the pancreas, <2 cm Tumor limited to the pancreas, 2–4 cm Tumor limited to the pancreas, >4 cm invading the duodenum or bile duct Tumor invading adjacent organs or the wall of large vessels	
N stage		
N0 N1	No regional LN involvement Regional LN involvement	
M stage		
M0 M1	No distant metastasis Distant metastasis	
Stage		
I II	T1, N0, M0 T2, N0, M0 T3, N0, M0	T1, N0, M0 T2,N0, M0 (IIA) T3, N0, M0 (IIB)
III	T4, N0, M0 Any T, N1, M0	T4, N0, M0 (IIIA) Any T, N1, M0 (IIIB)
IV	Any T, any N, M1	Any T, any N, M1

Stomach, spleen, colon, adrenal gland; celiac axis or superior mesenteric artery; *LN* Lymph node, *AJCC* American Joint Committee on Cancer, *ENETS* European Neuroendocrine Tumor Society, *PNENs* pancreatic neuroendocrine tumors

size according to sizes of 2 cm and 4 cm. However, the recently revised eighth Edition of the AJCC uses the same TNM staging criteria as ENETS. However, in the TNM stage, ENETS subdivided stages II and III into IIA, IIB, IIIA, and IIIB, but in the eighth Edition of AJCC, they were simply divided into II and III. These different classification and TNM staging systems can be considered the main variables in predicting prognosis and determining treatment direction, but to date no consistent standard is recommended, which limits actual clinical practice and research.

Management

Approximately two-thirds of malignant PNENs are metastatic at diagnosis; however, if possible, surgical resection including curative or cytoreductive operation has been advocated first. However, because systemic therapy plays an important role in controlling symptoms related to tumor growth and hormonal hypersecretion, most patients eventually require additional medical/systemic therapy [15–17].

Surgical Consideration

Surgical resection of the primary PNET and the resectable metastatic site is the cornerstone of PNEN management and has been associated with improved overall therapeutic outcomes [18]. In sporadic PNETs, the curative resection of the primary tumor in localized, regional, and even metastatic disease could improve patient survival. The goal of surgery is to completely remove the tumor for cure or, in appropriate cases, to debulk the tumor burden. However, for patients with PNEC, surgery alone is rarely curative, even for patients with apparently localized disease. Nevertheless, resection may benefit selected patients when used in conjunction with chemotherapy and/or radiation therapy in a multimodal approach. Interestingly, the case of small, asymptomatic sporadic well-differentiated PNETs remains controversial for initial surgery versus observation. A recent retrospective multicenter Korean study including 158 patients with pathologically confirmed small PNENs demonstrated that WHO grade is responsible for the malignant potential of small PNENS ≤2 cm. Thus, when ~1–2 cm-sized suspicious PNENs were incidentally found, pathological confirmation using EUS-FNAB is a useful diagnostic approach to provide early treatment strategies for these patients [19].

Systemic Therapies: Well-Differentiated Pancreatic Neuroendocrine Tumors (G1 and G2 PNETs)

There are multiple active systemic treatments for patients with metastatic grade 1 and 2 PNETs: somatostatin analogs (SSAs), everolimus, sunitinib, streptozocin-based cytotoxic regimens, capecitabine/temozolomide, and 177Lu-DOTATATE. However, especially those with a low tumor volume can be safely observed with close monitoring using cross-sectional imaging (Fig. 1).

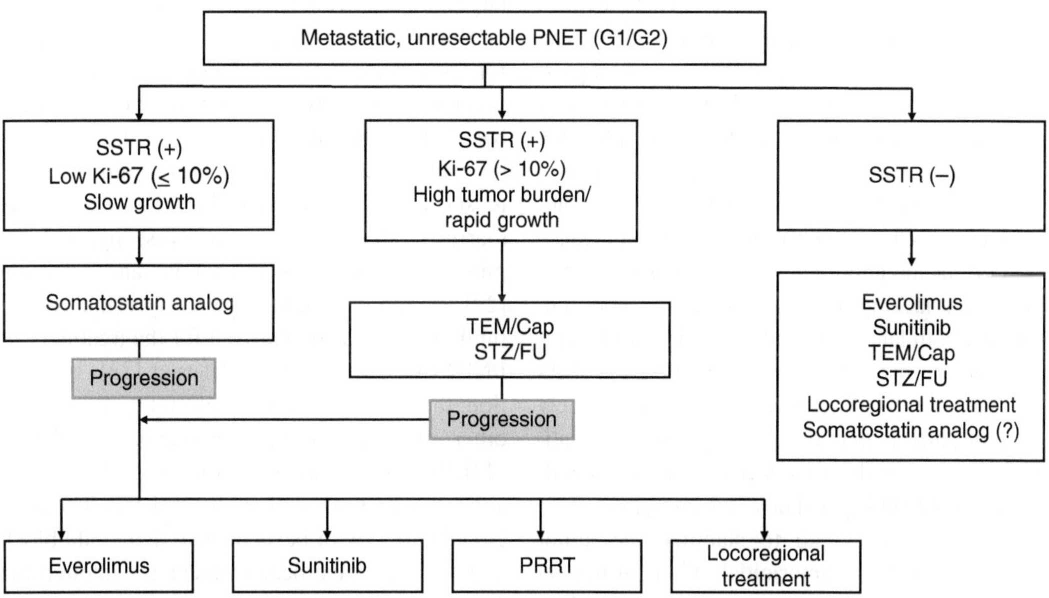

Fig. 1 Suggested therapeutic algorithm for metastatic/unresectable grade 1 or grade 2 pancreas neuroendocrine tumor
PNET Pancreatic neuroendocrine tumor, *SSTR* Somatostatin receptor, *PRRT* Peptide receptor radiotherapy, *Tem/Cap* Chemotherapy with temozolomide and capecitabine, *STZ/FU* Chemotherapy with streptozocin and 5-fluorouracil. Locoregional treatment: hepatic artery embolization, radioembolization, and radiofrequency ablation

Somatostatin Analogs

Somatostatin analogs (SSAs) are generally recommended as a first-line treatment option to slow disease progression in patients with advanced or metastatic PNETs. Currently, there are two approved SSAs such as octreotide and lanreotide. Both drugs have a similar mechanism of action and preferentially bind with similar affinity to somatostatin receptor subtypes 2 and 5. Historically, SSAs have been considered the initial treatment option for patients with PNETs with unresectable symptomatic functioning. SSAs are effective in controlling hormonal symptoms including VIPomas (diarrhea) and glucagonomas (rash); however, they are less effective in insulinoma and gastrinoma. In nonfunctioning PNETs, SSAs should be initiated for patients with high tumor burden or if tumor progression is documented after an observation period in patients with limited tumor burden. That is because SSAs can prolong periods of stability of PNETs and progression-free survival (PFS), and in less than 10% of the cases, objective tumor shrinkage has been reported. Of both SSAs, the antitumor activity of lanreotide in patients with PNET was well established in the CLARINET trial [20], while evidence supporting the antitumor activity of octreotide is somewhat lacking. However, there was a consensus that both lanreotide and octreotide are acceptable for the first-line treatment of PNETs. SSAs are generally well-tolerated, but approximately 25% of patients may develop asymptomatic gallstones or sludge due to reduced postprandial gallbladder contractility and delayed emptying.

Because SSAs tend to stabilize the tumor rather than have a tumoricidal effect, in tumors with a higher proliferation rate, SSA should be complemented or combined with other local therapeutic modalities such as hepatic arterial embolization and radiofrequency ablation. Furthermore, a trial of SSAs may also be considered in patients with negative octreoscan.

Interferon Alpha

Patients with advanced PNETs have been treated with interferon alpha (IFNα) for many decades, but its use has been limited by the severity of side effects, including fatigue, myelosuppression, depression, influenza-like symptoms, weight loss, and changes in thyroid function. The European Neuroendocrine Tumor Society (ENETS) and the North American Neuroendocrine Tumor Society (NANETS) guidelines specify the use of IFNα as a second-line therapy for functioning NETs after failure of SSAs. The combination of INFα with SSAs has been evaluated, but the results have been inconsistent.

Molecular Target Therapy

The current understanding of the molecular pathogenesis of PNETs has introduced molecular target therapy by modulating tumor angiogenesis, growth factor receptors, and the mammalian target of rapamycin (mTOR) pathway.

Everolimus (mTOR inhibitor) was approved for the treatment of PNET in patients with unresectable local, advanced, or metastatic disease based on the RADIANT-3 trial that showed a significant benefit of PFS [21]. Everolimus is related to several side effects, including rash, fatigue, diarrhea, stomatitis, pneumonitis, hyperglycemia, thrombocytopenia, anemia, and infection [22]. Sunitinib (multitargeted tyrosine kinase inhibitor) was also approved for the treatment of PNETs based on a phase III trial [23]. In addition, there have been many efforts to use various other molecular target treatments for PNETs [24]. Tyrosine kinase inhibitors such as sorafenib and pazopanib as well as the anti-VEGF monoclonal antibody of bevacizumab that could block angiogenesis have been evaluated. Although the efficacy of these agents has been established, a definitive conclusion has not been reached based on the lack of phase III trial.

Cytotoxic Chemotherapy

PNETs have been shown to respond to STZ-based combinations, STZ plus doxorubicin or STZ plus 5-FU. Dacarbazine is an alkylating agent that is similar to streptozocin with its activity against PNET but also with associated toxicity. More recently, temozolomide is an oral analogue of dacarbazine that is better tolerated. In a retrospective series of patients with NETs, temozolomide was demonstrated in PNETs with a reported objective tumor response of 34%. Furthermore, temozolomide in combination with capecitabine has shown promise in metastatic PNETs with a response rate of 70%. However, the benefit of cytotoxic chemotherapy is less clear with rare objective radiologic responses and a lack of substantial PFS or overall survival (OS) benefit in clinical trials. Therefore, the many guidelines indicate that chemotherapy may be considered in patients with progressive disease for whom no other treatment options are available.

Peptide Receptor Radionuclide Therapy

Peptide receptor radionuclide therapy (PRRT) with 177Lu-DOTATATE is an effective treatment option for progressive somatostatin receptor-positive PNETs after initial therapy [25]. The median overall response rate (ORR) was 58% and the median disease control rate (DCR) was 83%, with the median PFS ranging from 25–34 months. Furthermore, PRRT with 177Lu-DOTATATE is associated with a significant improvement in quality of life, including symptomatic improvement and a decrease of more than 80% in plasma hormone levels in patients with functional PNETs. Adverse effects included grade 3/4 hematologic toxicity in 10% (G3/4 thrombocytopenia in 5%, G3/4 leukopenia in 5%, and G3/4 anemia in 4%). The long-term risk of PRRT-induced myeloid neoplasms, including myelodysplastic syndrome and/or acute leukemia, appears to be 2%–3%.

Systemic Therapies: Poorly Differentiated Neuroendocrine Carcinomas

Poorly differentiated PNECs (G3 PNECs) carry a worse prognosis given the rapid progression and high probability of metastatic spread, even in patients with localized tumors. As surgery is necessary for localized disease but rarely curative, chemotherapy is the mainstay of treatment. Platinum-based chemotherapy of cisplatin or carboplatin plus etoposide for 4–6 cycles has been recommended for initial systemic therapy [26]. Alternatively, the combination of irinotecan plus cisplatin may be used. In a study of 18 patients with metastatic NEC, etoposide (130 mg/m^2, days 1–3) and cisplatin (45 mg/m^2, days 2 and 3), 12 (67%) patients presented an objective response and 3 complete regressions. In another retrospective analysis (etoposide 100 mg/m^2 on days 1–3 and cisplatin 100 mg/m^2 on day 1), 42% of the patients had an objective response and four complete responses. The median duration of the response was 9.2 months, with a median survival of 15 months. Interestingly, Ki-67 higher than 55% was predictive of response to chemotherapy, since tumors with Ki-67 below 55% were less responsive to platinum-based chemotherapy, with a response rate of 15% versus 42% in high Ki-67 tumors. Furthermore, median OS was significantly longer in high Ki-67 tumors (14 versus 10 months). Temozolomide-based treatment is also used as a second-line treatment. A study evaluating 25 patients with gas troenteropancreatic NEC who treated temozolomide with or without capecitabine and bevacizumab reported a response rate of 33%, stable disease in 38%, and a median OS of 22 months.

As noted above, several studies have challenged the assumption that poorly differentiated histology and high tumor grade are equivalent. It seems that a small subset of patients with neuroendocrine tumors that appear histologically well or moderately differentiated are grade 3 PNETs that have Ki-67 proliferation indices in the 20%–55% range. In these typical subsets, low response was demonstrated to platinum plus etoposide regimens. Although the appropriate systemic therapy remains unclear in grade 3 PNET, possible treatment options may include SSAs, molecularly targeted therapy, temozolomide, or chemotherapy (Fig. 2).

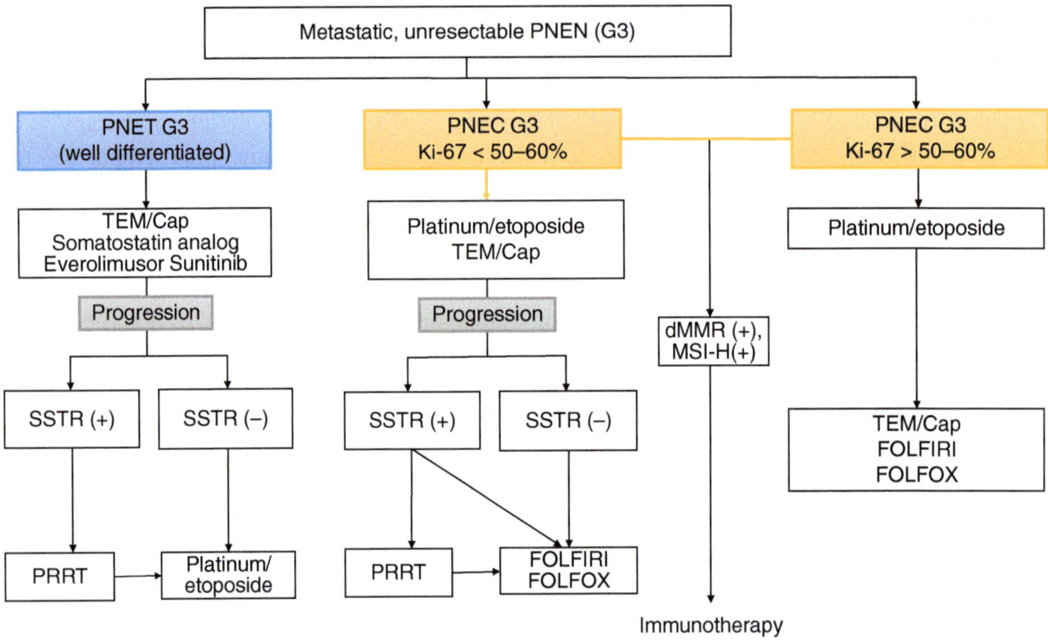

Fig. 2 Suggested therapeutic algorithm for metastatic/unresectable grade 3 pancreatic neuroendocrine neoplasm *PNEC* Pancreatic neuroendocrine carcinoma, *PNET* Pancreatic neuroendocrine tumor, *SSTR* Somatostatin receptor, *PRRT* Peptide receptor radiotherapy, *Tem/Cap* Chemotherapy with temozolomide and capecitabine, *FOLFIRI* Chemotherapy with irinotecan, folinic acid, and infusional 5-fluorouracil, *FOLFOX* Chemotherapy with oxaliplatin, folinic acid, and infusional 5-fluorouracil, *MSI* Microsatellite instability

Other Treatments

For patients with low-volume metastatic PNENs, surgical resection of metastatic sites in conjunction with adjuvant therapies such as ablation, embolization, or long-acting somatostatin analogs can prolong and improve quality of life. Of these, hepatic arterial embolization is a reasonable alternative approach to systemic therapy for patients with predominant hepatic disease, particularly those who are symptomatic but not surgical candidates. As part of another recent effort, radioembolization using 90Y-radiolabeled microspheres via the hepatic artery is used for local radioactive ablation. The role of immunotherapy with immune checkpoint inhibitors is only beginning to be studied in patients with PNENs. An early study suggested that anti-programmed cell death 1 (PD-1) antibodies have minimal activity as single agent therapy; however, ongoing trials are in progress to evaluate checkpoint inhibitors in combination with other immunomodulatory agents, including inhibitors of the vascular endothelial growth factor (VEGF) pathway.

Prognosis

Even when advanced, survival times for patients with well-differentiated PNETs are generally better than those of patients with other malignancies, although prognosis can be highly variable. The median survival for patients with distant metastases from grade 1/2 PNETs was 50 months. The main prognostic factors are the TNM stage and histologic grade, which is assigned based on the mitotic rate or the Ki-67 labeling index. Recently, longer survival of patients with advanced/metastatic PNENs has been increasingly observed, suggesting improved efficacy of therapy. Unfortunately, high-level evidence is still lacking for most interventions and follow-up. Therefore, there remains considerable debate on many topics, especially with regard to the sequencing of systemic therapy and surveillance. Given the limitations of the data and the heterogeneity of this patient population, optimal management is best determined in the context of multidisciplinary team support.

Conclusion

PNENs are diverse diseases with different prognosis. Among the therapeutic options available, curative resection should be considered for localized tumors and in some selected cases of metastatic disease. In unresectable disease, SSAs are regarded as first-line treatment not only to control hormonal symptoms but also to inhibit tumor progression. Molecular-targeted agents, such as sunitinib and everolimus, are also effective treatments for metastatic WHO Grade 1/Grade 2 PNETs. Chemotherapy is generally used in highly symptomatic and rapidly growing Grade 3 PNEC. In addition, local ablative therapy and PRRT could be applied after failure of initial medical therapy. Most importantly, a multidisciplinary team approach is essential to optimal management of PNENs.

References

1. Falconi M, Eriksson B, Kaltsas G, Bartsch DK, Capdevila J, Caplin M, et al. ENETS consensus guidelines update for the management of patients with functional pancreatic neuroendocrine tumors and non-functional pancreatic neuroendocrine tumors. Neuroendocrinology. 2016;103:153–71.
2. Berna MJ, Hoffmann KM, Serrano J, Gibril F, Jensen RT. Serum gastrin in Zollinger-Ellison syndrome—I. Prospective study of fasting serum gastrin in 309 patients from National Institutes of Health and comparison with 2229 cases from the literature. Medicine (Baltimore). 2006;85:295–330.
3. Jensen RT, Cadiot G, Brandi ML, de Herder WW, Kaltsas G, Komminoth P, et al. ENETS consensus guidelines for the management of patients with digestive neuroendocrine neoplasms: functional pancreatic endocrine tumor syndromes. Neuroendocrinology. 2012;95:98–119.
4. Cryer PE, Axelrod L, Grossman AB, Heller SR, Montori VM, Seaquist ER, et al. Evaluation and management of adult hypoglycemic disorders: an endocrine society clinical practice guideline. J Clin Endocrinol Metab. 2009;94:709–28.
5. Modlin IM, Gustafsson BI, Moss SF, Pavel M, Tsolakis AV, Kidd M. Chromogranin A—biological function and clinical utility in neuro endocrine tumor disease. Ann Surg Oncol. 2010;17:2427–43.
6. Kang CM, Park SH, Kim KS, Choi JS, Lee WJ, Kim BR. Surgical experiences of functioning neuroendocrine neoplasm of the pancreas. Yonsei Med J. 2006;47:833–9.
7. Khashab MA, Yong E, Lennon AM, Shin EJ, Amateau S, Hruban RH, et al. EUS is still superior to multidetector computerized tomography for detection of pancreatic neuroendocrine tumors. Gastrointest Endosc. 2011;73:691–6.
8. Chang FJ, Chandra A, Culora G, Mahadeva U, Meenan J, Herbert A. Cytologic diagnosis of pancreatic endocrine tumors by endoscopic ultrasound-guided fine-needle aspiration: a review. Diagn Cytopathol. 2006;34:649–58.
9. Cho JH, Ryu JK, Song SY, Hwang JH, Lee DK, Woo SM, et al. Prognostic validity of the American Joint Committee on Cancer and the European Neuroendocrine Tumors Staging Classifications for pancreatic neuroendocrine tumors a retrospective nationwide multicenter study in South Korea. Pancreas. 2016;45:941–6.
10. Basturk O, Yang ZH, Tang LH, Hruban RH, Adsay V, McCall CM, et al. The high-grade (WHO G3) pancreatic neuroendocrine tumor category is morphologically and biologically heterogenous and includes both well differentiated and poorly differentiated neoplasms. Am J Surg Pathol. 2015;39:683–90.
11. Sorbye H, Welin S, Langer SW, Vestermark LW, Holt N, Osterlund P, et al. Predictive and prognostic factors for treatment and survival in 305 patients with advanced gastrointestinal neuroendocrine carcinoma (WHO G3): the NORDIC NEC study. Ann Oncol. 2013;24:152–60.
12. Guilmette JM, Nose V. Neoplasms of the neuroendocrine pancreas: an update in the classification, definition, and molecular genetic advances. Adv Anat Pathol. 2019;26:13–30.
13. MB A, Cancer AJCo. AJCC cancer staging manual. 8th ed. Springer; 2017.
14. Pavel M, Valle JW, Eriksson B, Rinke A, Caplin M, Chen J, et al. ENETS consensus guidelines for the standards of care in neuroendocrine neoplasms: systemic therapy—biotherapy and novel targeted agents. Neuroendocrinology. 2017;105:266–80.
15. Halfdanarson TR, Strosberg JR, Tang L, Bellizzi AM, Bergsland EK, O'Dorisio TM, et al. The north American neuroendocrine tumor society consensus guidelines for surveillance and medical management of pancreatic neuroendocrine tumors. Pancreas. 2020;49:863–81.
16. Pavel M, O'Toole D, Costa F, Capdevila J, Gross D, Kianmanesh R, et al. ENETS consensus guidelines update for the management of distant metastatic disease of intestinal, pancreatic, bronchial neuro-

endocrine neoplasms (NEN) and NEN of unknown primary site. Neuroendocrinology. 2016;103:172–85.
17. Rinke A, Auernhammer CJ, Bodei L, Kidd M, Krug S, Lawlor R, et al. Treatment of advanced gastroentero-pancreatic neuroendocrine neoplasia, are we on the way to personalised medicine? Gut. 2021;70:1768–81.
18. Howe JR, Merchant NB, Conrad C, Keutgen XM, Hallet J, Drebin JA, et al. The north American neuroendocrine tumor society consensus paper on the surgical management of pancreatic neuroendocrine tumors. Pancreas. 2020;49:1–33.
19. Paik WH, Lee HS, Lee KJ, Jang SI, Lee WJ, Hwang JH, et al. Malignant potential of small pancreatic neuroendocrine neoplasm and its risk factors: a multicenter nationwide study. Pancreatology. 2021;21:208–14.
20. Caplin ME, Pavel M, Cwikla JB, Phan AT, Raderer M, Sedlackova E, et al. Lanreotide in metastatic enteropancreatic neuroendocrine tumors. N Engl J Med. 2014;371:224–33.
21. Yao JC, Shah MH, Ito T, Bohas CL, Wolin EM, Van Cutsem E, et al. Everolimus for advanced pancreatic neuroendocrine tumors. N Engl J Med. 2011;364:514–23.
22. Lee KJ, Cho JH, Lee SH, Song SY, Lee KH, Jeong S, et al. Clinical outcomes of everolimus in patients with advanced, nonfunctioning pancreatic neuroendocrine tumors: a multicenter study in Korea. Cancer Chemother Pharmacol. 2017;
23. Raymond E, Dahan L, Raoul JL, Bang YJ, Borbath I, Lombard-Bohas C, et al. Sunitinib malate for the treatment of pancreatic neuroendocrine tumors. N Engl J Med. 2011;364:501–13.
24. Kim EJ, Kim YJ, Lee HI, Jeong SH, Nam HJ, Cho JH. Upregulation of peroxiredoxin-2 in well-differentiated pancreatic neuroendocrine tumors and its utility as a biomarker for predicting the response to Everolimus. Antioxidants (Basel). 2020:9.
25. Strosberg J, El-Haddad G, Wolin E, Hendifar A, Yao J, Chasen B, et al. Phase 3 trial of (177)Lu-dotatate for midgut neuroendocrine tumors. N Engl J Med. 2017;376:125–35.
26. Garcia-Carbonero R, Sorbye H, Baudin E, Raymond E, Wiedenmann B, Niederle B, et al. ENETS consensus guidelines for high-grade gastroenteropancreatic neuroendocrine tumors and neuroendocrine carcinomas. Neuroendocrinology. 2016;103:186–94.

Part XI

GIST (Gastrointestinal Stromal Tumor)

Epidemiology, Clinical Presentation and Diagnosis, Staging, Treatment, and Prognosis

Key Points

- GIST is a type of submucosal tumor of the gastrointestinal tract most commonly seen in clinics and is known to originate from the interstitial cell of Cajal (ICC).
- It is known that a large size and high mitotic index have a high tendency to malignancy. However, even when the size is small and the mitotic index is low, the course of a malignant tumor with metastasis may follow, so GIST should always be considered a potentially malignant tumor.
- GIST is generally diagnosed through immunochemical staining for the expression of stem-cell growth factor receptor or KIT protein, a receptor tyrosine kinase protein known as CD117, present in ICC, and is expressed in about 95% of cases.
- Surgical resection is the treatment of choice for localized or potentially resectable tumors. However, when the lesion is borderline resectable or when surgically removed, the scope of surgery is extensive and there is a possibility that the function of the cut organ may be affected, the initial treatment using imatinib is preferred.
- For advanced/metastatic GIST, adjuvant or neoadjuvant chemotherapy using imatinib can be used according to the molecular classification.

Tae Ho Kim is the lead author of this chapter.

Introduction

GIST is a type of submucosal tumor of the gastrointestinal tract most commonly seen in clinics and is known to originate from the interstitial cell of Cajal (ICC), which acts as a pacemaker for gastrointestinal motility. GIST is mainly caused by oncogene mutations in the tyrosine kinase receptor KIT and platelet-derived growth factor receptor-α (PDGFR-α) [1, 2]. About 20%–30% of GISTs follow the course of a malignant tumor. It is known that large size and high mitotic index have a high tendency to be malignant. However, even when the size is small and the mitotic index is low, the course of a malignant tumor with metastasis may follow, so GIST should always be considered a potentially malignant tumor [3, 4].

Epidemiology

Globally, the incidence of GIST is estimated to be 10–15 people/1,000,000, and the prevalence is estimated to be about 13/100,000. However, most GISTs are asymptomatic and are rarely detected by symptom-based tests and are often discovered incidentally through tests such as health check-ups [5]. According to autopsy studies, when closely observing the gastrointestinal tract, up to 20%–35% of all autopsy cases for GIST smaller than 1 cm are reported, so the frequency of asymptomatic GIST is estimated to be much higher. GIST occurs at any age, but it is diag-

H. J. Chun et al., *Gastrointestinal Cancer*, https://doi.org/10.1007/978-981-99-0815-8_66

nosed most often in people over 60 years of age, and the sex ratio is similar for men and women. The most common organ is the stomach, with a frequency of 50%, the small intestine 35%, the large intestine 7%, the rectum 5%, and the esophagus 1%. At the time of discovery, the median tumor size was about 6 cm, and its incidence has increased every year since 2000. This is believed to be due to the increase in GIST, which is found with an increase in examinations such as upper gastrointestinal endoscopy and capsule endoscopy [6, 7].

The incidence of GIST varies by geographical location. According to a systematic review based on 30 studies conducted in about 20 countries, Hong Kong, Shanghai, Taiwan, Korea, and Norway had the highest incidence rate at 19–22 cases/1,000,000 per year. Shanxi province in China and the Czech Republic/Slovakia showed low incidence rates of 4.3 cases/1,000,000 per year and 5.2 cases/1,000,000 per year, respectively. In the United States and Canada, GIST occurs at a frequency of 7–8 cases/1,000,000 per year [8, 9].

Clinical Presentation and Diagnosis

In the case of small GIST, there are many asymptomatic cases, and it is discovered incidentally in the form of a hard, cushion-sign negative submucosal tumor that protrudes into the lumen with normal mucosa on endoscopy. However, it is difficult to accurately differentiate GIST from other submucosal tumors such as leiomyoma with endoscopy alone. If irregular borders, surface ulcers, and size increases are observed during follow-up endoscopy, it is clinically suggestive of malignancy. Through EUS, the exact size and location of the tumor can be confirmed, and it is possible to differentiate it from a lipoma or cyst [10]. Follow-up testing is also safe and accurate using EUS. The findings of the EUS examination, such as a size greater than 2 cm, irregular borders, heterogeneous echo patterns, anechoic spaces, and echogenic foci, are also known suggestive of malignancy. However, lesions observed as hypoechoic solid masses in EUS include malignant tumors such as malignant lymphoma, metastatic cancer, neuroendocrine tumor, and submucosal tumor type, and benign tumors such as leiomyoma, neurinoma, and ectopic pancreas. Since it is difficult to differentiate by EUS image alone, it is necessary to make a diagnosis by collecting samples for histological diagnosis including immunochemical staining [11]. Through EUS-guided fine-needle aspiration biopsy (EUS-FNA) or incision biopsy, a histological diagnosis can be made before surgery or chemotherapy. If EUS or endoscopic access is difficult, a biopsy can be performed using image-guided percutaneous biopsy for primary or metastatic lesions. However, percutaneous biopsy is not preferred because it has the potential to spread metastatic lesions or rupture of the primary tumor [12]. In addition to EUS, imaging studies such as computed tomography (CT scan), positron emission tomography/CT (PET-CT), and magnetic resonance imaging (MRI) are useful for diagnosing GIST. The CT scan is a very useful and accurate test for diagnosing relatively small GIST, but there are concerns about radiation exposure, so caution is required for some adults, young children, and women of childbearing age. GISTs larger than 5 cm are typically observed as exophytic and hypervascular lesions on CT, but smaller ones often appear as endoluminal polypoid masses. CT scan has the advantage of obtaining additional information on local invasion or metastasis. In PET-CT, GIST showed characteristically strong F-fluorodeoxyglucose uptake, which is helpful for diagnosis. On MRI, small GISTs show strong homogeneous arterial enhancement, while large GISTs have the form of lobulated tumors with gradual heterogeneous enhancement, and internal cystic changes are often observed [13].

GISTs larger than 5–6 cm often have well-developed blood vessels and are often diagnosed by examination with symptoms such as abdominal pain and accompanying bleeding. Bleeding occurs in the intestinal tract or intraperitoneal cavity and, in about 20% of patients, it is diagnosed as having metastasized at the time of diagnosis. Metastases to the liver are the most common and metastases to the abdominal cavity or lymph nodes are also common. In addition to abdominal pain and bleeding, it is often diagnosed with symptoms such as nausea, pleuritic chest pain, pelvic pain, and small bowel obstruction. The majority (>97%) of GIST are sporadic, but there are rare cases associated with family history. These cases are associated with neurofibromatosis type 1, Carney-Stratakis syndrome (GIST and paraganglioma due to germline mutation in the succinate dehydrogenase (SDH) mitochondrial tumor suppressor gene pathway), and Carney triad (GIST, pulmonary chondroma, and extra-adrenal paraganglioma). Carney-Stratakis syndrome has an autosomal dominant inheritable tendency due to epigenetic hypermethylation of the SDH complex genes. In this case, unlike general GIST, symptoms such as hyperpigmentation, urticaria pigmentosa, and increase in nevi are often accompanied. SDH-deficient GIST occurs almost always in the stomach, has the characteristic of growing in nests of tumor cells divided into septa of smooth muscle cells, and tends to follow an indolent course [14–16].

GIST is diagnosed at any age from 10 to 100 years old, but it is mainly diagnosed in those 50–70 years old or older. About 0.4%–2% of GIST is diagnosed in adolescents or children younger than 20 years of age. However, in the case of GIST diagnosed at an early age, it usually has a genetic predisposition to tumorigenesis [17].

Morphologically, GIST can be classified mainly as the spindle-shaped cell type (70%), epithelial cell type (20%), and mixed type (10%). GIST is generally diagnosed by immunochemical staining for the expression of stem-cell growth factor receptor or c-KIT protein, a receptor tyrosine kinase protein known as CD117, present in ICC, and is expressed in about 95% of cases. In addition to GIST, the c-KIT protein is also expressed in hematopoietic stem cells, mast cells, melanocytes, and germ cells. The main mechanism of GIST development is oncogenic activation by mutations in KIT (~90%) and PDGFR (~10%), and in less than 10%, mutational inactivation of the neurofibromatosis 1 protein (NF1) or mutational activation of RAS or BRAF occurs. In 70% of GIST, CD34, a transmembrane phosphoglycoprotein observed in hematopoietic stem cells, is expressed. In addition to CD117 and CD34, DOG1 is also expressed in 98%, which is very useful for diagnosis. DOG1 is a gene encoding the chloride channel protein anoctamin-1 and is independent of KIT or PDGFR mutational status. In most GIST, the smooth muscle markers desmin, actin, and myosin are not expressed [18, 19].

Staging

If GIST is confirmed, staging is performed using the American Joint Committee on Cancer (AJCC) eighth Edition and the Union for International Cancer Control (UICC) tumor, node, metastasis (TNM) staging system (Table 1) [20, 21]. In the AJCC staging system, the same criteria are applied regardless of the primary tumor site, but if the stomach and omentum are the primary sites, a separate staging system is applied.

Table 1 GIST TNM staging AJCC UICC eighth edition [20]

Definitions for TNM	
Primary tumor (T)	
Tx	Primary tumor cannot be assessed
T0	No evidence of primary tumor
T1	Tumor 2 cm or less
T2	Tumor more than 2 cm, but not more than 5 cm
T3	Tumor more than 5 cm, but not more than 10 cm
T4	Tumor more than 10 cm in greatest dimension
Regional LN (N)	
N0	No regional LN metastasis or unknown LN status
N1	Regional LN metastasis
Distant metastasis (M)	
M0	No distant metastasis
M1	Distant metastasis
Grade X	Grade cannot be assessed
Low	5 or fewer mitoses/50 HPF
G2	Over 5 mitoses/50HPF

(continued)

Table 1 (continued)

Definitions for TNM		
Anatomic stage/prognostic groups		
Gastric GIST (also used for omentum)		
IA	T1 or T2, N0, M0	Low mitotic rate
IB	T3, N0, M0	Low mitotic rate
II	T1, N0, M0 T2, N0, M0 T4, N0, M0	High mitotic rate High mitotic rate Low mitotic rate
IIIA	T3, N0, M0, G2	High mitotic rate
IIIB	T4, N0, M0, G2	High mitotic rate
IV	Any T, N1, M0 Any T, any N, M1	Any rate Any rate
Small intestinal GIST (also for esophagus, colorectal, mesenteric, peritoneal)		
I	T1 or T2, N0, M0	Low mitotic rate
II	T3, N0, M0	Low mitotic rate
IIIA	T1, N0, M0 T4, N0, M0	High mitotic rate Low mitotic rate
IIIB	T2, N0, M0 T3, N0, M0 T4, N0, M0	High mitotic rate High mitotic rate High mitotic rate
IV	Any T, N1, M0 Any T, any N, M1,	Any rate Any rate

Treatment and Prognosis

GIST can exhibit various biological disease behaviors, and in all cases, it has the potential to progress to metastatic lesions. Therefore, the treatment of GIST is based on available clinical risk factors such as preoperative diagnosis, tumor location and size, range of lesions or metastasis, and clinical symptoms such as bleeding, obstruction, and perforation. It is determined based on the prognostic model for the prediction of relative risk.

In general, a histological diagnosis is made, but if GIST is strongly suspected and surgery is possible, a biopsy before surgery or a preoperative biopsy may not be necessary. However, if metastatic lesions are suspected or if preoperative imatinib treatment is considered, EUS or endoscopic or radiographic biopsy is required prior to treatment. All GISTs ≥2 cm should be resected, but consensus has not yet been established for lesions smaller than this. Surgical resection is the treatment of choice for potentially resectable tumors. However, when the lesion is borderline resectable or when surgically removed, the scope of surgery is extensive and there is a possibility that the function of the cut organ may be affected, the initial treatment with imatinib, a tyrosine kinase inhibitor is preferred. The goal of surgical treatment for GIST is to completely excise the lesion without damaging the pseudocapsule. Segmental resection of the stomach or intestine may be necessary to secure sufficient negative resection margin. However, since local recurrence is relatively common, extensive resection of the tissue surrounding the tumor without invasion at the time of surgery is not recommended because the additional benefit is not high. Because nodal metastases are also very rare, routine lymphadenectomy is not necessary [10, 22, 23].

Although complete resection is possible in most local GISTs, only about half of them remain relapse-free for more than 5 years. Data from the representative ACOSOG Z9001 trial provided evidence that adjuvant imatinib therapy was effective in reducing GIST recurrence in the first year of treatment after 1 year of surgery. It has been approved by the United States Food and Drug Administration (FDA). Postoperative adjuvant imatinib treatment is recommended for patients with resected primary GIST at significant risk of recurrence, according to the European Medicines Agency, a European regulatory body. However, postoperative adjuvant imatinib treatment is not recommended for very low/low risk GIST [13, 24].

For advanced or metastatic GIST, neoadjuvant therapy with imatinib is also available. If the GIST is borderline resectable locally advanced disease, unresectable but nonmetastatic, potentially resectable primary tumor if a reduction in tumor size would significantly decrease the morbidity of surgical resection, neoadjuvant therapy with imatinib for 10–12 months can be applied [25].

According to the kinase mutational status of KIT and PDGFRA, GIST can be subclassified. Depending on the sensitivity to imatinib, the type and dose of the drug are determined according to this classification. The usual dose of imatinib is 400 mg daily for GIST with exon 11 KIT mutation. For GIST with exon 9 KIT mutation, 800 mg daily is recommended. GIST with PDGFRα D842V mutation or SDH-deficient or neurofibromatosis-related GIST is not recommended neoadjuvant imatinib. Besides imatinib, avapritinib (for GIST with PDGFRA exon 18 D842V mutation), sunitinib, regorafenib can also be available [26, 27].

KIT gene or platelet-derived growth factor receptor-α (PDGFR-α) gene mutations were absent in about 10%–15% of GISTs. This KIT/PDGFR-α wild-type GIST is the primary form of GIST that occurs in children and rarely occurs in adults. For wild-type GIST, evidence-based treatment strategies have not yet been established. In general, progression and recurrence are common, but the natural course is known to be relatively indolent. Although repeated surgery due to frequent relapse is associated with a decrease in event-free survival, if there is no approved drug yet due to a low response to drugs such as imatinib, and if there are symptoms due to a continuous increase in tumor size, surgical treatment is recommended as the most reasonable option [1, 14, 19, 28].

Both tumor size and mitotic rate are independent prognostic factors and are used to predict aggressive tumor behavior. These two factors were identified using data from three large-scale retrospective studies conducted at the Armed Forces Institute of Pathology (AFIP) in GIST diagnosed and treated before the era of tyrosine kinase inhibitors along with the primary tumor site. However, as the role of targeted therapies specific to tumor mutational status has evolved, it has become less clear how the presence or absence of gene mutations affects these prognostic factors. In general, primary tumors originating in the stomach show better survival outcomes than tumors originating in the small intestine, colon, rectum, or mesentery. However, large tumors with a high mitotic rate have a similarly poor prognosis regardless of the primary site, and more than 85% of such tumors progress to metastatic disease. However, intermediate tumors (large tumors with low mitotic rate or small tumors with high mitotic rate) that occur in the stomach have a better prognosis with a metastasis rate of 10%–15%, whereas tumors originating in the small intestine show a metastasis rate of 50% or more. Patients with colorectal GIST are reported to have similar or slightly reduced recurrent-free survival compared to patients with small intestine GIST. It is known that recurrence is more common even when GIST occurs outside the gastrointestinal tract. However, because these tumors are very rare, it is very difficult to determine the effect of the primary location on the prognosis [21, 29].

Intraoperative or spontaneous tumor rupture is as an independent risk factor negatively affecting disease-free survival. However, tumor rupture has a limitation that it is not reflected in the TNM staging system of the American Joint Committee on Cancer (AJCC). In addition to the AJCC staging system, various prognostic models or risk stratification schemes such as the AFIP prognostic model (Table 2) and the NIH

Table 2 AFIP prognostic model: progression-free survival for gastrointestinal stromal tumors (GISTs) of the stomach, small intestine, and rectum by mitotic rate and tumor size [21]

	Percent of patients progression-free during long-term follow-up by primary site			
Tumor size (cm)	Gastric	Jejunum/ileum	Duodenum	Rectum
Mitotic rate (HPF): ≤5/50				
≤2	100	100	100	100
2–5	98.1	95.7	91.7	91.5
5–10	96.4	76	66	43
>10	88	48		
Mitotic rate (HPF): >5/50				
≤2	100	50	–	46
2–5	84	27	50	48
5–10	45	15	14	29
>10	14	10		

HPF High power field

Table 3 Modified NIH risk stratification criteria for GIST with rupture included [30]

	Size (cm)	Mitotic count (/50 HPF)	Primary tumor site
Very low risk	≤2	≤5	Any site
Low risk	2.1–5	≤5	Any site
Intermediate risk	≤5	6–10	Any site
	2.1–5	>5	Gastric
	5.1–10	≤5	Gastric
High risk	>5	>5	Any site
	>10	Any mitotic rate	Any site
	Any size	>10/	Any site

risk stratification scheme (Table 3) have been developed and presented [21, 30]. It is widely used, based on various risk factors, to determine treatment policy and predict the prognosis of patients. Among them, the modified National Institutes of Health (NIH) risk stratification scheme based on tumor size, mitotic counts, and the addition of tumor rupture is more useful in predicting the 10-year risk of recurrence of GIST than before.

Conclusion

GIST is a relatively rare gastrointestinal submucosal tumor and is increasingly detected and diagnosed as the number of people undergoing endoscopy increases. Because it exists in the submucosal area, histological examination is not easy. However, GIST is a tumor that has malignant potential, and it is necessary to predict its possibility using the diagnostic modality of various methods such as EUS and CT, and to conduct a histological examination if necessary to actively diagnose and treat it. In terms of treatment, the tyrosine kinase inhibitor imatinib has been used, the survival rate of patients with metastatic lesions or inoperable lesions has significantly improved compared to the past. In the future, effective management could be achieved with the development of diagnostic methods or treatment in GIST.

References

1. Rubin BP, Fletcher JA, Fletcher CD. Molecular insights into the histogenesis and pathogenesis of gastrointestinal stromal tumors. Int J Surg Pathol. 2000;8:5–10.
2. Streutker CJ, Huizinga JD, Driman DK, Riddell RH. Interstitial cells of Cajal in health and disease. Part II: ICC and gastrointestinal stromal tumours. Histopathology. 2007;50:190–202.
3. Gheorghe G, Bacalbasa N, Ceobanu G, Ilie M, Enache V, Constantinescu G, et al. Gastrointestinal stromal tumors-a. Mini Review J Pers Med. 2021:11.
4. Miettinen M, Lasota J. Gastrointestinal stromal tumors: review on morphology, molecular pathology, prognosis, and differential diagnosis. Arch Pathol Lab Med. 2006;130:1466–78.
5. Søreide K, Sandvik OM, Søreide JA, Giljaca V, Jureckova A, Bulusu VR. Global epidemiology of gastrointestinal stromal tumours (GIST): a systematic review of population-based cohort studies. Cancer Epidemiol. 2016;40:39–46.
6. Miettinen M, Lasota J. Gastrointestinal stromal tumors (GISTs): definition, occurrence, pathology, differential diagnosis and molecular genetics. Pol J Pathol. 2003;54:3–24.
7. Ma GL, Murphy JD, Martinez ME, Sicklick JK. Epidemiology of gastrointestinal stromal tumors in the era of histology codes: results of a population-based study. Cancer Epidemiol Biomark Prev. 2015;24:298–302.
8. Patel N, Benipal B. Incidence of gastrointestinal stromal tumors in the United States from 2001-2015: a United States cancer statistics analysis of 50 states. Cureus. 2019;11:e4120.
9. Perez EA, Livingstone AS, Franceschi D, Rocha-Lima C, Lee DJ, Hodgson N, et al. Current incidence and outcomes of gastrointestinal mesenchymal tumors including gastrointestinal stromal tumors. J Am Coll Surg. 2006;202:623–9.
10. Akahoshi K, Oya M, Koga T, Shiratsuchi Y. Current clinical management of gastrointestinal stromal tumor. World J Gastroenterol. 2018;24:2806–17.
11. Nishida T, Goto O, Raut CP, Yahagi N. Diagnostic and treatment strategy for small gastrointestinal stromal tumors. Cancer. 2016;122:3110–8.
12. Philipper M, Hollerbach S, Gabbert HE, Heikaus S, Böcking A, Pomjanski N, et al. Prospective comparison of endoscopic ultrasound-guided fine-needle aspiration and surgical histology in upper gastrointestinal submucosal tumors. Endoscopy. 2010;42:300–5.
13. Nishida T, Kawai N, Yamaguchi S, Nishida Y. Submucosal tumors: comprehensive guide for the diagnosis and therapy of gastrointestinal submucosal tumors. Dig Endosc. 2013;25:479–89.
14. Mussi C, Schildhaus HU, Gronchi A, Wardelmann E, Hohenberger P. Therapeutic consequences from molecular biology for gastrointestinal stromal tumor

patients affected by neurofibromatosis type 1. Clin Cancer Res. 2008;14:4550–5.
15. National Multi-Center Treatment Collaboration Group For Neurofibromatosis T, National Multi-Center Research Platform For P, Reconstructive S. Expert consensus on diagnosis and management of neurofibromatosis type 1 (2021 edition). Zhongguo Xiu Fu Chong Jian Wai Ke Za Zhi. 2021(35):1384–95.
16. Wada R, Arai H, Kure S, Peng WX, Naito Z. "Wwild type" GIST: clinicopathological features and clinical practice. Pathol Int. 2016;66:431–7.
17. Antonescu CR. Gastrointestinal stromal tumor (GIST) pathogenesis, familial GIST, and animal models. Semin Diagn Pathol. 2006;23:63–9.
18. Nishida T, Blay JY, Hirota S, Kitagawa Y, Kang YK. The standard diagnosis, treatment, and follow-up of gastrointestinal stromal tumors based on guidelines. Gastric Cancer. 2016;19:3–14.
19. Wu CE, Tzen CY, Wang SY, Yeh CN. Clinical diagnosis of gastrointestinal stromal tumor (GIST): from the molecular genetic point of view. Cancers (Basel). 2019:11.
20. American College of Surgeons. The original source for this information is the AJCC cancer staging manual, eighth edition. 4th ed. Chicago, IL: Springer International Publishing; 2018.
21. Rubin BP, Blanke CD, Demetri GD, Dematteo RP, et al. Protocol for the examination of specimens from patients with gastrointestinal stromal tumor (GIST): based on AJCC/UICC TNM. 7th ed. Washington: College of American Pathologists (CAP); 2013.
22. El-Menyar A, Mekkodathil A, Al-Thani H. Diagnosis and management of gastrointestinal stromal tumors: an up-to-date literature review. J Cancer Res Ther. 2017;13:889–900.
23. Mantese G. Gastrointestinal stromal tumor: epidemiology, diagnosis, and treatment. Curr Opin Gastroenterol. 2019;35:555–9.
24. Joensuu H, Eriksson M, Sundby Hall K, Hartmann JT, Pink D, Schütte J, et al. One vs three years of adjuvant imatinib for operable gastrointestinal stromal tumor: a randomized trial. JAMA. 2012;307:1265–72.
25. Seshadri RA, Rajendranath R. Neoadjuvant imatinib in locally advanced gastrointestinal stromal tumors. J Cancer Res Ther. 2009;5:267–71.
26. von Mehren M, Joensuu H. Gastrointestinal stromal Tumors. J Clin Oncol. 2018;36:136–43.
27. Rubin BP, Heinrich MC, Corless CL. Gastrointestinal stromal tumour. Lancet. 2007;369:1731–41.
28. Schaefer IM, Mariño-Enríquez A, Fletcher JA. What is new in gastrointestinal stromal tumor? Adv Anat Pathol. 2017;24:259–67.
29. Stamatakos M, Douzinas E, Stefanaki C, Safioleas P, Polyzou E, Levidou G, et al. Gastrointestinal stromal tumor. World J Surg Oncol. 2009;7:61.
30. Joensuu H. Risk stratification of patients diagnosed with gastrointestinal stromal tumor. Hum Pathol. 2008;39:1411–9.

Part XII

Special Clinical Considerations for Gastrointestinal Cancer

Palliative Care for Patients with Gastrointestinal Cancer. I-1. Palliative Care for Cancer-Related Problems

Key Points

- Early palliative care intervention can improve the quality of life of patients with GI cancer.
- Surgery is the treatment of choice for malignant bowel obstruction; however, if not applicable, intervention therapies and pharmacological approaches should be considered.
- Nausea and vomiting are associated with many different etiologies, and treatment should be considered based on its etiology.
- Drainage and decompression are the principles of treatment for malignant ascites and jaundice; a pharmacological approach is also required to manage associated symptoms.
- Cancer-related fatigue and anorexia-cachexia syndrome are frequently underestimated; thus, early intervention with an interdisciplinary approach is necessary.

Introduction

Gastrointestinal (GI) cancer is an umbrella term that covers cancers of many organs, including the esophagus, stomach, small bowel, large bowel, anus, gallbladder, liver, and pancreas. Thus, patients diagnosed with GI cancer can present many different distressing symptoms, depending on the type of cancer and stage. Symptoms may negatively affect patients' quality of life (QOL); therefore, early assessment of symptoms and intervention in palliative care can improve cancer patients' QOL [1]. Palliative care for cancer patients is based on an interdisciplinary and patient-centered approach rather than a disease-centered approach. Providing the best QOL for patients and their families until the last moment is the primary goal of palliative care. In this chapter, palliative care for managing symptoms related to GI cancer is discussed.

Malignant Bowel Obstruction

Malignant bowel obstruction (MBO) is a common complication in patients with advanced GI cancer; 25–40% in advanced colon cancer and 6–19% in gastric cancer [2, 3]. MBO causes symptoms including nausea, vomiting, constipation, and colicky pain.

Palliation of MBO

Surgery is the treatment of choice for patients expected to live for months. However, if surgical complications are anticipated due to poor performance status, advanced disease, multiple obstruc-

Wonkil Jung is the lead author of this chapter.

H. J. Chun et al., *Gastrointestinal Cancer*, https://doi.org/10.1007/978-981-99-0815-8_67

tions, and multiple comorbidities, surgery may be avoided [4, 5]. Interventional therapies, such as endoscopic stents, percutaneous endoscopic gastrostomy, and a venting gastrostomy tube, can be considered to palliate MBO. Pharmacological approaches should be used to relieve the symptoms caused by MBO. A combination of antiemetic (metoclopramide, haloperidol, olanzapine) and antisecretory agents (scopolamine (hyoscine) butylbromide, glycopyrrolate, octreotide, and somatostatin analog) may relieve distressing nausea and vomiting. Corticosteroids (dexamethasone), an anti-inflammatory agent, can also be used. If the estimated life expectancy is years to months, but surgical treatment is not applicable, total parenteral nutrition could be beneficial. Hydration should be considered to improve symptoms and prevent cognitive impairment due to dehydration.

Nausea and Vomiting

Nausea and vomiting are among the most common and distressing symptoms in patients with GI cancer. In advanced cancer, more than one cause and multiple pathways trigger nausea and vomiting (NV) [6, 7]. Particularly for patients with cancer, anticancer drugs and opioids used during treatment can cause NV as a side effect [8].

Palliation of NV

In the case of chemical causes of NV, for example, drugs (opioids, antibiotics), cytotoxic toxins (ischemic bowel, infection), and metabolic abnormalities (hypercalcemia), the underlying causes should be managed, and haloperidol can be used as an appropriate first-line antiemetic [9]. Delayed gastric emptying caused by gastroparesis and gastric motility disorders is a common complication of GI malignancies accompanied by NV [10, 11]. Various factors can impair gastric emptying, including tumor progression, hepatomegaly, drugs, infection, metabolic abnormalities, bowel obstruction, intracranial injury, and anxiety [12]. In this case, metoclopramide and domperidone could be considered the treatment of choice. Bowel obstruction can initiate NV, and surgery can be limited in most cases of mechanical obstruction by a cancerous mass. Palliative approaches, including the placement of stents and percutaneous gastrostomies, should not be delayed. Agents for reducing gastric juice including hyoscine butylbromide, glycopyrrolate, H2-blockers, and octreotide can be considered the first line. Haloperidol, cyclizine, and corticosteroids such as dexamethasone can be added. If partial obstruction is suspected, metoclopramide can be attempted [9]. Increased intracranial pressure due to primary and secondary intracerebral tumors, bone metastasis to the skull, intracranial bleeding, and cerebral edema can cause NV with headaches. The treatment of choice is a high-dose corticosteroid (dexamethasone) combined with cyclizine [9].

Ascites and Jaundice

Malignant ascites commonly occurs in GI cancers, with a prevalence of approximately 15% [13]. Ascites increases intra-abdominal pressure causing symptoms including discomfort, nausea, vomiting, edema, dyspepsia, etc. Jaundice is presented by intrahepatic or extrahepatic bile duct obstruction in GI malignancies with liver metastasis [14, 15]. Anorexia, indigestion, and sleep quality can be improved by treating jaundice and relieving pruritus [16, 17].

Palliation of Ascites and Jaundice

Paracentesis and diuretics are the common medical interventions used to palliate ascites. The insertion of percutaneous drainage catheters and drainage of ascites multiple times at regular intervals can relieve symptoms such as abdominal pain, nausea, vomiting, and dyspnea [18]. Peritoneal-venous shunting, radioisotopes, immunotherapy, anti-VEGF, and targeted therapies can be considered; however, further studies are required [19]. Decompression and drainage by surgical or nonsurgical procedures (insertion of metallic or plastic stents, insertion of a percutaneous bile drainage catheter) are required to relieve biliary obstruction followed by relieving jaundice and pruritus symptoms [15]. Intravenous naloxone infusion and oral naltrexone and nalmefene can improve cholestatic pruritus [20]. Mirtazapine, selective serotonin reuptake inhibitors, ondansetron, rifampin, and bile acid-lowering agents such as cholestyramine are widely used to control pruritus caused by jaundice.

Fatigue and Anorexia-Cachexia Syndrome

Cancer-related fatigue is distressing to patients, with a prevalence of 70–100%; however, it is frequently underestimated [21]. For patients with GI cancer, fatigue is commonly associated with a lack of appetite, insomnia, and pain, leading to a decreased overall quality of life [22, 23]. The prevalence of anorexia-cachexia syndrome (ACS) is 25–80% in advanced cancer patients, which is closely associated with patients' prognosis and survival rate [24]. However, this was also underdetected. Thus, early diagnosis and treatment intervention from the initial stages are important.

Palliation of Fatigue and ACS

The possible underlying causes, including metabolic or endocrine abnormalities and anemia, should be screened and treated. Additionally, depression, anxiety, pain, and insomnia should be managed to improve cancer-related fatigue. It is helpful to provide psychotherapy and physiotherapy to reduce fatigue. Dietary education and regular exercise are effective in managing cancer-related fatigue. Pharmacological approach should be considered in patients with severe fatigue. Corticosteroids such as methylprednisolone at a dose of 32 mg/day decrease fatigue [25]. Rapid improvement in fatigue can be expected with megestrol acetate at a dose of 160–480 mg/day [26]. Normal food intake is the best way to increase or maintain energy and protein levels, leading to ACS improvement. Education through professional nutritional counseling helps patients understand nutritional topics, resulting in changes in eating habits. In cases where oral nutritional administrations are difficult, enteral nutrition (EN) or parenteral nutrition (PN) should be considered to treat ACS. A previous study showed that in improving ACS, there was no significant difference between PN and EN, but more infections were observed with PN [27].

Conclusion

As more effective anticancer therapies are available, patients with GI malignancy can survive longer. It has been proven that there are positive associations between palliative care interventions and patients' QOL [28]. Thus, as survival time is extended, palliative care for GI malignancy should be provided to maintain patients' QOL. Early intervention and interdisciplinary-based approaches in palliative care can improve QOL significantly [1, 29]. Therefore, all possible palliative care measures should be considered at all levels of care for patients with GI cancer to avoid unnecessary suffering [30]. Clinicians dealing with GI malignancy should be well-prepared to assess and manage various symptoms related to GI cancer to improve patients' QOL.

References

1. Temel JS, Greer JA, Muzikansky A, Gallagher ER, Admane S, Jackson VA, et al. Early palliative care for patients with metastatic non-small-cell lung cancer. N Engl J Med. 2010;363:733–42.
2. Miller G, Boman J, Shrier I, Gordon PH. Small-bowel obstruction secondary to malignant disease: an 11-year audit. Can J Surg. 2000;43(5):353–8.
3. Baines M, Oliver DJ, Carter RL. Medical management of intestinal obstruction in patients with advanced malignant disease. A clinical and pathological study. Lancet. 1985;2(8462):990–3.
4. Laval G, Marcelin-Benazech B, Guirimand F. Recommendations for bowel obstruction with peritoneal carcinomatosis. J Pain Symptom Manag. 2014;48(1):75–91.
5. Francescutti V, Miller A, Satchidanand Y. Management of bowel obstruction in patients with

stage IV cancer: predictors of outcome after surgery. Ann Surg Oncol. 2013;20(3):707–14.
6. Hardy J, Daly S, McQuade B, Albertsson M, Chimontsi-Kypriou V, Stathopoulos P, et al. A double-blind, randomised, parallel group, multinational, multicentre study comparing a single dose of ondansetron 24 mg p.o. with placebo and metoclopramide 10 mg t.d.s. p.o. in the treatment of opioid-induced nausea and emesis in cancer patients. Support Care Cancer. 2022;10(3):231–6.
7. Kennett A, Hardy J, Shah S, A'Hern R. An open study of methotrimeprazine in the management of nausea and vomiting in patients with advanced cancer. Support Care Cancer. 2005;13(9):715–21.
8. Oosten AW, Oldenmenger WH, Mathijssen RH, van der Rijt CC. A systematic review of prospective studies reporting adverse events of commonly used opioids for cancer related pain: a call for the use of standardized outcome measures. J Pain. 2015;16(10):935–46.
9. Gordon P, Le Grand SB, Walsh D. Nausea and vomiting in advanced cancer. Eur J Pharmacol. 2014;722:187–91.
10. Donthireddy KR, Ailawadhi S, Nasser E, Schiff MD, Nwogu CE, Nava HR, et al. Malignant gastroparesis: pathogenesis and management of an under recognized disorder. J Support Oncol. 2007;5(8):355–63.
11. Davis MP, Walsh D, Lagman R, Yavuzsen T. Early satiety in cancer patients: a common and important but under recognized symptom. Support Care Cancer. 2006;14(7):693–8.
12. Warr DG. Chemotherapy and cancer related nausea and vomiting. Curr Oncol. 2008;15(Suppl 1):4–9.
13. Smith EM, Jayson GC. The current and future management of malignant ascites. Clin Oncol (R Coll Radiol). 2003;15(2):59–72.
14. Boulay BR, Parepally M. Managing malignant biliary obstruction in pancreas cancer: choosing the appropriate strategy. World J Gastroenterol. 2014;20(28):9345–53.
15. Ho CS, Warkentin AE. Evidence based decompression in malignant biliary obstruction. Korean J Radiol. 2012;13(S1):S56–61.
16. Ballinger AB, McHugh M, Catnach SM, Alstead EM, Clark ML. Symptom relief and quality of life after stenting for malignant bile duct obstruction. Gut. 1994;35(4):467–70.
17. Luman W, Cull A, Palmer KR. Quality of life in patients stented for malignant biliary obstructions. Eur J Gastroenterol Hepatol. 1997;9(5):481–4.
18. Fleming ND, Alvarez-Secord A, Von Grueningen V, Miller MJ, Abernetjy AP. Indwelling catheters for the management of refractory malignant ascites: a systematic literature overview and retrospective chart review. J Pain Symptom Manag. 2009;38(3):341–9.
19. Cavazzoni E, Bugiantella W, Graziosi L, Franceschini MS, Donini A. Malignant ascites: pathophysiology and treatment. Int J Clin Oncol. 2013;18(1):1–9.
20. Bergasa NV, Alling DW, Talbot TL, Swain MG, Yurdaydin C, Turner ML, et al. Effects of naloxone infusions in patients with the pruritus of cholestasis. A double-blind, randomized, controlled trial. Ann Intern Med. 1995;123(3):161–7.
21. Franc M, Michalski B, Kuczerawy I, Szuta J, Skrzypulec-Plinta V. Cancer related fatigue syndrome in neoplastic diseases. Prz Menopauzalny. 2014;13(6):352–5.
22. Arndt V, Merx H, Stegmaier C, Ziegler H, Brenner H. Restrictions in QOL in colorectal cancer patients over three years after diagnosis: a population based study. Eur J Cancer. 2006;42(12):1848–57.
23. O'Gorman C, Denieffe S, Gooney M. Literature review: preoperative radiotherapy and rectal cancer impact on acute symptom presentation and QOL. J Clin Nurs. 2013;23(3–4):333–51.
24. Strasser F, Bruera E. Cancer anorexia/cachexia syndrome: epidemiology, pathogenesis, and assessment. In: Ripamonti C, Bruera E, editors. Gastrointestinal symptoms in advanced cancer patients. New York: Oxford University Press; 2002.
25. Popiela T, Lucchi R, Giongo F. Methylprednisolone as palliative therapy for female terminal cancer patients. The Methylprednisolone Female Preterminal Cancer Study Group. Eur J Cancer Clin Oncol. 1989;25(12):1823–9.
26. De Conno F, Martini C, Zecca E, Balzarini A, Venturino P, Groff L, et al. Megestrol acetate for anorexia in patients with far-advanced cancer: a double-blind controlled clinical trial. Eur J Cancer. 1998;34(11):1705–9.
27. Chow R, Bruera E, Chiu L, Chow S, Chiu N, Lam H, et al. Enteral and parenteral nutrition in cancer patients: a systematic review and meta-analysis. Ann Palliat Med. 2016;5(1):30–41.
28. Kavalieratos D, Corbelli J, Zhang DI, Dionne-Odom JN, Ernecoff NC, Hanmer J, et al. Association between palliative care and patient and caregiver outcomes: a systematic review and meta-analysis. JAMA. 2016;316(20):2104–14.
29. Swami M, Case AA. Effective palliative care: what is involved? Oncology (Williston Park). 2018;32(4):180–4.
30. Brennan F. Palliative care as an international human right. J Pain Symptom Manag. 2007;33(5):494–9.

Palliative Care for Gastrointestinal Cancer Patients. I-2. Management of Treatment-Related Adverse Events

Key Points

- Adverse events related to cancer treatment often deteriorate patients' quality of life, leading to poor treatment outcomes.
- Individualized risk assessment of chemotherapy-related adverse events is necessary for appropriate management and prevention.
- Prevention is the best treatment for chemotherapy-related adverse events

Introduction

Antineoplastic drugs, including chemotherapy, are commonly used to treat malignancies, but they often cause adverse events. Adverse events are concerning because they can deteriorate a patient's quality of life, lead to poor treatment compliance, and possibly result in withdrawal from treatment. Thus, the National Cancer Institute Common Terminology Criteria for Adverse Events (NCI CTCAE) [1] has listed, defined, and graded the severity of adverse events associated with cancer treatment. In this chapter, we discuss common treatment-related adverse events and their management.

Eun Joo Bang and Hyuk Soon Choi are the lead authors of this chapter.

Chemotherapy-Induced Nausea and Vomiting

Chemotherapy-induced nausea and vomiting (CINV) can result in dehydration, electrolyte imbalance, and debilitation of the patient's functional ability and performance status [2]. The incidence of CINV is affected by multiple factors, such as the type and dosage of anticancer agents administered. Patients who are young, female, or those with a history of morning sickness and no alcohol history are more vulnerable to CINV [3].

CINV is categorized as acute, delayed, breakthrough, anticipatory, or refractory. Acute-onset CINV develops soon after antineoplastic agents are administered and usually resolves within 24 h. Delayed-onset CINV occurs after 24 h of drug administration and may last for 6–7 days. Delayed nausea is more severe and more difficult to control than acute-onset nausea, even with the proper use of antiemetic agents [4].

Over 90% of patients undergoing high emetogenic chemotherapy will experience vomiting; however, the rate of vomiting can be decreased to 30% with the help of antiemetics [2]. Currently, chemotherapeutic agents are categorized into four groups based on their emetogenic potential: high, moderate, low, and minimal; guidelines for the use of antiemetics are established based on this classification [2, 5, 6] (Table 1).

H. J. Chun et al., *Gastrointestinal Cancer*, https://doi.org/10.1007/978-981-99-0815-8_68

Table 1 Emetogenic potential of anticancer agents commonly used for gastrointestinal and biliary malignancies

Degree of emetogenic agents [2, 5, 6]	Anticancer agents
High risk (>90% of patients experience emesis)	Cisplatin Epirubicin >90 mg/m^2
Moderate risk (30%–90% of patients experience emesis)	Epirubicin ≤90 mg/m^2 Irinotecan Oxaliplatin
Low risk (10%–30% of patients experience emesis)	Capecitabine Docetaxel 5-fluorouracil Gemcitabine Paclitaxel Paclitaxel-albumin
Minimal risk (<10% of patients experience emesis)	Bevacizumab Cetuximab Nivolumab Pembrolizumab Ramucirumab Trastuzumab

Currently, the National Comprehensive Cancer Network (NCCN) guidelines recommend a four-antiemetic regimen for patients receiving chemotherapy with high emetogenic risk. The regimen includes a serotonin (5-HT3) receptor antagonist, neurokinin 1 (NK1) receptor antagonist, dexamethasone, and olanzapine. For patients receiving cancer therapy with moderate emetogenic risk, a three-drug combination including a 5-HT3 receptor antagonist, an NK1 receptor antagonist, and dexamethasone is offered. For patients receiving treatment with low emetogenic risk, single-agent antiemetic regimens are offered, including dexamethasone, metoclopramide, or oral 5 HT3 antagonists [2]. Clinicians should avoid the routine use of antiemetics for patients receiving minimal emetogenic risk therapy.

In addition to pharmacologic interventions, patients can adjust their eating habits to ameliorate nausea and vomiting. Choosing foods that are easy on the stomach, eating small and frequent meals instead of skipping meals, and not drinking abundant amounts of liquids during meals are recommended to ease nausea [7].

The goal of using antiemetics is to prevent CINV, improve the patient's quality of life, and help maintain treatment compliance, with prevention being the best treatment option. It is important to start antiemetic treatment before CINV because it is more difficult to control it after onset. Thus, proper and timely use of prophylactic antiemetic agents, while considering individual risk factors, is necessary.

Febrile Neutropenia

Febrile neutropenia (FN) is defined as an absolute neutrophil count (ANC) of <500 cells/mm^3 or an ANC that is anticipated to decrease to <500 cells/mm^3 within the next 48 hours with an oral temperature of ≥38.3 °C or a temperature of ≥38.3 °C lasting for an hour [8]. FN is the most common cause of relative dose intensity (RDI) reduction and prolonged hospitalization. Patients hospitalized for FN have been reported to have an approximately 10% mortality rate, which increased to 20% in those with multiple comorbidities [9]. Additionally, FN results in compromised outcomes due to treatment delays or dose reduction [10]. Thus, the management and prevention of FN is an important supportive care for cancer patients.

Myeloid growth factors (MGFs), including granulocyte colony-stimulating factor (G-CSF) and granulocyte-macrophage colony-stimulating factor (GM-CSF), are commonly used to prevent FN. Numerous studies have shown that appropriate use of MGFs substantially reduces the incidence and severity of FN, which improves the clinical outcomes of cancer patients [11].

The risk of FN depends on the dose and type of chemotherapy regimen as well as on the patient's individual risk factors. Risk evaluation should be performed before the first and every subsequent treatment cycle; this evaluation should take into consideration the types of disease, treatment regimen, intent, and individual factors. Accordingly, patients with FN are categorized into the high-risk (>20% risk of FN), intermediate-risk (10–20% risk of FN), and low-risk (<10% risk of FN) groups based on the treatment regimen they receive (Table 2) [11]. Patient-specific risk factors are closely associated with the risk of FN and may increase the risk from intermediate to high [12]. The NCCN

Table 2 Chemotherapy regimen for gastrointestinal and biliary malignancies with high and intermediate risk of febrile neutropenia [11]

	Types of cancer	Chemotherapy regimens
High risk of FN (>20%) [11]	Colorectal cancer	FOLFIXIRI (fluorouracil, leucovorin, oxaliplatin, irinotecan)
	Pancreatic cancer	FOLFIRINOX (fluorouracil, leucovorin, irinotecan, oxaliplatin)
Intermediate risk of FN (10–20%) [11]	Colorectal cancer	FOLFOX (fluorouracil, leucovorin, oxaliplatin)
	Esophageal and gastric cancers	Irinotecan/cisplatin
		Epirubicin/cisplatin/5-fluorouracil
		Epirubicin/cisplatin/capecitabine

guidelines provide additional patient-specific risk factors for the development of severe FN; these include age >65 years, history of chemotherapy or radiation therapy, preexisting neutropenia, bone marrow involvement of the cancer, poor performance status, decreased renal or liver function, and immunocompromised state (such as HIV infection) [11]. Patients with the abovementioned risk factors require more cautious surveillance after initiation of anticancer treatment.

Prophylactic use of G-CSF has been shown to decrease the incidence, duration, and severity of FN, along with a reduction in antibiotic use and hospital stay [13]. Primary prophylaxis with G-CSF is recommended for patients with a 20% or higher risk of FN after the first cycle and every subsequent cycle [14]. Patients in the intermediate-risk group (10%–20% risk for FN) are offered G-SCF if they have one or more risk factors; routine use of G-CSF is not recommended for patients in the intermediate-risk group with no risk factors and for patients in the low-risk group with >10% risk of FN [11]. The types and uses of G-CSFs are listed in Table 3 [11].

Filgrastrim, tbo-filgrastim, and pegfilgrastim are all administered subcutaneously. Filgrastim and tbo-filgrastim can be used daily until ANC recovery, whereas pegfilgrastim has a relatively long half-life and is administered only once. Although G-CSFs improve the clinical outcomes of patients with FN, they may cause toxicities. The most common adverse event is bone pain, observed in 10%–30% of patients administered with G-CSF, which can be controlled with nonsteroidal anti-inflammatory drugs (NSAIDs) [11, 15]. Headache, fatigue, and myalgia are also commonly reported adverse events, and acute

Table 3 G-CSF dosage and administration

G-CSFs [11]	Dosage	Delivery schedule
Filgrastim or tbo-filgrastim	5 mcg/kg/day	Start the next day or 3–4 days after completion of chemotherapy until ANC recovers to normal levels
Pegfilgrastim	6 mg	Administer on the day after chemotherapy

respiratory distress syndrome and alveolar hemorrhage can occur in rare cases [16].

To summarize, prophylactic use of G-CSFs can prevent the development of FN and further improve the clinical outcomes of patients undergoing anticancer treatment. Individualized risk assessment of each patient for FN should be performed for appropriate G-CSF use.

Cancer-Related Anemia

Cancer-related anemia (CRA) has various causes, including direct cancer invasion of the bone marrow, treatment-induced anemia, and renal dysfunction. Treatment-induced anemia is associated with chemotherapy agents that suppress hematopoiesis [17]. Other factors, such as nutritional deficiency due to the loss of appetite, can contribute to the development of anemia. An overall decreased production of erythropoietin, increased destruction of RBCs, and spontaneous loss of blood cells by tumor-related bleeding can exacerbate CRA [17]. Additionally, myelosuppressive effects of anticancer agents accumulate through the course of repeated treatment, resulting in anemia aggravation [18]. CRA and fatigue diminish patients' quality of life and may influence clinical outcomes [19]. Anemia is an independent factor associated with a decreased survival rate of cancer patients; thus, management of anemia is an essential supportive care for cancer patients [18].

The NCI CTCAE has defined and graded anemia into five levels according to severity: Grade 1, hemoglobin (Hb) level <10 g/dL; Grade 3, Hb level <8 g/dL requiring urgent transfusion [1]. The NCCN guideline recommends immediate evaluation of anemia if a patient's Hb level becomes equal to or falls below 11 g/dL. The initial evaluation for anemia should include CBC, peripheral blood smear morphology, thorough medical history, and physical examination. Common symptoms of anemia include fatigue, exertional dyspnea, and dizziness [11].

Red blood cell transfusion is the best treatment for symptomatic anemia, and the NCCN guidelines categorize patients with CRA into three groups for appropriate treatment. The first group includes asymptomatic patients with no critical comorbidities, who did not require immediate transfusion. Patients with a high-risk of CRA or those with comorbidities should be considered for RBC transfusion. The last group includes patients with symptomatic anemia, which require immediate transfusion [11].

To prevent CRA aggravation in patients who refuse blood transfusion, physicians should try to minimize blood loss and use erythropoietin-stimulating agents (ESAs) to increase RBC production [20]. The initial and titration doses of ESAs are described in detail in Table 4 [11].

Cancer patients with CRA commonly experience iron deficiency. Iron estimations should be performed when evaluating CRA, and oral or IV iron supplementation is recommended for patients with iron deficiency [11].

Table 4 ESAs dosing for CRA [11]

Initial dose [11]	Response dose	No response dose
Epoetin alfa 150 units/kg 3 times/week	Reduce by 25% if Hb reaches sufficient level	Increase to 300 units/kg 3 times/week
Epoetin alfa 40,000 units/week		Increase to 60,000 units/week
Darbepoetin alfa 2.25 mcg/kg/week	Reduce by 40% if Hb reaches sufficient level	Increase to 4.5 mcg/kg/week

Hb Hemoglobin

Chemotherapy-Induced Peripheral Neuropathy

Chemotherapy-induced peripheral neuropathy (CIPN) is a complicated adverse event of anticancer treatment that reduces the quality of life of patients. However, CIPN is underreported because patients are hesitant about reporting the symptoms to clinicians, and there are no universally accepted assessment methods [21]. Thus, the diagnosis of CIPN is based on patient history, and neurological studies may be helpful.

CIPN has various clinical manifestations, and the peripheral sensory system is the most commonly affected. Usually, the distal parts of the limbs are symmetrically affected. CIPN can occur during or even after termination of chemotherapy [21]. Additionally, the incidence of CIPN usually depends on the chemotherapy agents used and the duration of therapy. Common chemotherapeutic agents that cause CIPN include platinum drugs, taxanes, vinca alkaloids, bortezomib, and thalidomide [22]; the agents used for gastrointestinal cancer are listed in Table 5 [23].

The most definitive treatment for CIPN is the reduction or removal of toxic agents, but it is not easy to cease anticancer treatment. Thus, when CIPN is diagnosed, adjuvant analgesics are used to control neuropathic pain. The adjuvant analgesics include anticonvulsants and antidepressants (Table 6) [24].

Table 5 Chemotherapeutic agents causing chemotherapy-induced peripheral neuropathy, and its clinical features

Chemotherapeutic agents [23]	Clinical features	Incidence
Cisplatin	Distal, symmetric, both upper and lower limbs	30%–40%
Oxaliplatin	Cold-induced dysesthesia in mouth and upper limbs	80%
Paclitaxel	Distal in lower limbs	10%–20%
Docetaxel		

Table 6 Adjuvant analgesics commonly used for chemotherapy-induced peripheral neuropathy

Adjuvant analgesics [24]			Dose
Antidepressants	TCAs	Nortriptyline desipramine	Initial: Low dose Increase every 5–7 days
		Amitriptyline Imipramine	
	SNRIs	Duloxetine	Initial: 20–30 mg daily Increase to 60 mg daily if tolerable
		Venlafaxine	Initial: 37.5 mg daily Increase up to 75–225 mg daily
Anticonvulsants		Gabapentin	Initial: 100–300 mg Increase up to 900–3600 mg daily in divided doses
		Pregabalin	Initial: 75 mg twice a day Increase up to 600 mg

SNRIs Serotonin-norepinephrine reuptake inhibitors

Chemotherapy-Induced Alopecia

Chemotherapy-induced alopecia (CIA), a consequence of the toxic effect of chemotherapy, is a significant adverse event that causes distress in patients undergoing cancer treatment. However, there is no established prevention or treatment guideline. Hair shedding usually begins at 1–3 weeks after the onset of chemotherapy, and the scalp is the area most affected [25]. The incidence and severity of CIA depends on the chemotherapeutic agent used. In particular, alkylating agents, anthracyclines, antibiotics, antimetabolites, vinca alkaloids, and taxanes are known to cause more rapid and severe hair loss than other agents (Table 7) [25, 26].

Hair loss is usually reversible, and hair regrows within 1–3 months after the termination of chemotherapy [26]. Although hair loss can be the most traumatic event of chemotherapy for patients, no definite treatment or prevention guidelines have been established yet. Few studies have shown that scalp cooling alleviates the severity of hair loss by slowing the cellular metabolism in the scalp and decreasing scalp perfusion to reduce the delivery of chemotherapeutic agents [27]. However, other studies have shown that scalp cooling causes discomfort and headache rather than hair loss prevention [25]. Topical minoxidil (2%) therapy was effective in shortening the period of CIA, but it is not recommended for its prevention because minoxidil induces vasodilation, which in turn allows greater exposure of chemotherapeutic agents to the hair follicles [28].

Table 7 Severity and frequency of CIA of chemotherapeutic agents commonly used for gastrointestinal malignancies

	Severity	Frequency
Chemotherapeutic agents [25, 26]	Paclitaxel Docetaxel	>80%
	5-fluorouracil plus leucovorin	10–50%

Clinicians can anticipate CIA; thus, it is best to educate patients about the inevitable hair loss that will occur and support them to be as comfortable as possible with the physical changes.

Conclusion

Although the goal of chemotherapeutic treatment is to alleviate cancer-related burdens of patients, chemotherapy-related adverse events have become a challenge to both clinicians and patients. Thus, it is important to provide proper and best management of the adverse events, which can improve quality of life for patients and further improve treatment outcomes.

References

1. National Cancer Institute. Common Terminology Criteria for Adverse Events (CTCAE) Version 5.0.2017. https://ctep.cancer.gov/protocoldevelopment/electronic_applications/docs/CTCAE_v5_Quick_Reference_8.5x11.pdf. Accessed 5 July 2021.
2. NCCN. Antiemesis (Version1.2021); 2021. https://www.nccn.org/professionals/physician_gls/pdf/antiemesis.pdf. Accessed 5 July 2021.
3. Dranitsaris G, Mazzarello S, Smith S, Vandermeer L, Bouganim N, Clemons M, et al. Measuring the impact of guideline-based antiemetic therapy on nausea and vomiting control in breast cancer patients with multiple risk factors. Support Care Cancer. 2016;24(4):1563–9.
4. Hickok JT, Roscoe JA, Morrow GR, Bole CW, Zhao H, Hoelzer KL, et al. 5-Hydroxytryptamine-receptor antagonists versus prochlorperazine for control of delayed nausea caused by doxorubicin: a URCC CCOP randomised controlled trial. Lancet Oncol. 2005;6(10):765–72.
5. Grunberg SM, Warr D, Gralla RJ, Rapoport BL, Hesketh PJ, Jordan K, et al. Evaluation of new anti-emetic agents and definition of antineoplastic agent emetogenicity—state of the art. Support Care Cancer. 2011;19(Suppl 1):S43–7.
6. Roila F, Herrstedt J, Aapro M, Gralla RJ, Einhorn LH, Ballatori E, et al. Guideline update for MASCC and ESMO in the prevention of chemotherapy- and radiotherapy-induced nausea and vomiting: results of the Perugia consensus conference. Ann Oncol. 2010;21(Suppl 5):v232–43.
7. National Cacner Institue. Eating hints: before, during and after cancer treatment; 2009. https://www.cancer.gov/publications/patient-education/eatinghints.pdf. Accessed 7 July 2021.
8. Freifeld AG, Bow EJ, Sepkowitz KA, Boeckh MJ, Ito JI, Mullen CA, et al. Clinical practice guideline for the use of antimicrobial agents in neutropenic patients with cancer: 2010 update by the infectious diseases society of America. Clin Infect Dis. 2011;52(4):e56–93.
9. Lalami Y, Klastersky J. Impact of chemotherapy-induced neutropenia (CIN) and febrile neutropenia (FN) on cancer treatment outcomes: an overview about well-established and recently emerging clinical data. Crit Rev Oncol Hematol. 2017;120:163–79.
10. Schwenkglenks M, Jackisch C, Constenla M, Kerger JN, Paridaens R, Auerbach L, et al. Neutropenic event risk and impaired chemotherapy delivery in six European audits of breast cancer treatment. Support Care Cancer. 2006;14(9):901–9.
11. NCCN. Hematopoietic Growth Factors (Version 4.); 2021. https://www.nccn.org/professionals/physician_gls/pdf/growthfactors.pdf. Accessed 8 July 2021.
12. Lyman GH, Abella E, Pettengell R. Risk factors for febrile neutropenia among patients with cancer receiving chemotherapy: a systematic review. Crit Rev Oncol Hematol. 2014;90(3):190–9.
13. Crawford J, Ozer H, Stoller R, Johnson D, Lyman G, Tabbara I, et al. Reduction by granulocyte colony-stimulating factor of fever and neutropenia induced by chemotherapy in patients with small-cell lung cancer. N Engl J Med. 1991;325(3):164–70.
14. Smith TJ, Bohlke K, Lyman GH, Carson KR, Crawford J, Cross SJ, et al. Recommendations for the use of WBC growth factors: American Society of Clinical Oncology Clinical Practice Guideline Update. J Clin Oncol. 2015;33(28):3199–212.
15. Kirshner JJ, Heckler CE, Janelsins MC, Dakhil SR, Hopkins JO, Coles C, et al. Prevention of pegfilgrastim-induced bone pain: a phase III double-blind placebo-controlled randomized clinical trial of the university of Rochester cancer center clinical community oncology program research base. J Clin Oncol. 2012;30(16):1974–9.
16. D'Souza A, Jaiyesimi I, Trainor L, Venuturumili P. Granulocyte colony-stimulating factor administration: adverse events. Transfus Med Rev. 2008;22(4):280–90.
17. Gilreath JA, Stenehjem DD, Rodgers GM. Diagnosis and treatment of cancer-related anemia. Am J Hematol. 2014;89(2):203–12.
18. Ludwig H, Van Belle S, Barrett-Lee P, Birgegård G, Bokemeyer C, Gascón P, et al. The European Cancer Anaemia Survey (ECAS): a large, multinational, prospective survey defining the prevalence, incidence, and treatment of anaemia in cancer patients. Eur J Cancer. 2004;40(15):2293–306.
19. Glaspy J. Anemia and fatigue in cancer patients. Cancer. 2001;92(6 Suppl):1719–24.
20. Panico ML, Jenq GY, Brewster UC. When a patient refuses life-saving care: issues raised when treating a Jehovah's Witness. Am J Kidney Dis. 2011;58(4):647–53.
21. Farquhar-Smith P. Chemotherapy-induced neuropathic pain. Curr Opin Support Palliat Care. 2011;5(1):1–7.
22. Kaley TJ, Deangelis LM. Therapy of chemotherapy-induced peripheral neuropathy. Br J Haematol. 2009;145(1):3–14.
23. Windebank AJ, Grisold W. Chemotherapy-induced neuropathy. J Peripher Nerv Syst. 2008;13(1):27–46.
24. NCCN. Adult Cancer Pain (Version 2.2021); 2021. https://www.nccn.org/professionals/physician_gls/pdf/pain.pdf. Accessed 9 Aug 2021.
25. Trüeb RM. Chemotherapy-induced alopecia. Curr Opin Support Palliat Care. 2010;4(4):281–4.
26. Chon SY, Champion RW, Geddes ER, Rashid RM. Chemotherapy-induced alopecia. J Am Acad Dermatol. 2012;67(1):e37–47.
27. Yeager CE, Olsen EA. Treatment of chemotherapy-induced alopecia. Dermatol Ther. 2011;24(4):432–42.
28. Rossi A, Caro G, Fortuna MC, Pigliacelli F, D'Arino A, Carlesimo M, et al. Prevention and treatment of chemotherapy-induced alopecia. Dermatol Pract Concept. 2020;10(3):e2020074.

Mental Health Care for Gastrointestinal Cancer Patients. II-1. Distress and Sleep Disorder Management

Key Points

- Half of cancer patients in Korea experience a significant level of distress during the diagnosis and treatment of cancer.
- Patients should be screened for distress using simple screening tools such as the Distress Thermometer and the NCC Psychological Symptom Inventory.
- Based on a triage system, distress should be managed by various psychological experts, including psychiatrists, clinical psychologists, social workers, and pastoral service providers.

Introduction

The diagnosis and treatment of cancer can affect patients and their families both emotionally and physically. Distress in cancer patients is a multifactorial, unpleasant emotional experience of a psychological, social, and/or spiritual nature that can interfere with the ability to cope effectively with cancer, its physical symptoms, and its treatment [1]. Distress has recently been considered the sixth vital sign in cancer care along with temperature, respiration, heart rate, blood pressure, and pain and should be recognized, monitored, documented, and treated promptly at all stages of the disease and in all settings [2].

Hyun Jung Lee is the lead author of this chapter.

H. J. Chun et al., *Gastrointestinal Cancer*, https://doi.org/10.1007/978-981-99-0815-8_69

Prevalence and Risk Factors

Overall, 35%–52% of patients show a significant level of distress throughout the path of the disease from the time of diagnosis to treatment, the termination of treatment, survivorship or recurrence, and palliation [3, 4]. Similar rates are reported in Korea that the prevalence of psychological distress was 56.5% in cancer patients [5]. In addition to general distress, psychiatric disorders such as depression, anxiety, sleep disorders, and delirium are often accompanied, and patients experience high levels of depression (15%–29%), anxiety (23%), and sleep disorders (30%–50%) [6]. Sleep disorders are also associated with pain, cancer-related fatigue, depression, and anxiety, which, in turn, reduces quality of life [7]. In particular, a recent Korean study found that 30% of patients with advanced gastrointestinal cancer had anxiety and depression [8], which implied the absolute importance of psychiatric intervention in these patients.

The prevalence of distress varies by type and stage of cancer and by patient age, sex, and race [9]. The characteristics associated with psychological distress are listed in detail in the NCCN guidelines [1]. Previous studies identified young age, female sex, poor performance status as predictors of distress. Furthermore, distress could also be affected by primary cancer type so that patients diagnosed with specific cancers of the breast, head and neck, colon, lung, brain, or pancreas particularly experience greater distress.

Meanwhile, distress is a risk factor for non-adherence to cancer treatment [10]. Patients with a high level of distress are more dissatisfied with overall care and experience a poorer quality of life. Untreated distress results in longer hospital stays and higher healthcare care, which may even negatively affect survival [11, 12].

Recognizing the impact of distress on the well-being of cancer patients, the current guidelines recommend screening for distress, identifying its sources, and properly manage distress.

Screening

The NCCN Guidelines for the management of distress in cancer patients were first published in 1999 and the latest update was made in 2021 [13]. Korean guidelines by the Korean Psycho-Oncology Society (KPOS) were developed for our own cancer patients that aimed at the health system in Korea in 2009 [14].

Ideally, patients should be screened for distress at every medical visit as a hallmark of patient-centered care. At a minimum, patients should be screened to determine their level of distress at the initial visit, at appropriate intervals, and as clinically indicated, especially with changes in disease status (e.g., remission, recurrence, progression, and treatment-related complications) [1].

Identification of a patient's psychologic needs is essential to develop a plan to manage these needs. Simple verbal questions can be used to detect distress in cancer patients, for example, "Are you depressed?" or "Have you lost interest?" [15]. However, it might be difficult in practice to identify psychological needs within the limited time of interviews, and patients may be reluctant to reveal their distress. Therefore, a rapid and simple screening method using a self-report questionnaire is critical to assess patients who require psychosocial care and/or referral to psychosocial resources.

The most well-known tool for initial screening is the Distress Thermometer (DT) developed by NCCN (Fig. 1) [1]. The DT and the accompanying problem list are recommended to assess the level of distress and to identify causes of distress. Patients are asked to indicate the number that best describes how much distress they have experienced in the past week, on a scale of 0–10. The DT has been validated in patients with different types of cancer, in different settings, and in different languages, cultures, and countries. Although the DT is not a screening tool for psychiatric disorders, it has also shown concordance with the Hospital Anxiety and Depression Scale and the Depression Anxiety and Stress Scale-21. The Korean version of the DT, NCC Psychological Symptom Inventory (NCCPSI) could be applied

NCCN distress thermometer

Distress is an unpleasant experience of a mental, physical, social, or spiritual nature. It can affect the way you think, feel, or act. Distress may make it harder to cope with having cancer, its symptoms, or its treatment.

Instructions: Please circle the number (0-10) that best describes how much distress you have been experiencing in the past week including today.

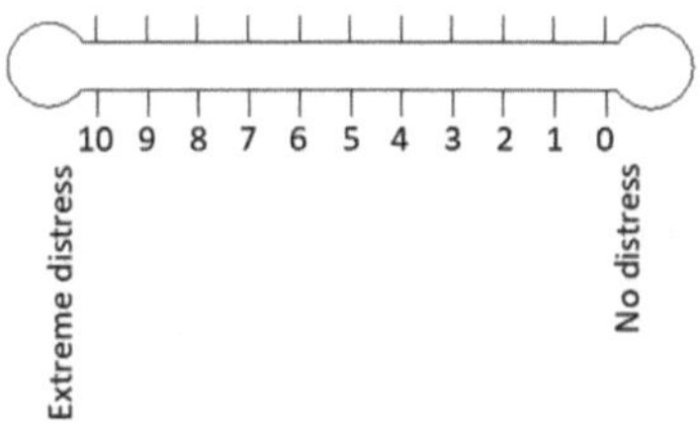

Problem list

Please indicate if any of the following has been a problem for you in the past week including today.
Be sure to check Yes or No each.

Yes	No	Practical problems
☐	☐	Child care
☐	☐	Food
☐	☐	Housing
☐	☐	Insurance/financial
☐	☐	Transportation
☐	☐	Work/school
☐	☐	Treatment decisions

Yes	No	Family problems
☐	☐	Dealing with children
☐	☐	Dealing with partner
☐	☐	Ability to have children
☐	☐	Family health issues

Yes	No	Emotional problems
☐	☐	Depression
☐	☐	Fears
☐	☐	Nervousness
☐	☐	Sadness
☐	☐	Worry
☐	☐	Loss of interest in usual activities

☐ ☐ **Spiritual/Religious Concerns**

Yes	No	Physical problems
☐	☐	Appearance
☐	☐	Bathing/dressing
☐	☐	Breathing
☐	☐	Changes in urination
☐	☐	Constipation
☐	☐	Diarrhea
☐	☐	Eating
☐	☐	Fatigue
☐	☐	Feeling swollen
☐	☐	Fevers
☐	☐	Getting around
☐	☐	Indigestion
☐	☐	Memory/concentration
☐	☐	Mouth sores
☐	☐	Nausea
☐	☐	Nose dry/congested
☐	☐	Pain
☐	☐	Sexual
☐	☐	Skin dry/itchy
☐	☐	Sleep
☐	☐	Substance use
☐	☐	Tingling in hands/feet

Fig. 1 NCCN distress thermometer and problem list (adapted from Saito, et al. [13])

to screen distress and psychosocial needs of patients, which suggested that a cutoff score of 4 was optimal [14].

Management

Distress management algorithms are divided into two levels depending on a triage system (Fig. 2) [14]. For patients with normal to mild distress (DT and/or a NCCPIS score <4), psychological support could be provided by the primary care team (e.g., oncologists and nurses). Referral to psychological experts would be recommended if the patient's distress did not decrease despite appropriate management by primary care providers. However, the guidelines recommend that moderate to severe distress (DT and/or NCCPSI score ≥4) should be managed by various psychological experts, including psychiatrists, clinical psychologists, social workers, and pastoral service providers. In Korean guidelines, symptom-specific management algorithms are suggested according to four major psychiatric symptoms: depression, anxiety, insomnia, and delirium.

For pharmacological interventions, selective serotonin reuptake inhibitors (e.g., fluoxetine, paroxetine) are widely used for depression and anxiety symptoms and tricyclic agents (e.g., desipramine, doxepin) may also be used in patients with depression. Non-pharmacological interventions including psychoeducation, supportive psy-

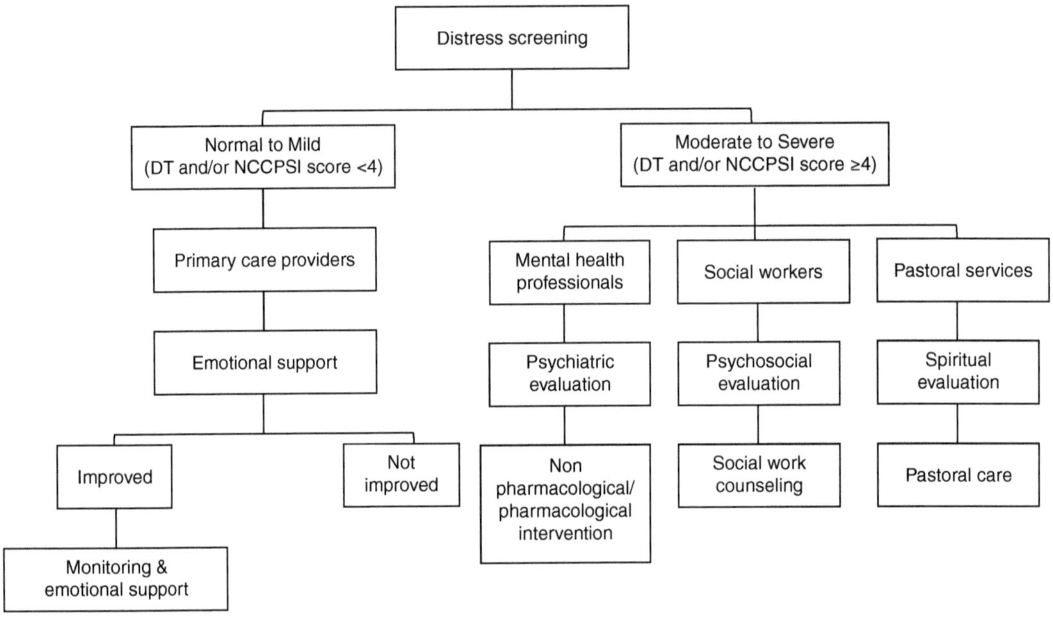

Fig. 2 Distress management algorithm (adapted from Yu, et al. [14]). *DT* Distress thermometer, *NCCPSI* National Cancer Center Psychological Symptom Inventory

chotherapy, cognitive behavioral therapy, and family and couple therapy need to be provided in combination with pharmacological treatments. Management of sleep disorder also consists of pharmacotherapy and psychological and behavior therapy such as sleep hygiene education and cognitive behavior therapy according to its severity.

Conclusion

Patients, families, and treatment teams should be informed that distress management is an integral part of total medical care and includes appropriate information on psychosocial services in the treatment center and in the community. Early evaluation and screening for distress leads to early and timely management of psychologic distress, which finally improves medical management.

References

1. Riba MB, Donovan KA, Andersen B, Braun I, Breitbart WS, Brewer BW, et al. Distress management, version 3.2019, NCCN clinical practice guidelines in oncology. J Natl Compr Cancer Netw. 2019;17:1229–49.
2. Bultz BD, Carlson LE. Emotional distress: the sixth vital sign in cancer care. J Clin Oncol. 2005;23:6440–1.
3. Zabora J, BrintzenhofeSzoc K, Curbow B, Hooker C, Piantadosi S. The prevalence of psychological distress by cancer site. Psychooncology. 2001;10:19–28.
4. Mehnert A, Hartung TJ, Friedrich M, Vehling S, Brähler E, Härter M, et al. One in two cancer patients is significantly distressed: prevalence and indicators of distress. Psychooncology. 2018;27:75–82.
5. Shim EJ, Shin YW, Jeon HJ, Hahm BJ. Distress and its correlates in Korean cancer patients: pilot use of the distress thermometer and the problem list. Psychooncology. 2008;17:548–55.
6. Park Y, Yu ES. Screening, assessment, and Management of Distress in cancer patients. Korean J Clin Psychol. 2019;38:257–74.
7. Büttner-Teleagă A, Kim YT, Osel T, Richter K. Sleep disorders in cancer-a systematic review. Int J Environ Res Public Health. 2021;18
8. Chung J, Ju G, Yang J, Jeong J, Jeong Y, Choi MK, et al. Prevalence of and factors associated with anxiety and depression in Korean patients with newly diagnosed advanced gastrointestinal cancer. Korean J Intern Med. 2018;33:585–94.
9. Ownby KK. Use of the distress thermometer in clinical practice. J Adv Pract Oncol. 2019;10:175–9.
10. Mausbach BT, Schwab RB, Irwin SA. Depression as a predictor of adherence to adjuvant endocrine therapy (AET) in women with breast cancer: a systematic review and meta-analysis. Breast Cancer Res Treat. 2015;152:239–46.

11. Nipp RD, El-Jawahri A, Moran SM, D'Arpino SM, Johnson PC, Lage DE, et al. The relationship between physical and psychological symptoms and health care utilization in hospitalized patients with advanced cancer. Cancer. 2017;123:4720–7.
12. Batty GD, Russ TC, Stamatakis E, Kivimäki M. Psychological distress in relation to site specific cancer mortality: pooling of unpublished data from 16 prospective cohort studies. BMJ. 2017;356:j108.
13. Saito M, Mori A, Irie T, Tanaka M, Morioka M, Ozasa M, et al. Endoscopic follow-up of 3 cases with gastrointestinal tract involvement of mantle cell lymphoma. Intern Med. 2010;49:231–5.
14. Yu ES, Shim EJ, Kim HK, Hahm BJ, Park JH, Kim JH. Development of guidelines for distress management in Korean cancer patients. Psychooncology. 2012;21:541–9.
15. Mitchell AJ. Are one or two simple questions sufficient to detect depression in cancer and palliative care? A Bayesian meta-analysis. Br J Cancer. 2008;98:1934–43.

Mental Health Care for Gastrointestinal Cancer Patients. II-2-1. Advance Care Planning

Key Points

- Interest and awareness of quality of life and well-being in seriously ill patients is increasing rapidly.
- Advance care planning (ACP) helps patients and their loved ones receive medical care according to their values and achieve greater satisfaction and peace of mind.
- It is necessary to discuss the start of ACP as soon as possible through accurate evaluation of patient eligibility and effective communication methods.

Introduction

The remarkable advances of recent medical technology have made it possible to treat diseases that were previously impossible to cure, and the life span of human beings has been extended dramatically. However, many patients still suffer during the course of treatment for incurable diseases, including cancer, while a prolonged treatment period and a serious deterioration in the patient's quality of life can occur in the process of life extension. For this reason, recently, as interest in "natural dying" has increased, awareness of advance care planning (ACP) is increasing. Here, we discuss ACP and end-of-life care in patients with cancer that is difficult to cure.

Definition and Background

Serious illness has been defined as "a condition that carries a high-risk of mortality, negatively affects quality of life and daily function, and/or is burdensome in symptoms, treatments, or caregiver stress" [1]. ACP is a process in which a patient with a serious disease decides on his future care considering personal values, preferences, and the purpose of treatment [2]. This is a comprehensive concept that includes a "living will" and a joint decision-making process in which patients share their opinions about medical care with others, including family and friends, reflecting their own values and wishes, in case the patient is faced with a situation where they cannot make decisions in the future [3]. A living will documents the wishes of an individual prospectively regarding the initiation, withholding, and withdrawal of certain life-sustaining medical interventions. It is effective when the patient becomes incapacitated and has certain medical conditions [4]. Advance Directives (AD) means writing down a legally binding preference or refusal for medical care in case a patient is faced with a situation where he or she cannot make a decision. Physician Orders for Life-Sustaining Treatment (POLST) or Medical Orders for Life-Sustaining Treatment (MOLST) is a process to determine the treatment range and make medical records that has the basic premise of specifying patient preferences as actionable medical orders regarding the emergent situation [3] (Fig. 1).

Dong Kyun Kim is the lead author of this chapter.

H. J. Chun et al., *Gastrointestinal Cancer*, https://doi.org/10.1007/978-981-99-0815-8_70

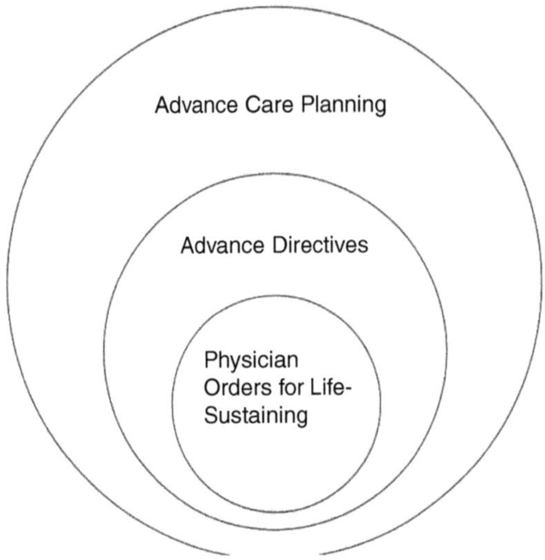

Fig. 1 Categories of advance care planning. Advance Care Planning (ACP), Advance Directives (AD), Physician Orders for Life-Sustaining Treatment (POLST) or Medical Orders for Life-Sustaining Treatment (MOLST) (adapted from Korean Society for Hospice and Palliative Care [3])

The concept of ACP evolved as a result of legal recognition of self-determination and the right of patients or their caregivers to decline life-sustaining treatment or intervention. Starting with the concept of "Do Not Resuscitate (DNR)" and "Living Will" in the 1960s, social interest in the death of dignity increased after the Karen Ann Quinlan and Nancy Cruzan cases that occurred in the United States in 1976 and 1983 over whether or not to stop life-sustaining treatment for patients with vegetative conditions. Since the late 1990s, the legal basis for AD has been prepared and applied in many countries in Europe, Japan, Singapore, and Taiwan [5].

Challenges of Incorporating ACP and Solutions

There are several challenges to overcome to implement an effective ACP [6] (Table 1) (Fig. 2).

1. **Poor illness understanding and uncertainty**

   Remarkable advances in cancer treatment and patient expectations for it can make it difficult for patients or caregivers to accurately understand the actual state or prognosis of the disease and, consequently, make meaningful ACP difficult [7]. An accurate understanding of realistic treatment goals and prognosis is necessary.

2. **Inappropriate timing of ACP**

   If the time for the end-of-life discussion is too late, the patient will not have enough time to reflect on his life and prepare for his last moments and suffer from prolonged aggressive care. ACP can be performed at any time during the clinical course of an incurable disease, but it is recommended to discuss as early as possible [8]. ACP can be started mainly when an advanced stage of cancer is diagnosed, when the medical condition worsens, when inpatient treatment begins to repeat, or when hospitalization is required in a nursing home or hospice ward and can be performed repeatedly. In the case of cancer patients, the timing of the onset of ACP is very important because the trajectory of death tends to show a rapid decline in the last few months after maintaining a relatively normal function [1] (Fig. 3).

3. **Who is a suitable subject for ACP?**

   All patients who are at a time when end-of-life discussion is necessary to discuss and who can fully understand their state of the dis-

Table 1 Barriers to advance care planning conversations [6]

Patient	Not wanting to have a conversation Physical deterioration/phase of illness Emotional unpreparedness
Capacity	Dose the patient have the capacity to make decisions?
Environment	Not conducive to sensitive conversations
Time	Not enough time (rushing a conversation), the wrong time (left it too late)
Health professionals	Lack of training, knowledge, skills, and confidence
Family	Unaware of need to have conversation
Public awareness	Improvements in health care changed the experience of illness, in postponing dying and offering hope and cure

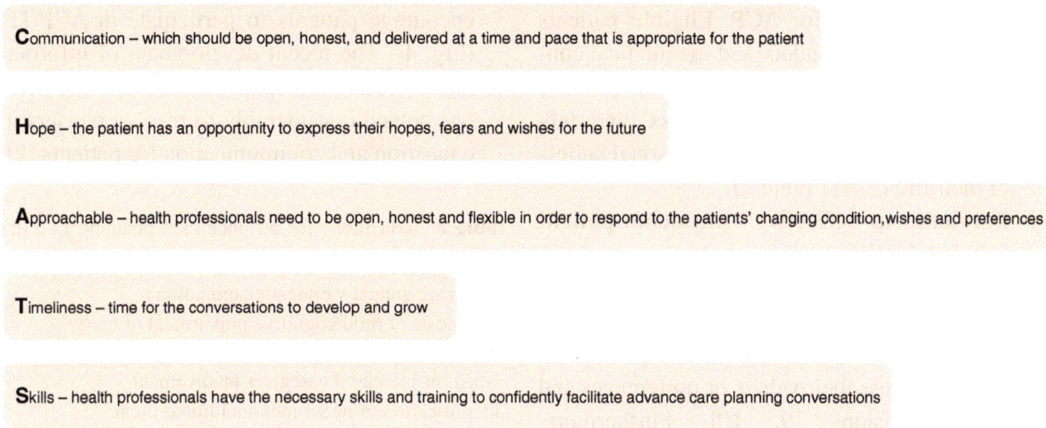

Fig. 2 The key components of facilitating advance care planning considerations (adapted from Merlane, et al. [6])

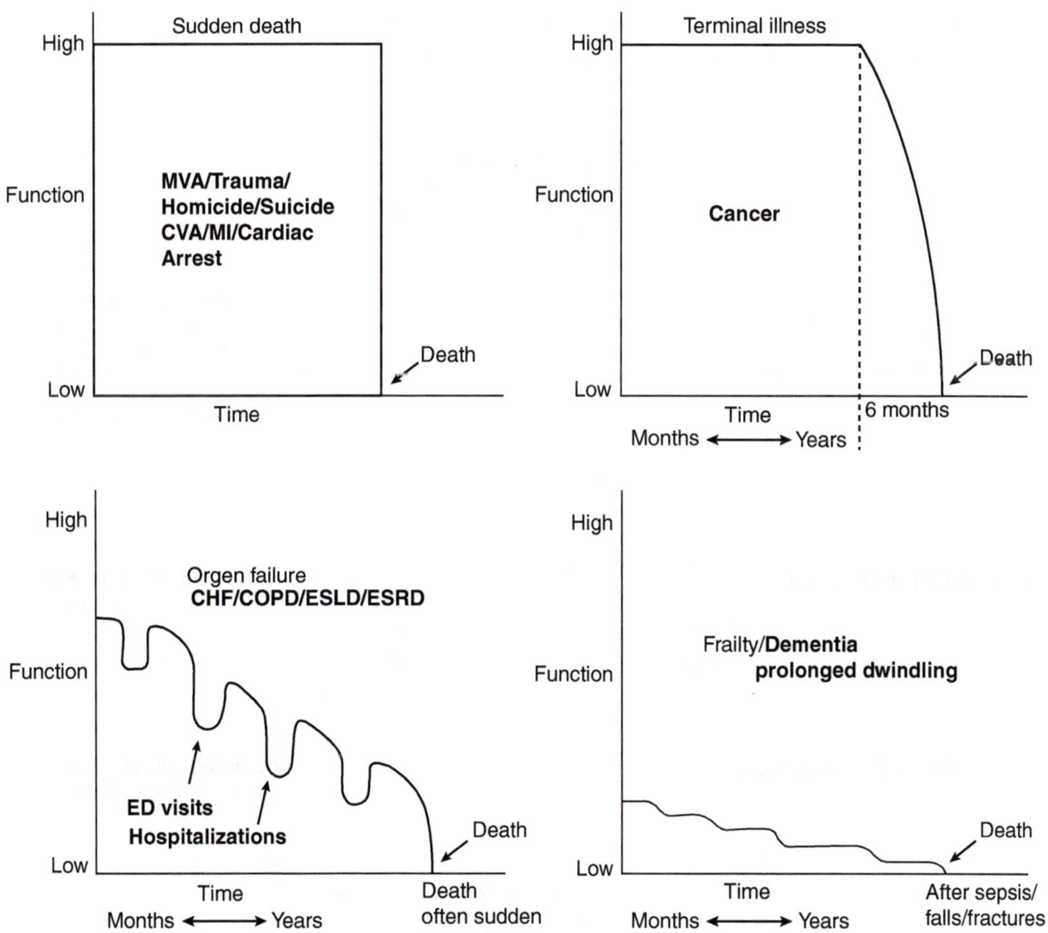

Fig. 3 Proposed trajectories of dying. *CHF* congestive heart failure, *COPD* chronic obstructive pulmonary disease, *CVA* cerebrovascular accident, *ESLD* end-stage liver disease, *ESRD* end-stage renal disease, *MI* myocardial infarction, *MVA* motor vehicle accident [1]

ease are eligible for ACP. Eligible patients should be able to understand the medical condition and possible complications, make choices in the treatment process, and talk about the purpose, values, and personal beliefs of their life [3, 4] (Table 2).

4. **Barriers to effective physician-patient communication**

   Communication barriers such as time constraints, poor health literacy, and misunderstanding can make it difficult for patients to clearly express their values or preferences and make decisions [9, 10]. Furthermore, concluding that end-of-life care discussions negatively affect patients' emotional and mental health and interfere with cancer treatment can also make effective ACP difficult [11, 12]. Accurate and candid information about the prognosis is an essential task that can further encourage patients to participate in ACP [1] (Fig. 4). The recent development of informational video tools and content from web sites has helped considerably to resolve barriers in education and communication for patients [2].

Table 2 Indications for advance care planning in older patients [4]

Medicare annual wellness examination
Diagnosis of mild cognitive impairment or early dementia
Need for increased caregiver involvement
Identification of new functional impairment
Transition to an assisted living facility or nursing home
Post-hospitalization, post-subacute rehabilitation, or other care transition
Change (decline or improvement) in health status
Changes in family or social situation, including death of loved ones

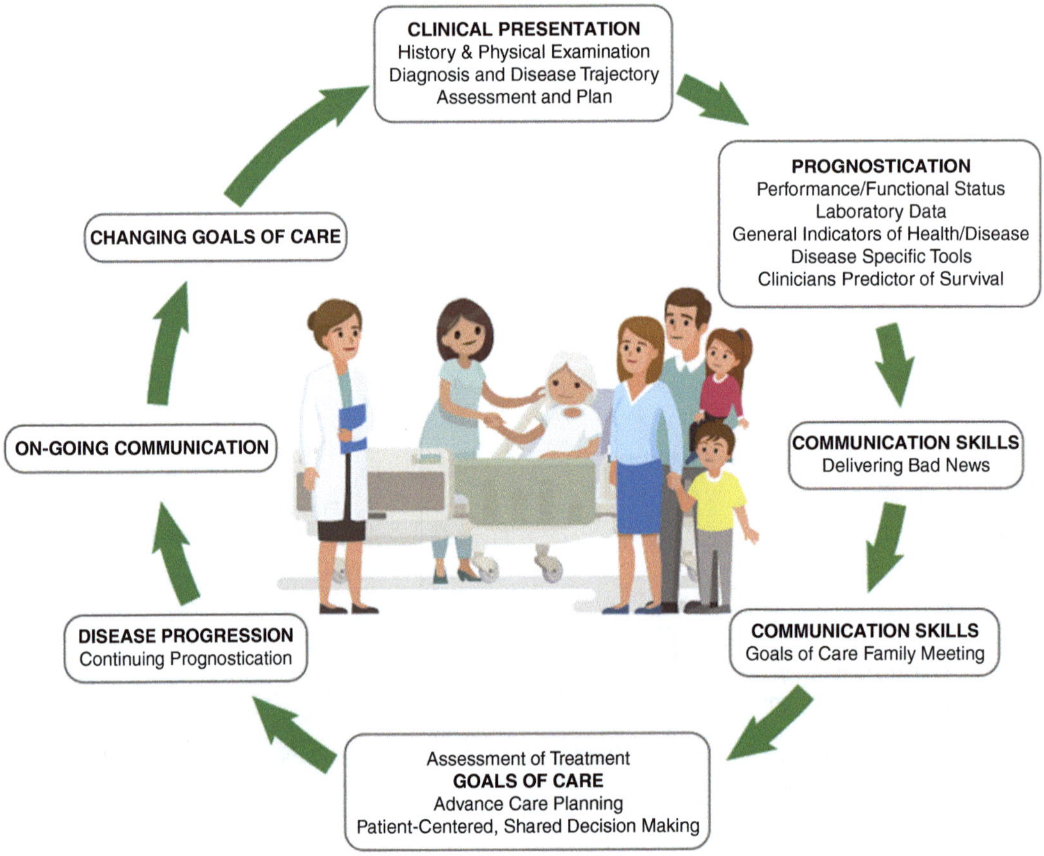

Fig. 4 Palliative goals of care model [1]

5. **Others**

   When the patient or clinician does not feel the need for ACP, when the patient's intention is distorted by different representatives, or when there is no consensus on ACP even within the patient's family members, effective ACP can create difficulties. In addition, decisions made by patients or caregivers may be influenced by cultural, racial, and religious factors.

Conclusion

For patients whose treatment is not expected to be no longer clinically meaningful, the decision to discontinue cancer-focused treatment and start ACP should be actively implemented as soon as possible. It is necessary to accurately evaluate the patient's end-of-life care eligibility, accurately inform patients and their families about the disease state based on effective communication methods, and provide sufficient information about end-of-life care. Although it is necessary to secure more human and institutional resources to meet the growing awareness and demand for the quality of life and well-being of patients, clinicians need to be aware of ACP and institutional protocols are needed.

References

1. Roth AR, Canedo AR. Introduction to hospice and palliative care. Prim Care. 2019;46:287–302.
2. Agarwal R, Epstein AS. Advance care planning and end-of-life decision making for patients with cancer. Semin Oncol Nurs. 2018;34:316–26.
3. Korean Society for Hospice and Palliative Care. Textbook of hospice and palliative care. 1st ed. Cham: Springer International Publishing; 2018.
4. Lum HD, Sudore RL, Bekelman DB. Advance care planning in the elderly. Med Clin N Am. 2015;99:391–403.
5. White ML, Fletcher JC. The patient self-determination act: on balance, more help than hindrance. JAMA. 1991;266:410–2.
6. Merlane H, Armstrong L. Advance care planning. Br J Nurs. 2020;29:96–7.
7. Fried TR, Bradley EH, Towle VR, Allore H. Understanding the treatment preferences of seriously ill patients. N Engl J Med. 2002;346:1061–6.
8. Mack JW, Cronin A, Taback N, Huskamp HA, Keating NL, Malin JL, et al. End-of-life care discussions among patients with advanced cancer: a cohort study. Ann Intern Med. 2012;156:204–10.
9. Christakis NA, Lamont EB. Extent and determinants of error in doctors' prognoses in terminally ill patients: prospective cohort study. BMJ. 2000;320:469–72.
10. Olson DP, Windish DM. Communication discrepancies between physicians and hospitalized patients. Arch Intern Med. 2010;170:1302–7.
11. Mack JW, Smith TJ. Reasons why physicians do not have discussions about poor prognosis, why it matters, and what can be improved. J Clin Oncol. 2012;30:2715–7.
12. Green MJ, Schubart JR, Whitehead MM, Farace E, Lehman E, Levi BH. Advance care planning does not adversely affect hope or anxiety among patients with advanced cancer. J Pain Symptom Manag. 2015;49:1088–96.

Mental Health Care for Gastrointestinal Cancer Patients. II-2-2. Hospice Care

Key Points

- Palliative care is for all patients with serious illness, as well as near-death patients, improving the quality of life of patients and their families.
- Hospice care is a subtype of palliative medicine and focuses on end-of-life care for patients with a life expectancy of less than 6 months.
- Palliative care and hospices also improve caregiver's experiences, including clinicians. It is also important to manage the caregiver's stress and burnout of the clinical personnel.

Introduction

Hospice care, a subtype of palliative care, focuses on end-of-life care for patients with a life expectancy of only a few months. Hospice care aims to control the painful symptoms of terminally ill patients and even help patients and their families with mental, social, and spiritual problems. In recent years, the importance of active application of advance care planning (ACP) and end-of-life care is emerging with increasing interest in life extension and dignity of death. Consequently, an accurate understanding of hospice care and a change in perception are necessary.

Dong Kyun Kim is the lead author of this chapter.

Definition and Background

Hospice is said to be derived from the Latin word "hospes," which means "host and guest." It is medical care to control the painful symptoms of terminally ill patients near the end of life and to help patients and their families with mental, social, and spiritual problems, and also refers to the philosophy of such care [1]. Historically, it is known to have originated during the Crusades in the eleventh century and has been revived in Europe centered in France from the seventeenth century and has been continuously developed in several countries worldwide including in England, Australia, and the United States. The modern hospice movement was started by Dame Cicley Saunders, who emphasized the concept of "total pain" or "total suffering" after World War II. From this hospice movement, the concept of "palliative care" was developed, which is for all patients suffering from life-threatening diseases, and is a broader concept than hospice [2–4] (Figs. 1 and 2). The National Consensus Project for Quality Palliative Care (NCP) defined palliative care as an interdisciplinary care delivery system designed to anticipate, prevent, and manage physical, psychological, social, and spiritual suffering to optimize quality of life for patients, their families, and caregivers. It is emphasized that palliative care is beneficial at any stage of a serious illness. Eight palliative care domains have been suggested [4] (Table 1).

H. J. Chun et al., *Gastrointestinal Cancer*, https://doi.org/10.1007/978-981-99-0815-8_71

Fig. 1 Similarities and differences of hospice and palliative care (adapted from Tatum, et al. [4])

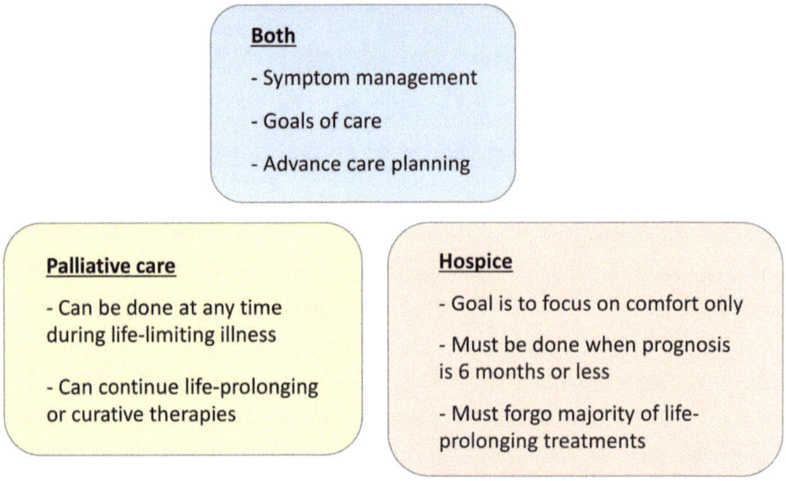

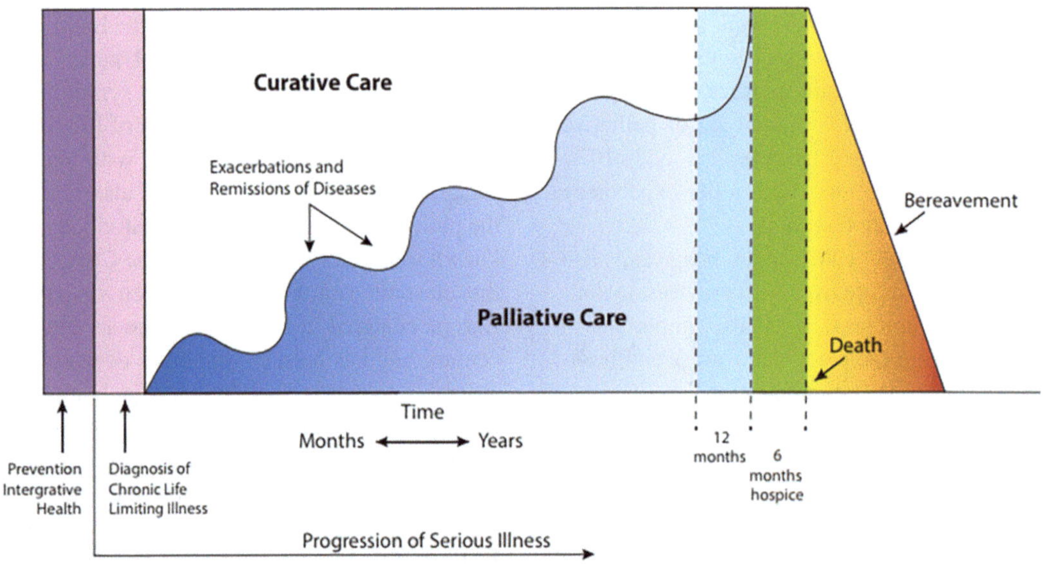

Fig. 2 Continuum of care model for patients with serious illness [2]

Table 1 National Consensus Project for Quality Palliative Care eight domains of palliative care delivery

Structure and process of care	Includes physicians, nurses, social workers, and pharmacists. Defined elements of assessment and care planning
Physical	Assessment and treatment of symptoms and care planning
Psychological and psychiatric	Psychological and psychiatric needed in context of serious illness
Cultural	Cultural context that influences both the way in which care is delivered and the experience of care by patient and family
Spiritual	Spiritual, religious, and existential needs, including the importance of screening for unmet needs
Social	Assessing and addressing patient and family social support needs
End of life	Symptoms and situations that focus on the final days and weeks of life
Ethical and legal	Advance care planning, surrogate decision-making, and regulatory and legal considerations, focusing on ethical imperatives

(adapted from Tatum, et al. [4])

Hospice and Palliative Care for Cancer Patients

Cardiac disease, dementia, and other noncancer diseases account for about 70% of patients admitted to hospice care, but cancer accounts for the largest proportion (about 27.2%) of patients receiving hospice care. Most cases are stage IV cancers that do not respond to treatment or have no further treatment options. However, patients with stage III cancer with complications such as airway obstruction or bleeding, or with Eastern Cooperative Oncology Group (ECOG) performance status 2 or higher, may also be eligible for hospice care [3].

Interdisciplinary Team

Working through the interdisciplinary team (IDT) is important in hospice and palliative care. It improves both the quantity and quality of services and has various advantages such as reduced hospital stay, reduced medical costs, and easier access for patients. IDT teams usually consist of 5–10 people and may include clinicians, nurses, social workers, pharmacists, and chaplains [4] (Fig. 3).

Models of Hospice and Palliative Care

1. **Home care (routine/continuous)**

   Although most terminally ill patients die in medical institutions such as hospitals, many patients tend to prefer to die at home. Although home care has several limitations and difficulties, it can make patients feel comfortable and free, reduce unnecessary visits to medical institutions, and reduce treatment costs. Depending on the patient's condition, the frequency and time of home visits by medical staff can be adjusted.
2. **Hospice and palliative care outpatient clinics**

   Although not yet active, it is a form of multidisciplinary palliative care in which patients and their families can easily see medical personnel or caregivers, identify problems, and establish a care plan.
3. **General inpatient care**

   General inpatient care is the highest level of hospice and palliative care services and is a form of management of symptoms that are difficult to control at home.

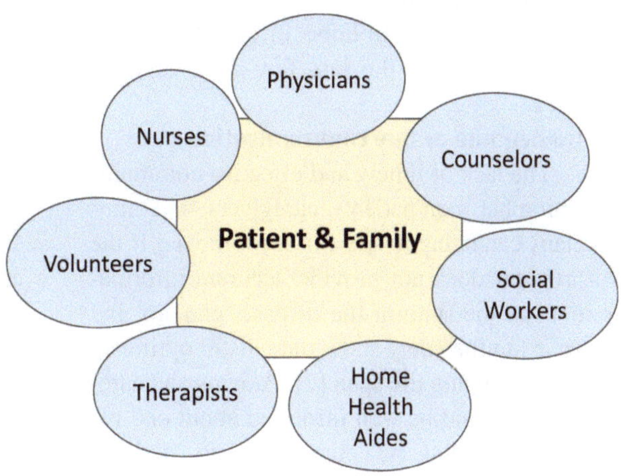

Fig. 3 Interdisciplinary team in hospice and palliative medicine (adapted from Tatum, et al. [4])

Benefits of Hospice Use

In terminal cancer patients, hospice use improves quality of life (QoL) by reducing intensity of pain, burden of symptoms, and psychological stress. It also reduces unnecessary aggressive care and provides an opportunity for patients to die where they want. In addition, the patient's family or caregiver exhibits less severe depressive symptoms, fewer mental health problems, less grief, and a lower risk of death during bereavement periods. In addition, cost savings can be expected by reducing unnecessary hospital visits and acute hospitalizations [5].

Barriers to Hospice Use and Future Directions

Despite the overwhelming benefits, there are several barriers to effective hospice care [5]

1. **Reluctance to acknowledge illness severity**
   Many cancer patients and their families are still reluctant to talk about the prognosis and death of the disease, and there is a tendency to view talking about death as a signal weakness, failure, or character flaw [6].
2. **Misperception about hospice**
   Still, many patients think of hospice as the abandonment of hope, or only for a brief period, such as the last few days of their lives.
3. **Inadequate or late communication**
   The lack of timely and effective communication between patients, caregivers, and clinicians can delay hospice use. Moreover, if the provider does not provide accurate information on the state of the disease, patients and their families may show unrealistic optimism for prolonging life span [7]. Patients and caregivers should be well informed about end-of-life care and be guaranteed to actively participate in the decision-making process. Recently, information related to hospice services can be easily obtained through the web or mobile application. The medical staff working in hospices must continuously apply and improve patient-centered communication skills. For this purpose, evidence-based communication tools such as VitalTalk, REMAP (Reframe, Expect Emotion, Map Future, Align Values, Plan Treatments), SPIKES (Set Up, Assess Perception, Obtain Invitation, Give Knowledge, Address Emotion, Summarize), and SICP (Serious Illness Care Program) can be appropriately used.
4. **Patient eligibility for hospice use**
   Due to the complexity of the nature of cancer and recent advances in cancer treatment, it is becoming increasingly difficult to find an appropriate time for prognostication and hospice initiation for a patient. Most of these problems lead to an overestimation of survival, resulting in patients receiving aggressive disease-focused treatment until their deathbed [8]. Clinicians should continuously assess patient hospice eligibility accurately by using validated prognostic and treatment risk tools [5].
5. **Stress, burnout, compassion fatigue, and compassion satisfaction**
   Hospice and palliative care workers are constantly exposed to problems from work-related stress and threats to the "values of life and death." Burnout and compassion fatigue, which consist of exhaustion, depersonalization, and reduced personal accomplishment, can negatively affect both the health care worker and the patient and family; therefore, appropriate management is required.
6. **Lack of resources**
   Physician participation in hospice care is still relatively low. To improve this, measures such as institutional improvement such as the establishment of a palliative care specialist system and the expansion of insurance coverage or reimbursement for hospice care, and the revitalization of education in academic societies and the education in palliative medicine in medical schools are necessary. Above all, it is essential to provide an efficient hospice service to develop a hospice infrastructure of various types, such as home care and general inpatient care, in a balanced way, and to establish a linkage system between each type of hospice [9].

Conclusion

Hospice and palliative care are not only for improving the quality of life and dying with dignity for terminally ill patients, but also to support the overall difficulties experienced by the patient's family. To provide a higher level of hospice and palliative care, it is important to form an interdisciplinary team with experts in various fields. It is necessary to change the perception of physicians and other medical personnel, improve the medical service system, and secure various resources. Furthermore, it is important to make an effort to relieve the psychological burden of medical personnel engaged in hospice-related work.

References

1. Korean Society for Hospice and Palliative Care. Textbook of hospice and palliative care. 1st ed. New York: Springer International Publishing; 2018.
2. Roth AR, Canedo AR. Introduction to hospice and palliative care. Prim Care. 2019;46:287–302.
3. Greenstein JE, Policzer JS, Shaban ES. Hospice for the primary care physician. Prim Care. 2019;46:303–17.
4. Tatum PE, Mills SS. Hospice and palliative care: an overview. Med Clin N Am. 2020;104:359–73.
5. Patel MN, Nicolla JM, Friedman FAP, Ritz MR, Kamal AH. Hospice use among patients with cancer: trends, barriers, and future directions. JCO Oncol Pract. 2020;16:803–9.
6. Mrig EH, Spencer KL. Political economy of hope as a cultural facet of biomedicalization: a qualitative examination of constraints to hospice utilization among U.S. end-stage cancer patients. Soc Sci Med. 2018;200:107–13.
7. Waldrop DP, Meeker MA, Kutner JS. Is it the difference a day makes? Bereaved caregivers' perceptions of short hospice enrollment. J Pain Symptom Manag. 2016;52:187–95.
8. Gramling R, Gajary-Coots E, Cimino J, Fiscella K, Epstein R, Ladwig S, et al. Palliative care clinician overestimation of survival in advanced cancer: disparities and association with end-of-life care. J Pain Symptom Manag. 2019;57:233–40.
9. Hong YS. Past, present and future of hospice in Korea. J Korean Med Assoc. 2008;51:509–16.

Nutritional Support for Gastrointestinal Cancer Patients. III-1. Management of Anorexia and Weight Loss

Key Points

- During the assessment of anorexia/cachexia, the underlying cancer-related symptoms that lead to anorexia and correctable metabolic abnormalities should be considered.
- For patients with short life expectancy, corticosteroids can be administered to improve appetite and sense of well-being.
- For patients with a longer life expectancy, progesterone analog (megestrol acetate) can be administered considering benefits (appetite stimulation and weight gain) and risks (edema, thromboembolism, and adrenal insufficiency).

Introduction

Anorexia is defined as a loss of appetite leading to a reduction in caloric intake. Anorexia is common in cancer patients especially in the advanced stage leading to weight loss. In addition to reduced oral intake, various factors in cancer patients (e.g., tumor cell metabolism, immune cell-released cytokines and tumor-derived substances) lead to weight loss and changes in body composition. Cancer cachexia is a multifactorial syndrome characterized by an ongoing loss of skeletal muscle mass leading to progressive functional impairment [1]. Several definitions of cachexia have been proposed so far, and in 2011 an international group of researchers published the most recent diagnostic criteria, which is weight loss >5% over the past 6 months (in the absence of simple starvation); or BMI <20 kg/m^2 and any degree of weight loss >2%; or appendicular skeletal muscle index consistent with sarcopenia and any degree of weight loss >2% [1].

Anorexia occurs in 30–60% of cancer patients [2, 3] and adversely affects nutritional status and quality of life. Anorexia and cachexia are also associated with length of survival [4]. Multiple factors contribute to cancer cachexia. These include altered hypothalamic control of appetite, cancer or treatment-related symptoms (e.g., nausea, vomiting, constipation, diarrhea, dumping syndrome, fatigue, pain, depression, dental problem, dysosmia, and dysgeusia), metabolic alteration (increased catabolism and resting energy expenditure). In this chapter, we discuss the current evidence in the management of anorexia and weight loss in cancer patients.

Patient Approach and General Aspects of Treatment

All cancer patients should be evaluated for nutritional status at diagnosis. There are several nutritional screening and assessment tools, including MUST (Malnutrition Universal Screening Tool), SGA (Subjective Global Assessment), and MNA

Seung-Joo Nam is the lead author of this chapter.

H. J. Chun et al., *Gastrointestinal Cancer*, https://doi.org/10.1007/978-981-99-0815-8_72

(Mini Nutritional Assessment). Screening tools aim to identify patients at risk, and assessment tools have been developed to diagnose malnutrition (Table 1) [5, 6]. Figure 1 shows an example of nutritional screening tool (MUST).

Symptoms related to underlying cancer that contribute to loss of appetite (e.g., pain, nausea, constipation, dysgeusia, and depression) and other

Table 1 Examples of nutritional screening and assessment instruments

Screening tools	Assessment tools
Simple screening tool	Mini nutritional assessment
Malnutrition universal screening tool	Subjective global assessment
Malnutrition screening tool	
Nutritional risk index	

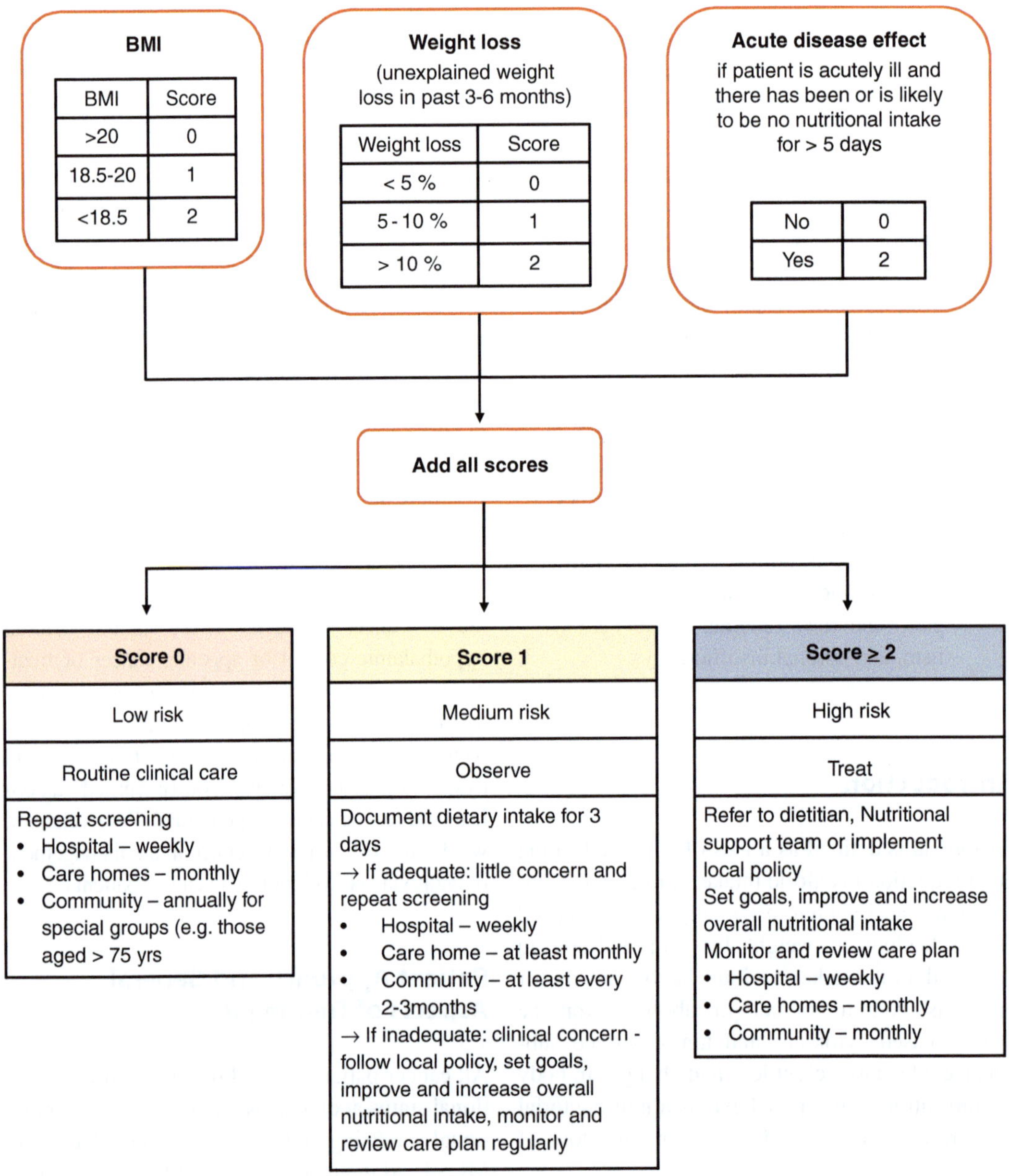

Fig. 1 The "MUST" flowchart. (Adapted from The 'MUST' report by the Malnutrition Advisory Group of the British Association for Parenteral and Enteral Nutrition, 2003)

correctable metabolic abnormalities (e.g., vitamin deficiencies, adrenal insufficiency, hypothyroidism, and hypogonadism) also need to be assessed and addressed [7]. A validated tool, such as the Edmonton Symptom Assessment System (ESAS), can be used to assess subjective symptoms [8].

After multidimensional assessment (nutritional, symptom, laboratory, and body composition), patients and caregivers should be informed about the current nutritional status together with cancer stage, comorbidities, and overall prognosis. Furthermore, treatment goals for anorexia/cachexia are established through discussions. Weight gain itself is not the goal of intervention. Instead, improving quality of life, physical function, or increasing lean body mass would be the desired result. Especially for patients with a short life expectancy (e.g., less than 3 months), the goal of nutritional care needs to change from nutritional evaluations and supply to ensure well-being and comfort [9].

Treatment can be classified into nutritional intervention, pharmacologic treatment, and other intervention [10]. The strength of the evidence for these interventions is low to intermediate. The risk of bias ranged from intermediate to high for most studies. None of the pharmacologic agents are approved by the United States Food and Drug Administration for cancer cachexia. This information is summarized in Table 2.

Table 2 Summary of recommendations for the treatment of cancer cachexia in patients with advanced cancer

Intervention	Strength of recommendation	Strength of the evidence	Benefits	Harms
Nutritional intervention				
Dietary counseling	Moderate in favor	Low	Moderate	Low
Parenteral or enteral nutrition (routine use)	Moderate against	Low	Low	Moderate to high
Omega-3 fatty acids	No recommendation	Low	Low	Low
Vitamins, minerals, and other dietary supplements	No recommendation	Low	Low	Low
Pharmacologic treatments				
Progesterone analogs	Moderate in favor	Intermediate	Moderate	Moderate
Corticosteroids	Moderate in favor	Intermediate	Moderate	Moderate
Anamorelin	No recommendation	Intermediate	Moderate	Low
Olanzapine	No recommendation	Low	Moderate	Low
Androgens	No recommendation	Low	Moderate	Low
Thalidomide	No recommendation	Low	Low	Low
NSAIDs	No recommendation	Low	Low	Low
Cyproheptadine	No recommendation	Low	None	Low
Cannabinoids	Weak against	Low	None	Low
Melatonin	Weak against	Low	None	Low
TNF inhibitors	Moderate against	Intermediate	None	Moderate
Hydrazine sulfate	Strong against	Intermediate	None	Moderate
Other interventions				
Exercise	No recommendation	Low	Unknown	Unknown

(Adopted and modified from Roeland et al. [10])
NSAIDs nonsteroidal anti-inflammatory drugs, *TNF* tumor necrosis factor

Nutritional Intervention

Patients who are able to eat can be advised to have frequent small amounts of high-calorie meals. However, forcing a patient to eat is never recommended. This is usually counterproductive and increases the distress of patients. Instead, caregivers simply need to listen to and support patients in other ways (e.g., giving a massage) [10]. There is limited scientific evidence of artificial nutrition (enteral or parenteral nutrition) in advanced cancer patients [9]. For most advanced cancer patients, providing extra calories does not improve outcomes. The discontinuation of previously initiated artificial nutrition can be considered in patients near the end of life [10].

Although there is inconclusive and limited evidence on the benefit of referring patients to a dietitian for nutritional evaluation and counseling, this can provide patients and caregivers with practical advice on the appropriate feeding (i.e., high-protein, high-calorie, and nutrient-dense food). In addition, counseling can prevent patients and caregivers from following unproven fad diets or treatments. About half of cancer patients have been reported to follow a fad diet or take dietary supplements [11, 12].

Pharmacologic Treatment

The effects of various pharmacologic agents on cancer anorexia/cachexia have been reported. However, there is insufficient evidence to support the use of any pharmacologic agent to manage cancer anorexia/cachexia as summarized in Table 2. Clinicians may choose not to prescribe any medication [10]. Some of the pharmacologic agents listed below have been reported to improve appetite and achieve a modest weight gain.

Progesterone Analogs

Several randomized controlled trials and systematic reviews have shown the efficacy of megesterol acetate in cancer anorexia/cachexia (i.e., appetite and weight gain) [13, 14]. The mechanisms associated with improved appetite are not clearly defined.

The appropriate dosage of megestrol acetate has not been clearly defined. The usual dose reported in previous studies was in the range of 160–1280 mg/day [13–18]. Mortality was reported to be more frequent with higher doses (≥800 mg/day) in a Cochrane systematic review, although this relationship was discarded by the updated version [14, 15]. Megesterol acetate can increase the risk of edema, thromboembolism, and suppression of the hypothalamic pituitary adrenal axis [14, 19, 20].

Corticosteroids

From the first report on the beneficial effect of corticosteroid (improvement of appetite and well-being sense) in advanced cancer-associated anorexia in 1974 [21], several clinical trials have shown similar beneficial effects [2]. The exact mechanism of action in cancer anorexia/cachexia has not been elucidated. The beneficial effect on appetite improvement seems to be similar to progesterone analogs [13]. Methylprednisolone, prednisolone, and dexamethasone all showed beneficial effects [2]. The optimal dose, the duration of treatment, and the time to start have not been clearly defined [2]. Short-term treatment (e.g., 2 weeks) is commonly recommended due to systematic adverse effects and a decrease in efficacy with long-term administration [2]. Therefore, usage is usually limited to the patients with short life expectancy (e.g., weeks to a couple of months).

Other Agents

Various pharmacological interventions have been reported so far, but the evidence supporting these agents is not conclusive or encouraging (Table 2) [10].

Other Interventions

For other interventions such as exercise, no recommendation can be made for the management of cancer anorexia/cachexia [10]. There is insufficient evidence to support or deny the effect of exercise on lean body mass, muscle strength, exercise capacity, and health-related quality of life [22].

Conclusion

Cancer-related anorexia/cachexia is a prevalent and multifactorial syndrome, which warrants systematic screening and management. Generally, the quality of evidence on the management is poor. The potential management options include nutritional support and pharmacological treatments (i.e., progesterone analogs and corticosteroids). The goal of management should focus on improving quality of life instead of providing additional calories. The treatment strategy should be determined through a discussion among the clinician, patients, and caregivers considering current nutritional status, stage of cancer, comorbidities, and overall prognosis.

References

1. Fearon K, Strasser F, Anker SD, Bosaeus I, Bruera E, Fainsinger RL, et al. Definition and classification of cancer cachexia: an international consensus. Lancet Oncol. 2011;12:489–95.
2. Yavuzsen T, Davis MP, Walsh D, LeGrand S, Lagman R. Systematic review of the treatment of cancer-associated anorexia and weight loss. J Clin Oncol. 2005;23:8500–11.
3. Van Lancker A, Velghe A, Van Hecke A, Verbrugghe M, Van Den Noortgate N, Grypdonck M, et al. Prevalence of symptoms in older cancer patients receiving palliative care: a systematic review and meta-analysis. J Pain Symptom Manag. 2014;47:90–104.
4. Reuben DB, Mor V, Hiris J. Clinical symptoms and length of survival in patients with terminal cancer. Arch Intern Med. 1988;148:1586–91.
5. Thomas DR. Nutrition assessment in long-term care. Nutr Clin Pract. 2008;23:383–7.
6. Mueller C, Compher C, Ellen DM, American Society for Parenteral and Enteral Nutrition (A.S.P.E.N.) Board of Directors. A.S.P.E.N. clinical guidelines: nutrition screening, assessment, and intervention in adults. JPEN J Parenter Enteral Nutr. 2011;35:16–24.
7. Del Fabbro E, Hui D, Dalal S, Dev R, Nooruddin ZI, Bruera E. Clinical outcomes and contributors to weight loss in a cancer cachexia clinic. J Palliat Med. 2011;14:1004–8.
8. Watanabe SM, Nekolaichuk C, Beaumont C, Johnson L, Myers J, Strasser F. A multicenter study comparing two numerical versions of the Edmonton symptom assessment system in palliative care patients. J Pain Symptom Manag. 2011;41:456–68.
9. Orrevall Y. Nutritional support at the end of life. Nutrition. 2015;31:615–6.
10. Roeland EJ, Bohlke K, Baracos VE, Bruera E, Del Fabbro E, Dixon S, et al. Management of cancer cachexia: ASCO guideline. J Clin Oncol. 2020;38:2438–53.
11. Luo Q, Asher GN. Use of dietary supplements at a comprehensive cancer center. J Altern Complement Med. 2018;24:981–7.
12. Zick SM, Snyder D, Abrams DI. Pros and cons of dietary strategies popular among cancer patients. Oncology (Williston Park). 2018;32:542–7.
13. Loprinzi CL, Kugler JW, Sloan JA, Mailliard JA, Krook JE, Wilwerding MB, et al. Randomized comparison of megestrol acetate versus dexamethasone versus fluoxymesterone for the treatment of cancer anorexia/cachexia. J Clin Oncol. 1999;17:3299–306.
14. Ruiz Garcia V, Lopez-Briz E, Carbonell Sanchis R, Gonzalvez Perales JL, Bort-Marti S. Megestrol acetate for treatment of anorexia–cachexia syndrome. Cochrane Database Syst Rev. 2013;3:CD004310.
15. Ruiz-Garcia V, Lopez-Briz E, Carbonell-Sanchis R, Bort-Marti S, Gonzalvez-Perales JL. Megestrol acetate for cachexia–anorexia syndrome. A systematic review. J Cachexia Sarcopenia Muscle. 2018;9:444–52.
16. Bruera E, Ernst S, Hagen N, Spachynski K, Belzile M, Hanson J, et al. Effectiveness of megestrol acetate in patients with advanced cancer: a randomized, double-blind, crossover study. Cancer Prev Control. 1998;2:74–8.
17. Loprinzi CL, Michalak JC, Schaid DJ, Mailliard JA, Athmann LM, Goldberg RM, et al. Phase III evaluation of four doses of megestrol acetate as therapy for patients with cancer anorexia and/or cachexia. J Clin Oncol. 1993;11:762–7.
18. Vadell C, Segui MA, Gimenez-Arnau JM, Morales S, Cirera L, Bestit I, et al. Anticachectic efficacy of megestrol acetate at different doses and versus placebo in patients with neoplastic cachexia. Am J Clin Oncol. 1998;21:347–51.

19. Leinung MC, Liporace R, Miller CH. Induction of adrenal suppression by megestrol acetate in patients with AIDS. Ann Intern Med. 1995;122:843–5.
20. Dev R, Del Fabbro E, Bruera E. Association between megestrol acetate treatment and symptomatic adrenal insufficiency with hypogonadism in male patients with cancer. Cancer. 2007;110:1173–7.
21. Moertel CG, Schutt AJ, Reitemeier RJ, Hahn RG. Corticosteroid therapy of preterminal gastrointestinal cancer. Cancer. 1974;33:1607–9.
22. Grande AJ, Silva V, Sawaris Neto L, Teixeira Basmage JP, Peccin MS, Maddocks M. Exercise for cancer cachexia in adults. Cochrane Database Syst Rev. 2021;3:CD010804.

Nutritional Support for Gastrointestinal Cancer Patients. III-2. Food and Nutritional Treatment

Key Points

- Eating plenty of whole grains, vegetables, and fruits will reduce the risk of gastrointestinal (GI) cancer.
- Dairy products and fish/marine omega-3 fatty acids may decrease the risk of colorectal cancer.
- Avoid alcohol, processed meat, and foods high in salt to prevent GI cancer.
- Consumption of raw freshwater fish should be avoided to prevent *Clonorchis sinensis* infection.

Introduction

Food and nutrition have long been identified as possibly important determinants of cancer risk. Several studies demonstrate significant associations between dietary habits and cancer risk [1, 2]. According to the 2018 World Cancer Research Fund/American Institute for Cancer Research (WCRF/AICR), various dietary habits are recommended for cancer prevention [3]. The main points of the recommendations on food and nutrition are: (1) eat foods rich in wholegrains, vegetables, fruits, and beans; (2) limit consumption of fast food and other processed foods high in sugars, starches, or fat; (3) limit consumption of red and processed meat; (4) limit consumption of sugar sweetened drinks; (5) limit alcohol consumption. Gastrointestinal cancer (including esophageal cancer, stomach cancer, colorectal cancer, and pancreatic biliary cancer) is an important disease with an incidence and mortality of more than one-fourth of all cancers worldwide [4]. The digestive system is the boundary to which food is directly exposed, and therefore it is considered to be more affected by the risk of cancer according to the dietary habit. In this chapter, we will look at the food and nutrition that affect each gastrointestinal cancer.

Su Young Kim is the lead author of this chapter.

Esophageal Cancer

According to recent meta-analysis, comparing the highest-intake participants with the lowest-intake participants of whole grains, the intake of whole grains was inversely related to esophageal cancer (relative risk [RR]: 0.54, 95% confidence interval [CI]: 0.44–0.67, $P < 0.001$) [5]. Similarly, research results were also published showing an inverse correlation with the risk of Barrett's esophagus and esophageal cancer as dietary fiber intake increased [6]. The potential mechanism by which whole grain and dietary fiber have a prevention effect on esophageal cancer is estimated as follows. It helps in weight control, neutralization of carcinogens contained in food, improves esophageal dysbiosis and gastroesophageal reflux [6–8]. Other meta-analysis studies demonstrate that veg-

H. J. Chun et al., *Gastrointestinal Cancer*, https://doi.org/10.1007/978-981-99-0815-8_73

etable and fruit intake may significantly reduce the risk of esophageal squamous cell carcinoma [9].

Alcohol intake is well known to increase the risk of esophageal cancer. Papadimitriou et al. showed that alcohol intake is highly associated with increased esophageal cancer (relative risk [RR] 1.33, 95% CI, 1.22–1.46) [10]. Compared to other organs, the cancerous effect on the esophagus was the greatest. Consumption of hot drinks and food also increases the risk of esophageal cancer [11]. These substances are believed to increase the risk of cancer because they cause long-term damage to cells in the esophagus.

Stomach Cancer

The incidence of stomach cancer is high in Eastern Asians, especially in the Korean and Japanese population. Kim et al. provided interesting results from a meta-analysis to determine whether the intake of fresh and pickled vegetables exert different effects on the risk of stomach cancer in Korean and Japanese populations [12]. In one study, a high intake of fresh vegetables was significantly associated with a decreased risk of stomach cancer (odds ratio [OR]: 0.62, 95% CI, 0.46–0.85); however, a high intake of pickled vegetables was significantly associated with an increased risk of stomach cancer (OR: 1.28, 95% CI, 1.06–1.53) [12]. Another two meta-analysis studies reported that increased consumption of *Allium* vegetables or fruits reduced the risk of stomach cancer [13, 14]. In particular, a higher intake of *Allium* vegetables reduced the risk of stomach cancer (OR: 0.54, 95% CI, 0.43–0.65) [13]. This study suggested that an increase in *Allium* vegetable intake of 20 g/day was associated with a statistically significant 9% decrease in the risk of stomach cancer. Because of flavonols and organosulfur compounds of *Allium* vegetables, they have anticancer effects [13, 15]. Recent meta-analysis showed that when comparing the highest-intake persons with the lowest-intake persons for whole grains, the intake of whole grains was inversely related to stomach cancer (RR = 0.64, 95% CI, 0.53–0.79) [5]. In addition to vegetables, allium, and whole grains, research results have reported that garlic supplementation reduces the risk of stomach cancer. The protective effect on stomach cancer mortality related to garlic supplementation was discovered only in people who did not drink alcohol [16].

High salt intake is well known as a risk factor for stomach cancer. According to the meta-analysis of prospective studies, dietary salt intake was directly associated with the risk of stomach cancer (high and moderately high versus low salt intake were associated with an increased risk of stomach cancer [RR: 1.68, $p = 0.005$ and RR: 1.41, $p = 0.032$]) [17]. Similarly, pickled food and salted fish were also found to increase the risk of stomach cancer (RR: 1.27, 95% CI, 1.09–1.49 and RR: 1.24, 95% CI, 1.03–1.50, respectively) [17]. Salt directly damages the gastric mucosa, produces N-nitroso, which is a known carcinogen, and promotes *Helicobacter pylori* infection [17]. Therefore, most experts recommend keeping sodium intake below 2.4 g per day.

Colorectal Cancer

The relationship between diet and colorectal cancer development has been a topic of great interest for more than a century. More studies have been conducted on the relationship between colorectal cancer and diet (including nutrients) than any other type of cancer.

Fiber and whole grains have long been known as a food that can reduce the risk of colorectal cancer. The mechanism for it has been known as follows. Fiber and whole grains induced bulking of the fecal stream and binding of fecal carcinogens; therefore, it limited the exposure of the epithelial mucosa to fecal carcinogens [18]. Furthermore, these diets increased the number of bacteria producing short-chain fatty acids (SCFA). Elevated SCFA facilitates the control of T-reg cells, leading to a strengthened intestinal barrier and reduced inflammation [19]. When 10 g of fiber and 50 g of wholegrains were consumed daily, the risk of colorectal cancer is decreased by 10% and 17%, respectively [20]. Another study showed very interesting findings. The study was carried out using two large prospective cohorts and demonstrated that higher fiber intake decreased colorectal cancer-specific mortality (HR: 0.54, 95% CI, 0.35–0.85) [21].

Dairy products have a high calcium and vitamin D content. Ionized calcium decreased tumor-promoting free fatty acids and bile acids in the colon [22]. Additionally, vitamin D has an anticancer effect that induces antiproliferation and apoptosis of cancer cells and suppresses tumor angiogenesis [23]. A meta-analysis showed that the summary RR for colorectal cancer was 0.83 (95% CI, 0.78–0.88) per 400 g/day of total dairy product [24].

Fruits and vegetables have several potential anticarcinogenic and antimutagenic compounds, including carotenoids, flavonoids, folate, multivitamins, minerals, and antioxidants [25]. Therefore, these compounds have multiple anticancer effects such as antioxidant activity, protection against DNA damage, modulation of DNA methylation, and promotion of apoptosis [25]. A weak but statistically significant inverse association between fruit and vegetable intake and colorectal cancer risk was observed (RR for high fruit and vegetable intake was 0.92 [95% CI, 0.86–0.99] for risk of colorectal cancer) [26].

Fish/marine omega-3 fatty acid decreased the inflammatory mediator and myeloid-derived suppressor cells, so it increased the antitumor immune response [27]. In the EPIC cohort study (European prospective investigation into cancer and nutrition) cohort study, including 521,324 participants, the intake of fish (HR: 0.88, 95% CI, 0.80–0.96) and long-chain polyunsaturated fatty acids n-3 (HR: 0.86, 95% CI, 0.78–0.95) were associated with a reduced risk of colorectal cancer [28]. In addition, another study indicated that colorectal cancer death was 35% decreased in higher omega-3 polyunsaturated fatty acid intake group compared to lower omega-3 polyunsaturated fatty acid intake group [29].

Alcohol includes acetaldehyde among its contaminants, and it acts as a carcinogen for colon cells. Alcohol increased reactive oxygen species, and also induced the cell penetration of dietary carcinogens [30]. A recent study demonstrated that alcohol intake is associated with an increased risk of colorectal cancer (15% increase in colorectal cancer with two drinks/day) [30, 31]. Red and processed meat is carcinogenic to humans. These foods produce heterocyclic amines while cooking at high temperatures, and they also produce N-nitroso compounds that induce mutations in DNA [32, 33]. Therefore, red and processed meat are associated with an increased risk of colorectal cancer (12–21% increase in colorectal cancer with a higher meat intake) [31]. The risk of colorectal cancer has been reported to increase by 17% when 100 g of red meat is consumed per day and when 50 g of processed meat are consumed per day, the risk of colorectal cancer increases by 18% [34, 35].

Pancreatobiliary Cancer

There are few studies showing which food and nutrition is helpful in the prevention of pancreatic cancer. According to a meta-analysis, a high intake of whole grains was associated with a reduced risk of pancreatic cancer (24% lower risk of pancreatic cancer when comparing the highest vs. lowest intake group) [36]. A recent large Danish cohort study also demonstrated that total whole grain intake was associated with a 75% lower incidence of pancreatic cancer per serving 50 g/day [37]. There are also reports that eating vegetables and fruits rich in lycopene may reduce the risk of pancreatic cancer [38]. As with other cancers, excessive consumption of alcohol and red/processed meat is known to increase the risk of pancreatic cancer [39]. Aune et al. showed interesting results that a positive association of pancreatic cancer was observed with fructose intake, summary RR = 1.22 (95% CI, 1.08–1.37) per 25 g/day [40].

Clonorchis sinensis causes mechanical damage and inflammation of the biliary tract after the diffusion of parasites in the human body after infection, and cholangiocarcinoma may occur due to genetic damage to epithelial cells in the biliary tract [41]. *Clonorchis sinensis* infection derives mostly from consumption of raw freshwater fish, and it is reported that the incidence and mortality of cholangiocarcinoma are also high in areas with high *Clonorchis sinensis* infection rates [42, 43]. Therefore, the most important way to prevent cholangiocarcinoma is not to eat raw freshwater fish.

Conclusions

Most studies investigating the effects of food and nutrition on cancer are observational studies. Therefore, caution is required in its interpretation and, in some studies, results that are different from those commonly known may be drawn. The cause of cancer is not fragmentary and is often determined by various factors, so the effect of food and nutrition is limited. However, the influence of dietary habits, which are consistently recommended in most studies so far, is meaningful. It is recommended to eat abundant whole grains, vegetables, and fruits and to eat limited processed meat, high-calorie foods, foods high in salt and alcohol for a healthy lifestyle and cancer prevention.

References

1. Lippman SM, Hawk ET. Cancer prevention: from 1727 to milestones of the past 100 years. Cancer Res. 2009;69:5269–84.
2. Norat T, Scoccianti C, Boutron-Ruault MC, Anderson A, Berrino F, Cecchini M, et al. European code against cancer 4th edition: diet and cancer. Cancer Epidemiol. 2015;39(Suppl 1):S56–66.
3. Malcomson FC, Willis ND, McCallum I, Xie L, Kelly S, Bradburn DM, et al. Adherence to the World Cancer Research Fund/American Institute for Cancer Research cancer prevention recommendations and WNT-pathway-related markers of bowel cancer risk. Br J Nutr. 2019;122:509–17.
4. Bray F, Ferlay J, Soerjomataram I, Siegel RL, Torre LA, Jemal A. Global cancer statistics 2018: GLOBOCAN estimates of incidence and mortality worldwide for 36 cancers in 185 countries. CA Cancer J Clin. 2018;68:394–424.
5. Zhang XF, Wang XK, Tang YJ, Guan XX, Guo Y, Fan JM, et al. Association of whole grains intake and the risk of digestive tract cancer: a systematic review and meta-analysis. Nutr J. 2020;19:52.
6. Sun L, Zhang Z, Xu J, Xu G, Liu X. Dietary fiber intake reduces risk for Barrett's esophagus and esophageal cancer. Crit Rev Food Sci Nutr. 2017;57:2749–57.
7. Tullio V, Gasperi V, Catani MV, Savini I. The impact of whole grain intake on gastrointestinal tumors: a focus on colorectal, gastric, and esophageal cancers. Nutrients. 2020;13:81.
8. Kubo A, Block G, Quesenberry CP Jr, Buffler P, Corley DA. Effects of dietary fiber, fats, and meat intakes on the risk of Barrett's esophagus. Nutr Cancer. 2009;61:607–16.
9. Liu J, Wang J, Leng Y, Lv C. Intake of fruit and vegetables and risk of esophageal squamous cell carcinoma: a meta-analysis of observational studies. Int J Cancer. 2013;133:473–85.
10. Papadimitriou N, Markozannes G, Kanellopoulou A, Critselis E, Alhardan S, Karafousia V, et al. An umbrella review of the evidence associating diet and cancer risk at 11 anatomical sites. Nat Commun. 2021;12:4579.
11. Andrici J, Eslick GD. Hot food and beverage consumption and the risk of esophageal cancer: a meta-analysis. Am J Prev Med. 2015;49:952–60.
12. Kim HJ, Lim SY, Lee JS, Park S, Shin A, Choi BY, et al. Fresh and pickled vegetable consumption and gastric cancer in Japanese and Korean populations: a meta-analysis of observational studies. Cancer Sci. 2010;101:508–16.
13. Zhou Y, Zhuang W, Hu W, Liu GJ, Wu TX, Wu XT. Consumption of large amounts of allium vegetables reduces risk for gastric cancer in a meta-analysis. Gastroenterology. 2011;141:80–9.
14. Wang Q, Chen Y, Wang X, Gong G, Li G, Li C. Consumption of fruit, but not vegetables, may reduce risk of gastric cancer: results from a meta-analysis of cohort studies. Eur J Cancer. 2014;50:1498–509.
15. Block E. The chemistry of garlic and onions. Sci Am. 1985;252:114–9.
16. Guo Y, Li ZX, Zhang JY, Ma JL, Zhang L, Zhang Y, et al. Association between lifestyle factors, vitamin and garlic supplementation, and gastric cancer outcomes: a secondary analysis of a randomized clinical trial. JAMA Netw Open. 2020;3:e206628.
17. D'Elia L, Rossi G, Ippolito R, Cappuccio FP, Strazzullo P. Habitual salt intake and risk of gastric cancer: a meta-analysis of prospective studies. Clin Nutr. 2012;31:489–98.
18. Ocvirk S, Wilson AS, Appolonia CN, Thomas TK, O'Keefe SJD. Fiber, fat, and colorectal cancer: new insight into modifiable dietary risk factors. Curr Gastroenterol Rep. 2019;21:62.
19. Desai MS, Seekatz AM, Koropatkin NM, Kamada N, Hickey CA, Wolter M, et al. A dietary fiber-deprived gut microbiota degrades the colonic mucus barrier and enhances pathogen susceptibility. Cell. 2016;167:1339–53.e21.
20. Aune D, Chan DS, Lau R, Vieira R, Greenwood DC, Kampman E, et al. Dietary fibre, whole grains, and risk of colorectal cancer: systematic review and dose-response meta-analysis of prospective studies. BMJ. 2011;343:d6617.
21. Song M, Wu K, Meyerhardt JA, Ogino S, Wang M, Fuchs CS, et al. Fiber intake and survival after colorectal cancer diagnosis. JAMA Oncol. 2018;4:71–9.

22. Norat T, Riboli E. Dairy products and colorectal cancer. A review of possible mechanisms and epidemiological evidence. Eur J Clin Nutr. 2003;57:1–17.
23. Feldman D, Krishnan AV, Swami S, Giovannucci E, Feldman BJ. The role of vitamin D in reducing cancer risk and progression. Nat Rev Cancer. 2014;14:342–57.
24. Aune D, Lau R, Chan DSM, Vieira R, Greenwood DC, Kampman E, et al. Dairy products and colorectal cancer risk: a systematic review and meta-analysis of cohort studies. Ann Oncol. 2012;23:37–45.
25. Zhang S, Jia Z, Yan Z, Yang J. Consumption of fruits and vegetables and risk of renal cell carcinoma: a meta-analysis of observational studies. Oncotarget. 2017;8:27892–903.
26. Aune D, Lau R, Chan DS, Vieira R, Greenwood DC, Kampman E, et al. Nonlinear reduction in risk for colorectal cancer by fruit and vegetable intake based on meta-analysis of prospective studies. Gastroenterology. 2011;141:106–18.
27. Song M, Chan AT. The potential role of exercise and nutrition in harnessing the immune system to improve colorectal cancer survival. Gastroenterology. 2018;155:596–600.
28. Aglago EK, Huybrechts I, Murphy N, Casagrande C, Nicolas G, Pischon T, et al. Consumption of fish and long-chain n-3 polyunsaturated fatty acids is associated with reduced risk of colorectal cancer in a large European cohort. Clin Gastroenterol Hepatol. 2020;18:654–66.e6.
29. Song M, Zhang X, Meyerhardt JA, Giovannucci EL, Ogino S, Fuchs CS, et al. Marine omega-3 polyunsaturated fatty acid intake and survival after colorectal cancer diagnosis. Gut. 2017;66:1790–6.
30. Vingeliene S, Chan DSM, Vieira AR, Polemiti E, Stevens C, Abar L, et al. An update of the WCRF/AICR systematic literature review and meta-analysis on dietary and anthropometric factors and esophageal cancer risk. Ann Oncol. 2017;28:2409–19.
31. Chapelle N, Martel M, Toes-Zoutendijk E, Barkun AN, Bardou M. Recent advances in clinical practice: colorectal cancer chemoprevention in the average-risk population. Gut. 2020;69:2244–55.
32. Bouvard V, Loomis D, Guyton KZ, Grosse Y, Ghissassi FE, Benbrahim-Tallaa L, et al. Carcinogenicity of consumption of red and processed meat. Lancet Oncol. 2015;16:1599–600.
33. Ferrucci LM, Sinha R, Huang WY, Berndt SI, Katki HA, Schoen RE, et al. Meat consumption and the risk of incident distal colon and rectal adenoma. Br J Cancer. 2012;106:608–16.
34. Carr PR, Walter V, Brenner H, Hoffmeister M. Meat subtypes and their association with colorectal cancer: systematic review and meta-analysis. Int J Cancer. 2016;138:293–302.
35. Chan DS, Lau R, Aune D, Vieira R, Greenwood DC, Kampman E, et al. Red and processed meat and colorectal cancer incidence: meta-analysis of prospective studies. PLoS One. 2011;6:e20456.
36. Lei Q, Zheng H, Bi J, Wang X, Jiang T, Gao X, et al. Whole grain intake reduces pancreatic cancer risk: a meta-analysis of observational studies. Medicine (Baltimore). 2016;95:e2747.
37. Schacht SR, Olsen A, Dragsted LO, Overvad K, Tjonneland A, Kyro C. Whole-grain intake and pancreatic cancer risk-the Danish, diet, cancer and health cohort. J Nutr. 2021;151:666–74.
38. Nkondjock A, Ghadirian P, Johnson KC, Krewski D, Canadian Cancer Registries Epidemiology Research Group. Dietary intake of lycopene is associated with reduced pancreatic cancer risk. J Nutr. 2005;135:592–7.
39. Lucas AL, Bravi F, Boffetta P, Polesel J, Serraino D, La Vecchia C, et al. Adherence to World Cancer Research Fund/American Institute for Cancer Research recommendations and pancreatic cancer risk. Cancer Epidemiol. 2016;40:15–21.
40. Aune D, Chan DSM, Vieira AR, Navarro Rosenblatt DA, Vieira R, Greenwood DC, et al. Dietary fructose, carbohydrates, glycemic indices and pancreatic cancer risk: a systematic review and meta-analysis of cohort studies. Ann Oncol. 2012;23:2536–46.
41. Rim HJ. Clonorchiasis: an update. J Helminthol. 2005;79:269–81.
42. Qian MB, Utzinger J, Keiser J, Zhou XN. Clonorchiasis. Lancet. 2016;387:800–10.
43. Kim TS, Pak JH, Kim JB, Bahk YY. *Clonorchis sinensis*, an oriental liver fluke, as a human biological agent of cholangiocarcinoma: a brief review. BMB Rep. 2016;49:590–7.

Survivorship Care for Gastrointestinal Cancer. IV-1. Daily Life After Cancer Treatment

Key Points

- In cancer survivors, impairment in the ability to complete activities of daily living (ADL) have been reported in up to a third of patients. The most frequently impaired ADLs include deficits in personal hygiene, walking, and transfers.
- It is recommended that the overall volume of weekly physical activity should be at least 150–300 min of moderate-intensity activity or 75 min of vigorous-intensity activity, which should be tailored to the individual survivor's abilities and preferences.
- Sexual dysfunction is common among cancer survivors. It can be managed by reducing risk and some medications.

Introduction

Most cancer survivors can return to normal life after the completion of cancer treatment. Most enjoy a high quality of life without cancer-related symptoms [1]. However, some survivors experience physical or psychosocial problems caused by cancer and its treatment [2]. The problems range from mild to severe, depending on the circumstances of the patients. Therefore, cancer survivors should lead their daily lives, considering various individual factors.

Activities of Daily Living

According to the National Cancer Institute, basic activities of daily living (ADLs) include eating, dressing, getting into or out of a bed or chair, taking a bath or shower, and using the toilet. Instrumental ADLs are related to independent living and include preparing meals, managing money, shopping, doing housework, and using a telephone [3]. In cancer survivors, impairments in the ability to complete ADLs have been reported with up to a third [4]. The most frequently impaired ADLs include deficits in personal hygiene, walking, and transfers.

First, clinicians should assess the ability of cancer survivors to perform routine and desired ADLs. In particular, screening for ADL impairments is more needed for older cancer survivors. Self-assessed health status and physical and functional limitations or an ADL index may be helpful [5, 6]. An earlier study suggested that a higher proportion of older cancer survivors used mobility devices (e.g., canes, walkers, wheelchairs, and scooters) than adults without a history of cancer [7]. Therefore, older survivors may require special attention to functional changes in survivorship. Caregivers should always pay attention to impaired ADLs of older survivors and consider the use of equipment or rehabilitation interventions.

Dong Kee Jang is the lead author of this chapter.

H. J. Chun et al., *Gastrointestinal Cancer*, https://doi.org/10.1007/978-981-99-0815-8_74

Physical Activity

Studies have shown that a higher level of physical activity after cancer diagnosis is associated with a reduced risk of cancer recurrence and improved overall mortality among multiple cancer survivor groups, including breast, colorectal, prostate, and ovarian cancer [8]. Among colorectal cancer survivors, studies have found an inverse association between physical activity after diagnosis and recurrence, colorectal cancer-specific mortality, or overall mortality [9, 10].

Aerobic and resistance exercises consistently show benefits for cardiopulmonary function, muscle strength, body composition, and body balance. In many studies, exercise improves quality of life, fatigue, psychosocial distress, depression, and self-esteem. The following recommendations are helpful for cancer survivors [8]. However, the recommendations for physical activity and exercise should be tailored to the abilities and preferences of the individual survivor.

- The overall volume of weekly activity should be at least 150–300 min of moderate-intensity activity (can talk, but not sing) activity or 75 min of vigorous intensity activity (can say a few words without stopping to catch a breath) activity or equivalent combination spread over the course of the week.
- Two to three sessions per week of strength/resistance training that include major muscle groups.
- Stretch the major muscle groups at least 2 days a week on the days that the other exercises are performed.

Sexual Activity

Sexual dysfunction is common among cancer survivors and can cause increased distress and have a significant negative impact on quality of life. However, sexual function is often not discussed with survivors. Among gastrointestinal cancers, rectal cancer is commonly associated with sexual dysfunction, which usually comes from surgery or radiotherapy. The prevalence of sexual dysfunction in women ranges from 65 to 80% after rectal cancer surgery [11]. Risk factors for sexual dysfunction after rectal cancer surgery are older age, tumors below peritoneal reflection, receiving preoperative radiotherapy [12]. Patients with such risk factors should be informed of sexual dysfunctions in preoperative consultations.

Erectile dysfunction is very common in male cancer survivors. Anticancer treatment used in various cancers has the potential to damage blood vessels, leading to a reduction in blood circulation to the penis or damage to the autonomic nervous system. The prevalence of erectile dysfunction in men survivors of colorectal cancer has been reported to range from 45 to 75% [13–15]. Treatment of male sexual dysfunction may require a multidimensional treatment plan. Referrals to specialists should be made if appropriate and available. Treatment for male sexual dysfunction includes modification of risk factors such as smoking cessation, weight loss, increased physical activity, and avoiding excess alcohol consumption. Treatment with oral phosphodiesterase type 5 inhibitors (PDE5i) has been shown to improve symptoms of erectile dysfunction [16]. Importantly, PDE5i are contraindicated in patients taking oral nitrates. Survivors receiving PDE5i should be monitored periodically for efficacy and side effects. If total morning testosterone is <300 ng/dL, then hypogonadism is diagnosed, and testosterone therapy may be helpful for male sexual dysfunction.

Female sexual dysfunction is often multifactorial in nature. Therefore, referrals to specialists should be considered if possible. Treatments depend on the type of sexual dysfunction and may include some medications, as well as pelvic physical therapy and integrative therapies such as yoga and meditation. Various oral medications (androgens, flibanserin, bremelanotide, bupropion, and buspirone) for low sex drive can be used, and topical agents (vaginal estrogen and vaginal androgens) for vaginal dryness can be used.

Work Life

Symptoms affecting work life may wax and wane with a survivor's treatments or disease status, especially if they are living with the consequences of cancer treatment. Employment helps protect survivors from financial burden, which may be the main reason they work even if they are not fully recovered. The psychosocial effects derived from work may include a sense of purpose, emotional well-being, identity link, improved quality of life, connection to others, and distraction [17]. Therefore, survivors should be offered information to help them understand their probable ability to work, consider their financial situation, and discuss potential work accommodations with their employers. If survivors have any work barriers, contributing symptoms including fatigue, pain, cognitive dysfunction, anxiety, depression, distress, and musculoskeletal issues should be treated.

Conclusion

For survivors who have finished their cancer treatment, it is much more important to return to normal life than to manage cancer after treatment. Survivors should be accurately assessed for their ability to carry out work and daily life and should have the opportunity to live accordingly. Clinicians should always be aware that even survivors are not completely healed. Clinicians should pay attention not only to the behavioral aspects of cancer survivors, but also to helping them through medications so that they can return to their normal lives.

References

1. Zucca AC, Boyes AW, Linden W, Girgis A. All's well that ends well? Quality of life and physical symptom clusters in long-term cancer survivors across cancer types. J Pain Symptom Manag. 2012;43(4):720–31.
2. Beckjord EB, Reynolds KA, van Londen GJ, Burns R, Singh R, Arvey SR, et al. Population-level trends in posttreatment cancer survivors' concerns and associated receipt of care: results from the 2006 and 2010 LIVESTRONG surveys. J Psychosoc Oncol. 2014;32(2):125–51.
3. NCI dictionaries—ADL: National Cancer Institute. https://www.cancer.gov/publications/dictionaries/cancer-terms/def/adl.
4. Neo J, Fettes L, Gao W, Higginson IJ, Maddocks M. Disability in activities of daily living among adults with cancer: a systematic review and meta-analysis. Cancer Treat Rev. 2017;61:94–106.
5. Chavan PP, Kedia SK, Mzayek F, Ahn S, Yu X. Impact of self-assessed health status and physical and functional limitations on healthcare use and mortality among older cancer survivors in US. Aging Clin Exp Res. 2021;33(6):1539–47.
6. Blackwood J, Karczewski H, Huang MH, Pfalzer L. Katz activities of daily living disability in older cancer survivors by age, stage, and cancer type. J Cancer Surviv. 2020;14(6):769–78.
7. Bluethmann SM, Flores E, Campbell G, Klepin HD. Mobility device use and mobility disability in U.S. Medicare beneficiaries with and without cancer history. J Am Geriatr Soc. 2020;68(12):2872–80.
8. Rock CL, Doyle C, Demark-Wahnefried W, Meyerhardt J, Courneya KS, Schwartz AL, et al. Nutrition and physical activity guidelines for cancer survivors. CA Cancer J Clin. 2012;62(4):243–74.
9. Meyerhardt JA, Heseltine D, Niedzwiecki D, Hollis D, Saltz LB, Mayer RJ, et al. Impact of physical activity on cancer recurrence and survival in patients with stage III colon cancer: findings from CALGB 89803. J Clin Oncol. 2006;24(22):3535–41.
10. Meyerhardt JA, Giovannucci EL, Ogino S, Kirkner GJ, Chan AT, Willett W, et al. Physical activity and male colorectal cancer survival. Arch Intern Med. 2009;169(22):2102–8.
11. Celentano V, Cohen R, Warusavitarne J, Faiz O, Chand M. Sexual dysfunction following rectal cancer surgery. Int J Color Dis. 2017;32(11):1523–30.
12. Li K, He X, Tong S, Zheng Y. Risk factors for sexual dysfunction after rectal cancer surgery in 948 consecutive patients: a prospective cohort study. Eur J Surg Oncol. 2021;47(8):2087–92.
13. Hendren SK, O'Connor BI, Liu M, Asano T, Cohen Z, Swallow CJ, et al. Prevalence of male and female sexual dysfunction is high following surgery for rectal cancer. Ann Surg. 2005;242(2):212–23.
14. Donovan KA, Thompson LM, Hoffe SE. Sexual function in colorectal cancer survivors. Cancer Control. 2010;17(1):44–51.
15. Ellis R, Smith A, Wilson S, Warmington S, Ismail T. The prevalence of erectile dysfunction in post-treatment colorectal cancer patients and their interests in seeking treatment: a cross-sectional survey in the west-midlands. J Sex Med. 2010;7(4 Pt 1):1488–96.
16. Fink HA, Mac Donald R, Rutks IR, Nelson DB, Wilt TJ. Sildenafil for male erectile dysfunction: a systematic review and meta-analysis. Arch Intern Med. 2002;162(12):1349–60.
17. National Comprehensive Cancer Network. Survivorship (Version 2.2021). https://www.nccn.org/professionals/physician_gls/pdf/survivorship.pdf.

Survivorship Care for Gastrointestinal Cancer. IV-2. Diseases Other Than Cancer

Key Points

- Cancer survivors have a higher prevalence of disease, including cardiovascular disease, compared to healthy people.
- The incidence rate of secondary primary malignancy is high, so regular checkups are necessary.
- In cancer survivors, the immune system is compromised and requires vaccinations, but not attenuated live vaccines.

Introduction

The incidence of cancer is gradually increasing, and at the same time, the proportion of cancer survivors is also increasing. A study from England showed that the overall survival increased and reported a recent 10-year survival rate of about 50% in 2010–2011 [1]. In South Korea, statistics showed that the incidence of cancer was 475.3 per 100,000 individuals in 2018. If people live to life expectancy (83 years in south Korea), the chance of being diagnosed with cancer is 37.4% and the 10-year survival rate was about 67% in 2009–2013 [2]. There were 15.5 million cancer survivors in 2016 and there will be 26.1 million in the United States by 2040 [3]. Cancer survivors are increasing every year, so it is time to pay greater attention to their health problems. In 2005, a publication of the landmark report of cancer survivors, "From Cancer Patients to Cancer Survivor: Lost in Transition" by the Institute of Medicine [4] introduced ten recommendations to strengthen care in the growing population of survivors transitioning to life after treatment (Table 1).

Cancer survivors are more likely to be affected by cancer-related treatments as well as other diseases. In a population-based study, 58% of cancer survivors had one or more comorbidities, a higher proportion than 45% of noncancer patients [5]. This may be because cancer patients had many comorbidities or comorbidity occurred by cancer treatment. The 5-year relative survival for stomach cancer is 77% and for colorectal cancer is 74.3% in South Korea [2]. If cancer was cured at the early stages, survivors are more likely to die from comorbidities rather than from cancer. A large cohort study enrolled 15,808 patients with 2025 cancer survivors. Comorbidity and degree of deterioration of health were investigated at 2-year intervals by interview. Cancer survivors have a significantly high percentage of comorbidities (34.02% vs 25.12%, $p < 0.001$) and a higher incidence of fair/poor status (34.79% vs 25.55%, $p < 0.001$) and a high 2-year mortality rate (7.6% vs 3.2%, $p < 0.001$) [6]. In a study comparing colorectal cancer patients by comorbidity, it was found that the survival rate in cancer, although early in the stage, also differed greatly depending on comorbidity. The hazard

Sung Yong Han is the lead author of this chapter.

H. J. Chun et al., *Gastrointestinal Cancer*, https://doi.org/10.1007/978-981-99-0815-8_75

Table 1 Institute of Medicine recommendations for cancer survivors (November 2005) [4]

Recommendations
1. Health-care providers, patient advocates, and other stakeholders should work to raise awareness of the needs of cancer survivors, establish cancer survivorship as a distinct phase of cancer care, and act to ensure the delivery of appropriate survivorship care
2. Patients that complete primary treatment should be provided with a comprehensive care summary and follow-up plan that is clearly and effectively explained. This survivorship care plan should be written by the principal provider(s) who coordinated oncology treatment. This service should be reimbursed by third-party payors of health care
3. Health-care providers should use systematically developed, evidence-based clinical practice guidelines, assessment tools, and screening instruments to help identify and manage late effects of cancer and its treatment. Existing guidelines should be refined and new evidence-based guidelines should be developed through public- and private-sector efforts
4. Quality of survivorship care measures should be developed through public/private partnerships and quality assurance programs implemented by health systems to monitor and improve the care that all survivors receive
5. The Centers for Medicare and Medicaid Services, National Cancer Institute, Agency for Healthcare Research and Quality, the Department of Veterans Affairs, and other qualified organizations should support demonstration programs to test models of coordinated, interdisciplinary survivorship care in diverse communities and across systems of care
6. Congress should support Centers for Disease Control and Prevention, other collaborating institutions, and the states in developing comprehensive cancer control plans that include consideration of survivorship care and promoting the implementation, evaluation, and refinement of existing state cancer control plans
7. The National Cancer Institute, professional associations, and voluntary organizations should expand and coordinate their efforts to provide educational opportunities to health-care providers to equip them to address the health care and quality-of-life issues that face cancer survivors
8. Employers, legal advocates, health-care providers, sponsors of support services, and government agencies should act to eliminate discrimination and minimize adverse effects of cancer on employment while supporting cancer survivors with short-term and long-term limitations in ability to work
9. Federal and state policymakers should act to ensure that all cancer survivors have access to adequate and affordable health insurance. Insurers and payors of health care should recognize survivorship care as an essential part of cancer care and design benefits, payment policies, and reimbursement mechanisms to facilitate coverage for evidence-based aspects of care
10. The National Cancer Institute, Centers for Disease Control and Prevention, Agency for Healthcare Research and Quality, Centers for Medicare and Medicaid Services, the Department of Veterans Affairs, private voluntary organizations, such as the American Cancer Society, and private health insurers and plans should increase their support of survivorship research and expand mechanisms for its conduct. New research initiatives that are focused on cancer patient follow-up are urgently needed to guide effective survivorship care

ratio was about 3.54 (95% CI, 2.88–4.35) when comparing the group with the lowest comorbidity and the group with the highest [7].

Major Cardiovascular Complication

Hypertension

In a large observational cohort study that included 17,712 patients, the most common comorbidity in cancer patients is hypertension, its prevalence is 38% [8]. Hypertension was considered a possible risk factor for malignancies such as renal cell carcinoma and others. Cancer survivors have increased cardiovascular risk, and anticancer therapy could increase the risk of hypertension. Antivascular endothelial growth factor (VEGF) and tyrosine kinase inhibitors are associated with hypertension. One-half of patients with anti-VEGF therapy have hypertension [9]. In addition, treatment with a tyrosine kinase inhibitor increased the risk of hypertension by approximately 3.78-fold (95% CI, 3.15–4.54) [10]. Erythropoietin stimulating agents [11] and corticosteroid [12] that were used as adjuvant therapies are related to hypertension. In addition, paraneoplastic syndrome or hormonal change due to malignancy were influenced by the risk of hypertension.

Diabetes

Thirteen population-based cohort studies were included in a meta-analysis that showed the risk ratio for the development of diabetes in cancer survivors was 1.39 (95% CI, 1.29–1.5, $p < 0.001$) compared to noncancer patients, particularly colorectal cancer among GI malignancies. This risk was higher with shorter duration of cancer survivor duration (<1 year) [13]. The mechanism of increasing the incidence of diabetes is unknown. Endocrine disruption due to corticosteroid treatment, which is used in adjuvant therapy for chemotherapy, may have been responsible or the chemotherapy agents itself [14, 15]. In addition, cancer cachexia was also associated with diabetes due to the release of cytokines such as interleukin 6 or tumor necrosis factor alpha [16].

Stroke

A meta-analysis showed that the relative risk of stroke in cancer survivors was 1.66 (95% CI, 1.35–2.04, $p < 0.001$) compared to noncancer patients, despite the heterogeneity of the type of cancer. Moreover, shorter cancer survivor duration was associated with a higher risk, immediately after cancer is cured [17]. Endothelial toxicity or coagulopathy caused by cancer or chemotherapy and the appearance of infections known to be related to stroke, such as *Chlamydia pneumoniae* and *Mycoplasma pneumoniae* due to reduced immunity, are thought to be the cause of stroke [18, 19].

Secondary Primary Malignancy

Cancers have several common risk factors, such as alcohol, tobacco, and old age. Treatment of cancer, such as chemotherapy and radiotherapy, could be a risk factor for secondary primary malignancy [20]. Therefore, a patient who has developed cancer could develop secondary primary malignancies. A large-scale study on gastric cancer that enrolled 33,720 patients revealed that the 7-year probability of developing secondary primary malignancy was 11% higher than general populations [21]. In another study on survivors with multiple myeloma survivors, the cumulative incidence of secondary primary malignancy was 14% over 25 years [22]. Thus, cancer survivors should perform routine checkups for other malignancies in addition to the primary cancer that has been treated.

Vaccination in Cancer Survivors

For cancer survivors, vaccination is important because the immune system has been weakened by cancer treatment. The Centers for Disease Control and Prevention (CDC) recommended vaccination schedule for immunocompromised individuals. Vaccines could be divided into live attenuated vaccines, inactivated vaccines, DNA or RNA vaccines. Above all, live attenuated vaccines such as varicella or measles, mumps, and rubella (MMR) should not be used to vaccinate cancer survivors. Influenza vaccination is recommended annually; however, an intranasal version of influenza vaccine is not recommended because it contains live viruses, so it is not safe for people with compromised immunity. Recombinant zoster vaccine should be administered to individuals 50 years of age and over, but a live attenuated vaccine is not recommended. Other vaccines such as pneumococcal, meningococcal, hepatitis A, hepatitis B, and tetanus, diphtheria, pertussis (Td/Tdap) are recommended in cancer survivors as scheduled.

Cancer Survivorship in Gastrointestinal Malignancy

Cancer survivor studies were conducted on cancer with many survivors, cancer with high 5-year survival rates, and high prevalence. Examples include breast cancer, prostate cancer, and colorectal cancer. In 2015, American Cancer Society published the Colorectal Cancer Survivorship Care Guideline. The guideline included not only cancer follow-up, but also complications and comorbidities that occur after cancer treatment [23]. The American Cancer Society provides cancer survivorship of each cancer on its homepage (https://www.cancer.org/treatment/survivorship-during-and-after-treatment.html). The Korean government provides information about cancer survivorship on the homepage of the National Center Information Center (https://www.cancer.go.kr/lay1/S1T786C784/contents.do).

Conclusion

Cancer survivors have many existing diseases, and a high-risk of developing new diseases subsequent to cancer and cancer treatments. Comorbidities in cancer survivors affect not only the quality of life, but also the life span; they should be carefully identified, evaluated, and managed especially in the early stages of cancer survival.

References

1. Quaresma M, Coleman MP, Rachet B. 40-year trends in an index of survival for all cancers combined and survival adjusted for age and sex for each cancer in England and Wales, 1971–2011: a population-based study. Lancet. 2015;385:1206–18.
2. Anonymous. National cancer information center. http://www.cancer.go.kr.
3. Shapiro CL. Cancer survivorship. N Engl J Med. 2018;379:2438–50.
4. Council NR. From cancer patient to cancer survivor: lost in transition. Washington, DC: National Academies Press; 2005.
5. Yabroff KR, Lawrence WF, Clauser S, Davis WW, Brown ML. Burden of illness in cancer survivors: findings from a population-based national sample. J Natl Cancer Inst. 2004;96:1322–30.
6. Bluethmann SM, Mariotto AB, Rowland JH. Anticipating the "silver tsunami": prevalence trajectories and comorbidity burden among older cancer survivors in the United States. Philadelphia: AACR; 2016.
7. Hahn EE, Gould MK, Munoz-Plaza CE, Lee JS, Parry C, Shen E. Understanding comorbidity profiles and their effect on treatment and survival in patients with colorectal cancer. J Natl Compr Cancer Netw. 2018;16:23–34.
8. Piccirillo JF, Tierney RM, Costas I, Grove L, Spitznagel EL Jr. Prognostic importance of comorbidity in a hospital-based cancer registry. JAMA. 2004;291:2441–7.
9. Pinkhas D, Ho T, Smith S. Assessment of pazopanib-related hypertension, cardiac dysfunction and identification of clinical risk factors for their development. Cardio-oncology. 2017;3:1–14.
10. Totzeck M, Mincu R-I, Mrotzek S, Schadendorf D, Rassaf T. Cardiovascular diseases in patients receiving small molecules with anti-vascular endothelial growth factor activity: a meta-analysis of approximately 29,000 cancer patients. Eur J Prev Cardiol. 2018;25:482–94.
11. Tonia T, Mettler A, Robert N, Schwarzer G, Seidenfeld J, Weingart O, et al. Erythropoietin or darbepoetin for patients with cancer. Cochrane Database Syst Rev. 2012;12(12):CD003407.
12. Goodwin JE, Geller DS. Glucocorticoid-induced hypertension. Pediatr Nephrol. 2012;27:1059–66.
13. Xiao Y, Wang H, Tang Y, Yan J, Cao L, Chen Z, et al. Increased risk of diabetes in cancer survivors: a pooled analysis of 13 population-based cohort studies. ESMO Open. 2021;6:100218.
14. Perez A, Jansen-Chaparro S, Saigi I, Bernal-Lopez MR, Miñambres I, Gomez-Huelgas R. Glucocorticoid-induced hyperglycemia (糖皮质激素诱导的高血糖). J Diabetes. 2014;6:9–20.
15. Ariaans G, De Jong S, Gietema J, Lefrandt J, de Vries E, Jalving M. Cancer-drug induced insulin resistance: innocent bystander or unusual suspect. Cancer Treat Rev. 2015;41:376–84.
16. Porporato P. Understanding cachexia as a cancer metabolism syndrome. Oncogenesis. 2016;5:e200.
17. Zhang F, Wang K, Du P, Yang W, He Y, Li T, et al. Risk of stroke in cancer survivors: a meta-analysis of population-based cohort studies. Neurology. 2021;96:e513–e26.
18. Chen J, Zhu M, Ma G, Zhao Z, Sun Z. *Chlamydia pneumoniae* infection and cerebrovascular disease: a systematic review and meta-analysis. BMC Neurol. 2013;13:1–13.
19. Chiang C-H, Huang C-C, Chan W-L, Chen Y-C, Chen T-J, Lin S-J, et al. Association between mycoplasma pneumonia and increased risk of ischemic stroke: a nationwide study. Stroke. 2011;42:2940–3.
20. Deniz K, O'Mahony S, Ross G, Purushotham A. Breast cancer in women after treatment for Hodgkin's disease. Lancet Oncol. 2003;4:207–14.
21. Shah BK, Khanal A, Hewett Y. Second primary malignancies in adults with gastric cancer—a US population-based study. Front Oncol. 2016;6:82.
22. Yang J, Terebelo HR, Zonder JA. Secondary primary malignancies in multiple myeloma: an old NEMESIS revisited. Adv Hematol. 2012;2012:801495.
23. El-Shami K, Oeffinger KC, Erb NL, Willis A, Bretsch JK, Pratt-Chapman ML, et al. American Cancer Society colorectal cancer survivorship care guidelines. CA Cancer J Clin. 2015;65:427–55.

If you have any concerns about our products,
you can contact us on
ProductSafety@springernature.com

In case Publisher is established outside the EU,
the EU authorized representative is:
Springer Nature Customer Service Center GmbH
Europaplatz 3, 69115 Heidelberg, Germany

Printed by Libri Plureos GmbH
in Hamburg, Germany